Fourth Edition

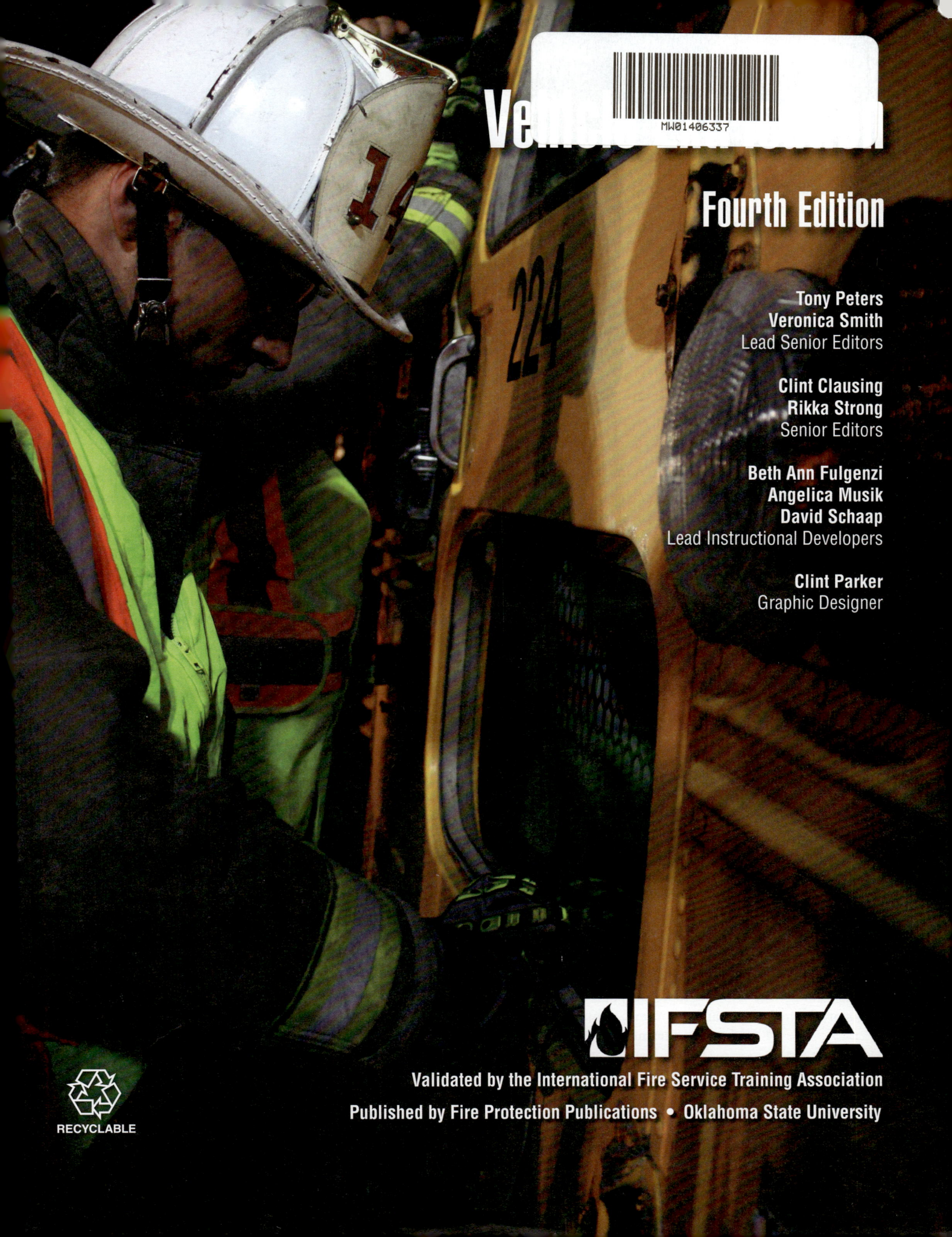

Tony Peters
Veronica Smith
Lead Senior Editors

Clint Clausing
Rikka Strong
Senior Editors

Beth Ann Fulgenzi
Angelica Musik
David Schaap
Lead Instructional Developers

Clint Parker
Graphic Designer

IFSTA

Validated by the International Fire Service Training Association
Published by Fire Protection Publications • Oklahoma State University

RECYCLABLE

IFSTA
INTERNATIONAL FIRE SERVICE TRAINING ASSOCIATION

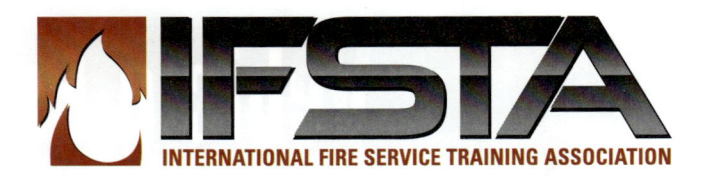

The International Fire Service Training Association (IFSTA) was established in 1934 as a *nonprofit educational association of fire fighting personnel who are dedicated to upgrading fire fighting techniques and safety through training.* To carry out the mission of IFSTA, Fire Protection Publications was established as an entity of Oklahoma State University. Fire Protection Publications' primary function is to publish and distribute training materials as proposed, developed, and validated by IFSTA. As a secondary function, Fire Protection Publications researches, acquires, produces, and markets high-quality learning and teaching aids consistent with IFSTA's mission.

IFSTA holds two meetings each year: the Winter Meeting in January and the Annual Validation Conference in July. During these meetings, committees of technical experts review draft materials and ensure that the professional qualifications of the National Fire Protection Association® standards are met. These conferences bring together individuals from several related and allied fields, such as:

- Key fire department executives, training officers, and personnel
- Educators from colleges and universities
- Representatives from governmental agencies
- Delegates of firefighter associations and industrial organizations

Committee members are not paid nor are they reimbursed for their expenses by IFSTA or Fire Protection Publications. They participate because of a commitment to the fire service and its future through training. Being on a committee is prestigious in the fire service community, and committee members are acknowledged leaders in their fields. This unique feature provides a close relationship between IFSTA and the fire service community.

IFSTA manuals have been adopted as the official teaching texts of many states and provinces of North America as well as numerous U.S. and Canadian government agencies. Besides the NFPA® requirements, IFSTA manuals are also written to meet the Fire and Emergency Services Higher Education (FESHE) course requirements. A number of the manuals have been translated into other languages to provide training for fire and emergency service personnel in Canada, Mexico, and outside of North America.

Copyright © 2017 by the Board of Regents, Oklahoma State University

All rights reserved. No part of this publication may be reproduced in any form without prior written permission from the publisher.

ISBN 978-0-87939-597-1   Library of Congress Control Number: 2017933496

Fourth Edition, First Printing, April 2017   *Printed in the United States of America*

10   9   8   7   6   5   4   3   2   1

If you need additional information concerning the International Fire Service Training Association (IFSTA) or Fire Protection Publications, contact:

Customer Service, Fire Protection Publications, Oklahoma State University
930 North Willis, Stillwater, OK 74078-8045
800-654-4055   Fax: 405-744-8204

For assistance with training materials, to recommend material for inclusion in an IFSTA manual, or to ask questions or comment on manual content, contact:

Editorial Department, Fire Protection Publications, Oklahoma State University
930 North Willis, Stillwater, OK 74078-8045
405-744-4111   Fax: 405-744-4112   E-mail: editors@osufpp.org

---

Oklahoma State University in compliance with Title VI of the Civil Rights Act of 1964 and Title IX of the Educational Amendments of 1972 (Higher Education Act) does not discriminate on the basis of race, color, national origin or sex in any of its policies, practices or procedures. This provision includes but is not limited to admissions, employment, financial aid and educational services.

Chapter Summary

Section A: Awareness Level Rescuer

Chapters
1 Vehicle Incident Safety 8

Section B: Operations and Technician Level Rescuers — Incident Tools, Skills and Responsibilities

2 Personal Protective Equipment, Hazards and Hazard Mitigation 55
3 Incident Management Responsibilities 92
4 Tools and Equipment 114
5 Victim Management 164

Section C: Operations Level Rescuer — Passenger Vehicle Extrication

6 Passenger Vehicles 188
7 Passenger Vehicle Stabilization Operations 232
8 Passenger Vehicle: Victim Disentanglement and Extrication 276

Section D: Technician – Heavy Vehicles Extrication

9 Commercial/Heavy Vehicles 336
10 Commercial/Heavy Vehicle Stabilization Operations 380
11 Commercial/Heavy Vehicle Disentanglement 398

Section E Ops/Tech: Special Passenger Vehicle Extrication Situations

12 Special Extrication Situations 436

Appendix   A   Chapter and Page Correlation to Chapter 8 of NFPA 1006 Requirements 489

Glossary 491

Index 499

Table of Contents

Acknowledgments xiii
Introduction 1
Purpose and Scope 1
Book Organization 2
Terminology 3
Key Information 3
Metric Conversions 4

Section A:
Awareness Level Rescuer

1 Vehicle Incident Safety 11
**Operational Capability and Training
    Requirements** 11
  Awareness Level 12
  Operations Level 12
  Technician Level 13
Preparation for Response 13
  Response Plans 14
  Hazard and Risk Assessment Surveys 16
  Extrication and Personal Protective
    Equipment 16
Scene Size-Up 16
  Environmental Considerations 17
    Weather 17
    Time of Day 17
    Terrain 18
  On-Scene Hazards 18
    Traffic Hazards 18
    Vehicle Stability 19
    Vehicle Contents 19
    *Downed Power Lines/
    Transformer Hazards* 20
    Fuel Spills 20
    Biohazards 21
    Vehicle Occupants 21
Safety Measures 22
  Training 22
  Crew Resource Management 22
  Medical Component 24
  Rehabilitation (Rehab) Station 24
  Potential Hazards 24
  Incident Safety Officer (ISO) 25
  Personnel Accountability 26
Scene Safety 26
  Incident Stability 27

  *Available Resource Capabilities and
    Limitations* 27
  Scene Control and Protection 27
  Vehicle Crash Dynamics 27
  Vehicle Stabilization and Access 28
  On-Scene Medical Care 28
  Restoring the Scene 29
  Personal Safety Equipment and Techniques 29
    Protecting Clothing and Equipment 29
    Shelter and Thermal Control 30
Safety Zones 30
  Types of Safety Zones 30
    Restricted (Hot) Zone 31
    Limited Access (Warm) Zone 32
    Support (Cold) Zone 32
    Zone Boundaries 32
  Staffing Requirements for Safety Zones 33
  Monitoring Hazard Zones 33
Traffic Control 35
  Traffic Control Concepts 35
    Control of Pedestrians 36
    Control of Rescuers 36
    *Control of Emergency Vehicles and
    Equipment* 36
  Traffic Control Devices 35
  Traffic Control Resources 40
Vehicle Incident Operations 40
  Operational Protocols 41
  Incident Action Plan (IAP) 42
    Verbal IAP 43
    *Communicating Rescue Strategy and
    Objectives* 43
    Assigned Incident Tasks 44
  Communication 44
    Dispatch 45
    Communicating Hazards 45
  Incident Support Operations and Resources 46
Chapter Review 48
Discussion Questions 48
Skill Sheets 49

iv

Section B:
Operations and Technician Level Rescuers — Incident Tools, Skills and Responsibilities

2   Personal Protective Equipment, Hazards and Hazard Mitigation 55
Personal Protective Equipment 55
- General Personal Protective Equipment 56
  - *Head, Eyes, and Face Protection* 56
  - *Hearing Protection* 57
  - *Body Protection* 57
  - *Foot Protection* 58
  - *Hand Protection* 58
  - *Respiratory Protection* 58
- Specialized Personal Protective Equipment 61

Hazards from Vehicle Energy Sources 61
- Hazards from Propulsion Power 62
  - *Conventional Fuels* 62
  - *Alternative Fuels* 63
  - *Hybrid Electric Vehicles* 64
- Hazards from Conventional Electrical Systems 65
- Hazards from Construction Materials 65
  - *Windows* 65
  - *Crushable Bumpers* 66
  - *Vehicle Components* 66

Hazards from Beneficial Vehicle Systems 67
- Hazards from Supplemental Restraint Systems 67
  - *Seat Belt Pretensioners* 68
  - *Airbags* 69
  - *Rollover Protection Systems* 73
- Hazards from Suspension Systems 73
- Hazards from Seat Adjustment or Positioning Controls 74

Fire and Explosion Hazards 74
- Fire Hazards 74
  - *Flammable and Combustible Substances* 74
  - *Ignition Sources* 75
- Explosion Hazards 76
  - *Shocks and Struts* 76
  - *Boiling Liquid Expanding Vapor Explosion (BLEVE)* 76

Fire Suppression Operations 77
- Establishing Fire Protection 77
  - *Fire Control Support* 77
  - *Fire Control Strategies* 78
  - *Extinguishing Devices and Agents* 79
- Alternative Energy Vehicle Fires 80
  - *Alcohol/Gasoline Blended Fuel Fires* 80
  - *Natural Gas Fires* 80
  - *Propane Fuel Fires* 81
  - *Hydrogen Fuel Fires* 81
  - *Biodiesel Fuel Fires* 81
  - *Hybrid and Electric Vehicle Fires* 81

Hazardous Materials 82
- Passenger Vehicle Haz Mat Incidents 82
- Medium and Heavy Truck Haz Mat Incidents ... 82
- Bus Haz Mat Incidents 85

Chapter Review 85
Discussion Questions 85
Skill Sheets 86

3   Incident Management Responsibilities 95
Initial and Ongoing Scene Size-up 95
- Initial Size-Up 95
- Scene Assessment 96
  - *Weather* 96
  - *Day of the Week* 97
  - *Time of Day* 97
  - *Vehicular Traffic* 97
  - *Pedestrians* 97
  - *Vehicles Involved* 97
  - *Hazards* 97
- Ongoing Size-Up 99

Incident Command System 99
- ICS Standards of Performance 99
- Command and Control 100
- Incident Operation Groups 100
  - *Extrication Group* 101
  - *Medical Group* 102
- Operating within the Incident Command System 103
- NIMS-ICS IAP Planning Process 104
- Situation Status Information 106
- Resource Status Information 106

Emergency Escape and Evacuation 106
- Escape and Evacuation Routes 107
- Emergency Evacuation and Safety Signals 107

Terminating an Incident 107
- Protecting Bystanders/Public 107
- Protecting Rescuers 108

Postincident Analysis 108
- Restoring Operational Readiness 109
- Conducting an After Action Review (AAR) 109
- Monitoring Critical Incident Stress (CIS) 109
- Completing Documentation 110

Chapter Review 110
Skill Sheets 111

4 Tools and Equipment 114

Rescue Vehicles, Vehicle Features, Equipment and Accessories 117
- Light Rescue Vehicles 117
- Medium Rescue Vehicles 118
- Heavy Rescue Vehicles................................... 118
- Rescue Engines.. 119
- Standard Engines 120
- Ladder Trucks.. 120
- Rescue Vehicle Chassis 121
- Rescue Vehicle Compartmentation 121
  - *Exclusive Exterior Compartmentation....... 121*
  - *Exclusive Interior Compartmentation 121*
  - *Combination Compartmentation............... 121*
- Rescue Vehicle Features and Equipment......... 122
  - *All-Wheel Drive 122*
  - *Rescue Vehicle Electrical Equipment......... 123*
  - *Vehicle Mounted Winches........................ 124*
  - *Gin Poles and A-Frames........................... 125*
  - *Hydraulic Cranes...................................... 125*
  - *Stabilizers.. 126*
  - *Air Supply Systems 126*

Stabilization Tools and Equipment 127
- Cribbing... 127
  - *Wooden Cribbing 127*
  - *Plastic Cribbing 128*
  - *Cribbing Applications 128*
- Step Chocks 129
- Struts 130
- Rigging 130
  - *Rope... 131*
  - *Chains.. 131*
  - *Webbing 132*
- Ratchet Straps and Tie Downs 132

Extrication Tools and Equipment 133
- Hand Tools.. 133
  - *Striking Tools 135*
  - *Prying Tools 136*
  - *Cutting Tools 137*
  - *Mechanic's Tools...................................... 139*
  - *Specialized Hand Tools 140*
  - *Lifting Tools 140*
  - *Trench Tools 142*
- Electric Tools and Equipment......................... 142
  - *Electric Spreaders and Cutters.................. 142*
  - *Electric Impact Wrenches......................... 143*
  - *Electric Drills and Drivers......................... 143*
  - *Portable Lights... 143*
  - *Auxiliary Electrical Equipment 144*
  - *Signaling Devices..................................... 144*
  - *Voltage Detection Devices 145*
- Power Saws 145
  - *Reciprocating Saws 146*
  - *Rotary Saws 147*
  - *Circular Saws... 147*
  - *Chain Saws 147*
  - *Portable Band Saws 148*
- Hydraulic Tools and Equipment 148
  - *Power-Driven Hydraulic Tools 148*
  - *Manuel Hydraulic Tools........................... 151*
- Pnuematic Tools and Equipment 152
  - *Pnuematic Chisels and Hammers 152*
  - *Pnuematic Wrenches............................... 153*
  - *Pnuematic Saws 153*
  - *Pnuematic Lifting Bags and Cushions 153*
- Lifting or Pulling Tools 156
  - *Griphoists.. 156*
- Come-Alongs... 156
  - *Mechanical Advantage Systems 157*
- Thermal Cutting Devices 158
  - *Exothermic Cutting Devices..................... 159*
  - *Cutting Flares 159*
  - *Plasma-Arc Cutters.................................. 160*
  - *Oxyacetylene Cutting Torches.................. 160*
  - *Oxygasoline Cutting Torches.................... 160*
- Routine Operational Checks and Maintenance 161

Chapter Review 162
Discussion Questions 162

5 Victim Management 164

Administering Care 167
- Mechanisms of Injury 168
  - *Head-On Impact Collision........................ 170*
  - *Side Impact Collision 171*
  - *Rear Impact Collision............................... 172*
  - *Rotational Impact 173*
  - *Rollover 173*
- Triage 173
- Preventing Further Injury............................... 175
- Common Vehicle Incident Injuries 176
  - *Fractures and Lacerations 176*
  - *Hypovolemia (Blood Loss)....................... 176*
  - *Hypothermia and Hyperthermia............... 177*
- Hazardous Materials Exposure 177
- Compartment/Crush Syndrome 177
- Field Amputations... 178
- Internal Injuries 178

Immobilization, Packaging, and Transfer 178
    Types of Immobilization, Packaging, and
        Transfer Devices 179
        Cervical Collar.. 179
        Seated Spinal Immobilization Device........ 179
        Long Board... 179
        Vacuum Mattress.. 179
    Immobilizing and Packaging a Patient............. 180
    Removing a Packaged Patient 181
    Transferring a Patient 182
        Communications with EMS............................ 182
        Patient Follow Up.. 182
Chapter Review... 183
Discussion Questions 184
Skill Sheets 185

Section C:
Operations Level Rescuer — Passenger Vehicle Extrication

6 Passenger Vehicles................................. 188
Types of Passenger Vehicles............................... 191
    Passenger Cars 194
        Minicompact Cars.. 194
        Subcompact Cars... 194
        Compact Cars... 195
        Midsize Cars... 195
        Large Cars... 195
        Specialized Passenger Vehicles 195
    Vans 196
        Minivans... 196
        Full-Size Vans 197
    Sport Utility Vehicles (SUVs) 197
    Pickup Trucks 197
Passenger Vehicle Anatomy 197
    Common Vehicle Terminology 198
    Vehicle Frame.. 200
        Full or Rigid Frame 200
        Unibody (Unitized Body)................................ 201
        Space Frame 201
    Vehicle Windows 201
        Laminated Safety Glass................................. 202
        Tempered Glass.. 202
        Enhanced Protective Glass (EPG)................ 202
        Polycarbonate.. 202
        Transparent Armo 204
Passenger Vehicle Construction 204
    Passenger Vehicle Construction Materials 204
        Passenger Vehicle Fuel Systems................. 206
        Conventional Fuels... 206
        Hybrid Electric Vehicles (HEV) 206

        Plug-In Hybrid Electric Vehicles (PHEV) ... 207
        Electric Vehicles (EV)..................................... 207
        Extended Range Electric Vehicles
        (EREV) 210
        Alternative Fuels... 211
        Fuel Tanks 212
    Passenger Vehicle Electrical Systems 213
        Keyless Entry and Smart Key Ignitions........ 214
        Headlights... 214
        Battery Systems.. 214
        Electric Engine Cooling Fans 215
        Electronic Front and Rear Defoggers........... 216
    Passenger Vehicle Exhaust Systems.................. 216
    Passenger Vehicle Powertrain Systems 216
    Passenger Vehicle Suspension Systems 218
        Springs 218
        Shock Absorbers... 218
        Suspension Struts 218
        Tires... 219
        Passenger Air-Suspension Systems 219
Passenger Vehicle Safety Features..................... 219
    Collision Avoidance Systems 219
        Forward-Looking Collision-Avoidance
        Systems 219
        Side-Sensing Collision-Avoidance
        Systems 220
        Rear-Looking Collision-Avoidance
        Systems 220
        Adaptive Cruise Control................................ 220
        Infrared Night Vision Systems..................... 220
    Passenger Vehicle Supplemental Restraint
        Systems 220
        Seat Belts, Seat Belt Pretensioners, and
        Load Limiters... 220
        Airbags.. 221
        Child Safety Restraint Devices 224
    Energy-Absorbing Features................................ 224
        Crushable Bumpers 225
        Bumper Struts... 225
        Steering Column... 227
        Collision Beams... 227
        Crumple Zones 228
    Passenger Vehicle Rollover Protection
        Systems 229
Chapter Review... 230

7 Passenger Vehicle Stabilization
    Operations 232
Introduction to Vehicle Stabilization 235
    Mechanisms of Movement................................ 236

vii

    Center of Gravity.................................. *236*
    Directional Movement *237*
  Stabilization Points and Surfaces/Terrain 238
    Stabilization Points *239*
    Stabilization Surfaces/Terrain *239*
  Lifting 239
Application of Stabilization Tools and Equipment..**242**
  Wheel Chocks 242
  Cribbing Materials 242
  Pnuematic Lifting Bags and Cushions............ 243
    High-Pressure Lifting Bags *244*
    Low- and Medium-Pressure Lifting Cushions.. *245*
  Jacks 245
  Levers 246
    Class I Lever *246*
    Class II Lever *247*
    Class III Lever *247*
  Hitches 247
    Vertical Hitch *247*
    Basket Hitch *248*
    Double Basket Hitch *248*
    Bridle Hitch *248*
    Choker Hitch *248*
    Double Choker Hitch *249*
  Chains 249
  Wire Rope 250
  Synthetic Slings 251
    Round Slings *252*
    Web Slings *253*
  Rigging 253
    Tighteners.. *255*
    Rigging Fittings *254*
  Struts 255
  Recovery Vehicles 255
Passenger Vehicle Stabilization Operations **255**
  Passenger Vehicle Structural and Damage Characteristics 256
  Maintaining Vehicle Stability 257
  Wheel-Resting Passenger Vehicle Stabilization 257
  Side-Resting Passenger Vehicle Stabilization 259
  Roof-Resting Passenger Vehicle Stabilization 261
  Passenger Vehicles in Other Positions Stabilization 261
Chapter Review **263**
Discussion Questions **263**
Skill Sheets **264**

8 Passenger Vehicle: Victim Disentanglement and Extrication 276
Victim Entrapment **279**
  Victim Locations 279
  Points of Entrapment 280
  Dynamics of Disentanglement 281
    Front-Impact Collisions *281*
    Rear-Impact Collisions......................... *282*
    Side-Impact (Lateral) Collisions *282*
    Rotational Collisions *283*
    Rollovers *283*
    Underride and Override *284*
  Multiple Vehicle Incidents 285
    MVI Considerations *285*
    MVI Operations *286*
  Minimizing Hazards to Victims 287
Passenger Vehicle Access and Egress Points......**287**
  Passenger Vehicle Access and Egress Routes... 288
  Passenger Vehicle Entry Points 288
    Windows *288*
    Doors.. *289*
    Floor Panels *290*
Passenger Vehicle Disentanglement and Extrication Operations **290**
  Techniques for Creating Access and Egress Openings on Passenger Vehicles 290
    Glass Removal *291*
    Door Removal.................................... *293*
    Factory Third/Fourth Doors *297*
    Total Sidewall Removal *298*
    Third-Door Conversion *298*
    Fourth-Door Conversion....................... *299*
    Roof Displacement and Removal *299*
    Kick Panel Removal............................. *300*
    Entry through the Floor *300*
    Trunk Tunneling................................. *301*
  Alternative Techniques for Creating Access and Egress Openings on Passenger Vehicles with Advanced Steel 301
    Pie Cut.. *302*
    B-Post Lift... *302*
    Cross Ramming *302*
    Ramming the Roof Off......................... *302*
    Partial or Total Sunroof *302*
  Techniques for Disentangling Victims from Passenger Vehicles.............................. 303
    Removing a Windshield from Around a Victim.. *303*
    Displacing a Steering Column *303*
    Displacing a Dashboard *303*

Dropping a Floor Plan 304
Displacing the B-Post 305
Displacing and Removing Seats ... 305
Displacing or Removing Pedals ... 306
Chapter Review 308
Discussion Questions 308
Skill Sheets 309

Section D:
Technician – Heavy Vehicles Extrication

9 Commercial/Heavy Vehicles 336
Medium and Heavy Trucks 339
Straight Trucks 340
Truck and Semitrailer Combinations 341
Specialty Trucks 341
Medium and Heavy Truck Anatomy 343
Cabs 343
Conventional Cabs 344
Air-Ride Cabs 344
Cab-Over Units 344
Cab-Beside Engine 344
Sleepers 344
Cab Doors 345
Cab Windows 346
Cab Roofs 346
Trailers 346
Box Trailers 348
Livestock Trailers 348
Tanker Trailers 348
Lowboys 349
Dump Trailers 349
Car Carrier/Hauler Trailers 349
Dry Bulk Trailers 349
Medium and Heavy Truck Construction 350
Medium and Heavy Truck Construction
   Components 350
Medium and Heavy Battery Systems 350
Medium and Heavy Truck Fuel Systems 350
Medium and Heavy Truck Conventional
   Electrical Systems 351
Medium and Heavy Truck Hazards Auxiliary
   Power and Hydraulics Systems 351
Mechanical Systems 352
Hydraulic Systems 352
Pnuemantic Systems 353
Medium and Heavy Truck Brake Systems 353
Medium and Heavy Truck Suspension
   Systems 354

Medium and Heavy Auxiliary Lift Axles 354
Medium and Heavy Truck Safety Features 355
Medium and Heavy Truck On-Board Safety
   Systems (OBSS) 355
Fifth Wheels 355
Buses 356
School Buses 356
Type A 356
Type B 357
Type C 357
Type D 357
Transit Buses 357
Commercial Buses 358
Specialty Buses 359
Type A and B School Bus Conversions 360
Commercial Bus Conversions 360
Bus Anatomy 360
Bus Doors 361
School Bus Front Doors 361
School Bus Rear Doors 362
Transit Bus Doors 362
Commercial Bus Doors 362
Bus Windows 363
School Bus Windows 363
Transit Bus Windows 364
Commercial Bus Windows 365
Bus Seats 365
School Bus Seats 365
Transit Bus Seats 365
Commercial Bus Seats 366
Bus Aisles 366
School Bus Aisles 366
Transit Bus Aisles 367
Commercial Bus Aisles 367
Bus Construction and Safety Features 367
School Bus Construction Components 368
School Bus Skeletal System 368
School Bus Floor and Undercarriage 369
Transit Bus Construction Components 370
Commercial Bus Construction
   Compenents 371
Hydraulic Lifts 371
Bus Battery Systems 371
School Bus Batteries 372
Transit Bus Batteries 372
Commercial Bus Batteries 372
Bus Electrical Systems 372
Bus Fuel Systems 374
Gasoline and Diesel 374
CNG, LPG, and LNG 374
Hydrogen Fuel Cells 375

Hybrid Electric Buses............................. *375*
Electric Buses *376*
Bus Suspension Systems 376
Chapter Review **378**
Discussion Questions **378**

10 Commercial/Heavy Vehicle Stabilization Operations 380

Operations Level Stabilization: Review **383**
Commercial/Heavy Vehicle Stabilization Considerations **385**
Medium and Heavy Truck Stabilization........... 385
Wheel-Resting Truck Stabilization *386*
Self-Resting Truck Stabilization................... *387*
Roof-Resting Stabilization *388*
Stabilization of Trucks in Other Positions .. *388*
Bus Stabilization...................................... 389
Wheel-Resting Bus Stabilization................ *389*
Self-Resting Bus Stabilization *392*
Roof-Resting Stabilization *392*
Buses in Other Positions Stabilization *393*
Chapter Review **394**
Discussion Questions **394**
Skill Sheets **395**

11 Commercial/Heavy Vehicle Disentanglement 398

Review: Operations Level Disentanglement and Extrication.. **401**
Medium and Heavy Truck Access and Egress Points.. **401**
Medium and Heavy Truck Access and Egress Routes... **402**
Medium and Heavy Truck Entry Points 402
Medium and Heavy Truck Extrication Operations 403
Techniques for Creating Access and Egress Openings on Medium and Heavy Trucks...................................... **404**
Medium and Heavy Truck Door Access and Egress *404*
Medium and Heavy Truck Window Access and Egress *405*
Medium and Heavy Truck Roof Access and Egress *406*
Medium and Heavy Truck Wall Access and Egress *406*
Techniques for Disentangling Victims from Medium and Heavy Trucks **407**
Bus Access and Egress Points........................ **408**
Bus Access and Egress Routes........................ 408
Bus Entry Points 408
Bus Extrication Operations **410**
Techniques for Creating Access and Egress Openings on Buses............................... **410**
Creating Openings through Bus Doors........ *411*
Creating Openings through Bus Windows *413*
Creating Openings through Bus Sidewalls *415*
Creating Openings through Bus Rear Walls *416*
Creating Openings through Bus Roofs *416*
Creating Openings through Bus Floor Panels... *417*
Techniques for Disentangling Victims from Buses.. **418**
Bus Driver Seat Disentanglement.............. *418*
Bus Steering Wheel Disentanglement......... *419*
Bus Interior Features (Seats and Partitions) Disentanglement *419*
Additional Bus Disentanglement Considerations..................................... *420*
Chapter Review **422**
Discussion Questions **422**
Skill Sheets **423**

Section E:
Ops/Tech: Special Passenger Vehicle Extrication Situations

12 Special Extrication Situations................ 436

Vehicles in a Structure **440**
Vehicles in a Structure — Considerations........ 440
Vehicles in a Structure — Operations.............. 441
Vehicles in Water...................................... **442**
Vehicles in Water — Considerations 442
Vehicles in Water — Operations 443
Hanging Vehicles **444**
Hanging Vehicles — Considerations 444
Hanging Vehicles — Operations 445
Recreational Vehicles (RVs)......................... **446**
RV Considerations 446
RV Operations 447
Industrial and Agricultural Vehicles **447**
Types of Industrial and Agricultural Vehicles................................ 447
Tractors *448*
Harvesters *450*
Graders... *451*

- *Booms*.. *451*
- *Cranes* *452*
- *Forklifts* *452*
- Industrial and Agricultural Vehicle Anatomy, Construction, and Features 453
  - *Drivetrain* *454*
  - *Operational Controls* *454*
  - *Tracked Vehicles* *454*
  - *Vehicle Tires* *455*
  - *Articulating and Telescoping Vehicles* *455*
  - *Industrial and Agricultural Vehicle Fuel Systems* *455*
  - *Industrial and Agricultural Vehicle Brake Systems* *455*
  - *Industrial and Agricultural Vehicle Auxiliary Power Sources* *456*
  - *Industrial and Agricultural Vehicle Rollover Protection Systems* *456*
  - *Jacks* *456*
- Industrial and Agricultural Incident Size-Up 457
- Industrial and Agricultural Vehicle Hazards 459
- Industrial and Agricultural Vehicle Stabilization 459
  - *Stabilization of Wheel-Resting Industrial and Agricultural Vehicles* *460*
  - *Stabilization of Side-Resting Industrial and Agricultural Vehicles* *460*
  - *Stabilization of Roof-Resting Industrial and Agricultural Vehicles* *460*
  - *Stabilization of Industrial and Agricultural Vehicles in Other Positions* *461*
- Industrial and Agricultural Vehicle Extrication 461
  - *Industrial and Agricultural Vehicle Access* *461*
  - *Industrial and Agricultural Vehicle Extrication Tactics* *462*
  - *Power Take Off (PTO) Incidents* *464*
  - *Railcars* *464*
- Types of Railcars 464
  - *Locomotives* *465*
  - *Passenger Cars* *466*
  - *Baggage Cars* *468*
  - *Freight Cars* *468*
  - *Material Handling Cars* *468*
  - *Lounge/Food Service Cars* *469*
- Railcar Anatomy, Construction, and Features 469
  - *Railcar Doors* *470*
  - *Railcar Windows* *470*
  - *Railcar Floors* *470*
  - *Railcar Walls and Roofs* *470*
  - *Railcar Trucks* *471*
  - *Railcar Brakes* *471*
  - *Railcar Electrical Systems* *472*
  - *Catenary Systems* *472*
  - *Third-Rail Systems* *475*
  - *Roadbeds* *475*
- Railcar Incident Size-Up 475
- Railcar Hazards 476
- Railcar Stabilization 477
  - *Stabilizing Wheel-Resting Railcars* *478*
  - *Stabilizing Side-Resting Railcars* *479*
  - *Stabilizing Roof-Resting Railcars* *479*
  - *Stabilizing Railcars in Other Positions* *479*
- Railcar Access and Egress 479
  - *Railcar Access* *480*
  - *Height Considerations* *480*
  - *Locomotive Entry* *480*
  - *Passenger Car Door Entry* *481*
  - *Passenger Car Window Entry* *481*
  - *Passenger Car Roof/Wall Entry* *482*
  - *Interior Door Locks/Latches* *482*
  - *Lounge/Food Service Car Entry* *483*
  - *Baggage Car Entry* *483*
  - *Material Handling Car Entry* *483*
- Railcar Extrication Situations 483
  - *Disentanglement/Tunneling* *484*
  - *Loading Platform Incidents* *484*
  - *Train/Highway Vehicle Collisions* *485*
  - *Train/Pedestrian Collisions* *485*
  - *Trams* *485*
- **Chapter Review** **486**
- **Discussion Questions** **487**
- **Appendices** **489**
- **Glossary** **491**
- **Index** **499**

List of Tables

Table 2.1	Examples of Supplemental Passenger Restraint Systems, Roll Over Protection Systems, and Components	68
Table 4.1	Hand Tools Listed By Categorization	134
Table 6.1	Examples of Passenger Vehicles, Cars, and Light Trucks	192
Table 6.2	Examples of Hybrid Cars (by automobile manufacturers)	208

Acknowledgements

The fourth edition of the **Principles of Vehicle Extrication** is designed to meet the objectives listed for the requirements from all of Chapter 8 of NFPA 1006, *Standard for Technical Rescuer Professional Qualifications, 2017 Edition*. The manual references relevant sections of NFPA 1670, *Standard on Operations and Training for Technical Search and Rescue Incidents*. The information in this manual also meets and exceeds sections 6.4.1 and 6.4.2 of the Fire Fighter II job performance requirements found in NFPA 1001, *Standard for Fire Fighter Professional Qualifications*.

Acknowledgement and special thanks are extended to the members of the IFSTA validating committee who contributed their time, wisdom, and knowledge to the development of this manual.

Contract Writer

The fourth edition of the **Principles of Vehicle Extrication** could not have been completed without the skill and hard work of contracted technical writer Kevin Kennedy. Captain Kennedy provided the early drafts of all manual chapters to the validation committee for their review, revision, and approval. He also assisted the committee and project manager with changes to chapter content and validation discussions.

IFSTA Principles of Vehicle Extrication Fourth Edition Validation Committee

Chair
Wes Kitchel
Assistant Chief
Sonoma County Fire and
Emergency Services Department
Santa Rosa, California

Vice Chair and Secretary
Alan Braun
Adjunct Instructor
University of Missouri Fire & Rescue
Training Institute
Jefferson City, Missouri

Committee Members

James Altman
Fire Captain/HazMat
Santa Monica Fire Department
Santa Monica, California

Sean Campbell
Lieutenant
Gainesville Fire Rescue
Newberry, Florida

David Caruana
Lieutenant
Prince William County Department of
Fire & Rescue
Fredericksburg, Virginia

Brian Cleland
Senior Firefighter
Bluffton Township Fire District
Ridgeland, South Carolina

Craig Cooper
Battalion Chief - Special Operations
Las Vegas Fire & Rescue
Las Vegas, Nevada

Anthony Correia
Active Instructor
Burlington Township
Burlington, New Jersey

Sandee Goulding-Harnum
Instructor/Program Chairperson
Safety & Emergency Response Training Centre,
Marine Institute
Stephenville, Newfoundland, Canada

Jeff Hakola
Firefighter
Merced City Fire Department
Atwater, California

IFSTA Principles of Vehicle Extrication
Fourth Edition Validation Committee
continued

Committee Members

Paul Januszewski
Deputy Chief/Training Officer/Fire Marshal
Enfield Fire Department
Enfield, Connecticut

Andrew McCullers
Captain
Wetumpka Fire Department
Wetumpka, Alabama

Jason Probst
Captain
Virginia Beach Fire Department
Virginia Beach, Virginia

Chris Ransom
Captain
Rock Springs Fire Department
Rock Springs, Wyoming

Alex Rivera
Station Captain
Ft. Jackson Fire Department
Columbia, South Carolina

Lane Sickles
Lieutenant
Jerome City Fire Department
Jerome, Idaho

John Sileski
Rescue Specialist
Municipal Emergency Services
Robesonia, Pennsylvania

Kevin Tobey
Lieutenant
Prince William County Department of
Fire & Rescue
Fredericksburg, Virginia

Ryan Webb
Fire Captain/Paramedic
Upland Fire Department
Upland, California

Much appreciation is given to the following individuals and organizations for contributing information, photographs, and technical assistance instrumental in the development of this manual:

Advanced Extrication Tech, Murrieta, California
- Randy Babbitt, Director of Training
- David Hudson, Operations Manager
- Darrel Anderson, Instructor
- Jim Gaboury, Instructor
- Jeff Hakola, Instructor
- Leo Ibarra, Instructor
- Eric Janert, Instructor
- Felipe Marcial, Instructor
- Chris Martinez, Instructor
- Rich Meline, Instructor
- Billy Milligan, Instructor
- Josh Randall, Instructor
- Jordan Wenner, Instructor

Avoca Fire Department, Avoca, Pennsylvania

Cottage Hose Ambulance Corporation, Carbondale, Pennsylvania

Commonwealth Health EMS, Scranton, Pennsylvania

Eastern Oklahoma City Fire Training Center, Choctaw, Oklahoma
- Alan Saunders, Instructor
- Roger Straka, Instructor

Dickson City Fire Department, Dickson City, Pennsylvania

Greenfield Township Volunteer Fire Department, Greenfield, Pennsylvania

Gouldsboro Volunteer Fire Department, Gouldsboro, Pennsylvania

Harding Fire Department, Harding, Pennsylvania

Jerimiah Hoffstatter, OKC Fire Department, Oklahoma City, Oklahoma

Kingston/Forty Fort Fire Department, Kingston, Pennsylvania

National Fire Protection Association

Northmoreland Township Volunteer Fire Department, Tunkhannock, Pennsylvania

Tarrant County Community College Fire Service Training Center, Fort Worth, Texas

Ron Moore, Prosper Fire Rescue

Christopher Gay, DFW Airport Fire Department

Steve Lopez, Dallas Fire Department

James R. Jones, Fort Worth Fire Department

Wade Williams, Irving Fire Department

William Walker Hose Company, Mayfield, Pennsylvania

Special thanks go to Joe Burke and Boots & Hanks Towing and Scrap, Scranton, Pennsylvania.

Last, but certainly not least, gratitude is extended to the following members of the Fire Protection Publications staff whose contributions made the publication of this manual possible:

Principles of Vehicle Extrication, Fourth Edition, Project Team

Project Manager
Tony Peters, Senior Editor
Veronica Smith, Senior Editor

Contract Writer
Kevin Kennedy
Captain
McKinney Fire Department
McKinney, Texas

Director of Fire Protection Publications
Craig Hannan

Curriculum Manager
Colby Cagle

Editorial Manager
Clint Clausing

Production Coordinator
Ann Moffat

Editors
Cindy Brakhage, Senior Editor
Lynne Murnane, Senior Editor
Michael Fox, Senior Editor

Illustrators and Layout Designer
Clint Parker, Senior Graphic Designer

Curriculum Development
Angelica Muzik, Instructional Developer
Beth Ann Fulgenzi, Instructional Developer
David Schaap, Instructional Developer

Photographer(s)
Jeff Fortney, Senior Editor
Veronica Smith, Senior Editor
Tony Peters, Senior Editor

Editorial Staff
Tara Gladden, Editorial Assistant

Indexer
Nancy Kopper

Dedication

This manual is dedicated to the men and women who hold devotion to duty above personal risk, who count on sincerity of service above personal comfort and convenience, who strive unceasingly to find better and safer ways of protecting lives, homes, and property of their fellow citizens from the ravages of fire, medical emergencies, and other disasters

...The Firefighters of All Nations.

The IFSTA Executive Board at the time of validation of the **Vehicle Extrication, Fourth Edition** was as follows:

IFSTA Executive Board

Executive Board Chair
Steve Ashbrock
Fire Chief
Madeira & Indian Hill Fire Department
Cincinnati, Ohio

Vice Chair
Bradd Clark
Fire Chief
Ocala Fire Department
Ocala, Florida

IFSTA Executive Director
Mike Wieder
Associate Director
Fire Protection Publications at OSU
Stillwater, Oklahoma

Board Members

Steve Austin
Past President
Cumberland Valley
Volunteer FF Association
Newark, Delaware

Mary Cameli
Assistant Chief
City of Mesa Fire Department
Mesa, Arizona

Dr. Larry Collins
Associate Dean
Eastern Kentucky University
Richmond, Kentucky

Chief Dennis Compton
Chairman
National Fallen Firefighters Foundation
Mesa, Arizona

John Hoglund
Director Emeritus
Maryland Fire & Rescue Institute
New Carrollton, Maryland

Scott Kerwood
Fire Chief
Hutto Fire Rescue
Hutto, Texas

Wes Kitchel
Assistant Chief
Sonoma County Fire & Emergency Services
Cloverdale, California

Brett Lacey
Fire Marshal
Colorado Springs Fire Department
Colorado Springs, Colorado

Robert Moore
Division Director
TEEX
College Station, Texas

Dr. Lori Moore-Merrell
Assistant to the General President
International Association of Fire Fighters
Washington, D.C.

Jeff Morrissette
State Fire Administrator
State of Connecticut Commission
on Fire Prevention and Control
Windsor Locks, Connecticut

Josh Stefancic
Division Chief
Largo Fire Rescue
Largo, Florida

Don Turno
Operations Chief
Savannah River Nuclear Solutions
Aiken, South Carolina

Paul Valentine
Senior Engineer
Nexus Engineering
Oakbrook, Illinois

Steven Westermann
Fire Chief
Central Jackson County Fire
Protection District
Blue Springs, Missouri

Introduction

Introduction Contents

Introduction 1	Resources 3
Purpose and Scope 3	Key Information 4
Book Organization 3	Metric Conversions 6
Terminology 3	

Introduction

Vehicle extrication incidents can occur everywhere that land-based vehicles operate — on streets and highways, on improved and unimproved rural roads, on railroads and light rail tracks, on farms and ranches, on industrial facilities and construction sites, and in remote wilderness areas. Often, victims are entrapped or entangled in the involved vehicles, requiring rescue personnel to perform vehicle extrication in order to free them. Response to vehicle extrication incidents is inherently dangerous and results in many injuries and deaths to response personnel because of exposure to vehicular traffic and other hazardous conditions.

Most vehicle extrication incidents are handled by firefighters, either career or volunteer. Others are handled by members of dedicated rescue squads or rescue companies, either public or private. Some are handled by law enforcement personnel. The concepts and techniques described in this manual can be applied by any or all of these groups provided that they are properly trained and equipped. Within the pages of this manual, safety and efficiency are recurring themes.

The term "extrication" means different things to different people, and in some jurisdictions it includes more or less than in others. According to NFPA 1670, *Standard on Operations and Training for Technical Rescue Incidents* (2009), extrication is defined as "the removal of trapped victims from a vehicle or machinery."

Purpose and Scope

Principles of Vehicle Extrication, Fourth Edition is designed to provide rescue personnel with an understanding of the current challenges, techniques, skills, and equipment available for the safe and effective extrication of victims trapped in land-based vehicles. This manual deals only with the mechanics of freeing victims from entrapment in vehicles and related machinery. It does not include specific emergency medical treatment protocols.

This manual is written for personnel who respond to vehicle extrication incidents including any of the following:

- Firefighters
- Law enforcement personnel
- Emergency Medical Services (EMS) personnel
- Industrial and transportation emergency response members
- Public works and utility employees
- Military responders
- Rescue personnel

The scope of this manual includes job performance requirements (JPRs) from all of Chapter 8 of NFPA 1006, *Standard for Technical Rescuer Professional Qualifications, 2017 Edition*. The manual references relevant sections of NFPA 1670, *Standard on Operations and Training for Technical Search and Rescue Incidents*. The information in this manual also meets and exceeds sections 6.4.1 and 6.4.2 of the Fire Fighter II job performance requirements found in NFPA 1001, *Standard for Fire Fighter Professional Qualifications*.

The tools, equipment, and techniques described in this manual represent the current best practices of rescuers, but they are not the only ways to perform extrication safely and effectively. No single tool or technique will be safe and effective in every situation. Readers are encouraged to master a wide variety of extrication tools and techniques.

Finally, the information in this manual must be combined with hands-on training. Simply reading this or any other book on extrication will not make an individual proficient at vehicle extrication. Training with qualified instructors who have experience on extrication incidents is essential to using this manual successfully.

Book Organization

The Fourth Edition of **Principles of Vehicle Extrication** gathers the knowledge, skills, and abilities listed above into 12 chapters divided into 3 sections as follows:

Section A: Awareness Level Rescuers

Chapter 1 — Vehicle Incident Safety

Section B: Operations and Technician Level Rescuers — Incident Tools, Skills, and Responsibilities

Chapter 2 — Personal Protective Equipment, Hazards and Hazard Mitigation

Chapter 3 — Incident Management Responsibilities

Chapter 4 — Tools and Equipment

Chapter 5 — Victim Management

Section C: Operations Level Rescuers — Passenger Vehicle Extrication

Chapter 6 — Passenger Vehicles

Chapter 7 — Passenger Vehicle Stabilization Operations

Chapter 8 — Victim Disentanglement and Extrication

Section D: Technician Level Rescuers — Heavy Vehicle Extrication

Chapter 9 — Medium and Heavy Vehicles

Chapter 10 — Commercial/Heavy Stabilization Operations

Chapter 11 — Commercial/Heavy Vehicle Disentanglement

Section E: Operations and Technician Level Rescuers – Special Vehicle Extrication Situations

Chapter 12 — Special Extrication Situations

Learning objectives, located at the beginning of each chapter, will assist the reader in focusing on the appropriate topic and knowledge. The numbers of the JPRs are also listed at the beginning of chapters where they are referenced. **Appendix A** contains a guide that correlates the JPRs to the specific page(s) of the chapter that relate to the requirements.

Terminology

This manual is written with an international audience in mind. For this reason, it often uses general descriptive language in place of regional- or agency-specific terminology (often referred to as *jargon*). Additionally, in order to keep sentences uncluttered and easy to read, the word *state* is used to represent both state and provincial level governments (or their equivalent). This usage is applied to this manual for the purposes of brevity and is not intended to address or show preference for only one nation's method of identifying regional governments within its borders.

The glossary at the end of the manual will assist the reader in understanding words that may not have their roots in the fire and emergency services. The sources for the definitions of fire-and-emergency-services-related terms will be the IFSTA **Fire and Emergency Services Orientation and Terminology** manual.

Key Information

Various types of information in this book are given in shaded boxes marked by symbols or icons. See the following definitions:

> **Information**
> Information boxes give facts that are complete in themselves but belong with the text discussion. It is information that needs more emphasis or separation. (In the text, the title of information boxes will change to reflect the content.)

A **key term** is designed to emphasize key concepts, technical terms, or ideas that rescue personnel need to know. They are listed at the beginning of each chapter and the definition is placed in the margin for easy reference. An example of a key term is on the right of this paragraph:

Three key signal words are found in the book: **WARNING, CAUTION,** and **NOTE**. Definitions and examples of each are as follows:

- **WARNING** indicates information that could result in death or serious injury to rescue personnel. See the following example:

> **WARNING**
> When dealing with an incident that involves a power pole, collapsed building, or other significant hazard, other agencies may need to be consulted before starting rescue operations.

Rehabilitation — Allowing firefighters or rescuers to rest, rehydrate, and recover during an incident; also refers to a station at an incident where personnel can rest, rehydrate, and recover. *Also known as* Rehab.

- **CAUTION** indicates important information or data that rescue personnel need to be aware of in order to perform their duties safely. See the following example:

> **CAUTION**
> Should an accidental deployment occur, having body parts positioned through an open window could result in serious injury. When reaching into the vehicle to remove or turn off the ignition, rescue members should reach from behind the steering hub.

- **NOTE** indicates important operational information that helps explain why a particular recommendation is given or describes optional methods for certain procedures. See the following example:

NOTE: It is highly desirable for all rescuers to have at least some formal basic first aid or emergency medical technician (EMT) training.

To find curriculum or study materials associated with this manual and its contents, please go to ifsta.org and use the search tool in the shop to find accompanying products. You can also search for IFSTA apps using your smartphone or tablet device.

Metric Conversions

Throughout this manual, United States units of measure are converted to metric units for the convenience of our international readers. Be advised that we use the Canadian metric system. It is very similar to the Standard International system but may have some variation.

We adhere to the following guidelines for metric conversions in this manual:

- Metric conversions are approximated unless the number is used in mathematical equations.
- Centimeters are not used because they are not part of the Canadian metric standard.
- Exact conversions are used when an exact number is necessary such as in construction measurements or hydraulic calculations.
- Set values such as hose diameter, ladder length, and nozzle size use their Canadian counterpart naming conventions and are not mathematically calculated. For example, 1½ inch hose is referred to as 38 mm hose.

The following two tables provide detailed information on IFSTA's conversion conventions. The first table includes examples of our conversion factors for a number of measurements used in the fire service. The second shows examples of exact conversions beside the approximated measurements you will see in this manual.

U.S. to Canadian Measurement Conversion

Measurements	Customary (U.S.)	Metric (Canada)	Conversion Factor
Length/Distance	Inch (in) Foot (ft) [3 or less feet] Foot (ft) [3 or more feet] Mile (mi)	Millimeter (mm) Millimeter (mm) Meter (m) Kilometer (km)	1 in = 25 mm 1 ft = 300 mm 1 ft = 0.3 m 1 mi = 1.6 km
Area	Square Foot (ft^2) Square Mile (mi^2)	Square Meter (m^2) Square Kilometer (km^2)	1 ft^2 = 0.09 m^2 1 mi^2 = 2.6 km^2
Mass/Weight	Dry Ounce (oz) Pound (lb) Ton (T)	gram Kilogram (kg) Ton (T)	1 oz = 28 g 1 lb = 0.5 kg 1 T = 0.9 T
Volume	Cubic Foot (ft^3) Fluid Ounce (fl oz) Quart (qt) Gallon (gal)	Cubic Meter (m^3) Milliliter (mL) Liter (L) Liter (L)	1 ft^3 = 0.03 m^3 1 fl oz = 30 mL 1 qt = 1 L 1 gal = 4 L
Flow	Gallons per Minute (gpm) Cubic Foot per Minute (ft^3/min)	Liters per Minute (L/min) Cubic Meter per Minute (m^3/min)	1 gpm = 4 L/min 1 ft^3/min = 0.03 m^3/min
Flow per Area	Gallons per Minute per Square Foot (gpm/ft^2)	Liters per Square Meters Minute (L/(m^2.min))	1 gpm/ft^2 = 40 L/(m^2.min)
Pressure	Pounds per Square Inch (psi) Pounds per Square Foot (psf) Inches of Mercury (in Hg)	Kilopascal (kPa) Kilopascal (kPa) Kilopascal (kPa)	1 psi = 7 kPa 1 psf = .05 kPa 1 in Hg = 3.4 kPa
Speed/Velocity	Miles per Hour (mph) Feet per Second (ft/sec)	Kilometers per Hour (km/h) Meter per Second (m/s)	1 mph = 1.6 km/h 1 ft/sec = 0.3 m/s
Heat	British Thermal Unit (Btu)	Kilojoule (kJ)	1 Btu = 1 kJ
Heat Flow	British Thermal Unit per Minute (BTU/min)	watt (W)	1 Btu/min = 18 W
Density	Pound per Cubic Foot (lb/ft^3)	Kilogram per Cubic Meter (kg/m^3)	1 lb/ft^3 = 16 kg/m^3
Force	Pound-Force (lbf)	Newton (N)	1 lbf = 0.5 N
Torque	Pound-Force Foot (lbf ft)	Newton Meter (N.m)	1 lbf ft = 1.4 N.m
Dynamic Viscosity	Pound per Foot-Second (lb/ft.s)	Pascal Second (Pa.s)	1 lb/ft.s = 1.5 Pa.s
Surface Tension	Pound per Foot (lb/ft)	Newton per Meter (N/m)	1 lb/ft = 15 N/m

Conversion and Approximation Examples

Measurement	U.S. Unit	Conversion Factor	Exact S.I. Unit	Rounded S.I. Unit
Length/Distance	10 in	1 in = 25 mm	250 mm	250 mm
	25 in	1 in = 25 mm	625 mm	625 mm
	2 ft	1 in = 25 mm	600 mm	600 mm
	17 ft	1 ft = 0.3 m	5.1 m	5 m
	3 mi	1 mi = 1.6 km	4.8 km	5 km
	10 mi	1 mi = 1.6 km	16 km	16 km
Area	36 ft^2	1 ft^2 = 0.09 m^2	3.24 m^2	3 m^2
	300 ft^2	1 ft^2 = 0.09 m^2	27 m^2	30 m^2
	5 mi^2	1 mi^2 = 2.6 km^2	13 km^2	13 km^2
	14 mi^2	1 mi^2 = 2.6 km^2	36.4 km^2	35 km^2
Mass/Weight	16 oz	1 oz = 28 g	448 g	450 g
	20 oz	1 oz = 28 g	560 g	560 g
	3.75 lb	1 lb = 0.5 kg	1.875 kg	2 kg
	2,000 lb	1 lb = 0.5 kg	1 000 kg	1 000 kg
	1 T	1 T = 0.9 T	900 kg	900 kg
	2.5 T	1 T = 0.9 T	2.25 T	2 T
Volume	55 ft^3	1 ft^3 = 0.03 m^3	1.65 m^3	1.5 m^3
	2,000 ft^3	1 ft^3 = 0.03 m^3	60 m^3	60 m^3
	8 fl oz	1 fl oz = 30 mL	240 mL	240 mL
	20 fl oz	1 fl oz = 30 mL	600 mL	600 mL
	10 qt	1 qt = 1 L	10 L	10 L
	22 gal	1 gal = 4 L	88 L	90 L
	500 gal	1 gal = 4 L	2 000 L	2 000 L
Flow	100 gpm	1 gpm = 4 L/min	400 L/min	400 L/min
	500 gpm	1 gpm = 4 L/min	2 000 L/min	2 000 L/min
	16 ft^3/min	1 ft^3/min = 0.03 m^3/min	0.48 m^3/min	0.5 m^3/min
	200 ft^3/min	1 ft^3/min = 0.03 m^3/min	6 m^3/min	6 m^3/min
Flow per Area	50 gpm/ft^2	1 gpm/ft^2 = 40 L/(m^2.min)	2 000 L/(m^2.min)	2 000 L/(m^2.min)
	326 gpm/ft^2	1 gpm/ft^2 = 40 L/(m^2.min)	13 040 L/(m^2.min)	13 000 L/(m^2.min)
Pressure	100 psi	1 psi = 7 kPa	700 kPa	700 kPa
	175 psi	1 psi = 7 kPa	1225 kPa	1 200 kPa
	526 psf	1 psf = 0.05 kPa	26.3 kPa	25 kPa
	12,000 psf	1 psf = 0.05 kPa	600 kPa	600 kPa
	5 psi in Hg	1 psi = 3.4 kPa	17 kPa	17 kPa
	20 psi in Hg	1 psi = 3.4 kPa	68 kPa	70 kPa
Speed/Velocity	20 mph	1 mph = 1.6 km/h	32 km/h	30 km/h
	35 mph	1 mph = 1.6 km/h	56 km/h	55 km/h
	10 ft/sec	1 ft/sec = 0.3 m/s	3 m/s	3 m/s
	50 ft/sec	1 ft/sec = 0.3 m/s	15 m/s	15 m/s
Heat	1200 Btu	1 Btu = 1 kJ	1 200 kJ	1 200 kJ
Heat Flow	5 BTU/min	1 Btu/min = 18 W	90 W	90 W
	400 BTU/min	1 Btu/min = 18 W	7 200 W	7 200 W
Density	5 lb/ft^3	1 lb/ft^3 = 16 kg/m^3	80 kg/m^3	80 kg/m^3
	48 lb/ft^3	1 lb/ft^3 = 16 kg/m^3	768 kg/m^3	770 kg/m^3
Force	10 lbf	1 lbf = 0.5 N	5 N	5 N
	1,500 lbf	1 lbf = 0.5 N	750 N	750 N
Torque	100	1 lbf ft = 1.4 N.m	140 N.m	140 N.m
	500	1 lbf ft = 1.4 N.m	700 N.m	700 N.m
Dynamic Viscosity	20 lb/ft.s	1 lb/ft.s = 1.5 Pa.s	30 Pa.s	30 Pa.s
	35 lb/ft.s	1 lb/ft.s = 1.5 Pa.s	52.5 Pa.s	50 Pa.s
Surface Tension	6.5 lb/ft	1 lb/ft = 15 N/m	97.5 N/m	100 N/m
	10 lb/ft	1 lb/ft = 15 N/m	150 N/m	150 N/m

SECTION A: AWARENESS LEVEL RESCUER

Vehicle Incident Safety

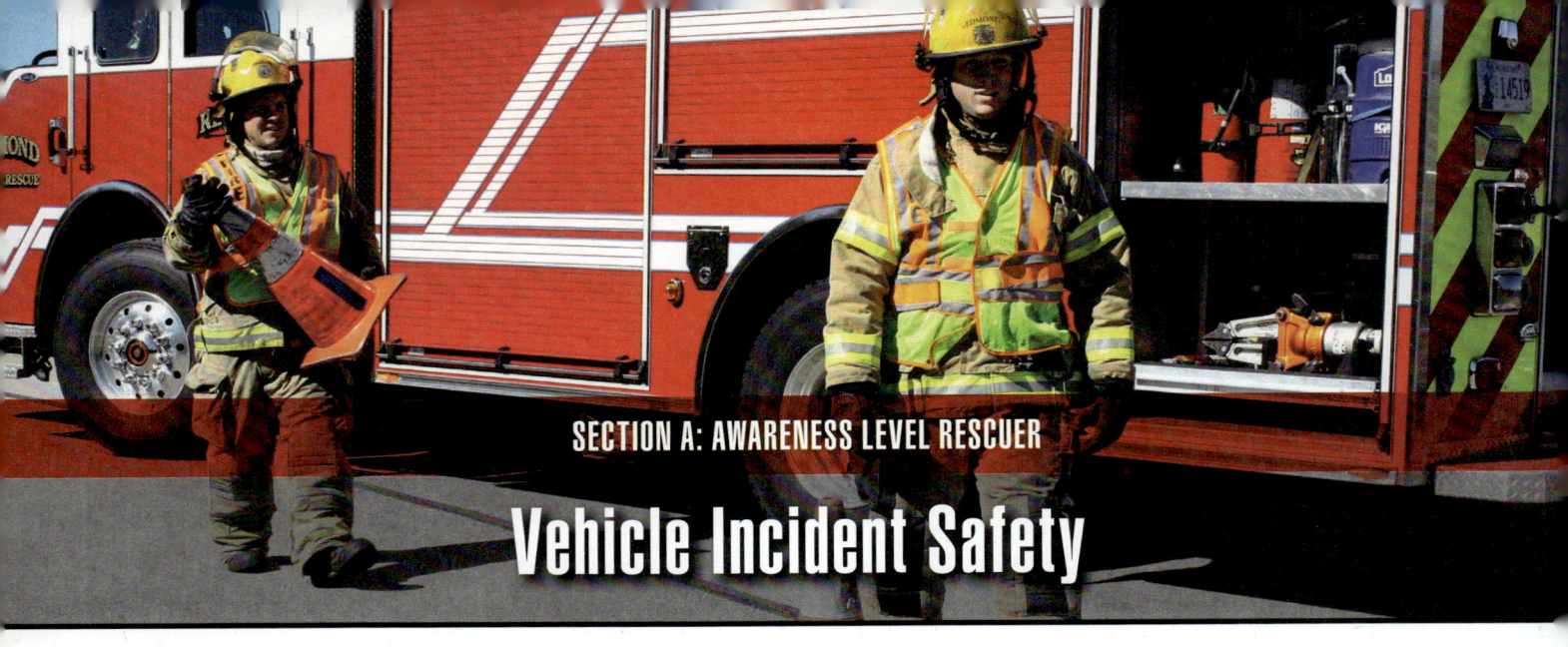

Chapter Contents

Operational Capability and Training Requirements 11
- Awareness Level 12
- Operations Level 12
- Technician Level 13

Preparation for Response 13
- Response Plans 14
- Hazard and Risk Assessment Surveys 16
- Extrication and Personal Protective Equipment 16

Scene Size-Up 16
- Environmental Considerations 17
- On-Scene Hazards 18

Safety Measures 22
- Training 22
- Crew Resource Management 22
- Medical Component 24
- Rehabilitation (Rehab) Station 24
- Potential Hazards 24
- Incident Safety Officer (ISO) 25
- Personnel Accountability 26

Scene Safety 26
- Incident Stability 27
- Personal Safety Equipment and Techniques 29

Safety Zones 30
- Types of Safety Zones 30
- Staffing Requirements for Safety Zones 33
- Monitoring Hazard Zones 33

Traffic Control 34
- Traffic Control Concepts 35
- Traffic Control Devices 35
- Traffic Control Resources 40

Vehicle Incident Operations 40
- Operational Protocols 41
- Incident Action Plan (IAP) 42
- Communication 44
- Incident Support Operations and Resources 46

Chapter Review 48
Discussion Questions 48
Skill Sheets 49

8   Section A • Chapter 1 – Vehicle Incident Safety

chapter 1

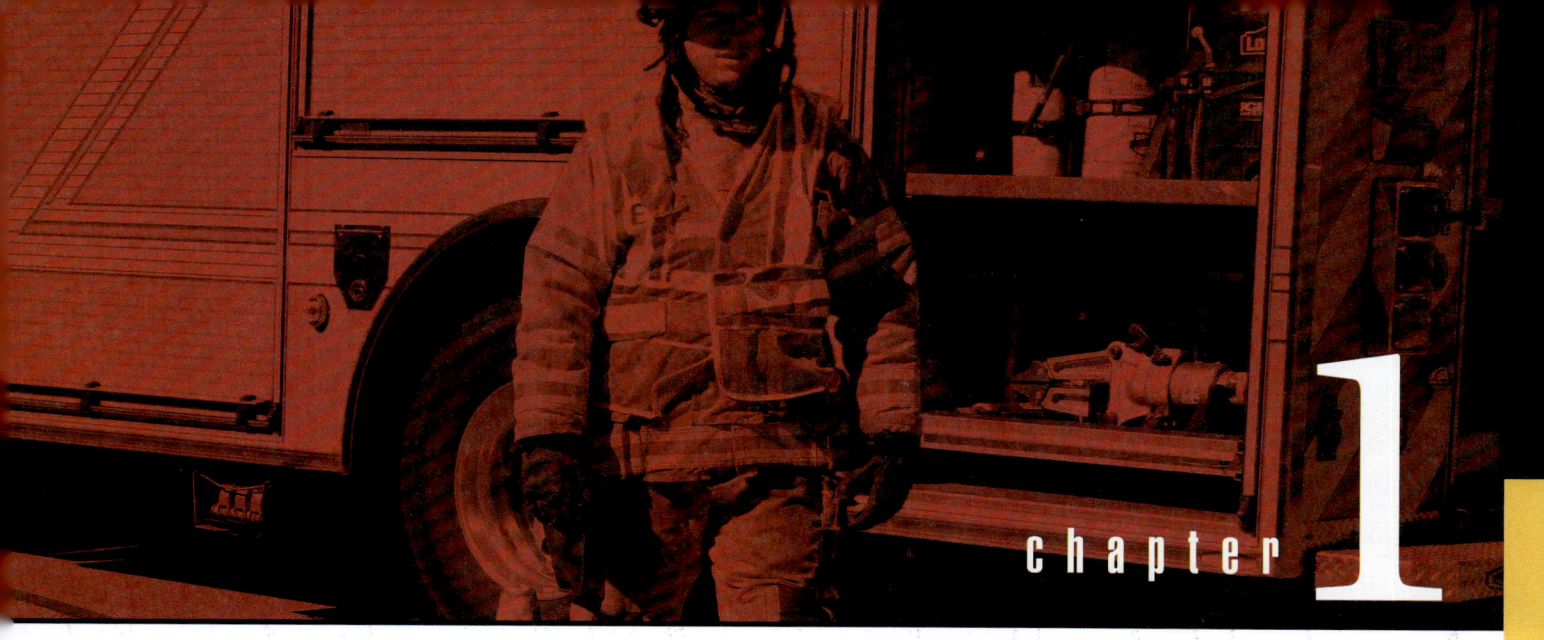

Key Terms

Assistant Incident Safety Officers (AISO) 33
Authority Having Jurisdiction (AHJ) 11
Basic Life Support (BLS) 41
Bloodborne Pathogens 21
Freelance 22
Incident Commander (IC) 25
Incident Safety Officer (ISO) 25
Limited Access (Warm) Zone 32

National Incident Management System - Incident Command System (NIMS-ICS) 40
Personnel Accountability System 26
Rehabilitation 24
Restricted (Hot) Zone 31
Risk-Benefit Analysis 17
Support (Cold) Zone 32
Tactical Worksheet 42
Traffic Control 34

JPRs addressed in this chapter

This chapter provides information that addresses the following job performance requirements of NFPA 1006, *Standard for Technical Rescuer Professional Qualifications (2016)*.

8.1.1   8.1.3
8.1.2   8.1.4

Vehicle Incident Safety

Learning Objectives

1. Differentiate among the duties of Awareness, Operations, and Technician level rescuers. [8.1.3]
2. Describe the types of planning that must occur for vehicle incidents. [8.1.1, 8.1.4]
3. Describe the process of completing size-up at a vehicle incident. [8.1.3, 8.1.4]
4. Identify factors that must be addressed in order to operate safely at a vehicle incident. [8.1.1, 8.1.2, 8.1.3]
5. Identify factors that must be addressed in order for an incident to successfully be carried out and stabilized. [8.1.1, 8.1.2, 8.1.3]
6. Describe personal safety equipment and techniques used at vehicle incidents. [8.1.2, 8.1.3]
7. Explain the use of scene safety zones at a vehicle incident. [8.1.1, 8.1.2, 8.1.3]
8. Describe traffic control flow and concepts for an incident location. [8.1.2]
9. Determine appropriate traffic control devices and methods based on incident information. [8.1.2]
10. Explain the purpose of operational protocols for vehicle incidents. [8.1.1, 8.1.2, 8.1.3]
11. Describe the role that communication plays at vehicle incidents. [8.1.1, 8.1.3, 8.1.4]
12. Identify incident support operations and resources for vehicle incidents. [8.1.1, 8.1.3, 8.1.4]
13. Skill Sheet 1-1: Provide support for a vehicle incident. [8.1.3]
14. Skill Sheet 1-2: Perform size up and initiate the response at a vehicle incident. [8.1.1, 8.1.4]
15. Skill Sheet 1-3: Establish scene safety zones at a vehicle incident. [8.1.2]

Chapter 1
Vehicle Incident Safety

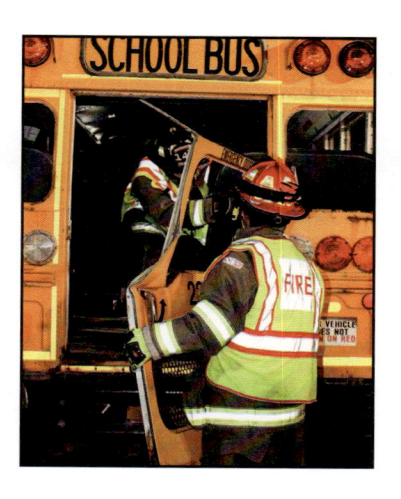

The safe and effective handling of vehicle incidents demands a well-organized extrication operation. This includes providing an appropriate response and using the adopted Incident Command System (ICS) to manage the scene and the available resources. In addition to NFPA 1670, *Standard on Operations and Training for Technical Search and Rescue Incidents,* and NFPA 1006, *Standard for Technical Rescuer Professional Qualifications*, on which this manual is based, the management of extrication operations is governed by NFPA 1561, *Standard on Emergency Services Incident Management System and Command Safety*, and NFPA 1500, *Standard on Fire Department Occupational Safety and Health Program*. In the United States, Homeland Security Presidential Directive-5 (HSPD-5) directs that all state and local governments and tribal entities adopt the National Incident Management System-Incident Command System (NIMS-ICS). Local emergency organizations should make sure that their command structure will interface with external organizations in an emergency.

Successful operation at a vehicle incident is defined by how effectively and safely it was conducted. These two criteria cannot be separated when assessing the outcome of a vehicle incident. However, because the subsequent chapters of this manual address the knowledge, skills, and abilities needed to conduct extrication operations effectively, the information in this chapter focuses on initiating effective operations and establishing safety at an incident scene.

Operational Capability and Training Requirements

The **authority having jurisdiction (AHJ)** should establish the level of capability at which the organization will perform technical rescue operations. This level should be selected based on:

- Types of hazards identified during the organization's hazard and risk assessment survey
- Level of personnel training
- Resources (internal and external) available to the organization

NOTE: Plans should also be developed for incidents that require a higher level of capability than the local jurisdiction provides.

> **Authority Having Jurisdiction (AHJ)** — An organization, office, or individual responsible for enforcing the requirements of a code or standard, or approving equipment, materials, an installation, or a procedure.

Rescue organizations should train all personnel to meet the organization's level of operational capability. NFPA 1006, *Standard for Technical Rescuer Professional Qualifications* provides requirements for three different operating levels:

- Awareness
- Operations
- Technician

Additionally, each member of the emergency response organization must be trained on the appropriate requirements of NFPA 472, *Standard for Competence of Responders to Hazardous Materials/Weapons of Mass Destruction Incidents* that correspond to the level of the organization's rescue capability. The organization should also provide for the continuing education necessary to maintain the organization's level of operational capability.

The organization should document all training and have a system for managing and maintaining this documentation. Authorized rescue team members and personnel should be available to review and inspect training documentation.

The organization should review its training program and its performance regularly. They should establish procedures for conducting an annual review of the organization's training program. This ensures that personnel are adequately trained to function in a variety of hazardous conditions and environments. Management should establish procedures for conducting an annual review of the organization's performance in relation to the appropriate standards.

Awareness Level

Organizations that wish to operate at the Awareness Level should train their personnel in accordance with the appropriate requirements of NFPA 1006. Some of these requirements may include the following:

- Conducting incident size-up
- Recognizing the need for rescue personnel and resources
- Establishing scene safety zones
- Initiating site and traffic control and scene management procedures **(Figure 1.1)**
- Identifying general hazards at an incident
- Reporting progress to Command
- Managing environmental concerns
- Facilitating personnel rehabilitation
- Supporting the Incident Action Plan (IAP) and operations/technician level rescuers during operations

Skill Sheet 1-1 describes the steps for providing support at a vehicle incident.

Operations Level

Organizations that wish to operate at the Operations Level should train their personnel in accordance with the appropriate requirements of NFPA 1006. In

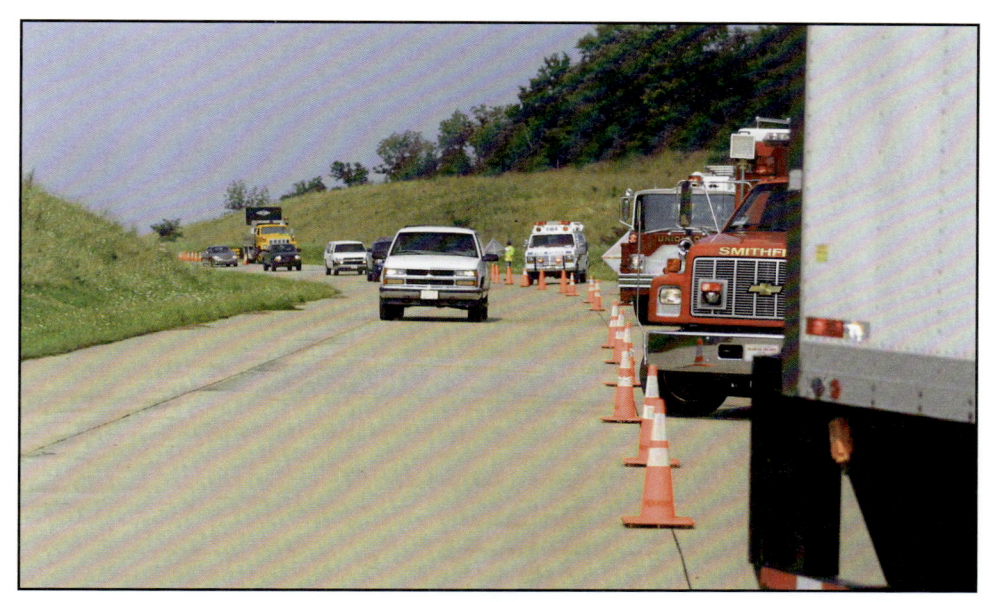

Figure 1.1 Vehicle traffic can pose a hazard to rescuers and patients during vehicle extrication operations.

addition to duties performed at the Awareness Level, Operations Level rescues should be able to perform the following at a vehicle extrication incident:

- Creating an Incident Action Plan for a vehicle incident
- Establishing fire protection for rescuers
- Stabilizing a passenger vehicle
- Isolating and managing hazards including harmful energy sources
- Accessing a passenger vehicle to extricate victims
- Operating extrication hand tools and equipment safely **(Figure 1.2)**
- Recognizing and controlling incident hazards
- Disentangling, packaging, and removing victims from a passenger vehicle without causing further harm to the victim
- Terminating a vehicle incident

Technician Level

Organizations that wish to operate at the Technician Level should train their personnel in accordance with the appropriate requirements of NFPA 1006. Technician Level rescuers must be able to perform all of the duties of Awareness and Operations Level rescuers. In addition, they must be able to apply all of the stabilization, extrication, disentanglement, and victim management techniques from the Operations Level to commercial or heavy vehicles **(Figure 1.3, p. 14)**. If an incident involves commercial or heavy vehicles, having Technician Level rescuers active at the scene is recommended.

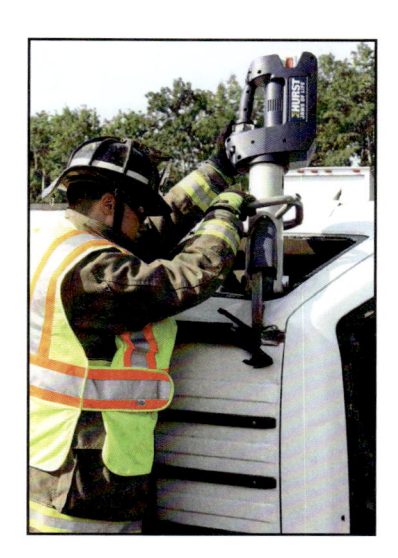

Figure 1.2 This responder is practicing the correct use of a hydraulic cutter tool.

Preparation for Response

Planning and training are the keys to effective response, organization, and management.

Section A • Chapter 1 – Vehicle Incident Safety

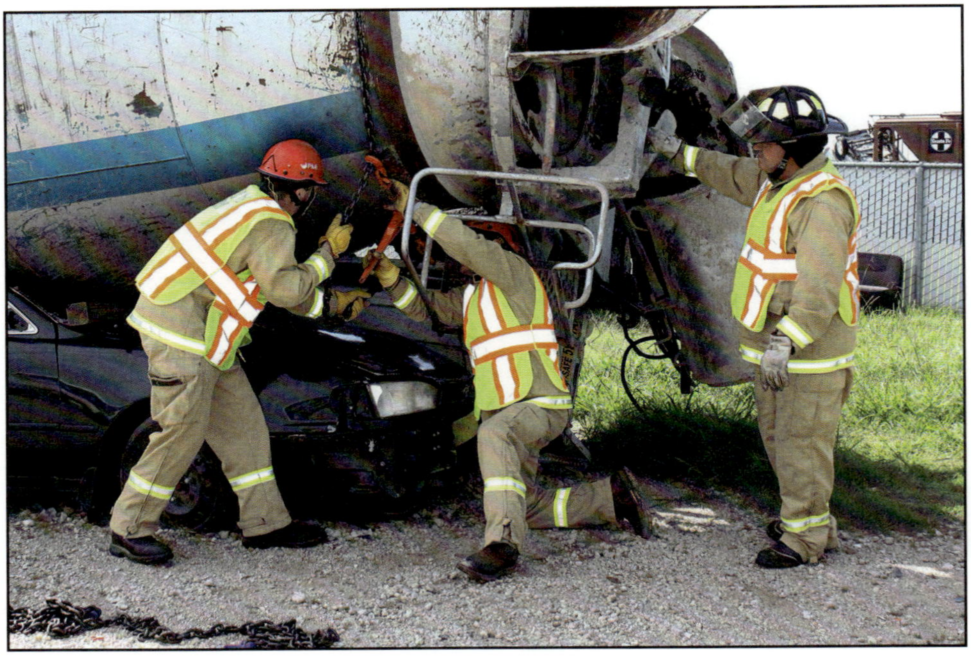

Figure 1.3 These Technician Level responders are applying chains to a commercial vehicle.

Preincident planning and realistic training enable emergency crews to gain familiarity on the following:

- Response district
- Local standard operating procedures (SOPs)
- Incident Command System
- Other agencies

Well-trained rescuers know what can and cannot be done with the resources available. Knowledge of the capabilities and limitations of equipment and personnel improves the decision-making of those in charge.

Topics covered in this section include:

- Response plans
- Hazard and risk assessment surveys
- Incident Action Plan
- Extrication and personal protective equipment

Response Plans

Part of incident action planning for a vehicle response is determining the initial response plan for each type of vehicle incident to any location within the district. Many emergency response organizations have predetermined response plans for specific types of incidents. If possible, organizations should develop standard response plans for vehicle incidents so that each responder knows which other resources can be expected to arrive at the scene. First-arriving personnel can use this knowledge to call for additional help or to cancel apparatus already en route. A predetermined, standardized response has many benefits and is an important step in organizing the vehicle incident.

Response plans generally include the resources that are likely to be needed for dealing with a variety of extrication incidents. Many response areas have predetermined Incident Management Coalition Teams. In these situations, the AHJ will determine the responders' role in these plans. Standardizing the response helps to ensure that all personnel and apparatus that may be needed will arrive soon enough to be used effectively.

The primary entities in a standard extrication response plan should understand their role and how they are expected to participate in emergency extrication activities. These entities include **(Figure 1.4)**:

- Extrication team
- Emergency medical services (EMS)
- Fire protection
- Law enforcement
- Relevant outside agencies

Proper communication is the key to a successful response plan. Organizations should incorporate communications into the response plan within ICS and other response agencies. Jurisdictions should ensure that radios and other communication equipment utilized are compatible with other assisting agencies.

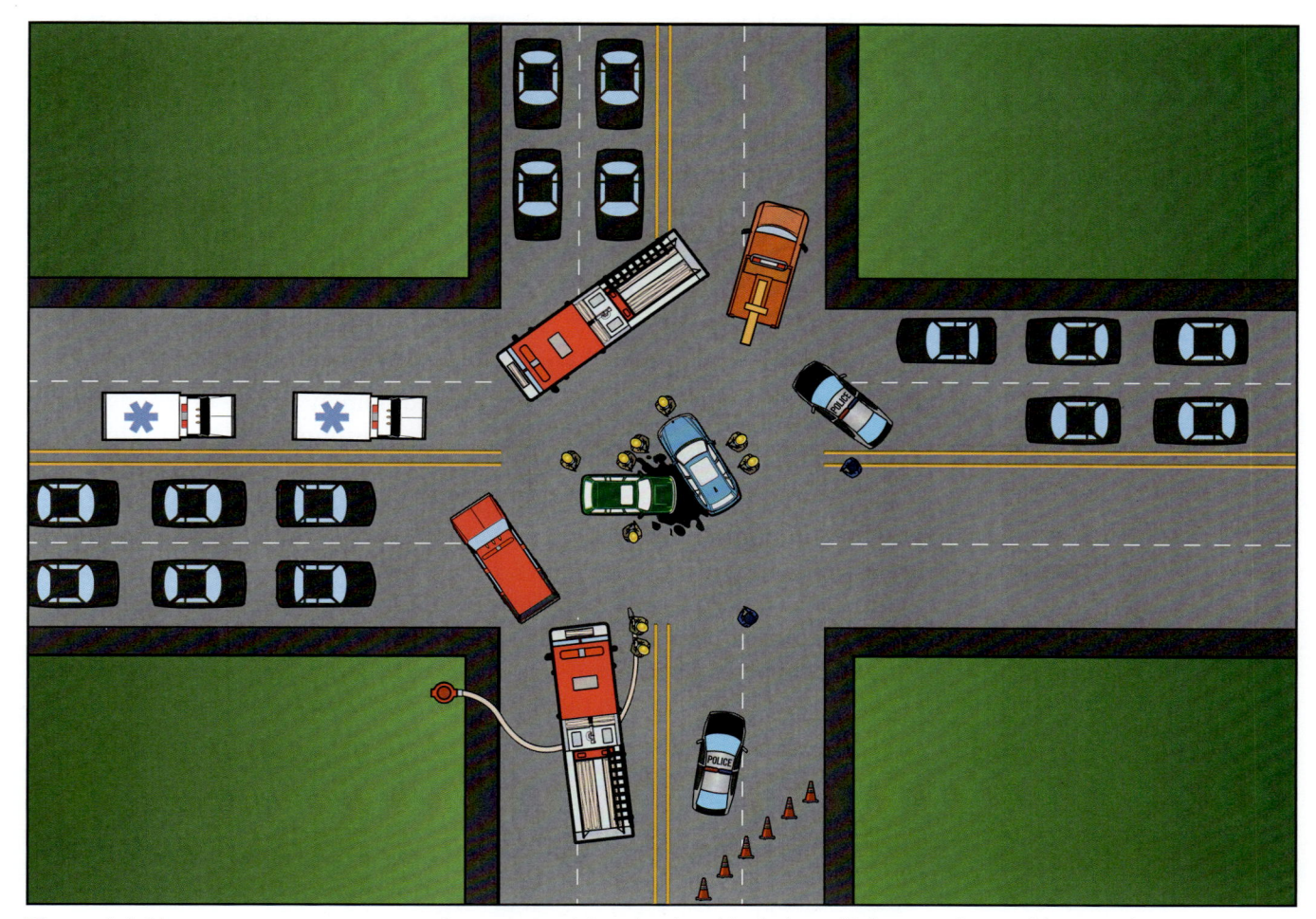

Figure 1.4 Many emergency response plans are predetermined and include multiple agencies working together.

Hazard and Risk Assessment Surveys

Before conducting rescue operations, a hazard and risk assessment survey of the response area should be conducted. In this survey, the organization will identify potential hazards, assess the level of risk within the locale, and determine possible rescue situations that may occur.

The organization should then examine the cultural, social, physical, and environmental factors that can influence the frequency, scope, or magnitude of possible incidents and compare them to the impact they may have upon the organization's ability to respond safely to an incident.

Information researched during preplanning is similar to information that will be assessed during scene size-up. The hazard and risk assessment survey should include:

- Traffic flows and patterns based on time of day
- Weather
- Terrain
- Construction
- Previously identified high-risk areas such as hairpin curves
- Locations with decreased visibility
- Alternate response routes and/or traffic diversion routes

The hazard and risk assessment survey should be documented, reviewed periodically, and updated regularly (or as needs arise). This process will help determine if additional types of rescue situations that require a higher level of response may occur within the local area.

The AHJ must assess the potential of an incident response involving nuclear and/or biological weapons, chemical agents, or weapons of mass destruction (WMDs). This assessment must include the potential of secondary devices at the incident scene. If the AHJ determines such risks exist, emergency response personnel must have appropriate training and equipment.

Extrication and Personal Protective Equipment

The rescue organization should identify the equipment and resources available (both internally and externally) and acquire equipment that is applicable to the organization's level of capability. The organization should list the types, quantities, and locations of this equipment in its SOPs or inventory control system. The SOPs should describe the procedures for accessing the equipment during emergency situations. Personnel should update the inventory list annually or when equipment is added or removed from service. The organization should maintain each piece of equipment in accordance with the manufacturer's recommendations. The rescue organization should properly train all rescue personnel in the use of each piece of equipment.

Scene Size-Up

Awareness level rescuers should be able to initiate size-up at a scene. Doing so mainly includes identifying hazards at the scene and communicating these hazards to an Operations or Technician level rescuer who will take command at the scene. Awareness level rescuers should also be able to perform a **risk-benefit analysis** of the hazards at the scene. Risk-benefit analysis entails comparing the risks to rescuers at the scene with the possible benefit of encountering those risks. For example, if it is likely that performing certain rescue tactics has a high likelihood that firefighters will be severely injured or killed, then different tactics to effect the rescue or delay operations until the scene can be made safer could be better options.

> **Risk-Benefit Analysis** – Comparison between the known hazards and potential benefits of any operation; used to determine the feasibility and parameters of the operation.

Environmental Considerations

Many agencies have identified certain environmental factors that may impact an extrication operation at specific locations. These factors may affect the agency's ability to safely mitigate an incident. Environmental factors that may influence a vehicle incident can include the following:

- Weather
- Time of day
- Terrain

Weather

Extended vehicle extrication operations during inclement weather, such as heat, cold, humidity, or heavy rain, pose a risk to rescuers and victims. Remain aware of potential heat- and cold-related emergencies at an extrication scene. Performing extrication operations during hot summer months can lead to heat-related stress. During cold winter months, victims are at greater risk of hypothermia or frostbite.

Time of Day

Incidents that occur at night or in low-light conditions require supplemental lighting provided by apparatus-mounted lights or portable lighting systems **(Figure 1.5)**. Illumination helps personnel identify safety hazards, such as downed power lines or trip hazards, and provides an adequate environment in which to operate.

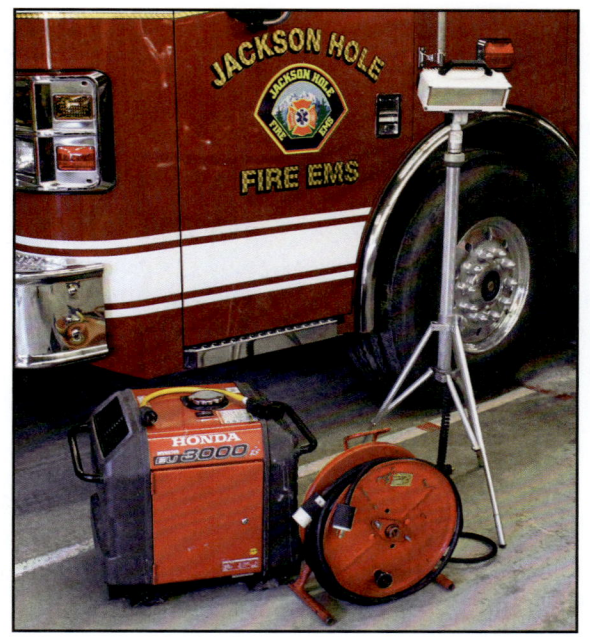

Figure 1.5 Incidents occurring at night often require additional lighting on the scene. Full-scene lighting equipment includes a portable generator, cord, and lights. *Courtesy of Shad Cooper/Wyoming State Fire Marshal's Office.*

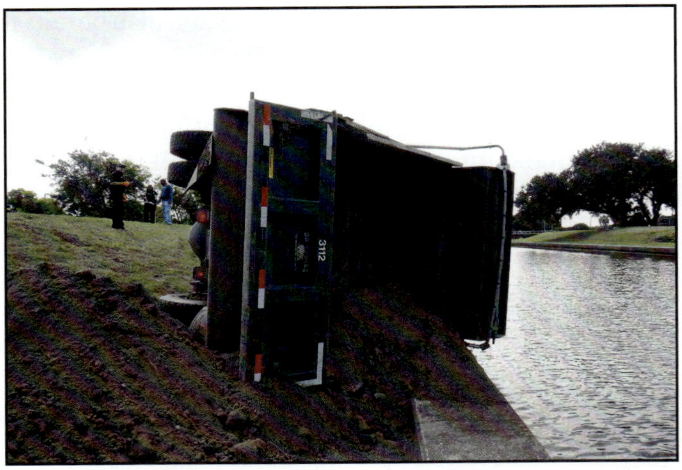

Figure 1.6 Vehicles that have left the roadway present unique challenges to rescuers. *Courtesy of Chris Mickal.*

Lighting units may produce extreme heat and can cause burns. Be careful when moving lights or turning them off. Bulbs can explode if they come in contact with water. Never direct lights toward moving traffic because this can blind drivers.

Terrain

Vehicle extrication does not always occur on flat and manageable surfaces. Often, vehicles may leave the roadway as a result of the accident **(Figure 1.6)**. Vehicles may come to rest in creeks, ravines, or canyons where the terrain can pose significant access and egress challenges. Hazards such as water, soil conditions, and uneven topography will all impact vehicle stabilization, spill containment, and victim removal.

On-Scene Hazards

Once emergency responders arrive on scene and position their apparatus for protection, they must identify and/or mitigate all scene hazards related to the incident. This section will describe the following on-scene hazards:

- Traffic hazards
- Vehicle stability
- Vehicle contents
- Transformers and downed power lines
- Fuel Spills
- Biohazards
- Vehicle Occupants

Vehicle hazards are not just a danger to response personnel, but also to victims. For more information on hazards and hazard mitigation.

NOTE: see Chapter 2.

Traffic Hazards

Every year, approximately six to eight firefighters die on roadways as a result of being struck by vehicles while working in or near moving traffic **(Figure 1.7)**. Proper scene protection with responding apparatus is imperative to a safe and effective extrication operation.

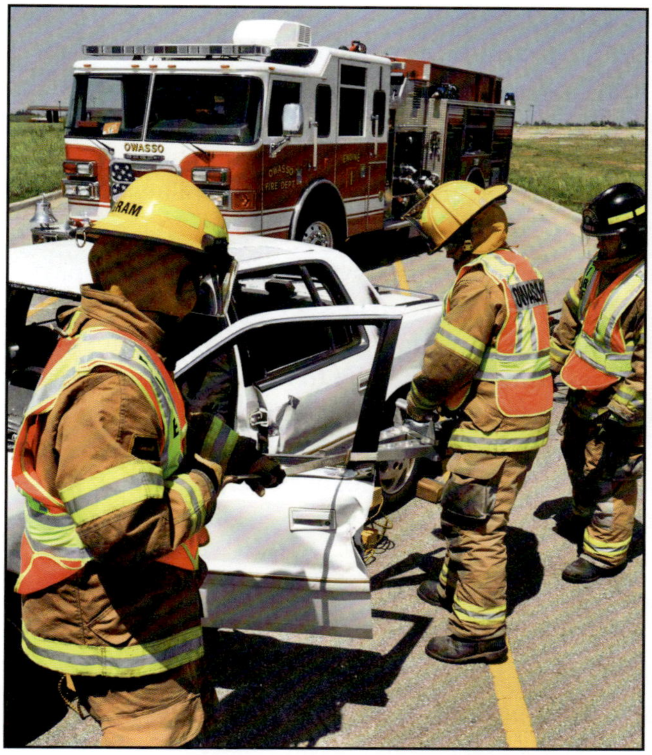

Figure 1.7 Fire and emergency service personnel practicing vehicle extrication techniques. *Courtesy of Sonrise Photography.*

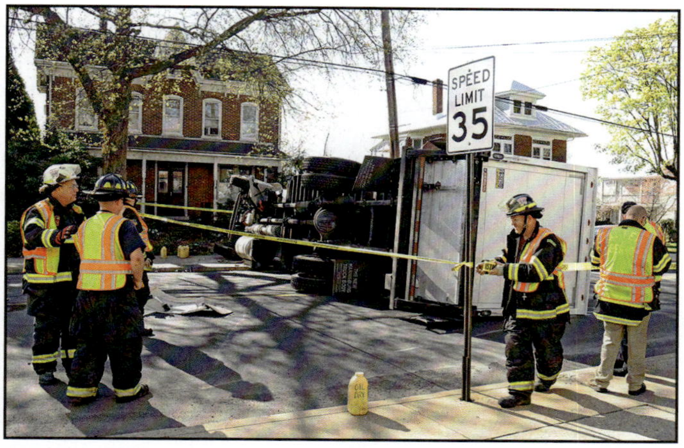

Figure 1.8 Responders cordoning off an overturned vehicle accident scene. *Courtesy of Bob Esposito.*

Practice constant situational awareness at any roadway incident. Position apparatus at the incident scene to form a protective barrier between the scene and all traffic. Implement signage and cones to detour approaching vehicles around the scene hazards **(Figure 1.8)**. Highway incident management procedures should reflect the Department of Transportation's *Manual on Uniform Traffic Control Devices* (MUTCD) and the appropriate AHJ procedures within the operational response area.

Vehicle Stability

Stabilize the vehicle before rescue personnel work around or enter a vehicle involved in a collision. This is necessary to prevent further injury to the victims, possible injuries to rescue personnel, and further degradation of the vehicle's structural integrity.

NOTE: For more information on vehicle stabilization operations, refer to Chapters 7 and 10.

Vehicle Contents

Additional hazards may be found in/on the vehicle. Rescuers commonly encounter flammable adhesives, pressurized solvents, or flammable liquids (such as gasoline) **(Figure 1.9)**. Illegal substances used to produce methamphetamine (meth) are also highly flammable. In extreme cases, vehicles have contained entire mobile meth laboratories. Medium and heavy trucks often transport bulky contents. These contents may be unstable and require rescuers to stabilize the contents in addition to the vehicle. Hazardous cargo in medium and heavy trucks will be covered later in this chapter.

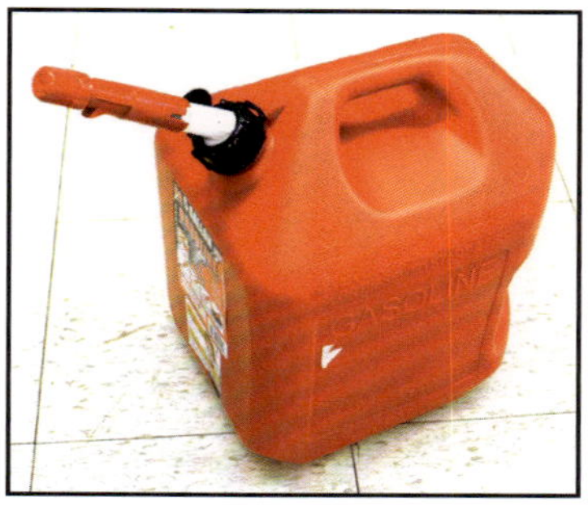

Figure 1.9 Responders should check vehicles involved in accidents for items such as plastic gas containers since they present a hazard.

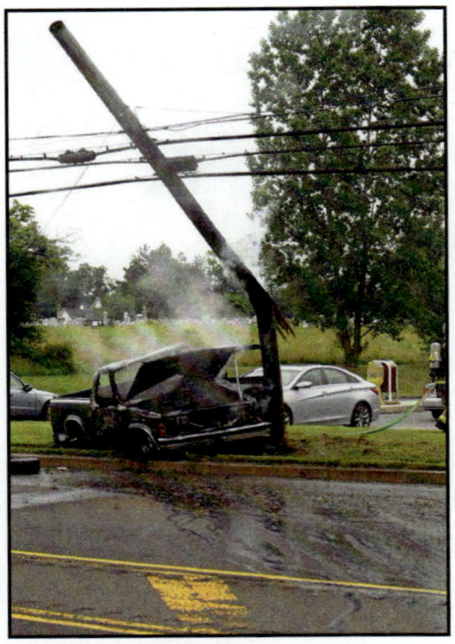

Figure 1.10 Downed power lines present life-threatening hazards. *Courtesy of Bob Esposito.*

Downed Power Lines/Transformer Hazards

Downed power lines add a life-threatening dimension to the incident. In areas with overhead electrical lines, vehicles may strike and damage utility poles causing power lines to fall near or on the vehicle(s) **(Figure 1.10)**. In some areas where electrical power lines are buried instead of being suspended, vehicles may come to rest on top of the electrical ground transformers. These vehicles may be energized and must be addressed as such.

One of the most frustrating and most dangerous vehicle extrication scenarios is one in which an injured vehicle occupant can be seen through the vehicle's windows but rescuers cannot touch the vehicle because it is in contact with a downed power line. Rescue personnel are trained to help those in need and the temptation to assume that the power line is no longer energized or to attempt to move the power line off the vehicle becomes almost overwhelming; resist this temptation. Assume that all power lines are energized until power has been shut off by utility service personnel.

> **WARNING!**
> Downed power lines will kill you. Ensure power lines are de-energized prior to working at a scene with downed power lines.

When performing a size-up, identify downed power lines and note any signs of a power outage near the incident, such as buildings without lighting or street lamps that are not working. Announce the presence of a downed power line over the radio to alert all emergency personnel and over public address systems or bullhorns to alert others. All personnel on the incident scene and responding to the incident scene should acknowledge the presence of downed power lines. While waiting for utility service personnel to arrive at the scene, rescuers should cordon off the area of the downed power line to protect themselves and others **(Figure 1.11)**.

Fuel Spills

Fuel leaks are common at vehicle accidents **(Figure 1.12)**. Modern vehicle plastic tanks puncture easily and fuel lines that run underneath the vehicle can sever during an accident. If vehicles come to rest on their side, gravity causes fuel, oil, and other fluids to flow into areas where they do not belong. These fluids may ignite if they come into contact with ignition sources such as hot exhaust system components or electrical components.

Be prepared to handle fuel spills at a vehicle incident **(Figure 1.13)**. Dependent upon the amount of fluids leaked, federal agencies may need to be notified for hazard disposal and/or clean-up. If larger spills or leaks are present, damming or diking to prevent runoff may be needed. Manage smaller spills with an approved adsorbent, or absorbent material.

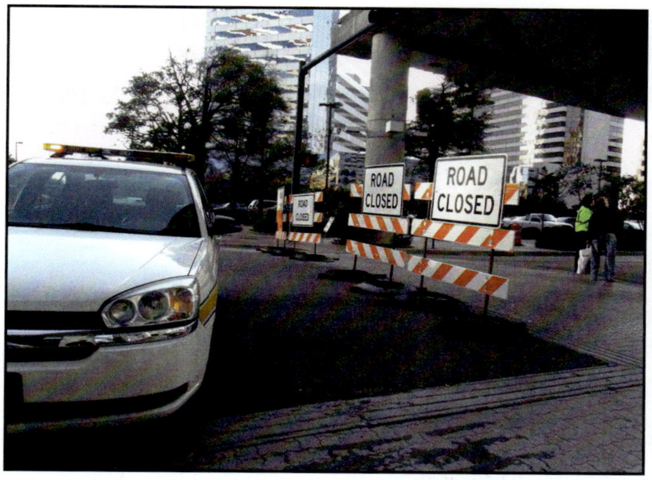

Figure 1.11 Streets and intersections can be blocked by vehicles and barricades.

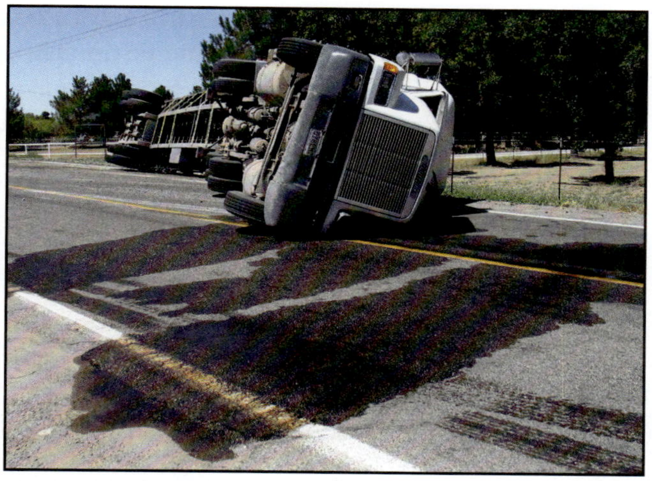

Figure 1.12 Hazardous Material incidents require responders with special training. *Courtesy of Rich Mahaney.*

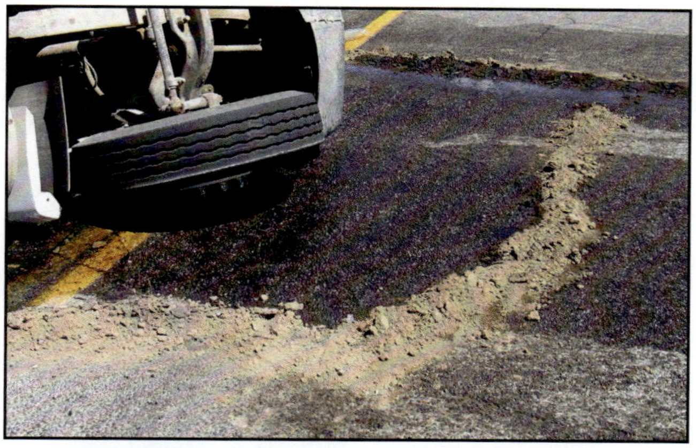

Figure 1.13 Some incidents include small fuel spills. *Courtesy of Rich Mahaney.*

Biohazards

Rescuers may encounter body fluids or biohazards resulting from victims during extrication operations. These can contaminate the interior and exterior of the vehicle involved. Rescuers should follow the AHJ's **bloodborne pathogen** procedures and wear appropriate protective clothing and equipment to avoid exposure to these materials.

Boots and the cuffs of protective trousers can become contaminated from standing in blood and other bodily fluids/ Take care to avoid possible contaminants when removing boots and protective trousers. Follow department SOPs for decontaminating this protective equipment.

Some jurisdictions may affix biohazard warning labels to the contaminated vehicle to warn others of the potential hazard **(Figure 1.14)**. On overturned vehicles, affix these labels so that they can be read by personnel approaching the vehicle.

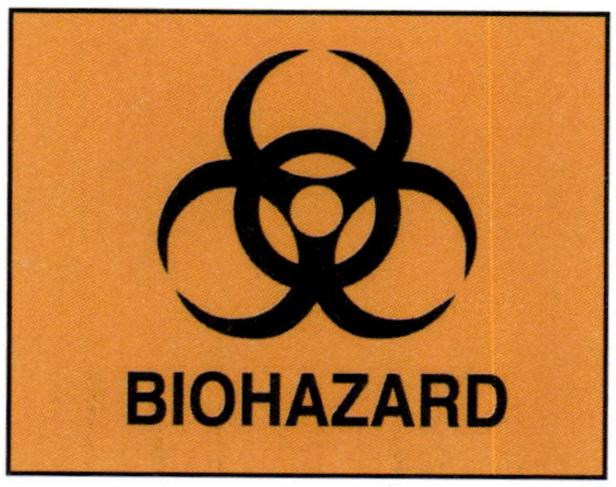

Vehicle Occupants

Vehicle accidents are often traumatic and emotional events for those involved. Occupants may be distraught and unmanageable, or even be angry and combative, posing a threat to emergency responders and bystanders. Alcohol or

Figure 1.14 This biohazard placard alerts responders to potential contamination.

Bloodborne Pathogens — Pathogenic microorganisms that are present in the human blood and can cause disease in humans. These pathogens include (but are not limited to) hepatitis B virus (HBV) and human immunodeficiency virus (HIV).

Section A • Chapter 1 – Vehicle Incident Safety **21**

drug use may cause unpredictable behavior of those affected. Law enforcement should be present at all vehicle accident and extrication events.

Safety Measures

Conducting extrication operations safely involves a number of different, but interrelated components. Each of the following components is important to incident safety:

- Training
- Crew resource management
- Medical component
- Rehabilitation (rehab) station
- Recognizing potential hazards
- Incident Safety Officer
- Personnel accountability

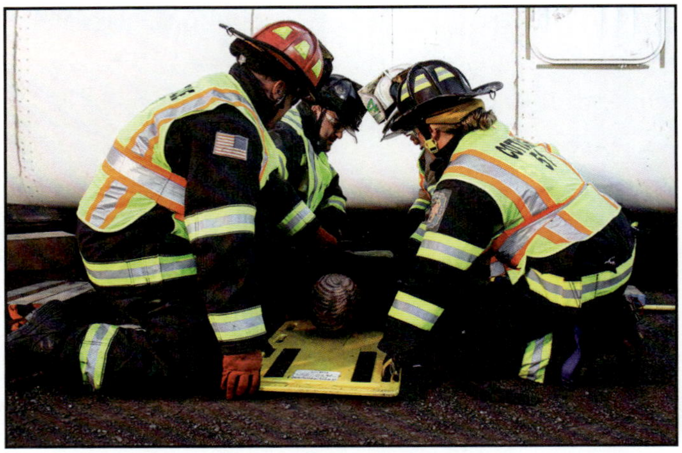

Figure 1.15 Teamwork is vital to successful extrication operations.

Training

Training firefighters and other rescuers to function safely during extrication operations involves a number of different considerations:

- Train personnel to use the most appropriate rescue tools and techniques for the task at hand so that all assignments are carried out safely.
- Teach personnel to function as a member of a rescue team **(Figure 1.15)**. Personnel should not **freelance**; that is, act individually without supervision and without coordination with other members of the team.
- Make personnel aware of the department's standard operating procedures (SOPs) and any other operational plans developed as part of the incident action plan. These individuals should also understand their roles within those plans. Operational plans and SOPs should be practiced during training until they become second nature.

Freelance — To operate independently of the Incident Commander's command and control.

Crew Resource Management

An integral part of all emergency operations is crew resource management. Before an Extrication Team Leader makes operational assignments, he or she must evaluate the situational requirements. When making these assignments,

22 Section A • Chapter 1 – Vehicle Incident Safety

the team leader must determine which rescuers have the knowledge, skills, and abilities to carry out the operations. The team leader should also consider which rescuers have the necessary:

- Experience and/or competence
- Physical strength and stamina
- Emotional strength and stability

This assessment can often be made instantly if the officer and the members of the crew have trained and worked together on other incidents. If the assessment is not done, or is done too casually, the results could be disastrous. The likelihood of failure or injury is increased by assigning a potentially hazardous task to someone who may be technically or physically incapable of completing the assignment safely. It is equally important to train with and assess the capabilities and limitations of mutual-aid resources that may be needed on vehicle incidents.

NOTE: If the organization has a system for certifying professional competencies, the likelihood of choosing the right subordinate for an assignment is greatly increased.

Every rescuer has the duty to report safety concerns and to stop unsafe operations:

- Discuss the safety concerns with the rescuer, Team Leader, or whoever is making the assignment and reach an agreement on how to alter the assignment to reduce the level of risk while still meeting the objective.
- Communicate with the Team Leader when rescuers are not qualified or lack the necessary resources to safely complete the task.

Turning Down Assignments

If a rescuer determines that an assignment is unsafe, he or she has the right to identify safer alternatives for completing that assignment. Sometimes, turning down assignments is the safest alternative. Rescuers may turn down an assignment under the following conditions:

- The assignment is a violation of safe work practices.
- The environmental conditions make the assignment unsafe.
- The rescuer does not possess the necessary qualifications or experience to complete the assignment.
- The equipment necessary to complete the assignment is defective or inoperable.

When making the decision to turn down an assignment, rescuers should inform their Team Leader, the Incident Safety Officer, and the Incident Commander. This communication allows necessary parties to identify the hazards present and develop a mitigation plan.

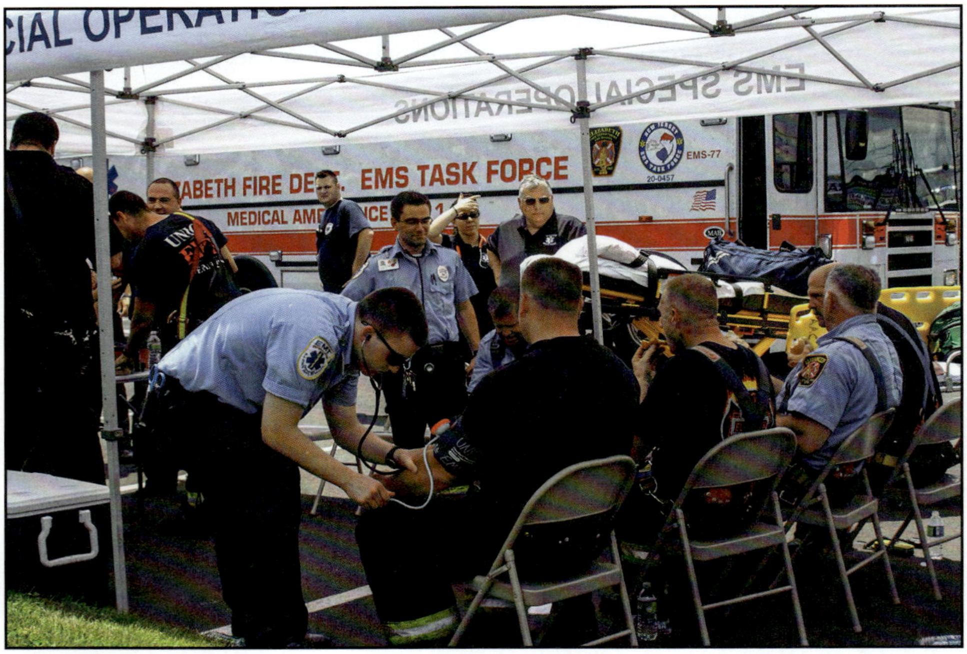

Figure 1.16 Responders recovering at a rehab station. *Courtesy of Ron Jeffers.*

Medical Component

Rescuers are often required to place themselves at risk in order to rescue someone in distress. The following items help to ensure that rescuers can complete their assignments safely:

- Training and experience
- Reliability of their equipment
- Safety margin built into their procedures

Despite the best efforts of rescuers to protect themselves, the unforeseen sometimes happens and rescuers get hurt. Because of this potential for injury, a suggested best practice is to have an ambulance available for the rescuers at every emergency incident in addition to any other ambulances that may be standing by to treat and/or transport the victim(s).

Rehabilitation (Rehab) Station

In every prolonged extrication operation, and especially those that are conducted in less than ideal weather conditions, there is a need to establish a **rehabilitation** (rehab) station for the rescue personnel **(Figure 1.16)**. Even in relatively hospitable conditions, rescuers often have to perform heavy physical labor, unrestrictive clauses (cms) such as operating power tools, struggling with debris, or installing cribbing. All of these activities can dehydrate and fatigue rescuers. Even under ideal circumstances, rescuers need to be relieved periodically for rest and rehydration. The frequency with which crews will need to be rotated will vary with the conditions, the type of personal protective equipment (PPE) being worn by the rescuers, and the types of activities in which they are engaged. For more information on this topic, refer to local SOPs.

Potential Hazards

Potential hazards can make extrication operations more difficult and can put rescuers at serious risk. These hazards must first be identified and addressed **(Figure 1.17)**. Therefore, the actual extrication operation might have to be de-

> **Rehabilitation** — Allowing firefighters or rescuers to rest, rehydrate, and recover during an incident; also refers to a station at an incident where personnel can rest, rehydrate, and recover. *Also known as* Rehab.

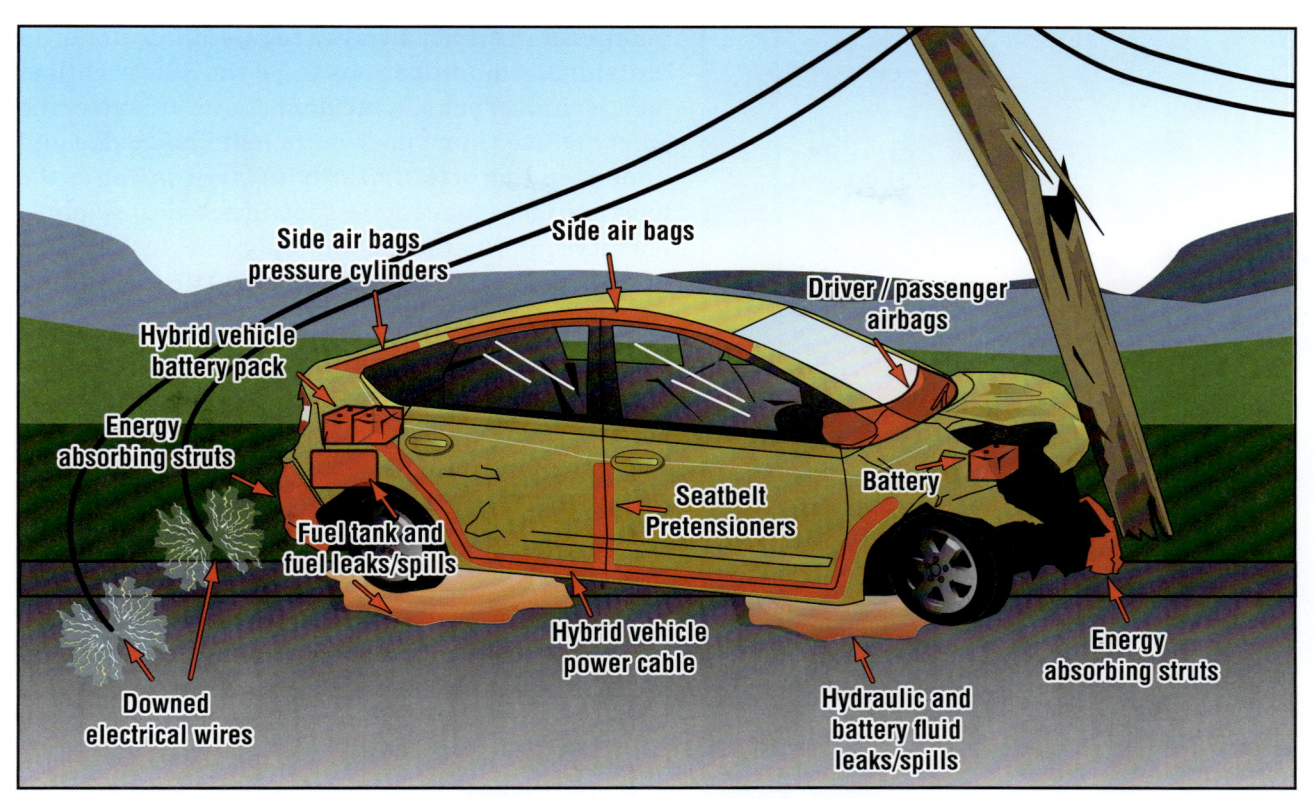

Figure 1.17 Examples of common hazards found at a motor vehicle and extrication scene.

layed until the hazards at the scene have been mitigated. Some of the hazards that rescuers may encounter during extrication operations include:

- Vehicular traffic
- Downed electrical power lines
- Leaking vehicle fluids
- Leaking flammable gas lines
- Unstable terrain
- Release of hazardous materials

NOTE: For more information on vehicle and vehicle incident hazards refer to Chapter 2.

Depending upon the nature of the hazard and its severity, what started as an extrication operation may turn into a recovery operation. Rescuers must exercise discipline and resist the temptation to enter the hazardous area prematurely in an attempt to conduct a recovery operation. It is not sound practice to put rescuers in serious jeopardy to recover the remains of people who have already lost their lives.

Incident Safety Officer (ISO)

Every extrication operation requires an **Incident Safety Officer (ISO)** (**Figure 1.18, p. 26**). On vehicle incidents that do not exceed the recommended span of control, the Incident Safety Officer functions remain with the **Incident Commander (IC)**. On larger incidents beyond the recommended span of control, the IC should assign an Incident Safety Officer whose only responsibility is to observe the operation and make sure that it is conducted in the safest possible

---

Incident Safety Officer (ISO) — Member of the Command staff responsible for monitoring and assessing safety hazards and unsafe conditions during an incident, and developing measures for ensuring personnel safety. The ISO is responsible for the enforcement of all mandated safety laws and regulations and departmental safety-related standard operating procedures. On very small incidents, the Incident Commander may act as the ISO.

Incident Commander (IC) — Person in charge of the Incident Command System and responsible for the management of all incident operations during an emergency.

Section A • Chapter 1 – Vehicle Incident Safety **25**

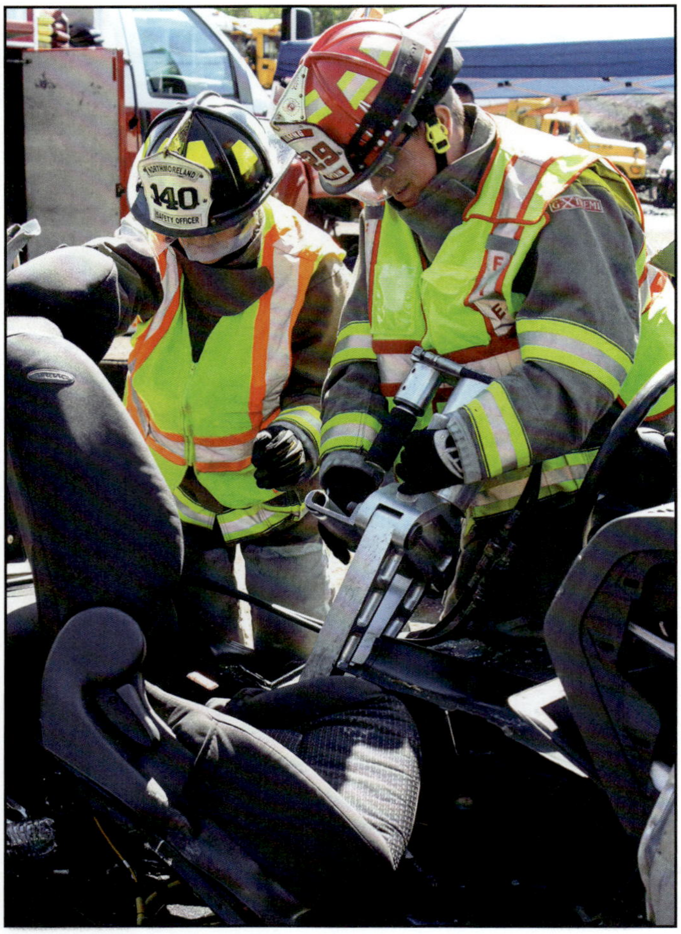

manner. Rank is not always a reliable indicator of an individual's qualifications to be the Safety Officer on a technical vehicle incident. To be effective, the Safety Officer must have sufficient knowledge and understanding of the hazards involved as well as the tools and techniques of the specific rescue discipline. For more information on this topic, refer to the IFSTA **Fire and Emergency Services Safety Officer** manual.

Personnel Accountability

Agencies use a number of different **personnel accountability systems**. Organizations that plan to implement a personnel accountability system during emergency incidents should make certain that the system is part of their SOPs. Organizations must ensure that it is used on every incident and is part of the organization's training plan.

A personnel accountability system is needed in any operation that requires rescuers or rescue crews to enter a hazard zone — especially a zone in which the rescuers are not visible from the Incident Command Post. To prepare for these incidents, organizations should stress the use of teamwork during training. Depending upon the organization of a particular vehicle incident, personnel accountability may or may not be a responsibility of the Incident Safety Officer. **Skill Sheet 1-2** describes the process of performing size-up and initiating the response at a vehicle incident.

Figure 1.18 A Safety Officer assists during a vehicle extrication training.

Personnel Accountability System — Method for identifying which emergency responders are working on an incident scene.

Scene Safety

One of the most important skills for rescue personnel at vehicle incidents is the ability to recognize existing and potential dangers to themselves and others. Rescue personnel are trained and equipped to help those who cannot help themselves, and they are willing to accept the risks involved in rescue operations. However, all on-scene rescue personnel should resist the urge to rush into the scene before it is safe to do so — and thereby add more victims to the incident. All rescuers must remember that they did not cause the problem and are not responsible for the victims being in that situation. A risk-benefit analysis should be performed before any rescue activities and is an ongoing process throughout the incident.

Victim and Patient Terminology

The terms victim and patient have different meanings depending on one's location, jurisdiction, and/or experience level. For the purposes of this manual, the term *victim* will refer to persons who are involved with a vehicle incident and may have suffered injury or death, and the term *patient* will refer to persons who are receiving medical care.

Incident Stability

To safely and successfully stabilize an incident, rescuers should be able to:

- Assess the situation (perform size-up)
- Make informed decisions about how to stabilize the situation
- Have the ability to devise and implement a plan of action that protects the rescuers and victims from further injury

To fulfill these general requirements, rescuers should have the knowledge, skills, and abilities to perform the necessary operations associated with the following topics:

- Available resource capabilities and limitations
- Scene control and protection
- Vehicle crash dynamics
- Vehicle stabilization and access
- On-scene medical care
- Restoring the scene

Available Resource Capabilities and Limitations

Rescuers should know the capabilities and limitations of all resources that would be immediately available and those that would be available with some delay. One of the best ways of learning this information is through realistic joint training exercises held on a regular basis. With this knowledge, personnel can work with outside agencies to increase the capabilities and reduce the limitations as much as possible.

Gaining access to those resources is another challenge. Regardless of where the additional resources come from, rescuers should be aware of how to activate the emergency response system and request assistance.

Scene Control and Protection

Procedures should be implemented for mitigating general and specific hazards at the scene and for maintaining scene control and protection. If the wrecked vehicles are still on the roadway, protect the scene from oncoming traffic. There may be other hazards, such as spilled fuel or downed power lines, which threaten those at the scene. Controlling a crash scene is critical to the safety of rescuers, trapped victims, and bystanders.

Vehicle Crash Dynamics

Understanding the construction of a vehicle and its systems is critical to the safety of rescuers, trapped occupants, and bystanders. Knowing the operational characteristics and locations of supplemental restraint systems (SRS), such as airbags and seat belt pretensioners, can protect both rescuers and trapped occupants. Being familiar with vehicle construction and its systems is also an important element in freeing trapped vehicle occupants as quickly and safely as possible.

To understand the nature of the extrication problem involved, it is important to know what happens to vehicles and their occupants when they collide with stationary objects or other vehicles. For example, knowing how vehicles designed with crumple zones react to impact compared to those without such features helps in assessing how occupants may be trapped in the wreckage. Different types of collisions may also indicate the types of injuries that occupants may have suffered.

Rescuers should combine their knowledge of vehicle construction with the dynamics of vehicle crashes to understand how and why occupants are entrapped in their vehicles. This knowledge can be obtained through years of experience or by studying data and video footage of controlled crash tests conducted by research organizations.

Understanding how the inertial forces produced during vehicle crashes result in injuries to occupants helps rescuers determine the proper packaging and handling techniques in a given situation. Matching the packaging and handling techniques to the victim's potential injuries minimizes trauma and maximizes their chance for survival.

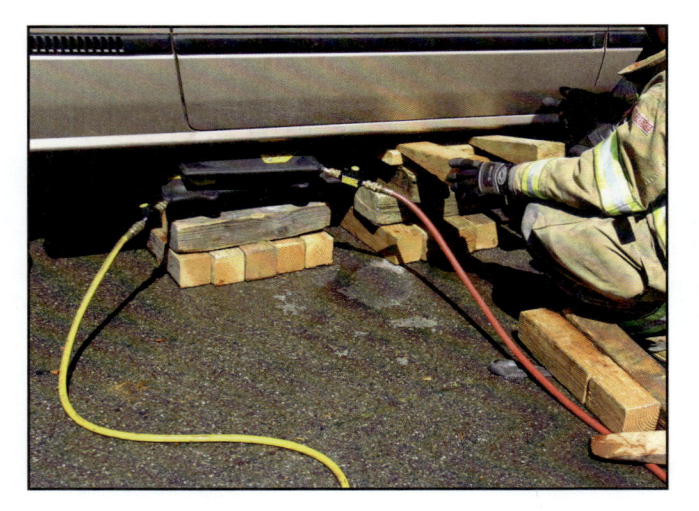

Figure 1.19 A solid crib is used to provide a stable base for air bag deployment.

Vehicle Stabilization and Access

A variety of equipment and techniques are commonly used to stabilize and access crashed vehicles. Rescuers should be well trained in the following:

- Knowing the procedures for accessing victims trapped in a vehicle and freeing them successfully
- Using a variety of tools and equipment to manipulate and/or remove major vehicle components
- Selecting and using the most appropriate tools and equipment to perform these operations **(Figure 1.19)**
- Using tools and equipment safely

On-Scene Medical Care

Before transporting trapped victims to a medical facility, they should be medically assessed to determine the nature and extent of any injuries suffered during the crash. From the standpoint of survival, assessment can be one of the most critical steps in the entire extrication operation. An injury overlooked during this assessment can develop into a life-threatening problem because of the movement and manipulation of the victim during extrication.

Rescuers should be able to properly protect and package victims in accordance with the findings of their medical assessment and within their medical training and capability. Packaging can include everything from simple bandaging to applying a cervical collar with full spinal immobilization and traction devices to prepare a victim for transport to further medical care.

Rescuers should be able to transfer victims to EMS personnel for transportation to an appropriate medical facility. This includes properly preparing the victim for transfer as well as following local protocols and passing on critical information about the victim's condition.

NOTE: For more information about assessing and transporting trapped victims, refer to Chapter 8.

Restoring the Scene

Rescuers should restore the vehicle extrication scene so that it is in a safe and environmentally stable condition. Rescuers should perform the following:

- Remove wrecked vehicles from the scene.
- Mitigate any hazards before the scene is abandoned.
- Isolate any hazards that cannot be immediately mitigated in order to prevent members of the public from inadvertently entering a hazardous area.

Personal Safety Equipment and Techniques

To safely perform extrication, rescuers should have adequate personal safety equipment and practice safety techniques appropriate for the hazards they will face. The organization should identify and acquire the appropriate personal protective clothing and equipment needed to provide this protection. The organization should also incorporate safety techniques, such as providing shelter and other thermal control methods, into their local SOPs.

Protective Protective Equipment (PPE)

To safely perform vehicle extrication, rescuers should have adequate personal protective equipment (PPE) suited to the hazards the rescuers will face. All personnel should be trained in and knowledge of the capabilities and limitations of each piece of PPE.

All personnel should be trained in the capabilities and limitations of each piece of protective clothing or equipment. They should also be trained to perform proper inspection, care and maintenance, selection and use of the personal protective clothing and equipment issued to them or made available for their use. To be effective, personal protective clothing and equipment must be worn properly when conducting emergency operations or training exercises **(Figure 1.20)**.

When needed, NFPA 1981, *Standard on Open-Circuit Self-Contained Breathing Apparatus (SCBA) for Emergency Services* compliant self-contained breathing apparatus (SCBA) or other approved respiratory protection should be available for use and worn by rescue team members during rescue incidents. At a minimum, the air for these systems should meet ANSI/CGA G7.1, *Commodity Specification for Air*, for Grade D air. SAR equipment must be equipped an emergency supply of self-contained breathing air to be used during egress should the primary air supply fail.

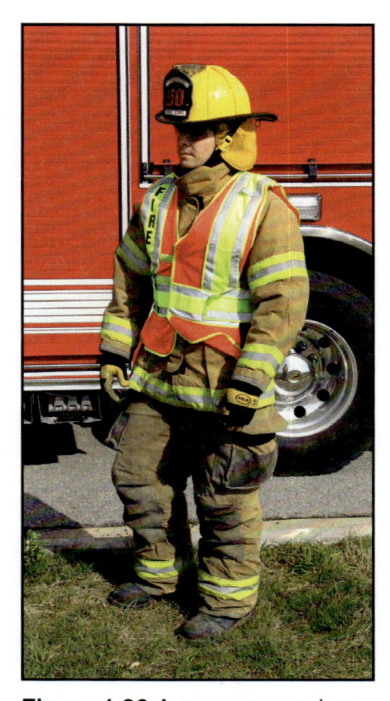

Figure 1.20 A rescuer wearing personal protective equipment.

NOTE: For more information on personal protective clothing and equipment used at a vehicle incident, refer to Chapter 4, Tools and Equipment.

Shelter and Thermal Control

Inclement weather can be a problem at any vehicle incident. In extremes of heat or cold or during heavy precipitation, such as rain, snow, or sleet, extended vehicle extrication operations pose a risk to rescuers and victims. Personnel at a vehicle accident may experience heat-related stress during the summer months or suffer hypothermia or frostbite during the winter. It is important that rescuers be outfitted properly and rotated into sheltered areas on a routine basis to prevent such injuries.

There are a variety of ways to provide protection during an incident:

- Large tents, canopies, gazebos, and temporary shelters often used for rehab or personnel decontamination areas
- Covered trailers and air-conditioned apparatus cabs
- Enclosed temporary structures or trailers equipped with portable heating and cooling units
- Permanent structures such as houses, storage facilities, barns, or other structures located near the incident

When creating the preincident plan, the AHJ should identify the need for such resources. If needed, these resources should be purchased and stored so they are readily accessible for use at an incident. If it is not possible to purchase these resources, every opportunity should be made to establish an aid agreement with an organization that possesses them.

Whenever necessary, rescuers should make every effort to protect accident victims from inclement weather conditions. Rescuers can use resources such as canvas salvage covers, fire resistant or extrication blankets or rapidly erected canopies to protect the victims. Blankets and heating or cooling packs may be used to control the temperature directly around the victim. Communication with victims is critical to their survival.

NOTE: Providing care for victims will be further described in Chapter 8.

Safety Zones

Proper scene management reduces congestion and confusion around the vehicle incident. Safety zones provide necessary organization to a hectic vehicle incident because each zone will likely be staffed by personnel from a variety of agencies. Keeping the operations and personnel within each zone safe is an essential part of managing every vehicle incident. Refer to **Skill Sheet 1-3** for steps on establishing scene safety zones at a vehicle incident

Types of Safety Zones

The most common method of organizing a rescue scene is to establish three operating safety zones: restricted, limited access, and support **(Figure 1.21)**. The safety zones are necessary to operating a safe and efficient extrication scene and should have a well-maintained perimeter or barrier, which is intended to:

- Provide a controlled work space
- Protect bystanders from hazards at the incident

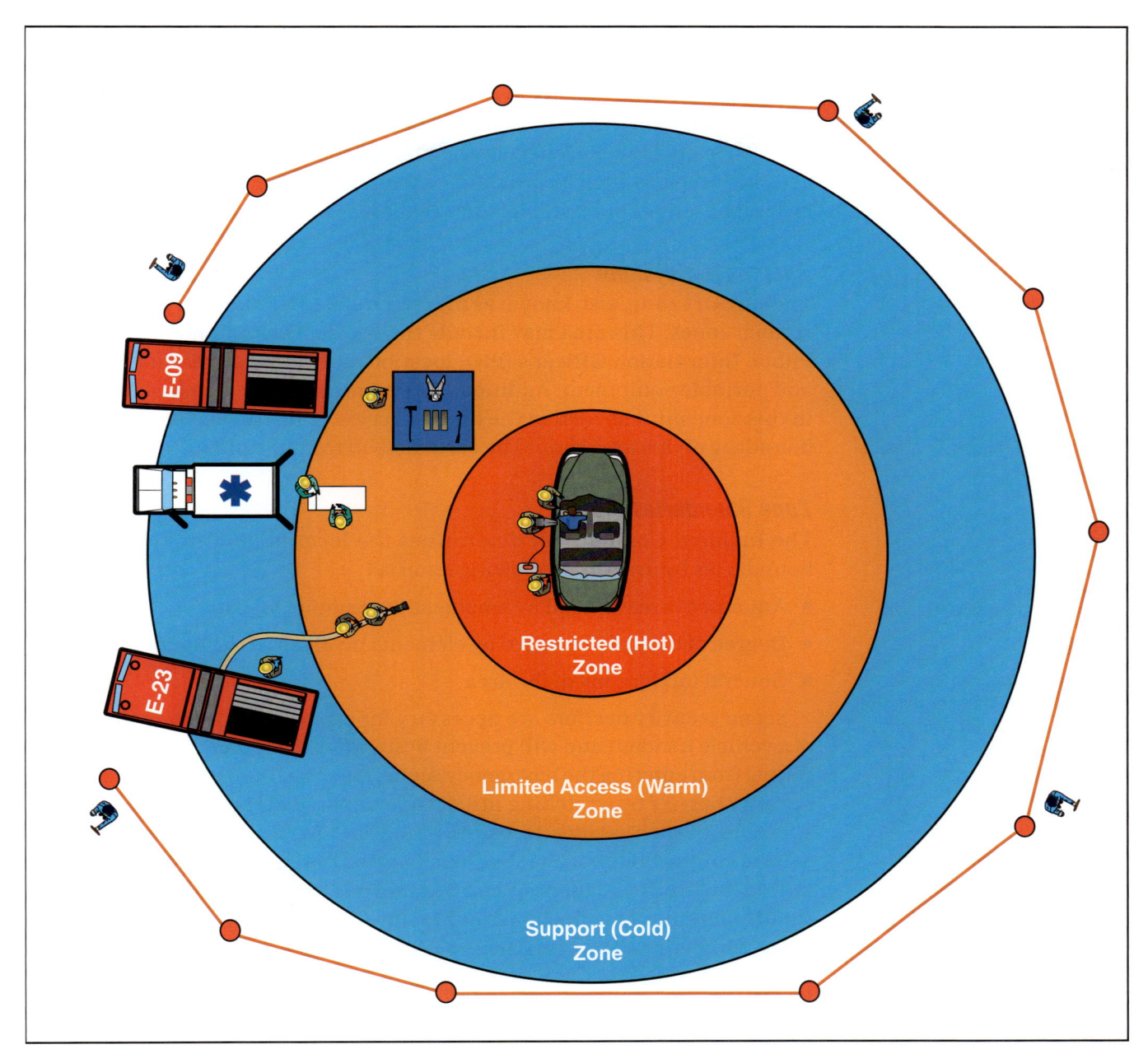

Figure 1.21 Examples of emergency control zones

- Ensure the use of the personnel accountability system
- Ensure that the location of victims is known
- Protect evidence in the event of a suspicious incident

Restricted (Hot) Zone

The **restricted zone**, also known as the hot zone, is where the rescue is taking place. Only personnel who are dealing directly with treating or freeing the victims are allowed in this zone. The restricted zone limits crowding and confusion at the scene. The size of this zone may vary greatly depending upon the nature and extent of the rescue incident.

> **Restricted (Hot) Zone** — In a rescue or extrication operation, the area where the extrication is taking place. Only personnel who are attending directly to the victims should be in this zone; this avoids crowding and confusion among rescuers.

Section A • Chapter 1 – Vehicle Incident Safety 31

> **Limited Access (Warm) Zone** — Large geographical area between the support zone and the restricted zone, for personnel who are directly aiding rescuers in the restricted zone. This includes personnel who are handling hydraulic tool power plants, fire personnel handling standby hoselines, and so on. Personnel in this zone should not get in the way of rescuers working in the restricted zone.

> **Support (Cold) Zone** — Area that surrounds the limited access (warm) zone and is restricted to emergency response personnel who are not working in either the restricted (hot) zone or the limited access (warm) zone. This zone may include the portable equipment and personnel staging areas and the Command Post; cordon off the outer boundary of this area to the public.

Limited Access (Warm) Zone

The **limited access zone**, also known as the warm zone, is immediately outside the restricted zone. Access to this zone should be limited to personnel who are not needed in the restricted zone but who are directly aiding rescuers in the restricted zone. Rescuers in the limited access zone may be involved in activities such as such as providing emergency scene lighting and standing by with hoselines or hydraulic tools that are ready for use.

Support (Cold) Zone

The **support zone**, also known as the cold zone, surrounds the previously described zones. This area may include the Incident Command Post (ICP), the Public Information Officer's (PIO) location, and staging areas for personnel and portable equipment. Additional rescuers and other resources are staged in this zone until needed in the limited access or restricted zones. The outer boundary of this area should be cordoned off from the public.

Zone Boundaries

The Incident Commander determines the location and establishes zone boundaries by using the following criteria:

- Amount of area needed by emergency personnel to work
- Degree of hazard presented by elements involved in the incident
- General topography of the area

Scene security barriers are necessary for establishing an outer perimeter of a vehicle incident and will prevent bystanders and other nonessential personnel from entering the emergency scene. Personnel can establish a physical security barrier by stretching utility rope or barrier tape between any available objects, such as signs, trees, utility poles, or parking meters. Any material used to cordon off the scene should not be tied to vehicles that may need to be moved during the incident. When the area has been cordoned off, personnel should communicate the boundary to the IC and all incident personnel. The Safety Officer monitors this area to make sure that unauthorized people do not cross the line.

When establishing a scene security barrier, personnel should leave a controlled opening near the ICP. An entry/egress corridor should be established to control the movement of vehicles and personnel into and out of the controlled areas.

The Accountability Officer should monitor this entry point to allow only authorized personnel to enter the scene. Another opening may be necessary to provide access for ambulances and other emergency equipment.

In smaller incidents where no evacuation is necessary, cordoning off the area where activity is happening keeps bystanders a safe distance from the scene and out of the way of emergency personnel. There is no specific distance or area that should be cordoned off; this should be determined by the IC.

Staffing Requirements for Safety Zones

Vehicle incidents involve a number of separate and distinct functions that should often be performed simultaneously. These functions can be and sometimes are performed by members of a single response agency. However, to perform these functions most efficiently, groups of personnel from more than one agency are usually required. Any personnel or agency that enters or leaves the hazard area must be allowed in/out and accounted for by the Accountability Officer. These groups and their roles and responsibilities are as follows:

- **Rescue Group** — Personnel directly responsible for stabilizing crashed vehicles. Responsibilities include accessing, stabilizing, disentangling, and packaging victims for removal from wrecked vehicles, and transferring them to EMS personnel.

- **Law Enforcement** — Responsible for directing traffic and providing crowd control at vehicle incident scenes and investigating these incidents if they occurred on public streets or highways.

- **Medical Group** — Emergency medical services (EMS) personnel who are responsible for evaluating, treating, and transporting (if necessary) victims to appropriate medical facilities once victims are removed from wrecked vehicles. If local protocols permit, the EMS group may begin its work prior to the victim(s) being extricated from the vehicle(s).

- **Suppression Group** — Personnel responsible for providing fire protection at an incident.

- **Other response agencies** — Personnel or agencies that can be of assistance during vehicle incidents by providing support to the extrication organization. Some of these agencies include, but are not limited to:
  — Utility companies
  — State/Provincial Department of Transportation
  — Private industrial response teams
  — Towing and recovery companies

Monitoring Hazard Zones

Through continual risk assessment, the ISO evaluates and suggests effective safety measures that provide a successful outcome of the incident while ensuring the safety of the members operating at the incident. In this role, the ISO must not circumvent the ICS chain of command. The only time the ISO intervenes at the tactical level is to stop an unsafe act or prevent an injury. All other suggestions on operations must be communicated to the IC.

As the ISO evaluates the incident, the strategies and tactics employed, and the available resources to achieve a successful outcome, he or she should forecast additional needs. This review may include requesting **Assistant Incident Safety Officers (AISOs)**. The ISO must conduct a risk management assessment and be able to recognize when assistance is needed. The technical ability of the ISO must meet the technical nature of the operation or a Technical Safety Officer (TSO) must be assigned to assist or assume safety officer duties.

Other duties of the ISO as outlined in NFPA 1521, *Standard for Fire Department Safety Officer Professional Qualifications,* include the following:

- Ensure that incident scene rehabilitation is established.
- Monitor the scene and report the status of conditions, hazards, and risks to the incident commander.
- Ensure that a personnel accountability system is being used.

Assistant Incident Safety Officer (AISO) — Individual(s) who reports to the Incident Safety Officer and assist with monitoring hazards and safe operations for designated portions of the operation at large or complex incidents.

- Ensure that all personnel understand the IAP.
- Provide the IC with a risk assessment of the IAP.
- Ensure a plan for the treatment and transport of any ill or injured member is in place, and ensure appropriate medical facilities are identified.
- Suggest safety zones, collapse zones, a hot zone, and other designated hazard areas.
- Evaluate motor vehicle traffic hazards.
- Monitor radio transmissions to ensure proper and effective communications.
- Identify the need for additional AISOs.
- Evaluate hazards associated with helicopter landings.

Tactical-level supervisors must be aware that the ISO is not a commander at the scene. He or she monitors the scene but is not responsible for providing orders to Divisions or crews. While both the tactical-level supervisor and the ISO report to the IC, they serve two different purposes. If serving as a Division Supervisor, the tactical-level supervisor will remain in a single location that funnels personnel in and out of the operational area. On the other hand, the ISO must be able to move freely around the incident scene and monitor operations to ensure the safety of all personnel.

Traffic Control

Fire and rescue personnel should be trained in the basics of traffic management and safety in accordance with the AHJ. Upon arrival at a vehicle accident, the IC must take into account a number of conditions and factors that will influence **traffic control** and scene safety. These conditions and factors include, but are not limited to, the following:

- Type of roadway, such as single lane, two lanes, or four lanes
- Location of the incident in relation to the road, such as on the road, on the median, on the shoulder, or off the road
- Number of lanes that might need to be closed and their locations
- Length of time that the incident may last
- Volume and speed of oncoming traffic
- Available line of sight leading up to the scene
- Need to restrict, detour, or stop traffic flow
- Available traffic control resources
- Environmental factors such as weather and roadway conditions
- Time of day

Traffic Control Concepts

To protect rescuers and victims during extrication operations, traffic must be routed into unobstructed lanes around the accident scene. While shutting down the roadway may be the only safe option, every effort should be made to detour traffic around the accident site **(Figure 1.22)**.

> **Traffic Control** — Important function of scene management that helps to control scene access and vehicular traffic in and out of the area. This function is generally handled by law enforcement personnel.

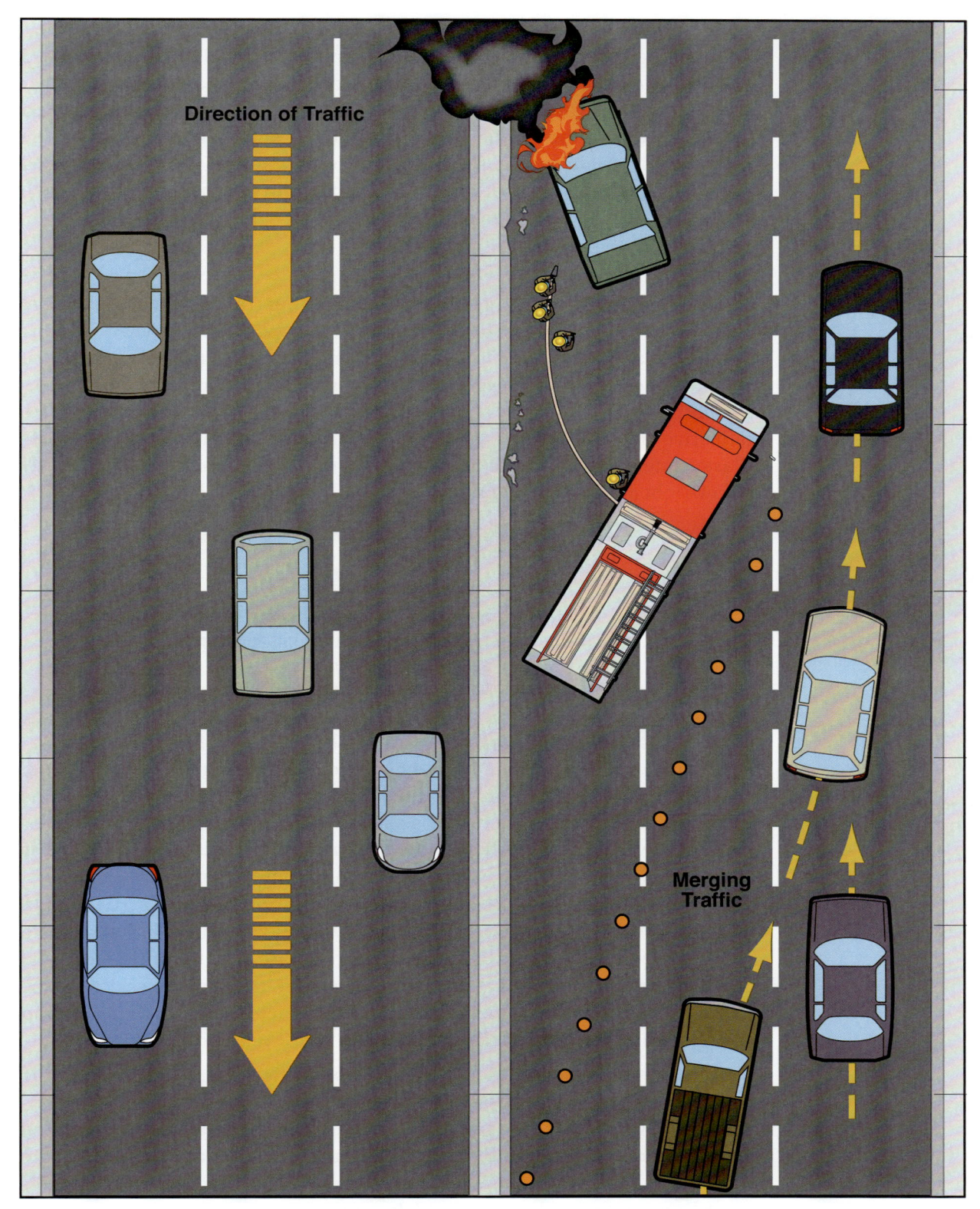

Figure 1.22 Apparatus can be positioned to block the roadway to offer protection to rescuers and victims.

Control of Pedestrians

Control of pedestrians and bystanders is essential to managing a well-organized extrication operation. As previously stated, it is important to keep nonessential persons away from the incident scene to keep them safe and to avoid interference with the rescue operation. The law enforcement agency at the scene usually manages this function, but sometimes rescue personnel may need to manage the scene. It is the IC's responsibility to ensure that the scene is secured and properly managed.

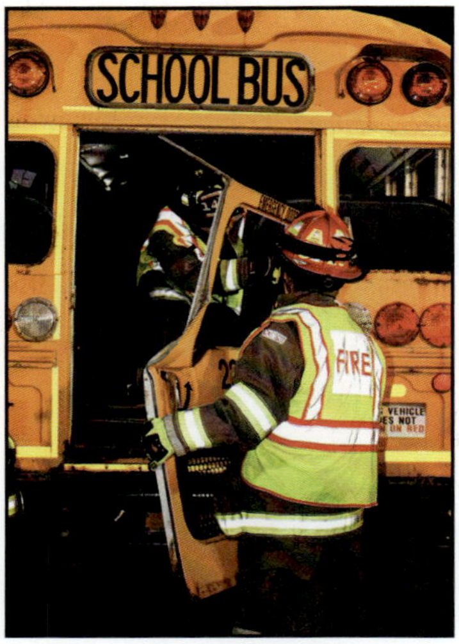

Control of Rescuers

To avoid the danger of being struck by oncoming traffic, rescue personnel should exercise extreme caution when exiting apparatus and when working around apparatus to gather tools and equipment for the extrication operation. Personnel need to keep an eye on traffic flow and always stay within the protective barrier provided by the apparatus. All personnel should wear appropriate reflective clothing, such as ANSI/U.S. Department of Transportation (DOT) Class 3 safety vests to make themselves more visible to motorists, especially in low-light conditions **(Figure 1.23)**.

Figure 1.23 Reflective vests make responders more visible at night.

> **CAUTION**
> Rescuers must also protect themselves from traffic hazards by maintaining constant situational awareness.

Control of Emergency Vehicles and Equipment

Proper placement of apparatus at emergency scenes is an important part of safe and effective extrication operations. Vehicles that need to be closest to the operation should be positioned as such. However, a path of entry and egress should be left clear for additional apparatus in case needs and responsibilities change during the incident. Apparatus, such as engine companies, that do not need to be close to the rescue area should leave room for later-arriving EMS and rescue vehicles. Rescue vehicles need to be close enough to the scene to operate effectively, especially if these apparatus are used to supply electrical power or operate hydraulic tools. To some extent, those at the scene can be protected by positioning emergency response vehicles between the scene and any oncoming traffic to act as blocking or shadow vehicles.

Many agencies have adopted a policy of shutting off unnecessary lighting on vehicles positioned in traffic lanes to avoid blinding and/or confusing oncoming drivers. Most modern fire apparatus are constructed with warning lights intended to alert motorists to the fact that the apparatus is blocking the traffic lane. In all cases, vehicle drivers should follow their agency's protocols regarding emergency lights on vehicles parked at the scene.

Traffic Control Devices

After appropriately positioning responding apparatus, the IC must determine what traffic control devices and methods will be used. The emergency responder or responders positioning traffic control devices must wear reflective clothing or vests. While positioning these devices, these personnel must be extremely cautious and constantly observe traffic around them to prevent being struck by oncoming vehicles.

> **CAUTION**
> Do not turn your back on traffic while positioning traffic control devices. Maintain visual contact with traffic at all times.

Traffic control devices include signs, channeling devices (traffic cones and flares), lighting devices, and shadow/advance warning vehicles that rescue organizations and personnel should use to help control traffic near an incident. The *Manual on Uniform Traffic Control Devices (MUTCD)* identifies the types of traffic control devices that should be used to establish work areas and identify incident scenes as well the methods for deploying these devices. The types of traffic control devices used and the methods in which they are applied will depend on the following:

- Size of the incident
- Posted speeds on the roadway
- Availability of personnel and equipment
- Amount of time spent mitigating the incident

Emergency responders now use signs that are collapsible, small, easy to carry, and easy to erect. Common warning signs used during vehicle extrication operations include:

- Accident/Emergency Ahead **(Figure 1.24)**
- Right/Left Lane Closed **(Figure 1.25)**
- Be Prepared to Stop **(Figure 1.26, p. 38)**
- The Flagger Symbol **(Figure 1.27, p. 38)**

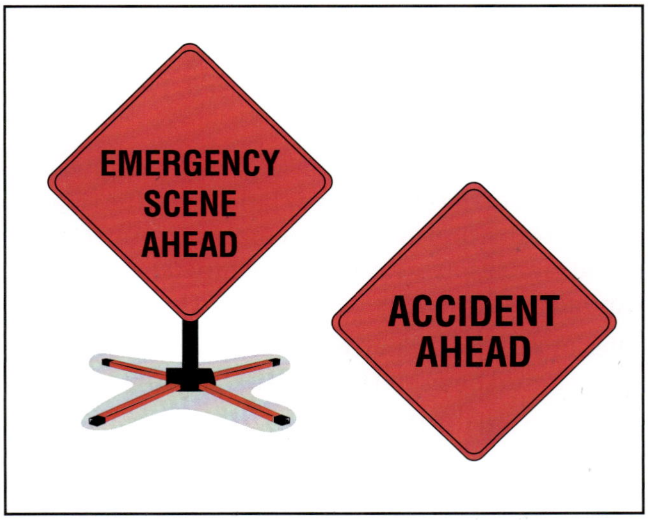

Figure 1.24 An example of an "Accident/Emergency Ahead" warning sign.

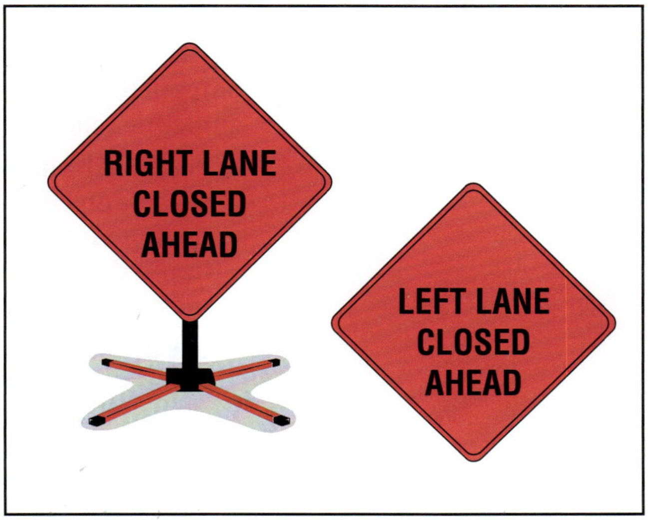

Figure 1.25 This sign lets oncoming traffic know that the "Right (or Left) Lane" is closed ahead.

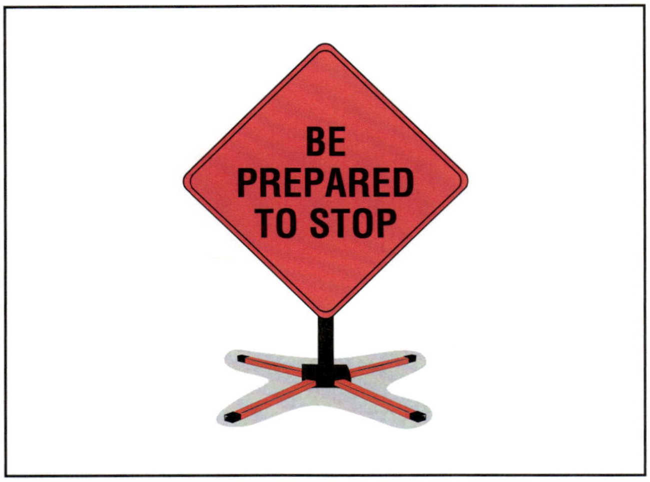

Figure 1.26 An example of a "Be Prepared to Stop" sign.

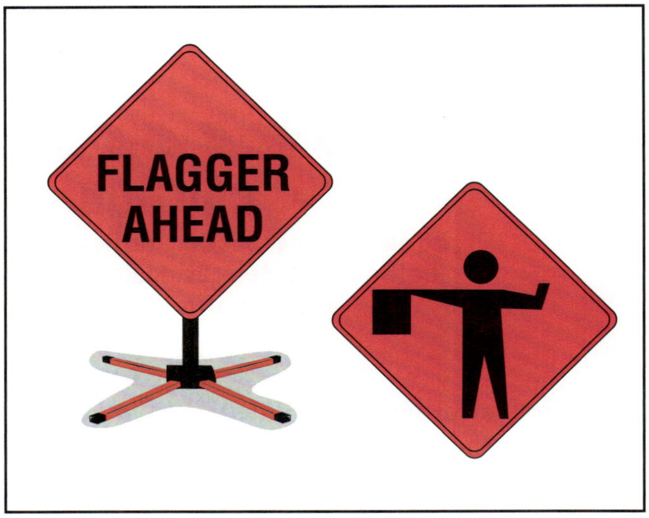

Figure 1.27 The "Flagger Symbol" sign.

Position signs well in advance of the accident site, on the right side of the roadway (no closer than 24 inches [600 mm] from the road edge) facing oncoming traffic. A combination of signs may be employed to warn oncoming traffic of the emergency ahead.

Use a flagger or flaggers to direct, slow, or stop traffic as needed. The flagger(s) may use a Stop/Slow paddle, red or orange flag, or red wand or flare to direct traffic. Flaggers should exercise extreme care during flagging operations. Flaggers should:

- Wear reflective protective clothing or a reflective vest.
- Stand on the shoulder of the roadway where he or she will be visible to oncoming traffic but not directly in front of such traffic.
- Identify an escape route to ensure personal safety.
- Locate a position based on the speed of traffic flow.
- Use light wands or flares during darkness.
- Monitor the flow of traffic and movement of vehicles at all times.

If adequate time, resources, and personnel are available, traffic channeling devices such as traffic cones, reflective triangles, flashing lights, and/or flares (if they do not pose an additional fire hazard) may be used. The following guidelines should be followed:

- Position the devices used in a tapered line from the edge of the roadway on the side of the accident to the edge of the clear lane or lanes of traffic (**Figure 1.28**). This taper establishes a transition area for oncoming traffic to move in the desired direction and transition away from the lane(s) containing the accident vehicles, responding apparatus, rescuers, and victim(s).
- Use a minimum of six cones or reflective devices. The longer the taper, the more traffic control devices should be used (**Figure 1.29, p. 40**).
- Place the first taper cone just behind the flagger along the inner edge of the pavement or the pavement edge marker line.
- Place the next device several feet (meters) closer to the accident site and a couple of feet (meters) further into the traffic lane.
- Continue this process until all cones are positioned forming the taper.

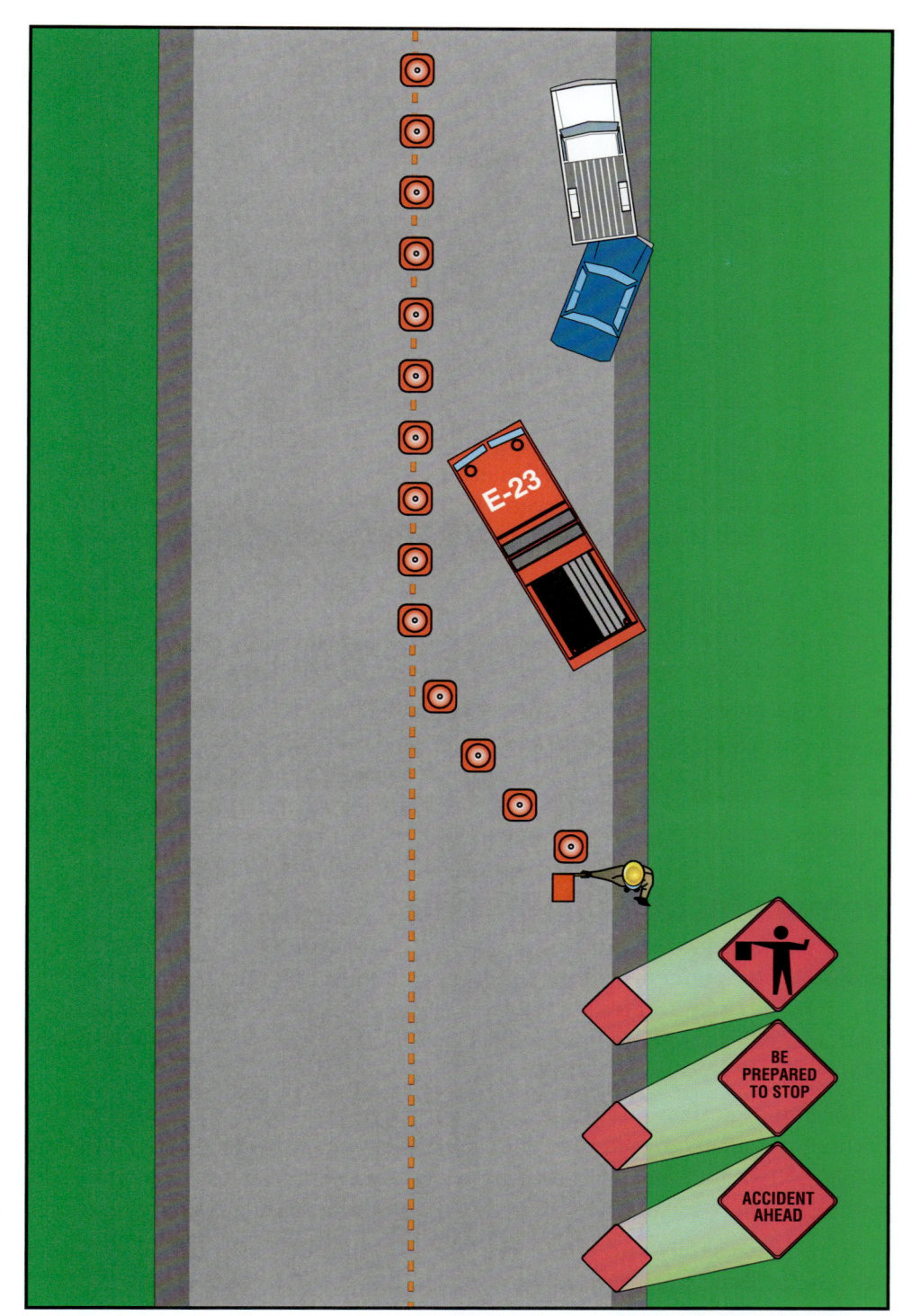

Figure 1.28 An example of how warning signs and traffic cones would be set up to create a traffic channeling taper.

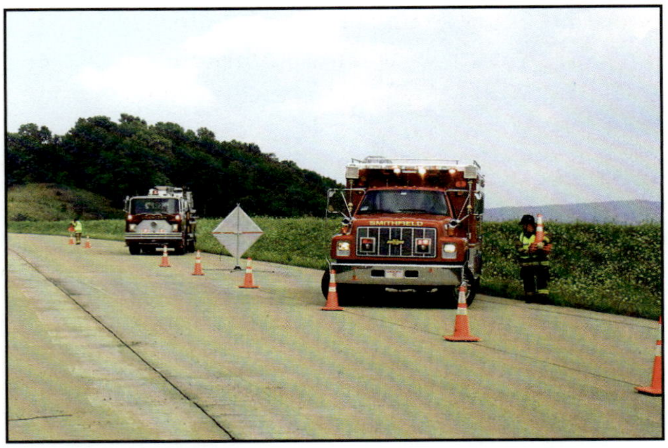

Figure 1.29 Examples of traffic control devices being set up at a motor vehicle accident.

If needed and available, warning vehicles with flashing or reflective arrows may be used to redirect traffic. Generally, these types of vehicles are highway department vehicles. Warning vehicles should be positioned well ahead of the incident scene to warn oncoming traffic of the incident.

Traffic Control Resources

In addition to the traffic control devices previously mentioned, rescuers may also use outside resources to control traffic flow. These resources include:

- Law enforcement
- Fire services personnel
- Department of Transportation
- Other agencies

Vehicle Incident Operations

The organization should train members of the organization to implement appropriate components of local, state/provincial, or federal/national response plans. In the United States, for example, these plans would include the National Search and Rescue Plan, the Federal Response Plan, and the **National Incident Management System (NIMS)**.

Rescue organizations should also conform to national standards of performance such as those created by the National Fire Protection Association (NFPA). NFPA 1006 and NFPA 1670 both identify a number of responsibilities the rescue organization or AHJ should meet in order to conduct rescue operations.

In order to safely and effectively operate at a vehicle and/or machinery vehicle incident, personnel should be familiar with the following:

- Operational protocols
- Communication
- Incident support operations and resources

Operational Protocols

The organization should develop SOPs, or operational protocols, in accordance with the operational capability level of the organization as described previously. These SOPs should be in a written format, and all personnel should become familiar with their content. The organization should review the SOPs

---

National Incident Management System - Incident Command System (NIMS-ICS) — The U.S. mandated incident management system that defines the roles, responsibilities, and standard operating procedures used to manage emergency operations; creates a unified incident response structure for federal, state, and local governments.

on a recurring basis and update as needed to meet its needs. The SOPs should address a broad range of topics related to vehicle and industrial machinery rescue to ensure these operations are conducted in the safest possible manner for victims and rescuers.

The AHJ should establish a policy for the adoption and implementation of an Incident Management System and a Personnel Accountability System as outlined in NFPA 1561 *Standard on Emergency Services Incident Managment System*. This policy will provide training for all rescue personnel in the activation and implementation of both systems at each incident. This policy also addresses the Incident Commander's responsibility to brief rescuers on the appropriate safety considerations at each incident and to establish a personnel rotation that will reduce rescuer fatigue and stress. In the United States, the policy should conform to the NIMS-ICS.

The organization's SOPs should also address emergency medical care. The minimum level of emergency medical care that should be provided during technical search and rescue operations is **basic life support (BLS)**. BLS personnel should be standing by whenever training exercises or rescue operations are underway (in which there is a high potential for injury). Some organizations may choose to provide advanced life support (ALS).

NOTE: Chapter 8 of this manual contains additional information regarding providing care to victims.

A key component of any rescue organization is a safety program. A safety program ensures that all personnel are trained to recognize and control the hazards and/or risks associated with vehicle rescue operations in order to minimize danger posed to victims and rescuers. Rescue organizations must train rescuers performing tasks at vehicle rescue incidents to meet the safety requirements for emergency operations, special operations, and protective clothing and protective equipment sections of NFPA 1500. The organization's safety program should be described in the SOPs. This SOP should also incorporate national, regional, or local safety standards if and when applicable.

The AHJ's SOPs should address the role of an Incident Safety Officer. The Incident Commander assigns the Incident Safety Officer at each incident and during training exercises. The Incident Safety Officer should meet the appropriate requirements of NFPA 1521, *Standard for Fire Department Safety Officer Professional Qualifications*, and should be able to identify, evaluate, and mitigate, if possible, any hazardous situations or conditions, and unsafe procedures found at an incident **(Figure 1.30, p. 42)**.

NOTE: Additional information on the roles and responsibilities of the safety officer can be found in IFSTA's **Fire and Emergency Services Safety Officer** manual.

In imminent danger situations, the rescue team must follow the AHJ's procedures or guidelines for evacuation and accountability measures. These SOPs should address the methods used to notify rescue personnel of an evacuation such as a radio notification and/or using visual and/or audible warning signal devices.

In the SOPs, the AHJ outlines the minimum entrance and fitness requirements for personnel to perform their duties during training exercises and

> **Basic Life Support (BLS)** — Emergency medical treatment administered without the use of adjunctive equipment; includes maintenance of airway, breathing, and circulation, as well as basic bandaging and splinting.

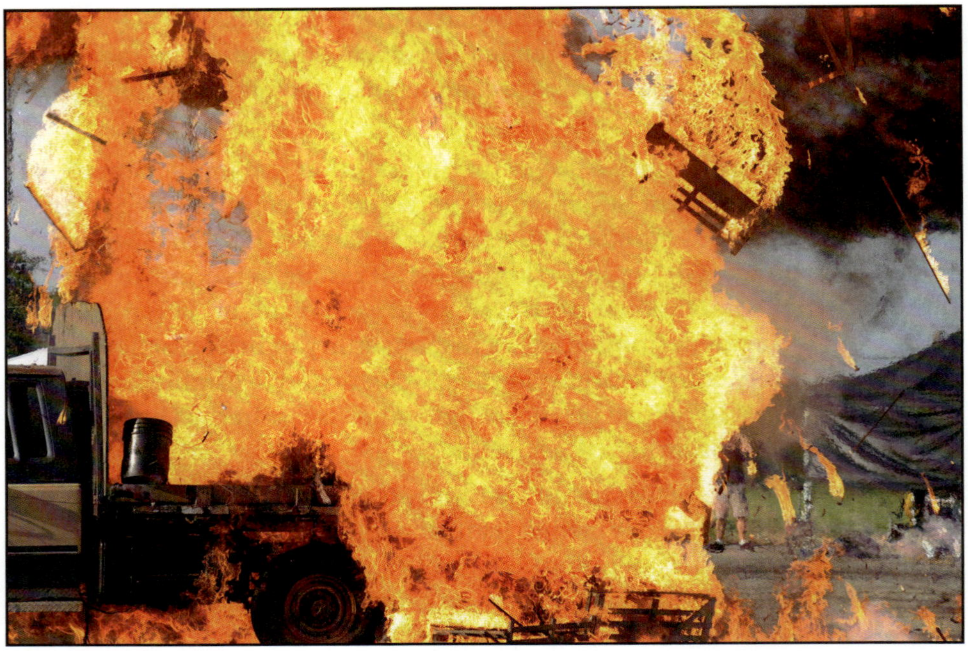

Figure 1.30 Hazardous items on a vehicle should be identified before they cause harm. *Courtesy of Chris Mickal.*

actual emergencies. Because of the inherent dangers posed by vehicle rescue situations, rescuers must be psychologically, physically, and medically able to perform their duties. The minimum requirements for rescue personnel may include the following items:

- Minimum age
- Medical condition(s)
- Physical and psychological fitness
- Level of emergency medical care training
- Level of technical rescue training
- Educational level
- Hazardous materials incident and contact control training

Incident Action Plan (IAP)

Incident Action Plans (IAPs) are created for all vehicle incidents, and may be verbal or in written form. The IC is responsible for creating the IAP, but Awareness level rescuers must understand the components of the IAP as well as their responsibilities within the IAP. IAPs usually contain the following elements:

- **Tactical worksheet** — Basis for the development of an IAP
- **Incident briefing** — Serves as an initial action worksheet
- **Incident objectives** — Objectives should be SMART: Specific, Measurable, Action-oriented, Realistic, and Time frame
- **Organization** — Description of the ICS table of organization, including the units and agencies that are involved
- **Assignments** — Specific unit tactical assignments divided by branch and division

> **Tactical Worksheet** — document that the IC may use on the fireground to track units and record field notes during an incident; could evolve into a written IAP if an incident escalates in size or complexity.

- **Support materials** — Includes site plans, access or traffic plans, locations of support activities (staging, rehabilitation, logistics, and others), and similar resources
- **Safety message** — Information concerning personnel safety at the incident; may also be part of the incident safety plan that the incident safety officer develops

A variety of planning forms are available that support the information taken from the hazard and risk assessment surveys. Some agencies develop their own planning forms, while others use generic forms.

Verbal IAP

The IC will communicate the incident objectives of the IAP to units and individuals operating at the scene who are tasked with a specific work assignment. This communication is done in person or over designated radio frequencies. All incident personnel must function within the scope of the IAP. Incident personnel should direct their actions toward achieving the incident objectives, strategies, and tactics specified in the plan. When all members understand their positions, roles, and functions in the ICS, the system can safely, effectively, and efficiently use resources to accomplish the plan.

All verbal instructions should be communicated to responders at the scene and to the assigned Incident Safety Officer (ISO). The ISO should ensure that all SOPs are followed, such as the establishment of an accountability system or rapid intervention in the verbal orders. If the IC's instructions do not follow established procedures, the ISO should discuss this issue with the IC and recommend changes to assignments. Other responders are expected to follow the assigned plan and act within the safety guidelines provided.

Communicating Rescue Strategy and Objectives

Rescue strategy and objectives must be communicated with all responding personnel during vehicle and machinery extrication operations. These include the following incident priorities:

- Personnel protection and life safety
- Incident stabilization
- Property and environmental conservation

Personnel Protection and Life Safety. This priority involves protecting the victims involved in the incident, the bystanders in the immediate area, and the emergency response personnel operating on the scene. Meeting this priority involves the following:

- A safe response by emergency personnel
- Implementing the Incident Command System
- Providing scene safety by controlling and protecting the scene from oncoming traffic or interference from curious bystanders
- Determining the condition of victims and how their condition may impact the types of tools and procedures used
- Conducting the operation in a safe manner
- Protecting trapped victims during the operation

Incident Stabilization. This priority involves taking the necessary steps to prevent the situation from getting any worse than it was when emergency response personnel arrived. Some of these steps are as follows:

- Maintaining scene control and protection
- Stabilizing the vehicles
- Stabilizing and removing trapped victims
- Eliminating sources of ignition
- Providing fire protection and hazardous materials control as needed

Property and Environmental Conservation. This priority involves preventing unnecessary damage to property during and immediately after the operation. Personnel can meet this priority by performing the following:

- Developing and adopting procedures that result in as little property damage as possible and are consistent with achieving incident objectives
- Using nondestructive techniques that accomplish the objective as fast or faster than other more destructive techniques
- Providing security for unprotected property at the conclusion of the operation
- Protecting the environment by preventing gasoline, hydraulic fluids, battery acids, coolants, or other contaminants from running into sewer drains or streams **(Figure 1.31)**

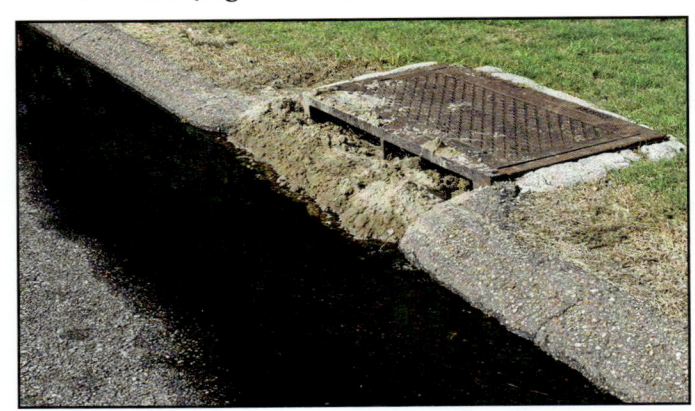

Figure 1.31 Personnel should prevent hazardous fluids or chemicals from running into a sewer drain. *Courtesy of Chris Mickal.*

Assigned Incident Tasks

The IC should brief all responders at the scene on all assigned incident tasks. The ISO will provide a safety briefing to accompany the assignments. The ISO can then independently verify incident operations are proceeding as designed. All personnel should be working towards the common goal of the IAP. Personnel operating outside the established IAP or freelancing are a danger to themselves and all other personnel on scene. A properly implemented ICS structure with clear incident objectives should be sufficient to address this concern.

Communication

An effective vehicle incident operation can be achieved in part through good communication practices. This communication starts with the dispatcher and is continued throughout the incident. Some things that may be communicated at an incident include hazards present and rescue strategies and objectives.

Dispatch

Dispatchers, also called telecommunicators, need to communicate effectively with both callers and responding rescue personnel. Dispatchers need to be familiar with the district and with field operations to be effective. The enhanced 9-1-1 emergency phone system allows the dispatcher to have the location of the telephone from which the call is being made if a caller is too excited to speak coherently or if the caller does not speak English fluently. Of course, this assumes that the call is being made from a land-based telephone at a fixed location. If the call is coming from a cellular phone, the dispatcher may have to rely upon the caller to supply as much information as possible. However, improvements in global positioning system (GPS) technology are making it possible to locate cell phone callers through a system of triangulation by signal alone.

In some cases, excited or confused callers provide incorrect information about the location of an incident, such as mistakenly describing the location to be at the intersection of two parallel streets. However, if the dispatcher knows the district, he or she should be able to recognize the discrepancy and question the caller further to get more accurate information.

Effectively handling the initial response is the first step toward efficiently organizing a vehicle incident. Therefore, dispatchers must attempt to determine the nature and extent of the emergency so that they can dispatch the most appropriate response. To do this, dispatchers receiving the call should:

- Follow their agency's standardized procedures, guidelines, or checklist for taking information from the reporting party.
- Determine the nature and extent of the problem, because it may not be an emergency.
- Determine if the problem involves more than one agency, or if it is an incident that is appropriate for an extrication agency.
- Request essential information about the location of the problem — Street address, business name, or some nearby landmark.
- Ask how many people are involved and what their status is — Injured, trapped, or in immediate mortal jeopardy.

The dispatcher should try to get as much information as possible, giving priority to the nature of the problem and the location of the incident. The dispatcher can then use this information to dispatch emergency crews based on predetermined response levels and on what appears to be needed.

Communicating Hazards

Personnel operating at the scene of a vehicle incident need to communicate hazards to fellow rescuers and to the Incident Commander (IC). For small incidents, this communication can be verbal, using face-to-face communication **(Figure 1.32, p. 46)**. If there is too much ambient noise to allow unaided verbal communication between the rescuers and the IC, the Incident Commander must establish some alternative means of effective communication. This is also necessary if the extrication area is remote from the ICP; that is, far enough away that the victim cannot be seen from the ICP. Depending upon conditions, personnel can use portable radios, hard-wired telephones, and cell phones. However, each form of communication has its limitations, such as concrete

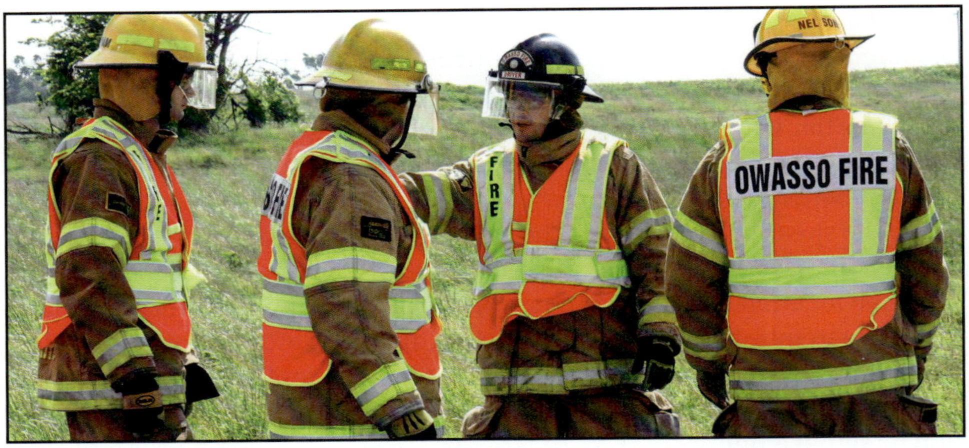

Figure 1.32 Face-to-face communications may be used in small incidents.

walls, which make radios and cell phones unreliable. Organizations should determine what form of communication works best for their organization, and implement the most effective means of communication.

Incident Support Operations and Resources

While personnel are operating at a vehicle incident, they may determine that additional support and resources are necessary. Personnel usually make this determination during scene size-up while taking into account the incident scene as well as the on-scene and responding resources. The IC will have to consider the following questions:

- What has happened?
- What is happening?
- What is likely to happen?
- Are the current resources going to be enough to mitigate the incident?
- What additional resources may be necessary?

The answers to these questions will assist the IC in identifying what support operations and resources are needed at the incident. Oftentimes, the following support and resources that are necessary at a vehicle incident:

- EMS **(Figure 1.33)**
- Law enforcement
- Department of Transportation
- Additional rescue/extrication resources

Some incidents may present complicated scenarios that go beyond the expertise of the IC and on-scene personnel. Therefore, in the process of developing rescue strategy and objectives, the IC should obtain whatever expert assistance is necessary. Examples of the types of experts whose advice the IC may need during vehicle incidents include:

- Structural or mechanical engineers
- Chemists or hazardous materials specialists
- Railroad officials
- Farmers or agricultural extension agents

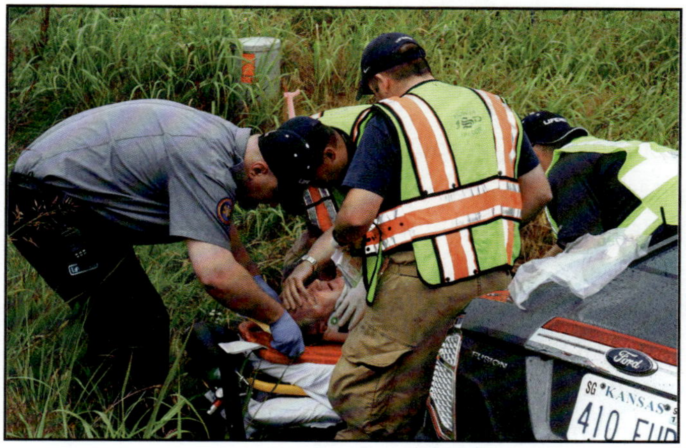

Figure 1.33 The support of EMS is frequently needed at vehicle incidents. *Courtesy of Mike Wieder.*

- Industrial plant maintenance or engineering personnel
- Elevator mechanics or building engineers
- Mine, cave, or tunnel rescue experts
- Heavy equipment operators
- Construction engineers
- Physicians
- Military specialists

Experts or professionals in a specialized field can be brought to the ICP to advise the IC. These resources may be able to better predict the consequences of a particular action and to suggest alternatives. When dealing with unfamiliar situations, an effective IC will take advantage of every resource available. In some cases, it may be advantageous to implement a Unified Command to more effectively manage the incident.

NOTE: The IC should request these support resources in accordance with local standard operating procedures.

Once these resources arrive at the vehicle incident, they should be deployed in a support role of the rescue operations. EMS personnel are used to provide medical care and transport. Law enforcement assists with traffic control and any investigation(s). The Department of Transportation is responsible for coordinating the operation of the roadways. Additional resources and specialists are utilized to best maximize their abilities.

Support operation resources will fall into the Incident Command structure described previously. The IC provides these operational directives to assist in the accomplishment of the primary rescue objective(s). The IC coordinates all these support operations with extrication and rescue operations. Rescue personnel should conduct all operations in accordance with local SOPs.

Chapter Review

1. How do the duties of Awareness, Operations, and Technician level vehicle rescuers differ from one another?
2. Describe the use of standardized response plans for vehicle incidents.
3. What factors should be considered when conducting a hazard and risk assessment survey for vehicle incidents?
4. What should the rescue organization consider when identifying and acquiring personal protective equipment?
5. What environmental considerations and on-scene hazards must be identified during initial size-up?
6. List the seven main components that are vital to ensuring safety at a vehicle incident.
7. What must rescuers be able to do in order to safely stabilize a vehicle incident?
8. What personal protective clothing and equipment can rescuers use to provide protection for themselves and victims?
9. What are the three scene safety zones used by rescuers?
10. What personnel and resources are located within each of the scene safety zones?
11. What are the responsibilities of the rescue group, law enforcement, medical group, and suppression group at an incident?
12. What are the duties of the Incident Safety Officer with regards to monitoring hazard zones at a vehicle incident?
13. What types of traffic must be controlled in order to ensure scene safety?
14. How are traffic control devices used to ensure scene safety
15. What types of operational protocols should a jurisdiction have in place for vehicle incidents?
16. What elements are usually contained within an Incident Action Plan?
17. What are the three major incident priorities that must be communicated to personnel on scene?
18. What role does communication play at a vehicle incident?
19. What factors must be considered in order to determine the need for resources at a vehicle incident?
20. What are five examples of outside resources that may be necessary at a vehicle rescue?

Discussion Questions

1. Your crew is the first to arrive on scene at a vehicle incident. You are trained to the Awareness level, and a more highly-qualified rescuer will not arrive for several minutes. What actions should you take prior to their arrival?
2. What type of preincident planning for vehicle incidents occurs in your jurisdiction?
3. In addition to common support resources such as law enforcement and EMS, what types of specialized resources are available to support vehicle incident operations in your jurisdiction?

1-1
Provide support for a vehicle incident.

SKILL SHEETS

NOTE: Personnel must follow the Incident Action Plan according to local SOPs.

Step 1: Don the appropriate PPE.

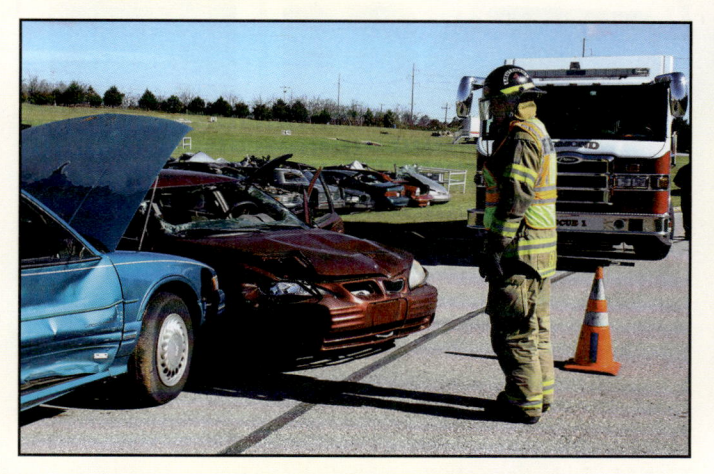

Step 2: Identify whether the incident is an operations-level or technician-level incident.

Step 3: Provide support as directed by the Incident Commander. Support actions may include, but are not limited to the following:

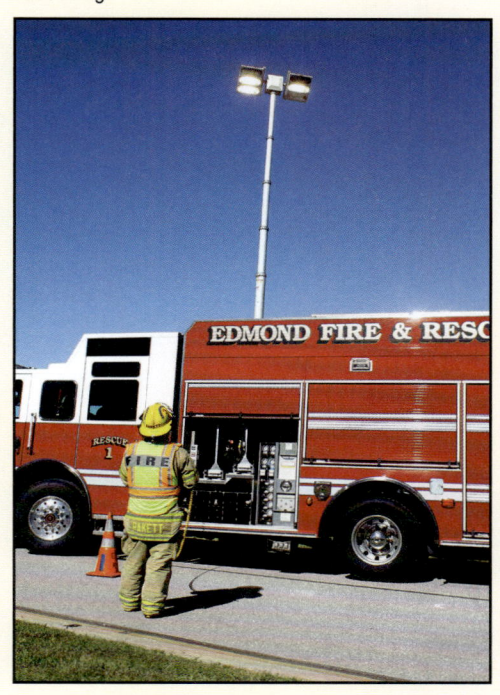

a. Scene lighting setup
b. Monitoring hazard zones
c. Ventilation
d. Facilitation of personnel rehabilitation
e. Resource selection and management
f. Management of environmental concerns

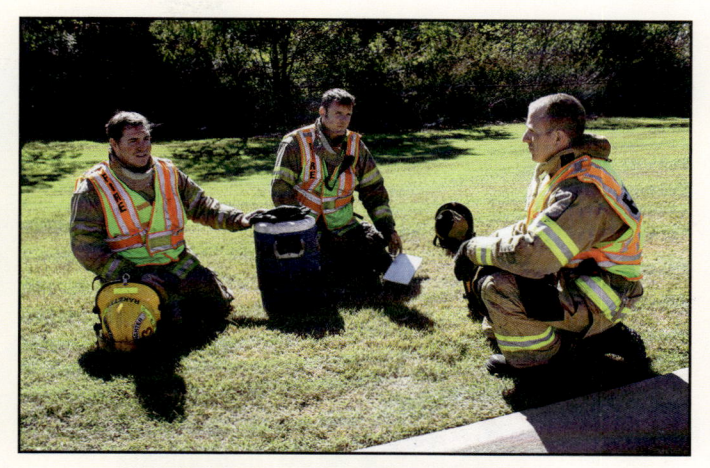

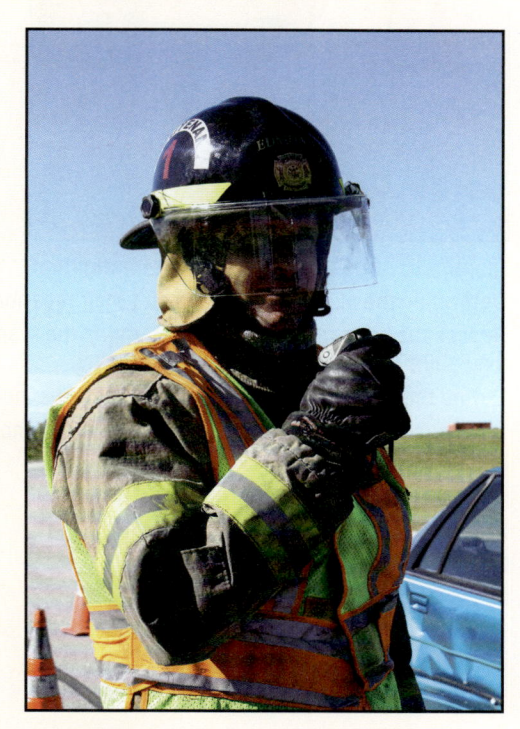

Step 4: Report progress to Command as directed.

Section A • Chapter 1 – Vehicle Incident Safety 49

SKILL SHEETS

1-2

Perform size up and initiate the response at a vehicle incident.

NOTE: This skill sheet covers one method of conducting size up and initiating response. Always follow local SOPs.

Step 1: Establish communication and initiate the response system.
Step 2: Secure the scene.

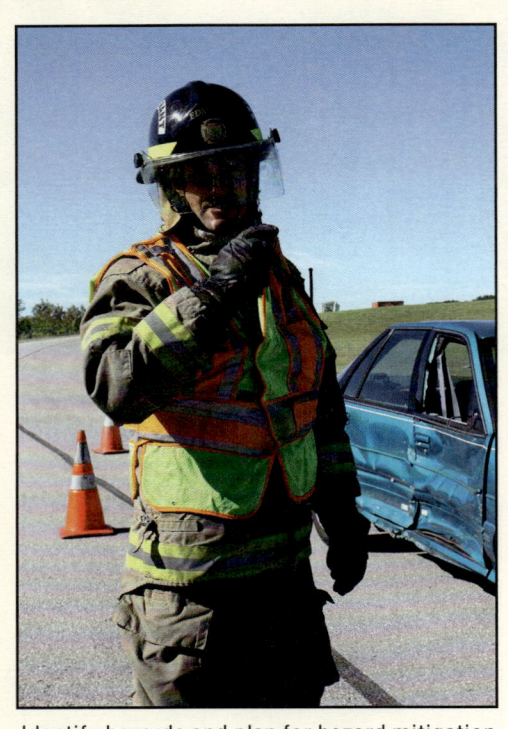

Step 3: Identify hazards and plan for hazard mitigation.
Step 4: Determine the number of victims and their location.
Step 5: Assess the need for resources. Determine the resource availability and resource response time.
Step 6: Define the operational mode to be used for the incident.
Step 7: Determine the type of rescue to be carried out and make assignments as necessary.
Step 8: Establish search parameters.
Step 9: Refer to reference materials as necessary.

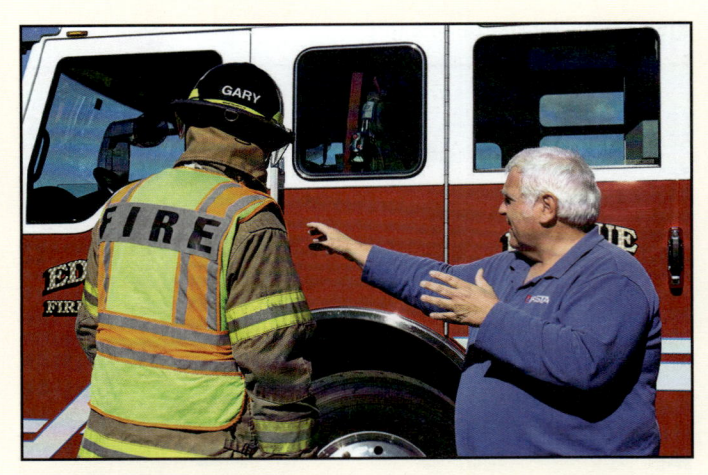

Step 10: Interview witnesses.
Step 11: Collect any other information required to develop an Incident Action Plan and select the appropriate planning forms to be used.
Step 12: Communicate size up information to other rescuers.

1-3
Establish scene safety zones at a vehicle incident.

Step 1: Don the appropriate PPE.

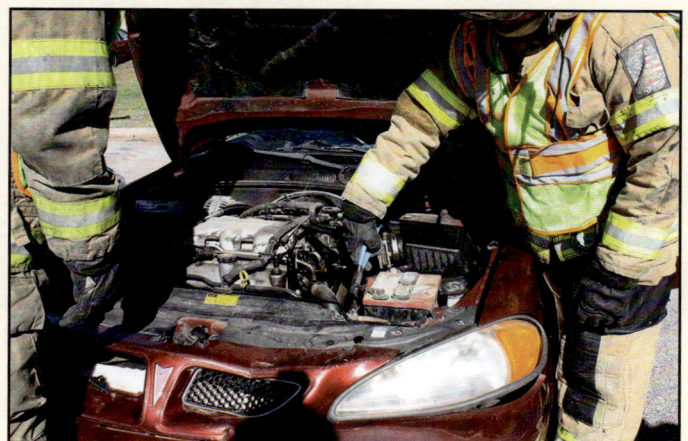

Step 2: Identify hazards.

Step 3: Position scene security barriers or control devices to designate scene safety zones.

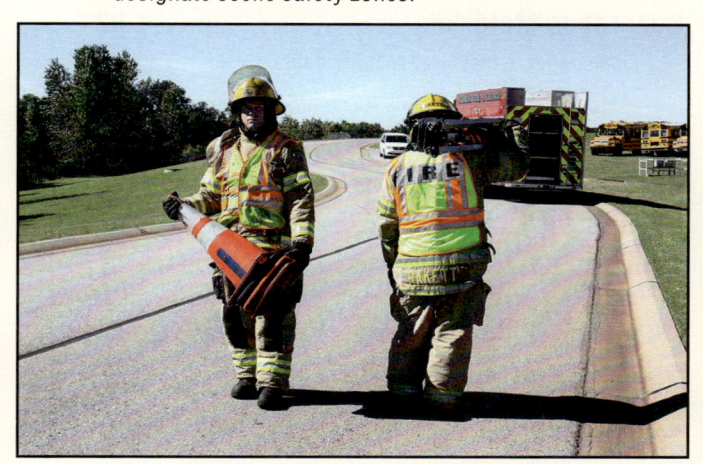

a. Ensure that the perimeters are consistent with the incident requirements.

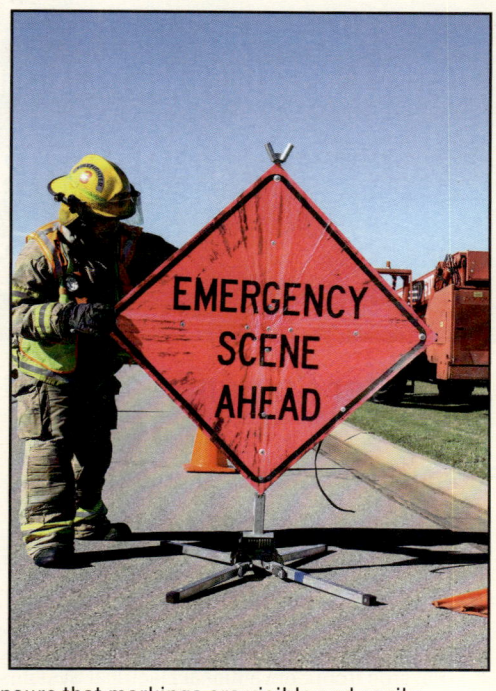

b. Ensure that markings are visible and easily recognizable.

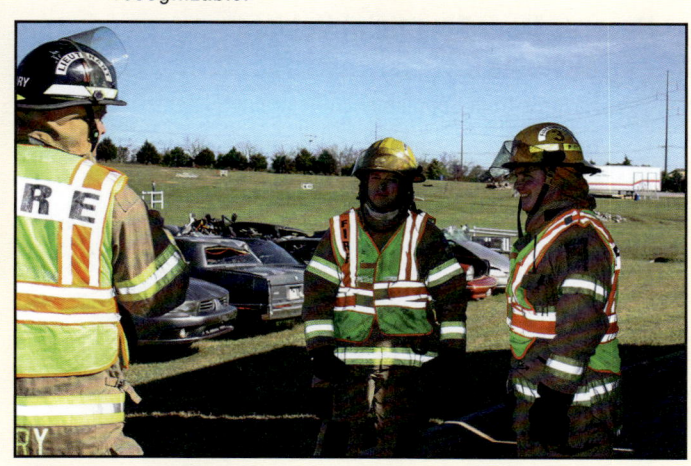

Step 4: Communicate zone boundaries to Command and other personnel.

Step 5: Restrict access to unauthorized personnel.

Step 6: Mitigate any hazards.

Section A • Chapter 1 – Vehicle Incident Safety

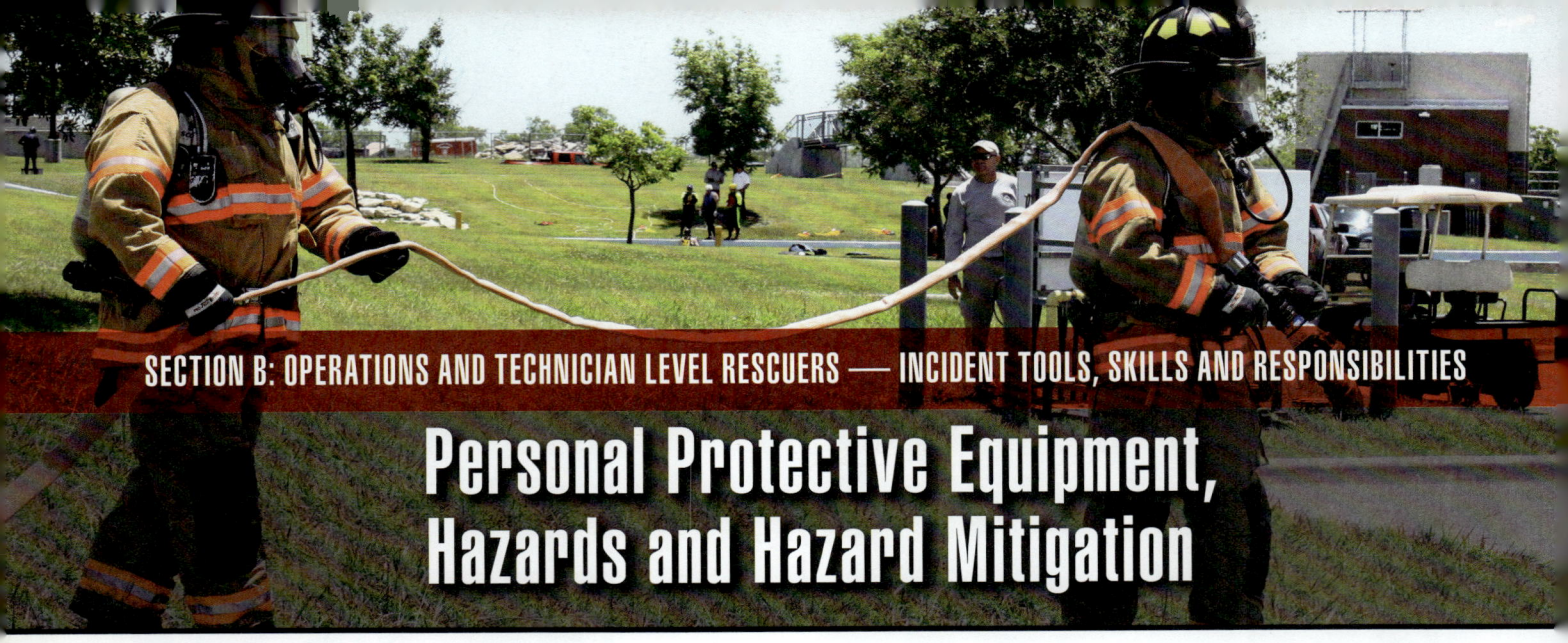

SECTION B: OPERATIONS AND TECHNICIAN LEVEL RESCUERS — INCIDENT TOOLS, SKILLS AND RESPONSIBILITIES

Personal Protective Equipment, Hazards and Hazard Mitigation

Chapter Contents

Personal Protective Equipment 55
    General Personal Protective Equipment..................... 56
    Specialized Personal Protective Equipment 61

Hazards from Vehicle Energy Sources 61
    Hazards from Propulsion Power 62
    Hazards from Conventional Electrical Systems 65
    Hazards from Construction Materials 65

Hazards from Beneficial Vehicle Systems 67
    Hazards from Supplemental Restraint Systems 67
    Hazards from Suspension Systems 73
    Hazards from Seat Adjustment or
        Positioning Controls...74

Fire and Explosion Hazards 74
    Fire Hazards..75
    Explosion Hazards..76

Fire Suppression Operations 77
    Establishing Fire Protection 77
    Alternative Energy Vehicle Fires 80

Hazardous Materials 82
    Passenger Vehicle Haz Mat Incidents 82
    Medium and Heavy Truck Haz Mat Incidents 82
    Bus Haz Mat Incidents.. 85

Chapter Review 85
Discussion Questions 85
Skill Sheets 86

chapter 2

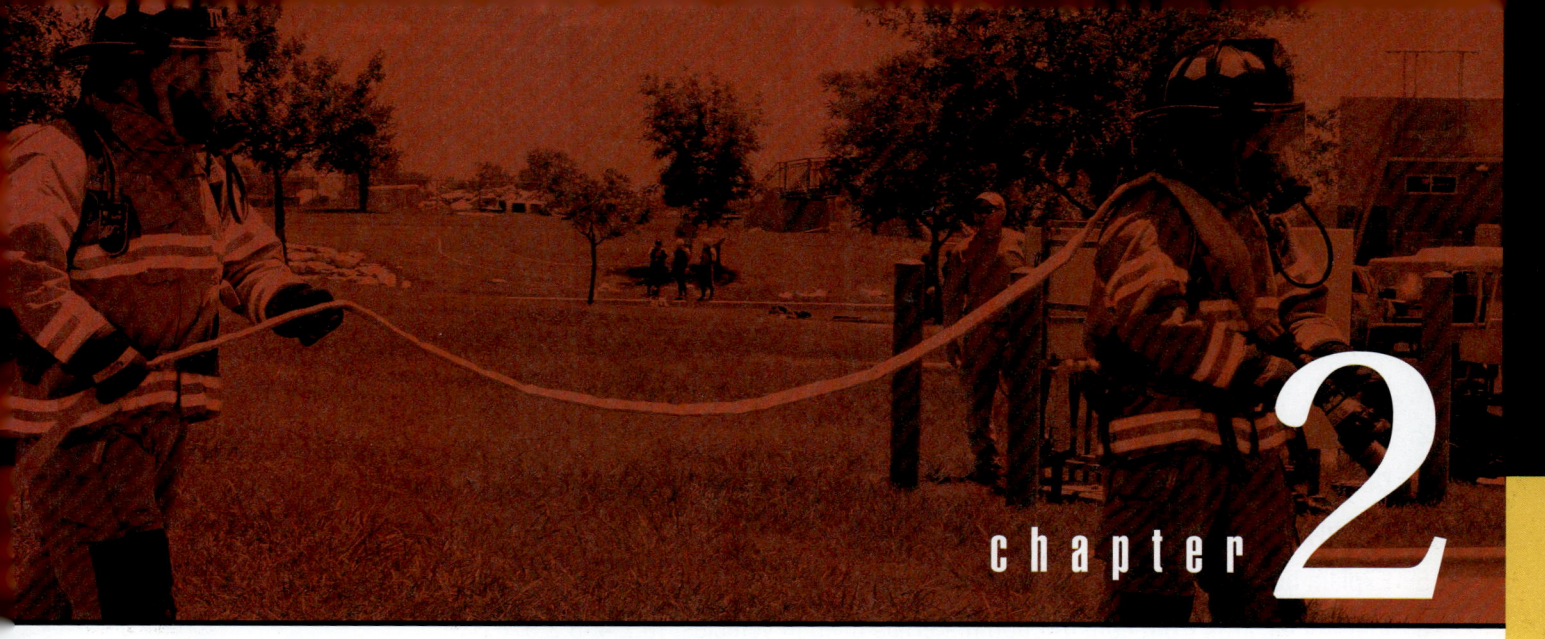

Key Terms

Boiling Liquid Expanding Vapor Explosion (BLEVE)	76
Compressed Natural Gas	81
Hazardous Material (Haz Mat)	82
Liquefied Natural Gas (LNG)	77
Liquefied Compressed Gas (LPG)	77
National Highway Traffic Safety Administration (NHTSA)	70
Standard Operating Procedure (SOP)	55

JPRs addressed in this chapter

This chapter provides information that addresses the following job performance requirements of NFPA 1006, *Standard for Technical Rescuer Professional Qualifications (2016)*.

8.2.1	8.3.1
8.2.2	8.3.3
8.2.4	8.3.4
8.2.9	8.3.6

Section B • Chapter 2 – Personal Protective Equipment, Hazards and Hazard Mitigation   53

Personal Protective Equipment, Hazards and Hazard Mitigation

Learning Objectives

1. Explain the use of personal protective equipment at vehicle incidents. [8.2.4, 8.2.9, 8.3.6]
2. Identify hazards associated with vehicle propulsion power. [8.2.4, 8.2.9, 8.3.6]
3. Describe the methods used to isolate and manage vehicle propulsion power hazards. [8.2.4, 8.3.6]
4. Identify hazards from conventional electrical systems in vehicles. [8.2.4, 8.2.9, 8.3.6]
5. Explain how to isolate and manage hazards caused by conventional electrical systems. [8.2.4, 8.3.6]
6. Identify hazards from construction materials used in vehicles. [8.2.4, 8.2.9, 8.3.6]
7. Describe the methods used to manage hazards caused by materials used in vehicle construction. [8.2.4, 8.3.6]
8. Identify hazards from supplemental restraint systems. [8.2.4, 8.2.9, 8.3.6]
9. Describe the methods used to manage supplemental restraint system hazards. [8.2.4, 8.3.6]
10. Identify hazards from vehicle suspension systems. [8.2.4, 8.2.9, 8.3.6]
11. Identify hazards from seat adjustment or positioning controls in a vehicle. [8.2.4, 8.2.9, 8.3.6]
12. Identify types of fire and explosion hazards that may be present at a vehicle incident. [8.2.2]
13. Explain how to establish fire protection at a vehicle incident. [8.2.1, 8.2.2, 8.3.1]
14. Describe fire protection considerations related to alternative energy vehicle fires. [8.2.1, 8.2.2, 8.3.1]
15. Identify potential hazards from hazardous materials at a vehicle incident. [8.2.1, 8.3.1]
16. Skill Sheet 2-1: Access a vehicle to secure and disable hazards. [8.2.4, 8.3.6]
17. Skill Sheet 2-2: Disconnect or disable a battery. [8.2.4, 8.3.6]
18. Skill Sheet 2-3: Secure suspension. [8.3.6]
19. Skill Sheet 2-4: Secure an air ride cab. [8.3.6]
20. Skill Sheet 2-5: Establish fire protection at a vehicle incident. [8.2.2]

Chapter 2
Personal Protective Equipment, Hazards and Hazard Mitigation

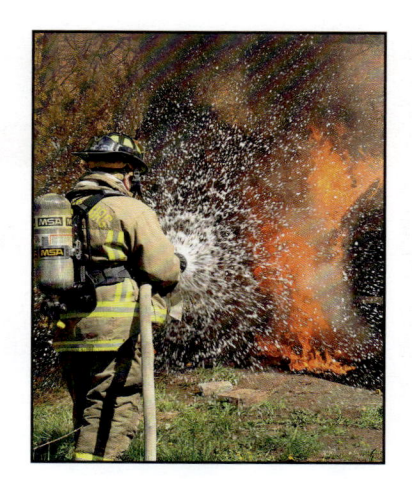

Identifying hazards and the measures needed to control those hazards forms the basis of a safe and effective vehicle rescue operation. Rescuers must first and foremost protect rescue personnel, victims, and bystanders. This chapter will detail specific hazards and control measures concerning a broad spectrum of extrication activities.

Personal Protective Equipment

Because rescuers work in hazardous environments, they should be provided with the best personal protective equipment (PPE) available. In many agencies, **standard operating procedures SOPs** specify the most appropriate type and level of PPE to be used based on temperature, humidity, environmental factors, and present hazards. During an incident, the Incident Commander (IC), or an appointed Incident Safety Officer (ISO), enforces the applicable SOPs and dictates any changes in the type and level of PPE as necessary. The ISO should ensure that all personnel working in the action area are wearing proper and appropriate PPE. Coveralls, street clothing, or station uniforms are usually not acceptable at extrication incidents.

> **Standard Operating Procedure (SOP)** — Formal methods or rules to guide the performance of routine functions or emergency operations. Procedures are typically written in a handbook, so that all firefighters can consult and become familiar with them. *Also known as* Operating Instruction (OI), Predetermined Procedures, *or* Standard Operating Guideline (SOG).

WARNING!
Rescue personnel not wearing appropriate PPE or not wearing it properly should not be permitted to operate on the scene of an emergency.

For most extrication incidents, standard structure fire turnout gear is sufficient. Special operations, such as extrication in a body of water or over a steep cliff, may require specialized personal protective equipment. The following sections describe the basic types of PPE and other equipment, including:

- General personal protective equipment
- Specialized personal protective equipment

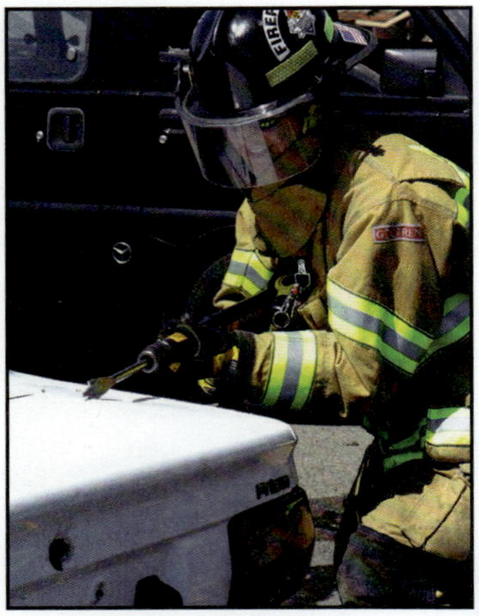

Figure 2.1 A responder wearing appropriate PPE for using an extrication tool.

General Personal Protective Equipment

Don PPE appropriate for the operations. Always comply with local policies and procedures **(Figure 2.1)**. Required PPE includes the following:

- Head, eye, and face protection
- Hearing protection
- Body protection
- Foot protection
- Hand protection
- Respiratory protection

Universal Precautions and Body Substance Isolation

Rescue personnel often work in close proximity to badly injured vehicle occupants. Take precautions to prevent contact with blood and other bodily fluids. Wear any PPE items necessary to isolate these substances. These protective clothing items include medical gloves and eye protection. Other necessary items may include appropriate respiratory protection and Tyvec® suits (disposable suits or garments) that are worn over rescuers' regular protective clothing.

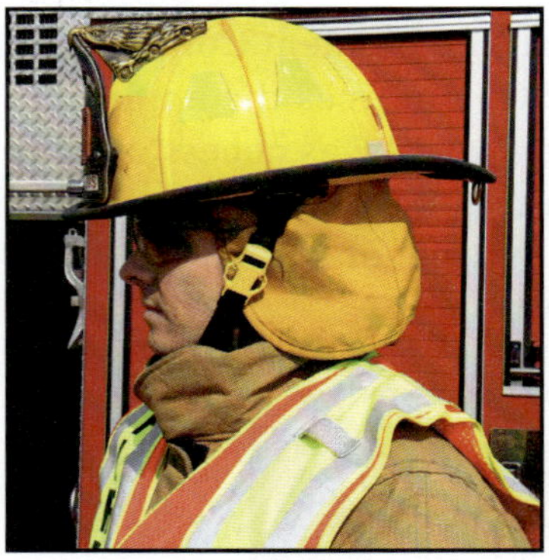

Figure 2.2 Helmet flaps prevent foreign objects from striking the wearer's ears or neck.

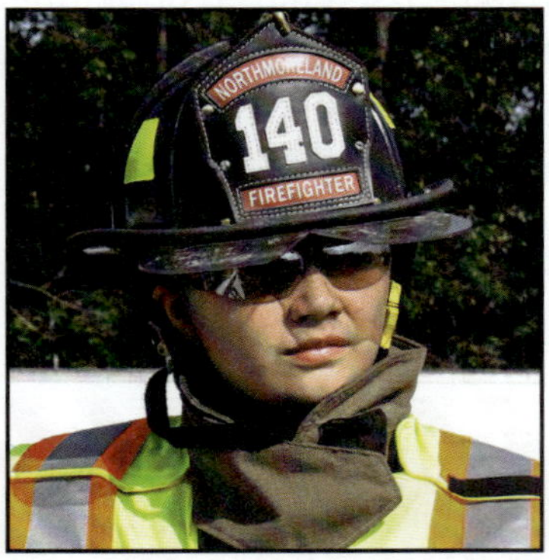

Figure 2.3 A responder wearing safety glasses for eye protection.

Head, Eyes, and Face Protection

Wear proper protective headgear at all extrication incidents **(Figure 2.2)**. Helmets protect the head and skull from injury that may be caused by tripping and falling, as well as being struck by flying or protruding objects. All helmets should meet the requirements set forth by NFPA 1971, *Standard on Protective Ensembles for Structural Fire Fighting and Proximity Fire Fighting.* Pull helmet flaps down over the ears to protect the ears from flying sparks or glass fragments.

Protect the eyes and face from flying objects and spraying liquids, such as battery acid or hydraulic fluid that may cause severe injury **(Figure 2.3)**. Unprotected eyes provide a pathway for infectious organisms. One of the most commonly used types of protection for the eyes and face is the protective shield of the helmet. Standard shield sizes are 4 and 6 inches (100 and 150 mm). Generally, the 6-inch (150 mm) shield is more desirable for extrication personnel because it covers a larger portion of the face.

NOTE: NFPA 1500, *Standard on Fire Department Occupational Safety and Health Program*, requires that helmet goggles or safety glasses be worn in addition to the helmet face shield when performing extrication tasks.

When selecting head protection, agencies should consider fire-resistant, protective hoods. These hoods provide excellent heat protection for the neck, ears, head, and sides of the face **(Figure 2.4)**. In addition to protecting against radiant heat and direct flame impingement, they provide warmth during cold weather. They may also prevent some cuts and scratches caused by brushing against sharp objects. These hoods are recommended on all vehicle extrication operations.

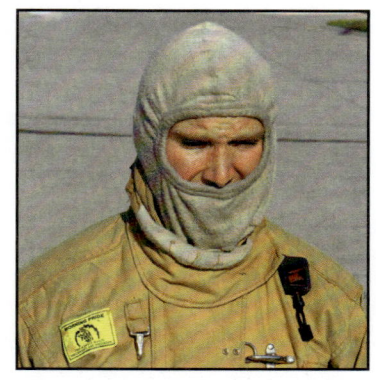

Figure 2.4 Flash hoods provide another layer of protection for rescuers.

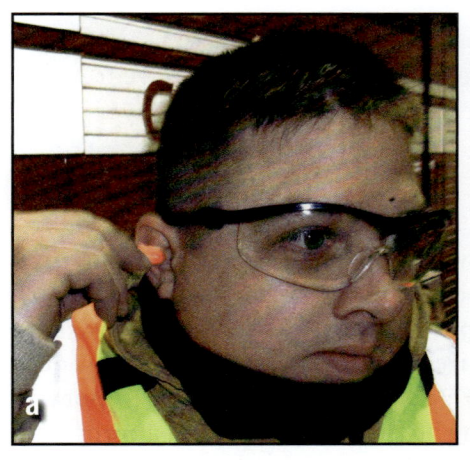

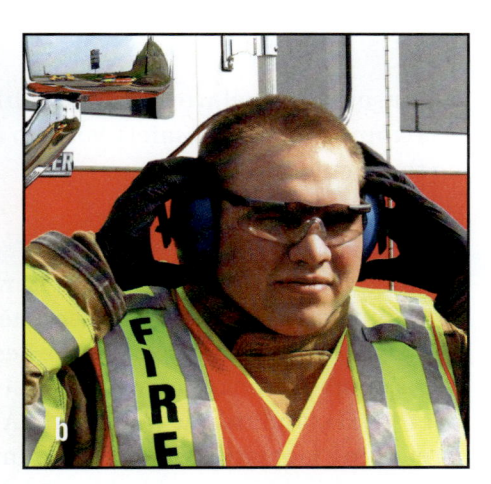

Figure 2.5 a. A rescuer inserting ear plug hearing protection into his ear. *Courtesy of Alan Braun, University of Missouri Fire and Rescue Training Institute.* **b.** Ear muffs are another type of hearing protection.

Hearing Protection

The operation of generators, hydraulic power units, and power tools makes vehicle extrication operations extremely noisy. The operators of these tools, and anyone nearby (including trapped victims), should wear appropriate hearing protection. This protection may be in the form of ear plugs inserted into the ear canal or external ear muffs **(Figure 2.5 a and b)**.

Body Protection

Appropriate protective clothing must be worn at all extrication incidents. Rescue company members should be in complete gear upon arrival at the scene. Any turnout gear should conform to the standards set forth by NFPA 1971. Turnout gear protects rescuers from fires and from sharp objects and many other hazards found on the extrication scene. This protection reduces the chance of injury.

Rescue personnel must be visible on the incident scene. Regardless of color, pants and coats should have adequate reflective striping **(Figure 2.6)**. NFPA 1971 gives specific requirements for the amount of striping. Helmets can also be outfitted with reflective strips or patches. It is best practice for emergency

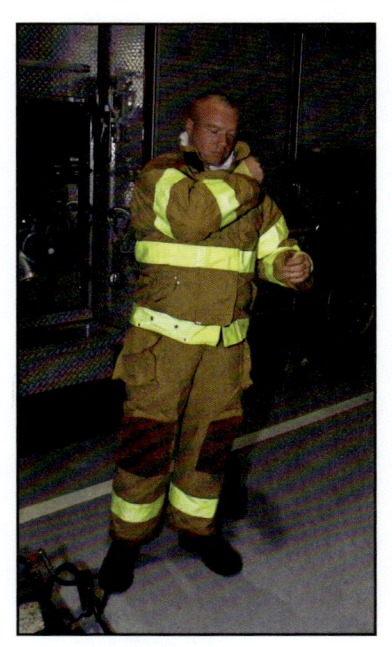

Figure 2.6 Reflective trim catches the light and reflects it to enhance the visibility of responders at night or in low-light conditions.

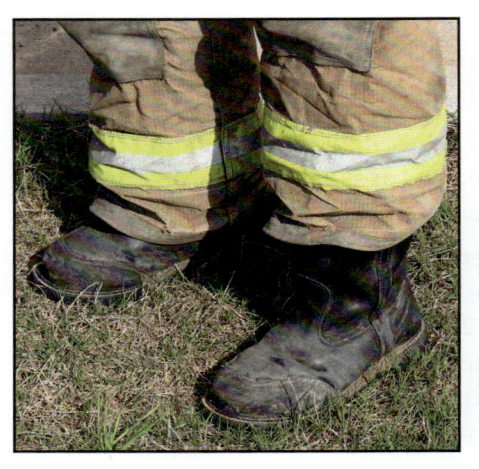

Figure 2.7 A rescuer wearing approved footwear.

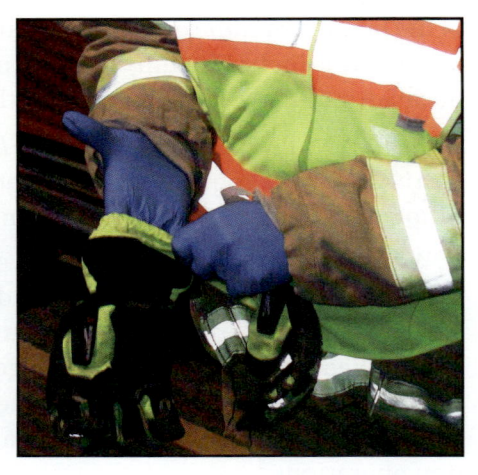

Figure 2.8 Rescue gloves may be worn over latex gloves.

response personnel working at a vehicle extrication incident to wear ANSI/DOT approved Class 3 safety vests to increase their visibility to drivers passing the incident area.

Foot Protection

Vehicle collision scenes are often strewn with broken glass and other potential hazards to the feet; therefore, adequate foot protection is essential **(Figure 2.7)**. Foot protection should provide the best protection against likely hazards that the rescuers will encounter: heat, punctures, and impact. All footwear should meet ANSI standards as well as NFPA 1971. Because a proper fit is important in reducing foot fatigue and in preventing blisters or other sores, appropriate footwear should be provided to each rescuer.

Hand Protection

Gloves are an important part of a rescuer's PPE **(Figure 2.8)**. The type of gloves will vary with the job they are doing and the type of protection required. When fighting fire, wear gloves that meet the standards set forth by NFPA 1971. However, this type of glove may be too bulky and restrictive to allow for the dexterity required to perform extrication functions that do not involve fire.

When performing most extrication functions, rescuers need gloves that protect their hands but allow freedom of movement. Therefore, in most situations, rescuers should wear close-fitting, specially designed and approved extrication gloves. In addition, gloves should be thin enough to allow dexterity but sturdy enough to protect hands from cuts, punctures, and abrasions.

NFPA 1500 requires that rescue personnel wear medical exam gloves inside their leather gloves or wear emergency medical work gloves, if they are likely to contact bodily fluids. These gloves must meet the requirements of NFPA 1999, *Standard on Protective Clothing for Emergency Medical Operations*.

Respiratory Protection

Hazardous vapors, fumes, smoke, and dust are often present at vehicle extrication incidents. Therefore, rescuers (and in some cases, trapped victims) often

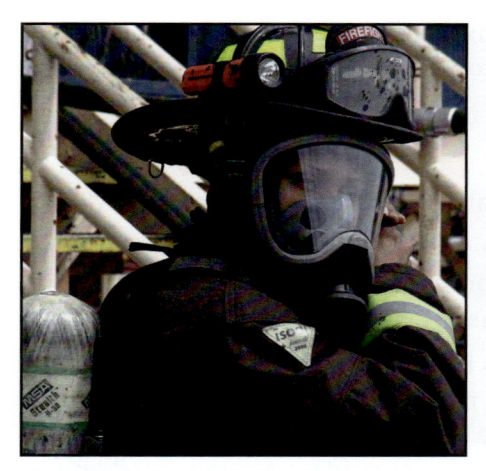

Figure 2.9 Since inhalation is one of the most dangerous routes of entry for many hazardous materials, respiratory protection is extremely important.

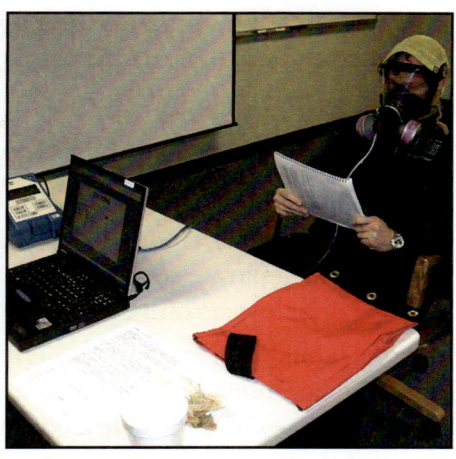

Figure 2.10 A rescuer undergoing a test to ensure a proper facepiece fit. *Courtesy of Alan Braun, University of Missouri Fire and Rescue Training Institute.*

require respiratory protection **(Figure 2.9)**. Rescue personnel should be well trained in the operation, use, capabilities, and limitations of all types of respiratory protection available to them. Achieving and maintaining this level of proficiency requires regular training and periodic testing. Rescue personnel typically use one of two types of breathing equipment: self-contained breathing apparatus (SCBA) and air-purifying respirators (APRs).

Self-contained breathing apparatus (SCBA). All self-contained breathing apparatus must be of the positive-pressure type and should meet the requirements of NFPA 1981, *Standard on Open-Circuit Self-Contained Breathing Apparatus (SCBA) for Emergency Services*. Because facial contours vary from person to person, facepieces are designed in different sizes in order to obtain a proper fit. Each rescuer should be issued a personal face piece that is fit-tested at the time of issue and annually thereafter **(Figure 2.10)**. NFPA 1500 expressly prohibits beards, long sideburns, or other facial hair that would interfere with the face piece seal or the operation of the unit.

SCBA come in 30-minute, 45-minute, or 60-minute ratings. These ratings are frequently misunderstood and personnel can be put in danger if the ratings are taken literally. These ratings are determined by timing a number of average, healthy individuals breathing at a relaxed, normal respiratory rate and averaging those times. The time-related ratings of SCBA cylinders represent the maximum amount of time the air supply will last under ideal circumstances.

The actual duration of support depends on the individual wearer's physiological and psychological conditioning. Training should be frequent enough and of sufficient duration to allow personnel to become comfortable and to overcome any tendency they may have toward claustrophobia. Given this type of training, rescuers who know their jobs and who are in good physical condition can remain calm during emergencies and make maximum use of the air supply in each cylinder.

Air-purifying respirator (APR). APRs contain an air-purifying filter, canister, or cartridge that removes specific contaminants found in ambient air as the air passes through the air-purifying element **(Figure 2.11)**. Based on

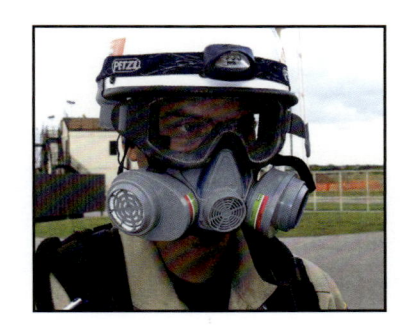

Figure 2.11 A rescuer wearing an APR.

what cartridge, canister, or filter is being used, these purifying elements are generally divided into the three following types:

- Particulate-removing APRs
- Vapor-and-gas-removing APRs
- Combination particulate-removing and vapor-and-gas-removing APRs

APRs may be powered (PAPRs) or non-powered. APRs do not supply oxygen or air from a separate source, and they protect only against specific contaminants at or below certain concentrations.

Respirators with air-purifying filters may have either full face pieces that provide a complete seal to the face and protect the eyes, nose, and mouth or half face pieces that provide a complete seal to the face and protect the nose and mouth. Disposable filters, canisters, or cartridges are mounted on one or both sides of the face piece. Canister or cartridge respirators pass the air through a filter, sorbent, catalyst, or combination of these items to remove specific contaminants from the air. The air enters the system either from the external atmosphere through the filter or sorbent or when the user's exhalation combines with a catalyst to provide breathable air.

APRs should be worn only in controlled atmospheres where the hazards present are completely understood and at least 19.5 percent oxygen is present. If oxygen contents are lower than prescribed, positive-pressure SCBA must be worn during emergency operations. No single canister, filter, or cartridge protects against all chemical hazards. Responders must know the hazards present in the atmosphere in order to select the appropriate canister, filter, or cartridge. Responders should be able to answer the following questions before deciding to use APRs for protection at a vehicle incident involving hazardous materials:

- What is the hazard?
- Is the hazard a vapor or a gas?
- Is the hazard a particle or dust?
- Is there some combination of dust and vapors present?
- What concentration levels are present?

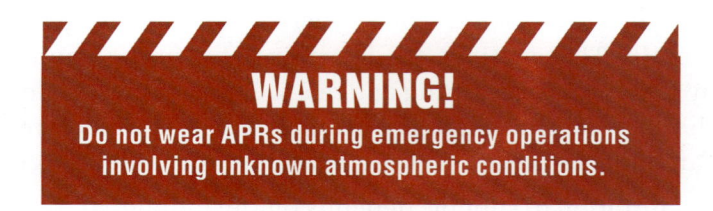

WARNING!
Do not wear APRs during emergency operations involving unknown atmospheric conditions.

APRs do *not* protect against oxygen-deficient or oxygen-enriched atmospheres. The three primary limitations of an APR are:

- Limited life of its filters and canisters
- Need for constant monitoring of the contaminated atmosphere
- Need for a normal oxygen content of the atmosphere before use

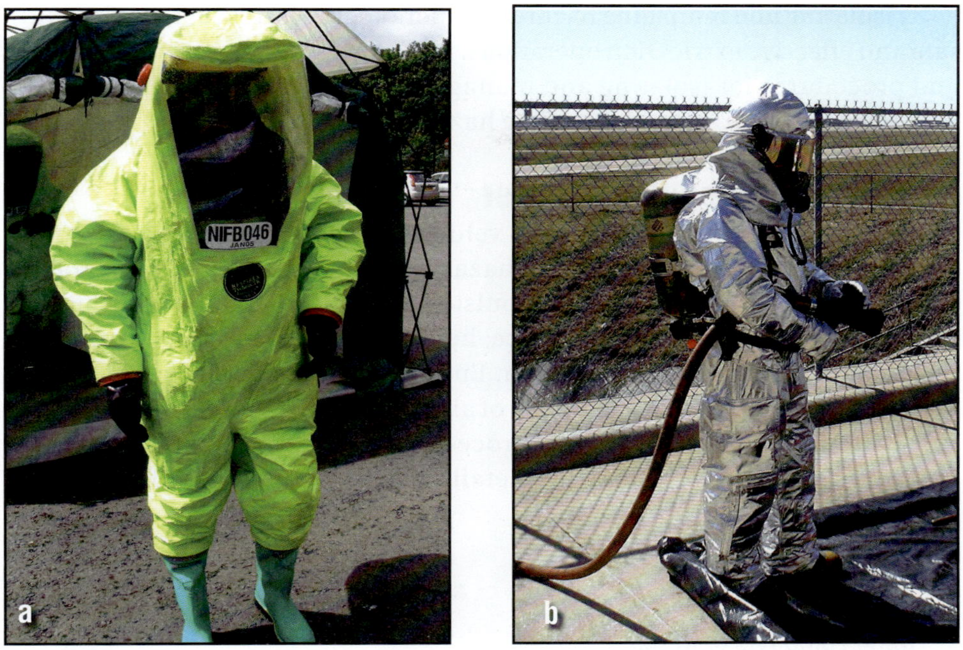

Figure 2.12 a. Resuer is wearing a haz mat vapor protective suit. *Courtesy of Brian Canady, DFWIA Department of Public Safety.* **b.** Rescuer is wearing proximity suit.

Take the following precautions before using APRs or PAPRs:

- Know what chemicals/air contaminants are in the air
- Know how much of the chemicals/air contaminants are in the air
- Ensure that the oxygen level is between 19.5 and 23.5 percent
- Ensure that atmospheric hazards are not immediately dangerous to life and health conditions

Specialized Personal Protective Equipment

In a small number of extrication incidents, the IC may have to call in technical rescue personnel who are specially trained and equipped to operate in extremely hazardous environments. The special protective equipment that these teams wear may include hazardous materials suits, proximity or entry suits, body armor, and wet suits **(Figure 2.12 a and b)**.

NOTE: More information on specialized personal protective equipment may be found in the IFSTA **Fire Service Technical Search and Rescue** and **Hazardous Materials for First Responder** manuals.

Hazards from Vehicle Energy Sources

Rescuers should familiarize themselves with the various vehicles and hazards common to their jurisdiction. Many vehicle hazards can be grouped into one of two categories: hazards from energy sources and hazards from beneficial systems.

Potential energy sources should be identified and evaluated at all vehicle incidents. These energy sources serve as a source of ignition for any flammable or combustible hazards, and have the potential to cause serious injury to emergency responders if not isolated and managed.

By isolating and managing hazardous energy sources, rescuers can perform safe and effective extrication operations. Personnel should follow AHJ policies and procedures for isolating and managing energy sources. **Skill Sheet 2-1** lists steps for securing and disabling hazards.

Hazards from Propulsion Power

The fuels or energy that propel the vehicles create hazards at vehicle incidents. Responders face additional hazards when attempting to control any consequential movement from propulsion power. Most vehicles still utilize conventional fuels as a power source; however, alternative fuels and hybrid technology are gaining momentum. Emergency responders should always be aware of the types and variations of all vehicles in their response area and stay up to date on the emergency procedures and measures to mitigate the associated hazards. This section details the following types of propulsion power hazards:

- Conventional fuels
- Alternative fuels
- Hybrid/electric vehicles

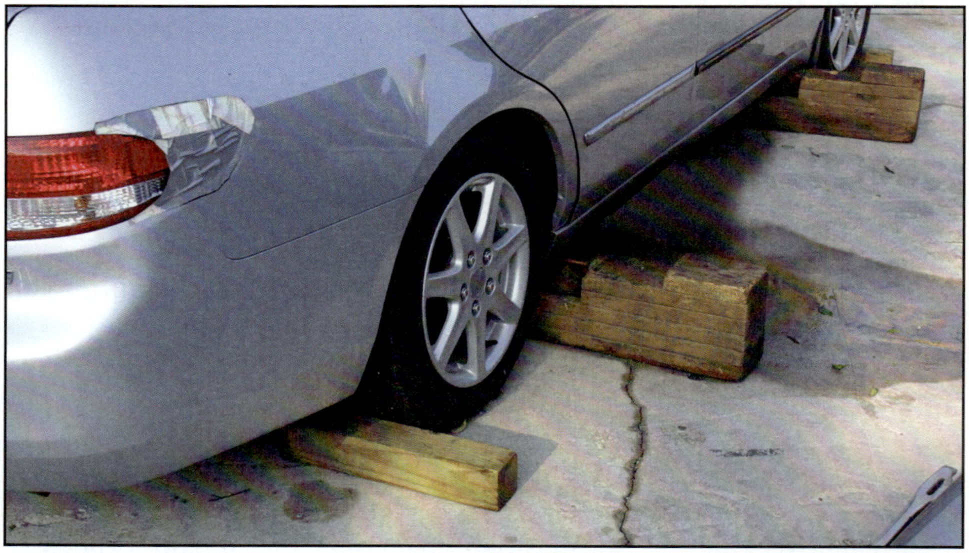

Figure 2.13 This vehicle has been chocked to prevent horizontal movement and step chocked to prevent vertical movement.

Conventional Fuels

Most passenger vehicles, medium and heavy trucks, and buses still utilize conventional fuels such as gasoline and diesel. Fuel tanks and systems may contain less than 15 gallons (60 L) for passenger vehicles, but may contain more than 500 gallons (2 000 L) in large buses and heavy trucks. Isolate and manage these systems using the following technique:

- Secure the vehicle by placing wheel chocks in front and behind tires to prevent unexpected movement **(Figure 2.13)**.
- Apply the emergency brake.
- If the vehicle has an automatic transmission:
  — Place the gear selector in park.

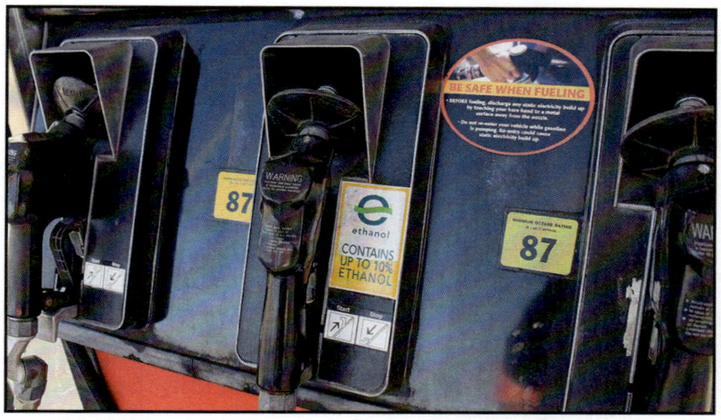

Figure 2.14 Ethanol is a readily available alternative fuel.

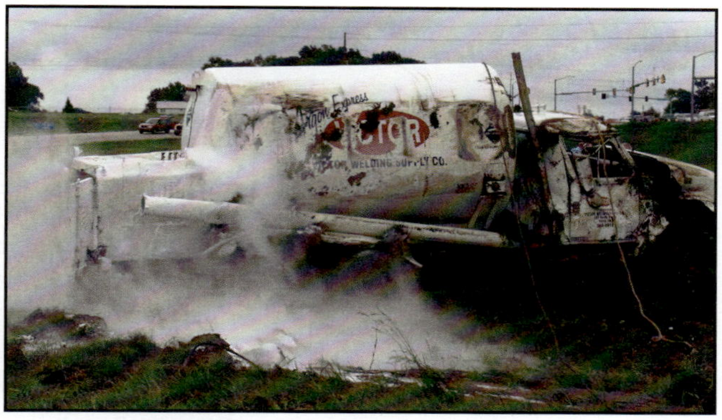

Figure 2.15 A spill or leak of cryogenic liquids typically results in a vapor cloud. Not only are these materials very cold, but they can be flammable, and responders should avoid coming into contact with them. *Courtesy of Steve Irby, Owasso Fire Department*.

- — Turn off the ignition.
- — Remove the key.
- If the vehicle has a manual transmission:
  - — Turn off the ignition.
  - — Remove the key.
  - — Place the gear shift in the lowest gear.
- Eliminate any ignition sources

NOTE: If the vehicle is equipped with a smart key system and rescuers are unable to disable the 12-volt battery, locate and remove the key from the area surrounding the vehicle. Personnel should be aware of the potential for a second smart key. **Skill Sheet 2-1** describes the steps to access a vehicle to secure and disable hazards.

Alternative Fuels

An alternative fuel is a fuel that is not entirely derived from petroleum products. Alternative fuels can be a mixture of petroleum with another fuel source, such as ethanol (alcohol/gasoline) **(Figure 2.14)**, and may have the same hazards as conventional fuels. Some alternative fuels may also be stored in pressurized cylinders in a gaseous or liquid state, which present combustible and explosive hazards when damaged in a collision. Examples of alternative fuels include the following:

- Propane/liquefied petroleum gas (LPG)
- Natural gas
- Auxiliary fuel cells
- Alcohol/gasoline blended mixtures
- Biodiesel
- Aircraft fuel

Rescuers have to exercise further mitigation techniques on vehicles using alternative fuels. Rescuers should monitor the atmosphere with a combustible gas indicator and stay clear of vapor clouds **(Figure 2.15)**. Once the vehicle is secured and ignition sources have been eliminated, rescuers should locate, access, and manually turn off the fuel at the tank shut-off valve.

> ### Monitoring the Atmosphere
>
> In many entrapment incidents, the atmosphere in the immediate rescue area can be contaminated by escaping gases or vapors from fluids leaking from the damaged vehicle. It can also become contaminated with the exhaust from gasoline-driven rescue equipment. Whatever the source of contamination, personnel should be assigned to monitor the atmosphere in the immediate rescue area. These personnel should use single or multi-gas detectors as dictated by the situation. For more information on atmospheric monitoring, refer to the IFSTA **Hazardous Materials for First Responders** manual.

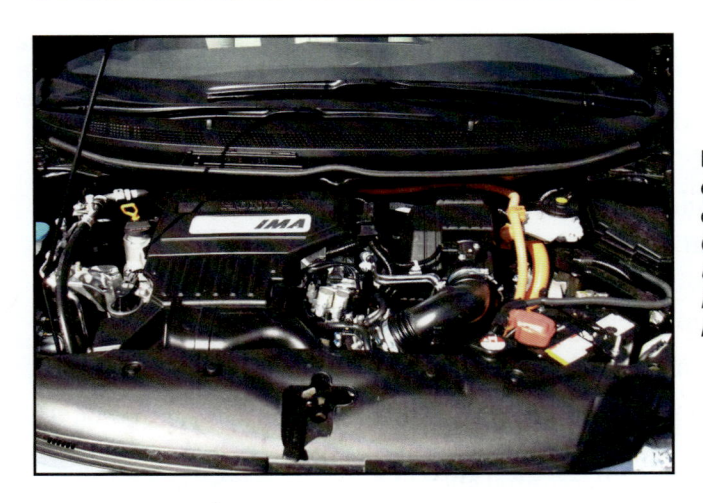

Figure 2.16 The gasoline engine and electric motor on a hybrid vehicle. *Courtesy of Alan Braun, University of Missouri Fire and Rescue Training Institute.*

Hybrid Electric Vehicles

The danger associated with hybrid vehicles is the high voltage stored within the propulsion batteries and running through wiring or cables connected to the vehicle's electric motor. Depending on the type of vehicle, these systems may contain as much as 800 volts of DC current **(Figure 2.16)**.

NOTE: Rescuers should always assume that every hybrid electric vehicle is powered up despite a lack of engine noise.

The techniques for isolating and managing the 12-volt electrical system in hybrid electric vehicles are similar to that of the fuel-driven vehicles. The most desirable method for disabling a hybrid electric vehicle is to shut down the vehicle with the switch and key system. Then rescuers should disable the 12-volt electrical system using the same methods used to disable the battery in a conventional vehicle. Disconnecting or cutting the 12-volt negative and positive cables will open relays to isolate the high-voltage system.

Shutting down the high-voltage battery system consists of a more detailed operation. On some vehicles, rescuers will simply remove a cover and flip a breaker-like switch. In other vehicles, rescuers will have to remove a fuse. Some manufacturers recommend the use of 10,000-volt lineman gloves for this procedure. **Skill Sheet 2-2** lists the steps for disabling a battery.

NOTE: Rescuers should consult manufacturer's Emergency Response Guides for more detailed information on isolating and managing hybrid electric vehicle's battery systems.

Hazards from Conventional Electrical Systems

Vehicle electrical systems are a likely ignition source. These include battery systems, window defoggers, and other systems. Battery systems can impart heat energy to various parts of a wrecked vehicle, that increases the risk of spark and ignition of spilled fuels and/or hydraulic fluids. Defoggers can produce sparks or shock a person during window removal.

Some modern passenger vehicles may have onboard power inverters that provide electricity to remote power outlet (RPO) sites. These allow the use of AC power for the operation of electrically powered equipment such as drills, saws, or other devices at various locations on or in the vehicle. Many work/service vehicles have higher capacity power inverters that are capable of high energy output.

Isolating and managing these electrical systems eliminates a potential source of ignition, deactivates the vehicle's supplemental restraint system, and de-energizes any additional accessories or power equipment that may still be running. Isolating the electrical system may require disconnecting or cutting the battery cables, or can be as simple as flipping a master disconnect switch.

> **WARNING!**
> When isolating the vehicle's electrical system, rescuers should ensure that all electrical cables have been disconnected or cut.

Rescuers should verify that the battery system has been isolated by observing systems that normally operate on battery power. Some jurisdictions perform this by activating the hazard lights and verifying their inoperability.

Hazards from Construction Materials

Various construction materials used in vehicles create hazards for rescuers. This section discusses the materials found in vehicle components including:

- Windows
- Bumpers
- Other components

Windows

Laminated safety glass consists of two sheets of glass bonded to a sheet of plastic sandwiched between them. Impact produces multiple long, pointed shards with sharp edges. In addition, any fine dust created from cutting this type of glass creates respiratory hazards for the emergency responders and victims.

Tempered glass is most commonly used in side windows and some rear windows. Tempered glass is designed to spread small fracture lines throughout the plate when struck. This decreases the hazards of long, pointed pieces of glass. However, tempered glass causes small nuisance lacerations to unprotected body parts. Open wounds and eyes may get contaminated with tiny bits of glass.

Rescuers can practice multiple methods to manage window hazards. For example, rescuers can apply a sheet of self-adhering contact paper to the surface of the glass. Once broken, the glass adheres to the contact paper. Another

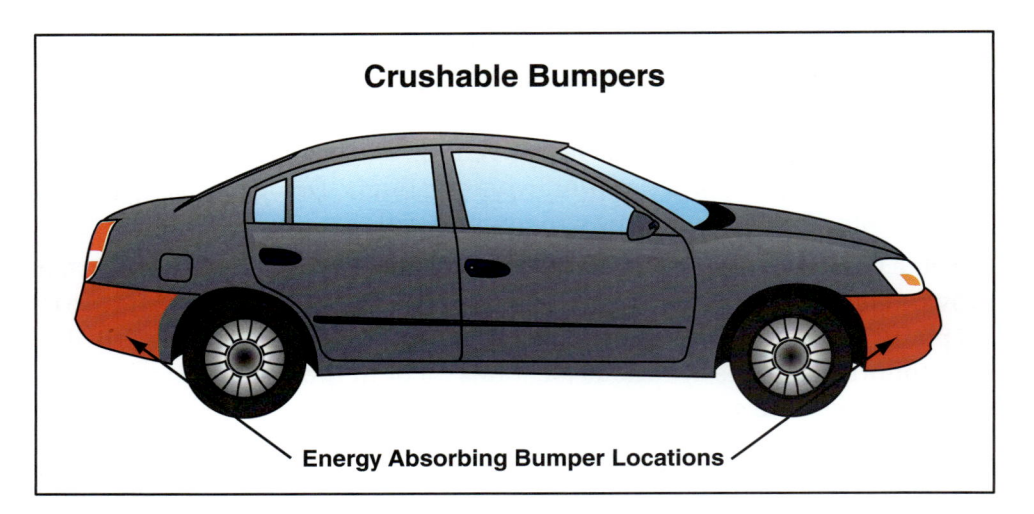

Figure 2.17 Locations of energy absorbing bumpers on passenger vehicles.

method of controlling breaking glass is to place duct tape on the windows and then spray the glass surface with an aerosol adhesive that forms a coating on the glass. This coating sets up in seconds and allows the glass to be broken and retained in a sheet.

Crushable Bumpers

Crushable bumpers absorb energy by flexing when struck **(Figure 2.17)**. Some bumpers are made of polystyrene foam molded into an egg crate structure covered by a flexible rubber shell. Others are made of synthetic rubber molded into a honeycomb structure covered with a flexible shell.

Crushable bumpers are not a hazard in a fire until the fire is out. As these bumpers cool after being exposed to the heat of a fire, beads of a clear liquid form on the surface of the bumper. This liquid appears to be water but is actually concentrated hydrofluoric acid (HF), which is a highly corrosive substance. Flush these bumpers with copious amounts of water to minimize the presence of HF.

Vehicle Components

Vehicle wheels and tires, either on the vehicle or in the trunk, may also create a hazard. When exposed to fire, alloy wheels made with magnesium (also known as mag wheels) can burn with intense heat. Wheels made from pure magnesium are no longer produced, but may still be encountered. High-pressure tires can also create an explosion hazard when punctured or exposed to fire.

Other magnesium vehicle components that can cause high heat fires include the following:

- Valve covers
- Steering columns
- Mounting brackets on antilock braking systems
- Transmission casings
- Engine blocks
- Frame supports
- Exterior body components

Hazards from Beneficial Vehicle Systems

For the purpose of this text, *beneficial vehicle systems* are defined as any system or component of a vehicle that provides benefit to and/or enhances the safety and comfort of the vehicle occupant(s). Although technology continues to improve vehicle safety and comfort systems, it also necessitates that emergency responders stay up-to-date on measures required to safely and effectively manage emerging beneficial technology during the vehicle incidents. Responders should maintain knowledge of AHJ policies and procedures involving hazards from beneficial vehicle systems. Beneficial systems acting as potential hazards include **(Table 2.1, p. 68)**:

- Supplemental restraint systems
- Suspension systems **(Figure 2.18)**
- Seat adjustment or positioning controls

Hazards from Supplemental Restraint Systems

Supplemental restraint systems (SRS) can be hazardous to rescuers who are working in or around a vehicle that has been compromised. The unintentional activation of one or more of these systems during extrication operations can severely injure occupants and rescuers.

The safest manner in which to deal with SRS devices is to give them space. The ABCs of dealing with SRS are as follows:

- **A**lways respect the deployment path of any type of airbags, rollover protection systems (ROPS), or SRS.
- **B**e aware that there is no way to make an undeployed airbag, ROPS, or SRS safe.
- **C**aution must be paramount in cutting or manipulating any vehicle equipped with airbags, ROPS, or SRS.

SRS, which are concealed within the vehicle's interior trim pieces, require rescuers to *peel and peek* behind the interior trim to identify stored gas and canister type inflators, and other components. Rescuers should look for and

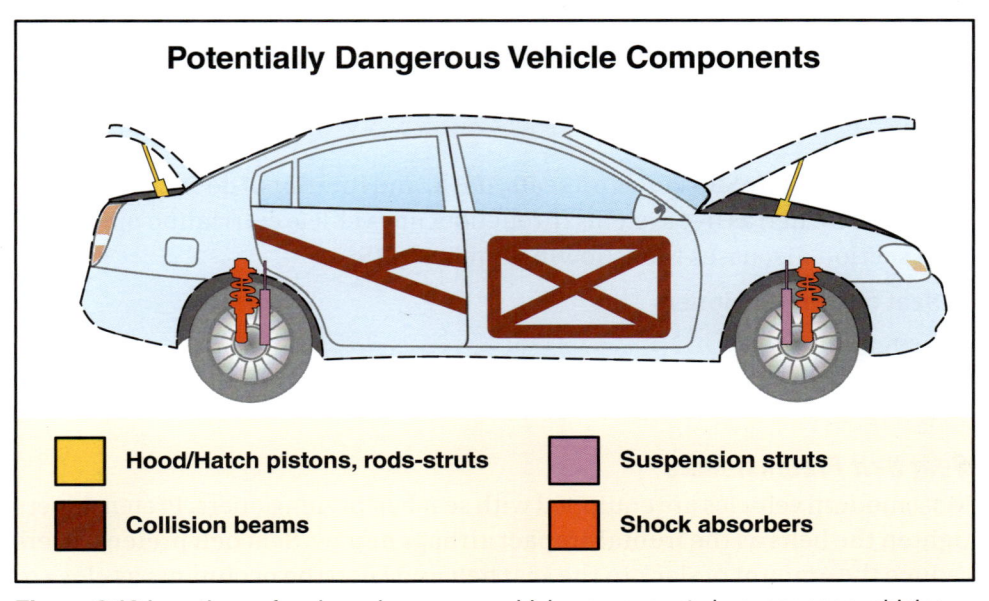

Figure 2.18 Locations of various dangerous vehicle components in passenger vehicles.

Table 2.1
Examples of Supplemental Passenger Restraint Systems, Roll Over Protection Systems, and Components
(as of date of publication)

AIR BAGS
- Driver's single and dual stage (frontal)
- Passenger single and dual stage (pyrotechnic inflated)
- Passenger single and dual stage (compressed gas inflated)
- Front side impact in the door (torso style)
- Front side impact in seat (head and torso types)
- Front side impact in seat (torso type)
- Front side impact (extending up from door)
- Rear side impact in the door
- Rear side impact in the seat (torso type)
- Rear side impact in seat (head and torso types)
- Rear occupant frontal in back of front seat
- Side curtain (front windows)
- Side curtain (full length)
- Head protection tube type
- Third row side curtain
- Driver's knee (bolster)
- Passenger knee (bolster)
- Carpet
- Seat belt
- Seat position

ROLL OVER PROTECTION
- Full bar
- Dual bar

PRE-TENSIONERS
- Pyrotechnic seat belt (spool and buckle types)
- Pyrotechnic seat belt (buckle type)
- Dual pyrotechnic seat belt

OCCUPANT POSITION SENSORS
- Strain gage
- Sonogram (Jaguar)
- Wireless antenna (Honda)

SEAT POSITION SENSORS (OCCUPANT WEIGHT SENSORS)
- Blatted
- Matt
- I-bolt strain gage

OTHER
- Back lash protection headrests
- Seat belt tension sensors
- Air bag cut-off switches
- Pre-accident sensing systems
- Post-accident reporting systems
- Multiple batteries
- Multiple battery locations
- Windows and door locks operated by air bag module

communicate any SRS labels on seats, dash, and interior of doors. SRS should always be treated as live systems throughout any vehicle extrication operation. This section discusses the following types of SRS:

- Seat belt pretensioners
- Airbags
- ROPS

Seat Belt Pretensioners

Most modern vehicles are equipped with seat belt pretensioners. Pretensioners tighten the belts as the frontal-impact airbags deploy. Seat belt pretensioners reduce the amount of slack in the seat belt and keep the occupants as close to the seat as possible during an impact.

In some cases, the belts may be tightened to the point that they restrict the wearer's ability to breathe normally. Simply releasing or cutting the seat belts will relieve this pressure. Once the seat belt is cut, remove the buckle and excess belt so that they cannot strike anyone if the system suddenly activates. Victims in a side-resting or roof-resting vehicle may be suspended by their seatbelts. Support these victims prior to cutting the seat belts.

The seat belt pretensioners in most modern vehicles deploy using pyrotechnic devices. The pyrotechnic device is usually located near the bottom of the B-post at the base of the seat belt. These pyrotechnic devices detonate and retract the seat belt upon receiving a signal from crash sensors placed throughout the vehicle. If the pretensioner is heated during a vehicle fire, it can explode, potentially causing injury to the rescuers and victims.

Avoid cutting the pyrotechnic devices when cutting the vehicle's B-posts during extrication. During extrication, remove any molding or trim to visualize the pretensioner. Make cuts into the B-post well above or well below the external seat belt retractor. Some automobile manufacturers enclose pretensioners within steel caissons or casings inside the B-post to protect them from being cut. Often, rescuers should only need to unbuckle or cut belts, and will not need to cut the posts containing seatbelt pretensioners.

Airbags

Often, airbags will not deploy during a vehicle collision. Most modern airbag systems detect the following:

- The occupant's weight and position
- If the seat belt is buckled
- The vehicle's speed and area of impact

Using this information, the system determines if an airbag needs to deploy to its full capacity or just simply deploy the pretensioner assembly. If the airbag does not detect an occupant in a seat, the airbag may not deploy.

Rescuers should maintain a safe working distance from all active airbags by using the 5-10-12-18-20-inch safe practice guideline. The following are suggested minimum safety zone distances:

- 5 inches (125 mm) for side impact airbags and knee bolsters
- 10 inches (250 mm) for driver frontal airbags
- 12 to 18 inches (300 to 450 mm) for impact curtains that deploy down from the head liner
- 20 inches (500 mm) for passenger frontal airbags

While these distances will not be appropriate for all airbags, they provide a general guideline. The same precautions must be used with knee bolsters as with other front-impact airbags. When mitigating supplemental restraint system during extrication operations:

- Do not cut inflators.
- Peel away interior trim and peek before cutting (peel and peek).
- Work with the safety systems that are not around them.
- Maintain situational awareness of airbag locations and appropriate airbag deployment zones while working in and around the vehicle.

> ⚠️ **CAUTION**
> Should an accidental airbag deployment occur, having body parts positioned through an open window could result in serious injury. When reaching into the vehicle to remove or turn off the ignition, rescuers should reach from behind the steering hub.

Always use caution when working around airbags. Treat them as live systems even after disconnecting the power source. Static electricity can cause these systems to detonate without an electrical source.

National Highway Traffic Safety Administration (NHTSA) — Agency within the U.S. Department of Transportation (DOT) that publishes annual summary reports of fatal highway accidents.

Airbag manufacturers, automobile manufacturers, and the **National Highway Traffic Safety Administration (NHTSA)** do not recommend cutting or restraining any airbag system. If there is an accidental airbag deployment or a failure of a device that a rescuer is using to restrain an airbag system, the rescuer and his or her department will be assumed liable for any injuries that result. Also, the injury from the device may be greater than the injury caused by the airbag itself.

Prying away trim and looking for SRS devices, also known as *peeling and peeking,* before cutting will reduce chances of injury from cutting into an inflator pressure chamber **(Figure 2.19)**. Knowing modern vehicle construction and airbag systems and practicing safe distancing should reduce the risk and severity of injury.

NOTE: Based on test data from controlled crashes and the investigative results from actual collisions, the information in the following sections is the most current available regarding airbags.

Frontal- and side-impact airbags. Driver and front passenger airbags can be single, dual-stage, or dual-depth systems. Single stage airbags deploy at a standard rate every time they deploy. Dual-stage airbags utilize sensors that will detect the rate of speed, impact, and weight of the occupant. It will then use this information to determine if the airbag should deploy using its full capacity or a diminished deployment (dual stage) to reduce the possibility of injuring a lighter, smaller occupant. Dual-depth systems work the same as

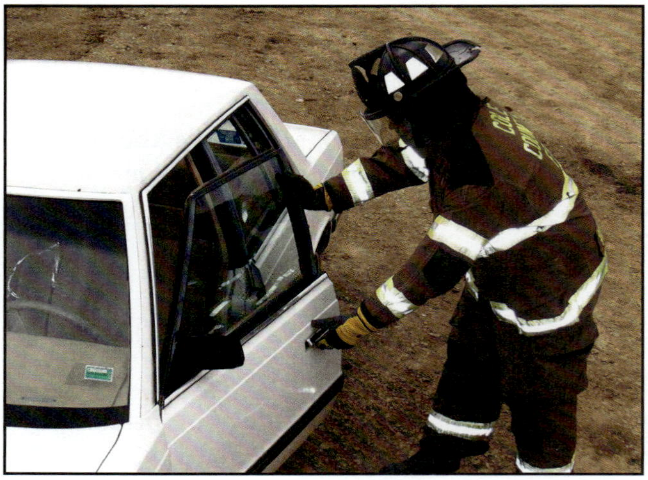

Figure 2.19 Just as in structural entry situations, rescuers should try to open doors normally before resorting to prying them open.

Section B • Chapter 2 – Personal Protective Equipment, Hazards and Hazard Mitigation

dual state systems, but have two airbags. One airbag is the normal size while the other one is smaller and located inside the larger bag. The purpose of the smaller airbag is to provide a shorter reaching bag if the system determines that a shorter reach is necessary. Single stage airbags can deploy only once. Dual-stage and dual-depth airbags are equipped with two inflator devices for each airbag unit that can each be deployed only once (twice for the inflator bag unit).

Front-impact airbags deploy in 0.05 seconds at speeds in excess of 200 mph (320 km/h) with an inflating force of over 3,000 psi (21 000 kPa). Side-impact airbags deploy at even higher rates than front-impact airbags. The sound of airbag deployment is loud, in the range of 165 to 175 decibels for 0.1 second. Hearing damage can result in some cases.

Electrically activated airbags continue to be armed even after the vehicle's battery has been disconnected until the reserve power has drained. The amount of time needed for the reserve power to drain varies from one second to thirty minutes depending upon the make and model of the vehicle involved. The current average time is less than five minutes. Many vehicles have after-market energy capacitors or amps installed for other electronic devices such as entertainment systems, computers, and video games. These may take longer to drain. Some of these devices may discharge or backfeed electricity through the vehicle's electrical system which will keep the airbags energized. Airbag and vehicle construction information can be found on websites, in reference books, and on different mobile applications that are available on the open market. Get the latest information directly from vehicle manufacturers regarding airbag deactivation times for vehicles.

Airbag inflation materials. When a vehicle's collision sensor signals an airbag to inflate, an igniter starts a rapid chemical reaction that generates gas to fill and deploy the airbag. Some systems employ gases such as nitrogen or argon gas, while others may use a variety of energetic propellants. Passenger frontal inflators containing sodium azide reach temperatures in excess of 1,200° F (650° C). Cutting the cushion to the airbag system will allow hot gases to be released unrestrained into the ambient atmosphere of the occupant cabin, and could direct them at a rescuer or victim. Cutting the inflator could result in the two ends becoming projectiles as has been demonstrated in bench tests.

When an airbag deploys, the interior of the vehicle and all those inside may be covered with a dusting of fine white powder. This powder contains sodium azide residue and the talcum powder or cornstarch that was used to lubricate the bag during deployment. In the chemical reaction that deploys an airbag, the sodium azide converts to sodium hydroxide, a highly alkaline powder that becomes ordinary lye when wet. Protect eyes and any open wounds from contamination by this residue or any other foreign material. This powder may cause minor irritation of the throat and eyes in most people if occupants remain in the vehicle for several minutes. The powder may cause asthma attacks.

Rescuers should exercise caution if the sodium azide canister has been opened without the airbag deploying. Sodium azide that has not been converted to sodium hydroxide is extremely toxic. Refer to the latest edition of the Department of Transportation's *Emergency Response Guidebook* for information on handling sodium azide.

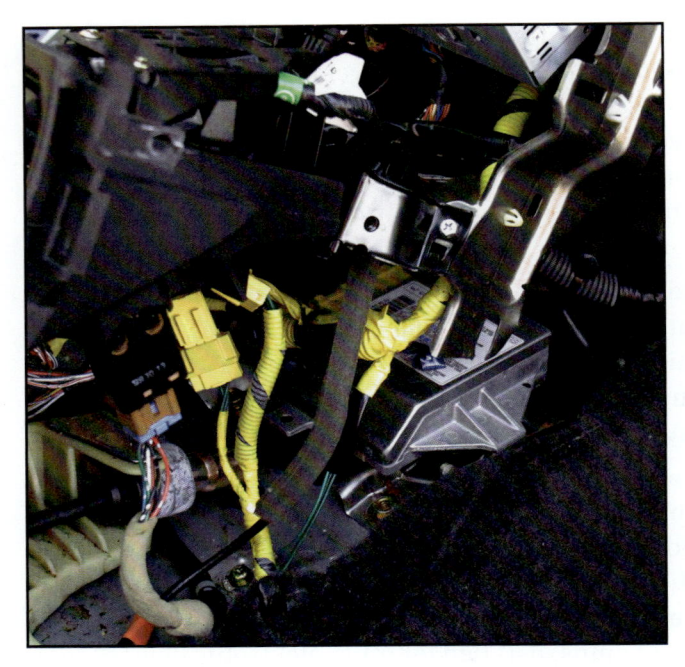

Figure 2.20 Electrical wiring for air bag systems is sometimes identified by yellow tape, insulation, or tags.

Mechanically activated airbags and supplemental restraint systems respond to shock or pressure. If rescue personnel strike the sensor unit or put too much pressure on it during extrication operations, the bag can suddenly deploy. Mechanically impacted side impact bags have sensor units located in various locations throughout the vehicle. Airbags can be activated if an object is between the sensor unit and the inside of the door as the door is closed. Each airbag operates independently, so accidentally activating one of them does not activate both **(Figure 2.20)**.

> **WARNING!**
> Do not cut yellow colored or yellow-tagged cables in an airbag system. Doing so may deploy armed airbags.

Head Protection Systems (HPS). Many vehicles are equipped with HPS. On vehicles equipped with side-impact protection systems (SIPS), HPS deploy from a narrow opening between the headliner and the top of the door frame. Unlike SRS and SIPS that deflate immediately after deployment, HPS airbags may remain rigidly inflated after activation. However, they are easily removed by cutting the nylon straps or deflating the airbag.

HPS typically use compressed gas inflators. Inert gases, such as argon or helium, are used as the propellant and stored in steel or aluminum cylinders at pressures of 2,500 to 4,000 psi (17 500 to 28 000 kPa), or higher. These compressed gas cylinders can be in a variety of locations within the vehicle, usually in the A-post, roof rail, and C-post; however, never assume the location of these cylinders. Before any cut or spread is attempted, the trim and molding must be removed to expose the area (peel and peek).

Rollover Protection Systems

Some manufacturers provide an extendable roll bar system on some of their newer convertible models. This pop-up style roll system activates and extends up behind the passengers when the vehicle exceeds 23 degrees from the horizontal, a lateral angle limit of 62 degrees, or a longitudinal angle of 72 degrees. Additionally, these systems can deploy if the vehicle experiences a 3G acceleration force or becomes weightless for at least 80 milliseconds. These devices pose a significant safety hazard to rescuers when they deploy.

Look for the presence of extendable ROPS and the potential for their deployment if not already deployed. Some ROPS will be behind the front seats of smaller sports cars and some will be found in the rear window deck. Assume a safe position within a vehicle equipped with an active ROPS when stabilizing a victim's cervical spine. To secure these devices, power down the vehicle as soon as possible.

NOTE: Some vehicles are equipped with a ROPS shut off system that may be equipped with a dedicated power source.

Hazards from Suspension Systems

Vehicle suspension systems provide a variety of hazards. Spring assemblies provide one such hazard. Coil springs are under significant tension and, if broken, can fly off the vehicle with great energy. Be aware of these potential projectiles when working near the spring assemblies, especially when pinching the fender or making relief cuts.

Also consider the hazards from a vehicle's shock absorbers and struts. If a rescuer were to cut one of these components during extrication operations, then the component may release pressurized hydraulic fluid. When heated, both shock absorbers and struts can become dangerous and possibly explode.

NOTE: Tires also pose an explosion hazard as they may blow up upon impact or when exposed to fire.

> **WARNING!**
> When exposed to fire, struts and shock absorbers pose an explosion hazard. Upon explosion, pieces of these suspension components become high-speed projectiles.

Some modern passenger vehicles are now equipped with air suspension systems. Air ride suspension systems give the vehicle self-leveling capability. The computer controls the adjustment of the individual air ride components in milliseconds. If the power is not interrupted by isolating the battery, the system may try to auto-level during stabilization and extrication efforts.

Depending upon the load of the vehicle and the condition of the road, the pressure within each bag automatically increases or decreases to maintain the vehicle in a level state. If the pressure in an air suspension bag is lost because of damage to the bag or its associated piping, the truck chassis can drop several inches without warning. For the necessary steps to secure a vehicle's suspension, refer to **Skill Sheet 2-3**.

NOTE: Some medium and heavy trucks are equipped with air-ride cabs. **Skill Sheet 2-4** lists the steps for securing an air-ride cab.

> **WARNING!**
> Never put any part of your body beneath a vehicle with an air suspension system without proper stabilization in place.

Hazards from Seat Adjustment or Positioning Controls

The seats of many newer automobiles may contain sensors or electronic controls. Seat backs often house side-impact airbags. These features can sometimes cause injuries to passengers and rescuers. When performing any action associated with seat removal, displacement, or floor pan removal near these systems, take care to avoid contact with the airbags or any electrical component.

> **WARNING!**
> Do not damage the electronic control modules for the front-impact airbags which are often located in various locations in the vehicle, such as under the front seats. De-energize these systems by disconnecting the battery(ies) prior to working around these systems.

Fire and Explosion Hazards

Fire and explosion hazards are common at vehicle incidents **(Figure 2.21)**. Be aware of these hazards as well as the various flammable and combustible substances and ignition sources. Rescuers should approach all vehicles with caution.

> **CAUTION**
> Approach vehicles from a 45 degree angle. Remain aware of the various fire and explosion hazards that are on/in a vehicle.

Fire Hazards

The primary hazard at most vehicle incidents is the potential for fire from the many different varieties of fuel sources that are used in today's modern vehicles. Fuel spills are common after crashes, and any ignition sources that may ignite those fuels should be recognized and isolated before addressing any other concerns. The following section describes common flammable and combustible substances and ignition sources.

Flammable and Combustible Substances

Many of the fuels used in vehicles are flammable and combustible substances. Responders should be aware of these liquids if they are leaking, as well as if there is a fire or other ignition source nearby. Examples of these flammable and combustible fuels include:

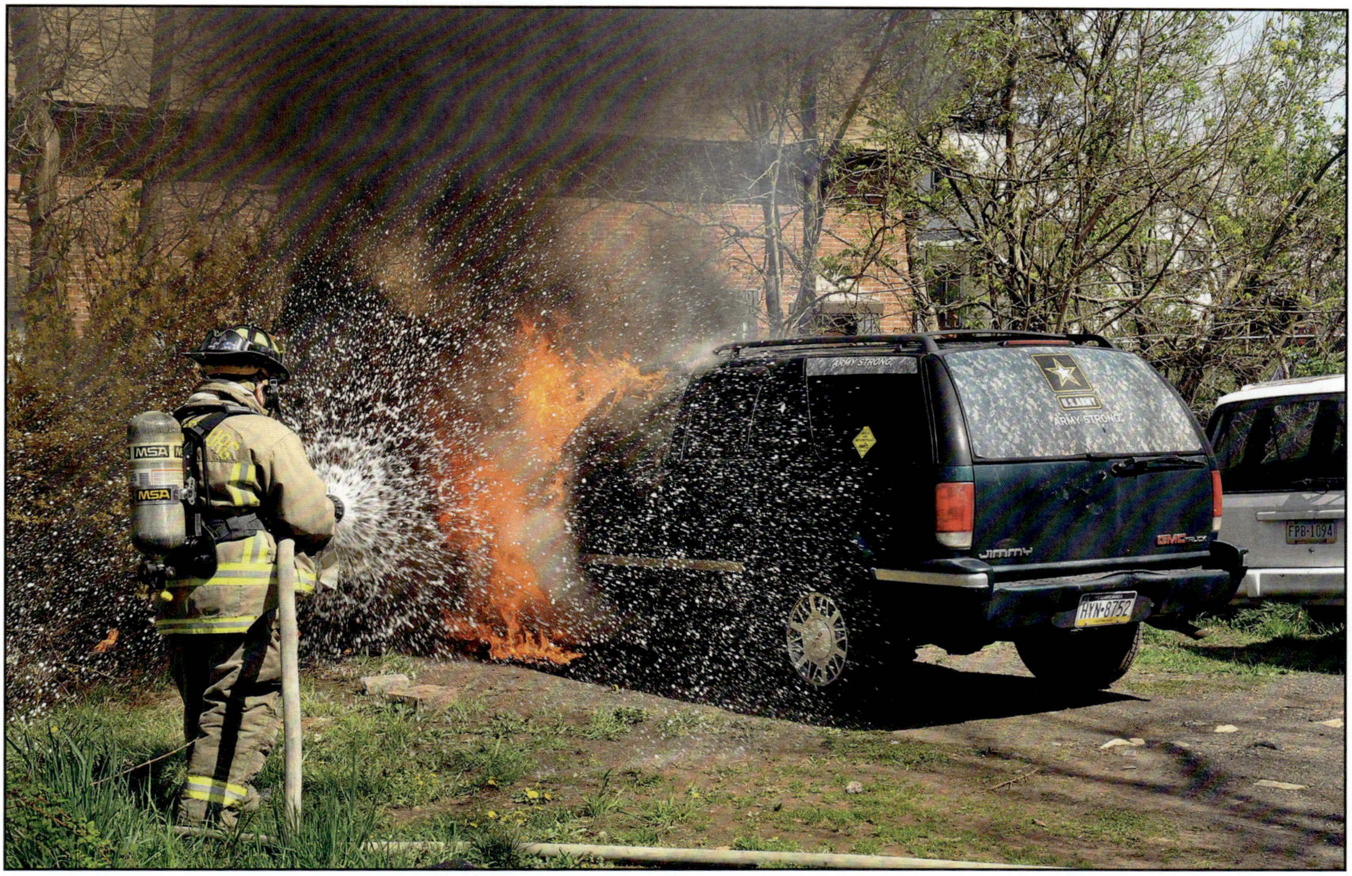

Figure 2.21 A rescuer using foam to put out a vehicle fire. *Courtesy of Bob Esposito.*

- Conventional fuels
- Propane/liquefied petroleum gas
- Natural Gas
- Auxiliary Fuel Cells

If a vehicle fuel tank or other type of tank becomes damaged or ruptured, the flammable and combustible substance inside could catch fire and potentially explode. Alternative fuels such as natural gas and the hydrogen found in auxiliary fuel cells are highly flammable. Rescuers should exercise caution when performing extrication operations around these substances in order to prevent their release and ignition.

Other flammable and combustible substances are present in a vehicle. Substances such as combustible metals (magnesium) and petroleum based materials (plastics) are typically used in interior finishes. When they burn, they create a significant health hazard to rescuers and victims.

Ignition Sources
The scene of a vehicle accident is full of possible ignition sources. Some of these ignition sources include:
- Downed power lines
- Vehicle batteries and electrical systems
- Static energy sources

Emergency responders introduce sources of ignition when they arrive. Portable engines that power hydraulic tools, lighting, and apparatus engines can act as an ignition source. The static energy from hydraulic tool hoses can also act as an ignition source.

Identify and manage these ignition sources. Cordon downed wires, disable battery and electrical systems, avoid pyrotechnic devices, and protect struts from excessive heat or physical damage. In addition, consider appropriate apparatus and tool placement and atmospheric monitoring.

Explosion Hazards

Although explosion hazards are not as prevalent as fire hazards, emergency responders should still be aware of the risk associated with these hazards. The following section discusses two potential explosion hazards: shocks and struts and fuels in a container.

Shocks and Struts

Many automobiles are equipped with energy-absorbing bumper struts. These struts make the vehicle less vulnerable to damage in low-speed collisions. Two struts are mounted between the front bumper and the vehicle frame or chassis, and two more are mounted on the rear of the vehicle. Similar to conventional shock absorbers, these sealed units contain hydraulic fluid and compressed gas.

When these struts are exposed to the heat of fire, they can explode with tremendous force. If both struts attached to a bumper explode simultaneously, they can launch the bumper and/or the struts 100 feet (30 m) or more from the vehicle. If only one strut explodes, the other acts as a pivot point and the bumper can swing in an arc across the front or rear of the vehicle. Anyone in the path of a bumper attached to an exploding strut is in serious jeopardy. Therefore, when the front or rear bumper of an automobile is exposed to heavy flame impingement, all personnel should stay out of the danger zone — directly in front of the bumper and to each side, a distance equal to the length of the bumper.

There are similar hazards associated with gas-filled struts used to support the hoods and hatchbacks on some vehicles. When exposed to the heat of a fire, these struts can explode and launch the components of the strut many yards (meters) from the vehicle at speeds sufficient to cause fatal injuries. Rescuers have been impaled when these struts have exploded and forcibly ejected strut components from the vehicle.

Suspension struts and shock absorbers are components of a vehicle's suspension system. They are designed to operate in a similar manner to the hood and hatch struts and thus present similar hazards.

Boiling Liquid Expanding Vapor Explosion (BLEVE)

Fuels that are stored in closed and pressurized containers have the potential to explode when exposed to fire. This **boiling liquid expanding vapor explosion (BLEVE)** occurs as internal pressure builds within the vessel (**Figure 2.22**). The vessel loses its structural integrity and ruptures, releasing massive amounts of pressure and the flammable contents. Large pieces of shrapnel are projected along with a fireball. This is a life-threatening situation to emergency responders and victims.

> **Boiling Liquid Expanding Vapor Explosion (BLEVE)** — Rapid vaporization of a liquid stored under pressure upon release to the atmosphere following major failure of its containing vessel. Failure is the result of over-pressurization caused by an external heat source, which causes the vessel to explode into two or more pieces when the temperature of the liquid is well above its boiling point at normal atmospheric pressure.

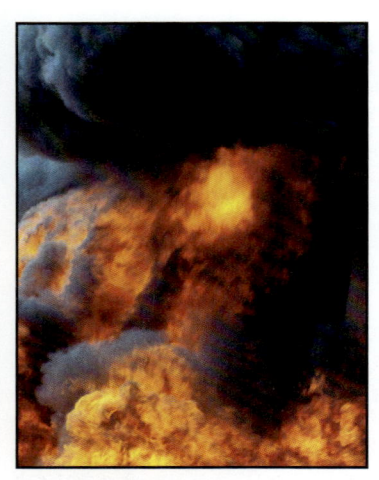

Figure 2.22 BLEVE can occur when a liquid in a container is heated to its boiling point. The expanding vapor inside the tank can increase the pressure to such a degree that the tank will fail catastrophically. Any compressed liquefied gas can BLEVE, so there may be a fireball.

Fire Suppression Operations

Fire suppression operations are common at vehicle incidents. If fire is visible, rescuers should extinguish the fire when appropriate and control the source of fuel. When dealing with special fire hazards such as a **liquefied natural gas (LNG)** or **liquefied compressed gas** tank or a combustible metal fire, personnel must control the hazards appropriately according to agency policies and procedures. For more information on fire fighting techniques, refer to the IFSTA **Essentials of Fire Fighting** manual. The following section discusses establishing fire protection and special precautions associated with alternative energy vehicle fires.

> **Liquefied Natural Gas (LNG)** — Natural gas that has been converted to a liquid form for storage or transport.
>
> **Liquefied Compressed Gas** — Gas that under the charging pressure is partially liquid at 70°F (21°C). *Also known as Liquefied Gas.*

Establishing Fire Protection

Rescuers must practice establishing fire protection to suppress fire hazards and prevent the ignition of fuel vapors. Fire protection can range from someone standing by with a portable fire extinguisher to a crew of firefighters ready with fully charged hoselines **(Figure 2.23)**. Follow local protocols, but it is recommended that at least one, 1 1/2-inch (38 mm) hoseline be charged and ready for use by at least two firefighters equipped with full PPE, including SCBA. **Skill Sheet 2-5** lists the steps for use of extinguishing devices. This section discusses the following procedures for establishing fire protection:

- Fire control support
- Fire control strategies
- Extinguishing devices and agents

Fire Control Support

Upon arrival at the scene, perform a size-up to determine the severity or magnitude of the incident **(Figure 2.24, p. 78)**. Some extrication events may require only one rescue team to perform the extrication and another team

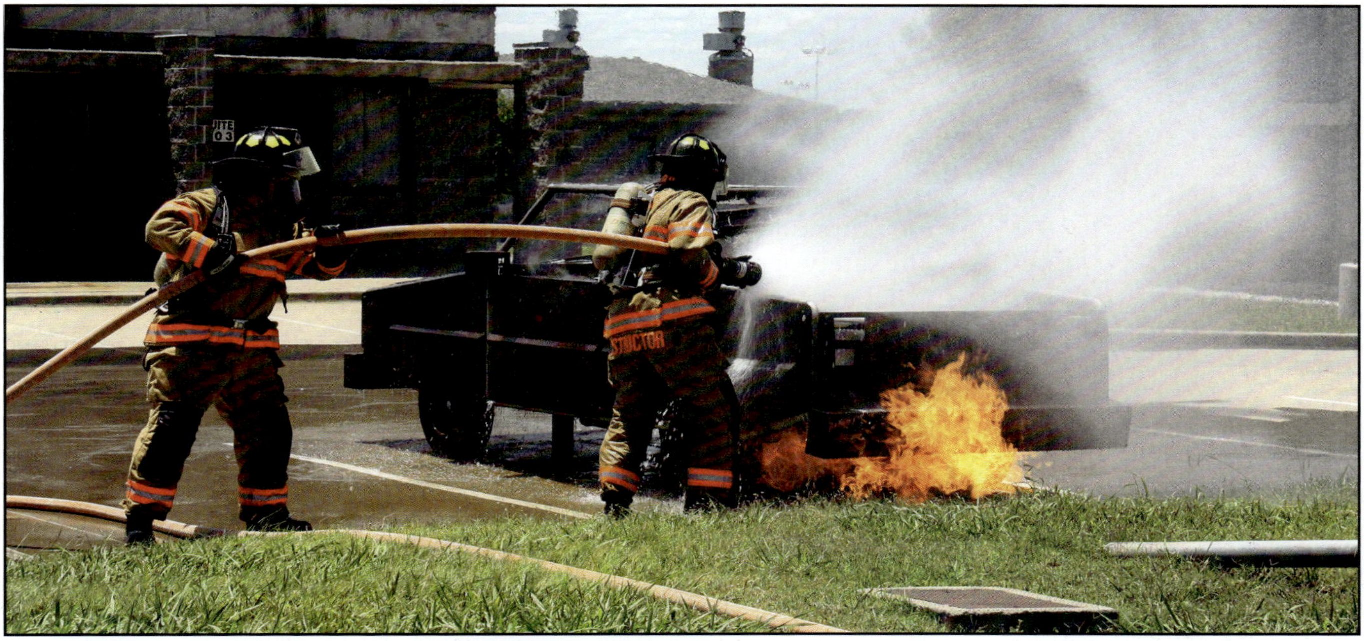

Figure 2.23 Responders practicing fire protection on a training vehicle.

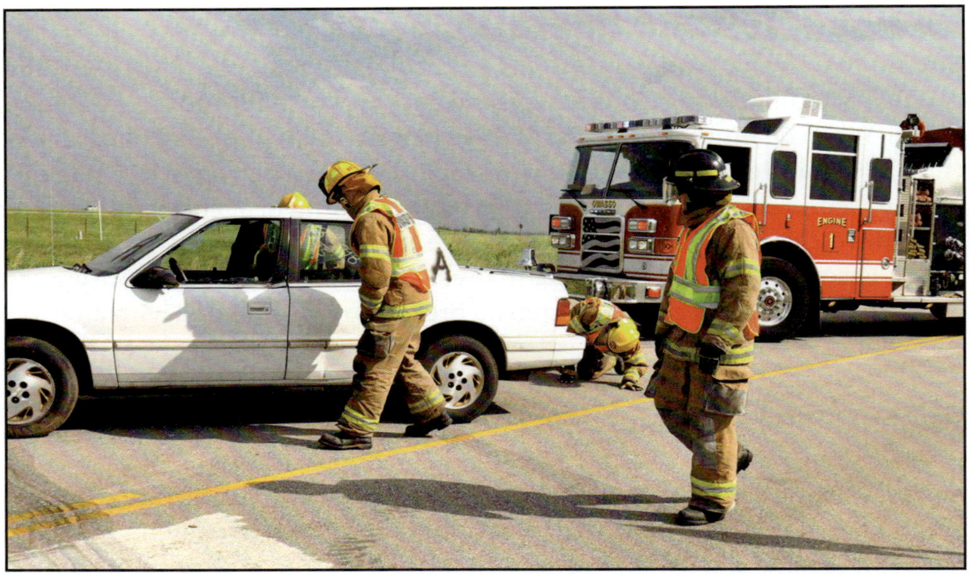

Figure 2.24 Rescuers beginning an assessment of the vehicle at an accident scene. *Courtesy of Sonrise Photography.*

for fire control. Other events will necessitate a host of rescuers to mitigate an extended incident. This includes: the number of vehicles and victims involved, fire potential, or the presence of hazardous materials. All these factors may require calling additional resources in a timely manner to get them on scene for the safety of all involved.

Fire Control Strategies

Fire control strategies should be pre-planned and SOPs should be in place for controlling hazards or fires at vehicle incidents. Every incident is different in terms of needs and types of strategy required; however, the following is an example of strategies and tactics that should be addressed:

- Establish Command
- Perform a 360-degree scene size-up
- Ensure that an apparatus is protecting the scene
- Ensure that personnel and apparatus are positioned uphill and upwind
- Determine hazards and initiate appropriate control measures while ensuring the safety of personnel and bystanders (the appropriate control measures will be determined by the type and amount of fuel that is involved)
- Monitor the atmosphere with a multi-gas detector if hazards are identified
- Advance the appropriate size hoseline (minimum of 1 1/2-inch) with the appropriate type of extinguishing agent (water, foam)
- Advance the hoseline at a 45-degree angle to the involved vehicle, avoiding strut and SRS explosion hazards
- Extinguish the fire using appropriate technique
- Overhaul and investigate

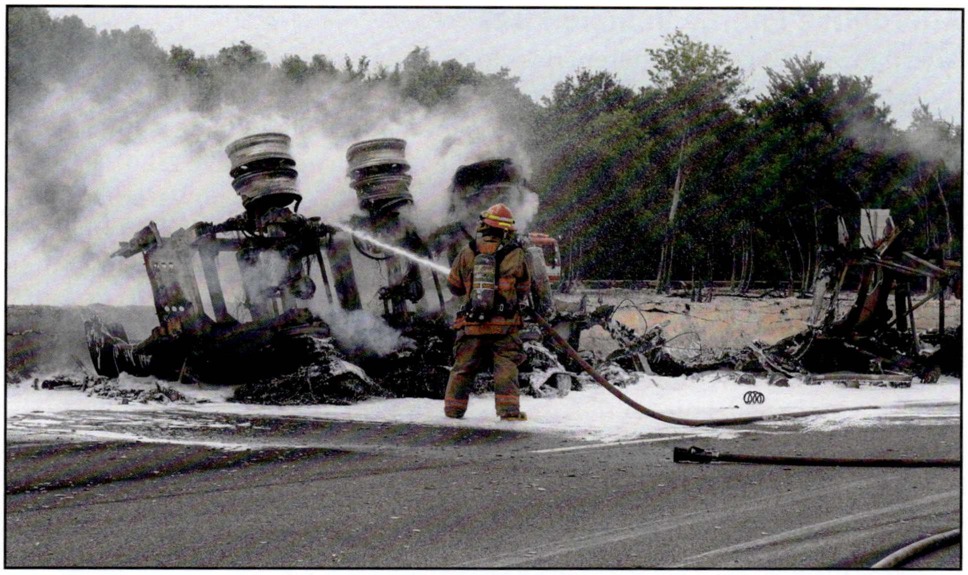

Figure 2.25 An incident fire requiring foam as an extinguishing agent. *Courtesy of Chris Mickal.*

Extinguishing Devices and Agents

A pre-connected hoseline, preferably foam capable, is the best and most appropriate form of fire protection at vehicle incidents. However, it may not always be readily available. In these situations, emergency personnel may use an ABC dry-chemical fire extinguisher. Use good judgment when determining if the fire is small enough to control with a portable fire extinguisher.

Emergency responders may use water for flash protection, controlling passenger compartment fires, or to cool ignition sources. Water may be also be used to suppress vapors from leaking or ruptured natural gas and propane cylinders in an effort to keep the atmosphere below the flammable range. Water is also used to cool these containers if involved in fire. If natural gas or propane cylinders are on fire, do not extinguish them until the containers are cooled and the valves and fuel source can be turned off.

Some vehicle incidents may require the use of foam as an extinguishing agent **(Figure 2.25)**. This foam will most likely be alcohol-resistant aqueous film forming foam (AR-AFFF), which is the extinguishing agent of choice for fires involving all types of hydrocarbon or solvent fuels. These solvents include ethanol and ethanol blended gasoline (E-10, E-85 and E-95), acetone, methanol, ethers, esters, and some acids.

Emergency personnel may also use aqueous film forming foam (AFFF), which rapidly extinguishes hydrocarbon fuel fires and forms an aqueous film on the fuel surface. This film prevents reignition of the fuel once it has been extinguished by the foam. The film has a unique, self-healing capability whereby scars in the film layer caused by falling debris or fire fighting activities are rapidly resealed.

Some vehicles have incorporated combustible metals into their construction. Firefighters should utilize copious amounts of water when dealing with a combustible metal fire.

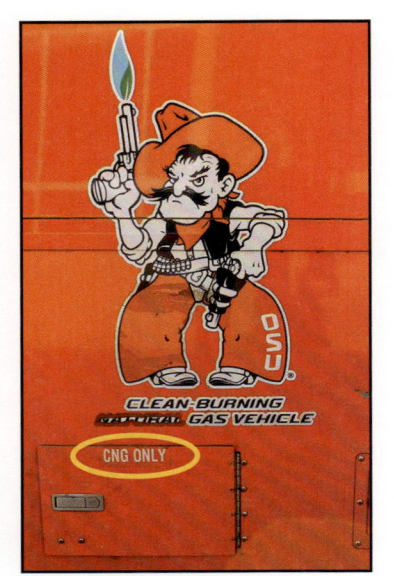

Figure 2.26 An example of a CNG label on a commercial vehicle.

Alternative Energy Vehicle Fires

Alternative fuels create different risks to emergency responders, making it even more important to accurately size-up every motor vehicle incident. Emergency responders should look for identification methods (logos or badges) that would indicate that an alternative fueled vehicle is involved **(Figure 2.26)**. Personnel can no longer assume that all vehicles are built and powered like one another. Dependent upon what portion of the vehicle is involved, for instance the passenger compartment, alternative energy vehicle fires can be fought in much the same manner as conventional fueled vehicle fires. However, when fuel systems are involved, differing extinguishing agents are often used. In some cases, the fire is allowed to burn, while only providing fire protection to nearby exposures. This section discusses fires in the following vehicle fuels:

- Alcohol/gasoline blended
- Natural gas
- Propane
- Hydrogen
- Biodiesel
- Hybrid and Electric

Alcohol/Gasoline Blended Fuel Fires

Alcohol/gasoline blended fuels are water soluble gasoline blends. Alcohol fuels do not react to standard fire fighting extinguishment methods. Water dilutes the alcohol, increasing the amount of liquid, and produces a running fuel fire. These fuels are electrically conductive clear liquids that have a slight gasoline odor. Ethanol and methanol fires burn bright blue and produce little smoke; therefore, they may be hard to see in daylight hours. Using a thermal imager can help locate the fire. Once the fire is located, use AR-AFFF to extinguish the fire.

Natural Gas Fires

In the presence of a natural gas fire, it is recommended to allow the fire to burn off all the fuel as long as no lives or exposures are threatened. When dealing specifically with liquefied natural gas (LNG), personnel should not spray water directly on an LNG fire. When water is applied, it warms the liquid, increasing the amount of vapor production, therefore increasing the intensity of the fire. Control an LNG fire by using Purple-K dry-chemical agent or high expansion foam on the surface of the fire.

CAUTION
Rescuers should exercise caution when performing extrication operations around these substances in order to prevent their release and ignition.

With **compressed natural gas (CNG)**, leaks and fires can occur during fueling, maintenance, and repair or as a result of traffic collisions. Use water or foam to extinguish a CNG fire. Use a fog stream to disperse vapor clouds. Avoid contact with any high-velocity jets of escaping gas.

> **Compressed Natural Gas** — Natural gas that is stored in a vessel at pressures of 2,400 to 3,600 psi (16 800 kPa to 25 200 kPa).

Propane Fuel Fires

Propane is the third most common vehicle fuel type after gasoline and diesel. LPG contains about 90 percent propane, with small concentrations of ethane, butane, propylene, and other gases. LPG expands rapidly when heated. Because it is stored in pressurized tanks, this rapid expansion creates the condition for a BLEVE when exposed to heat. Fires may be allowed to self-extinguish, but if extinguishment is necessary, use foam or water. Direct streams at the top of the tank to provide adequate cooling.

Hydrogen Fuel Fires

Hydrogen is colorless, odorless, non-toxic, and energy efficient. It has a self-ignition temperature of 550° F (290° C) with a flammability range between 4-75 percent. As with alcohol-blended fuels, the flame may be invisible during the day, so use a thermal imaging device to see the flame. Do not extinguish hydrogen fires in vehicles. Instead, protect any exposures and allow the fuel to burn off.

Biodiesel Fuel Fires

Biodiesel is a yellow liquid with an odor of cooking oil that is non-toxic, biodegradable, and sulfur free. It is slightly lighter than water. Biodiesel can be used in any vehicle designed to use diesel. Combustion of biodiesel fuel produces carbon monoxide and carbon dioxide along with thick smoke. Use dry chemical, foam, carbon dioxide, or water spray (fog) for extinguishment.

Hybrid and Electric Vehicle Fires

Hybrid electric and all electric vehicle fires are fought much the same as conventionally fueled vehicle fires. Most of the same construction components are utilized; therefore, the same agents are used for extinguishment. Hybrid vehicles have internal combustion engines that use battery power and also use gasoline, diesel, biodiesel, or natural gas to propel the engines. Electric vehicles operate solely on electricity stored in batteries. Unless the vehicle is plugged in and charging, use copious amounts of water and/or foam on electric vehicle fires.

Although many of the same tactics are used to fight fires in these types of vehicles, one key difference in hybrid and electric vehicle fires is the extinguishing agent to be used if the fire is confined to the battery packs or battery system. The following are the recommended extinguishing agents for specific battery types:

- Lead-acid batteries — Use carbon dioxide, foam, or dry chemical.
- Nickel metal hydride batteries — Use a Class D extinguisher (Metal-X or similar).
- Lithium-ion batteries — Use dry sand, sodium chloride powder, graphite powder, or copper powder.

Hazardous Material — Any substance or material that poses an unreasonable risk to health, safety, property, and/or the environment if it is not properly controlled during handling, storage, manufacture, processing, packaging, use, disposal, or transportation.

Hazardous Materials

One of the most important parts of a scene size-up of a vehicle incident is identifying any potential **hazardous materials (haz mat)** threats involved. Hazardous materials can be found in any accident, but should be a major concern in accidents involving commercial transportation such as medium and heavy trucks. Responders should know agency policies and procedures regarding hazardous materials. This section discusses the types of hazardous materials to look out for in:

- Passenger vehicle incidents
- Medium and heavy truck incidents
- Bus incidents

Passenger Vehicle Haz Mat Incidents

Among the most common hazardous materials found at passenger vehicle incident are the fuels that propel the vehicles. If a large amount of these fuels is released or spilled, specialty teams may need to be summoned to the scene to properly manage the hazard. In addition, hazardous materials may be stored in the trunk or transportation compartment of SUVs and pickup trucks **(Figure 2.27 a and b)**. Common items include pool chemicals, portable propane tanks, gas cans, and even clandestine drug labs.

Medium and Heavy Truck Haz Mat Incidents

Commercial medium and heavy trucks transport a tremendous amount of hazardous materials. Look out for large amounts of fuel and identify the cargo when sizing up incidents involving commercial medium and heavy trucks. Before approaching a crashed medium or heavy truck, stop a safe distance away and use binoculars to look for hazardous materials labels or placards.

Follow agency protocols for the material indicated on any labels or placards **(Figure 2.28)**. These protocols will usually follow the recommendations contained in the latest edition of the Department of Transportation's *Emergency Response Guidebook*. Rescuers should be aware that the absence of labels or placards does not indicate the absence of hazardous materials **(Figure 2.29, p. 84)**.

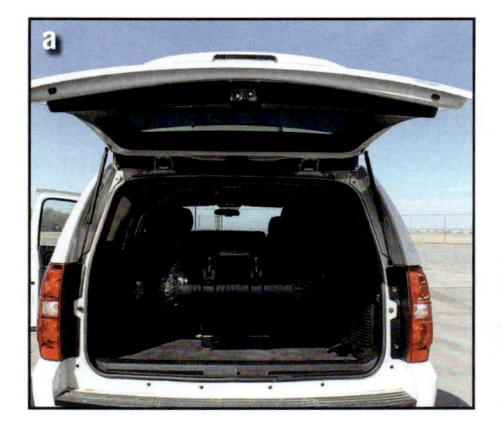

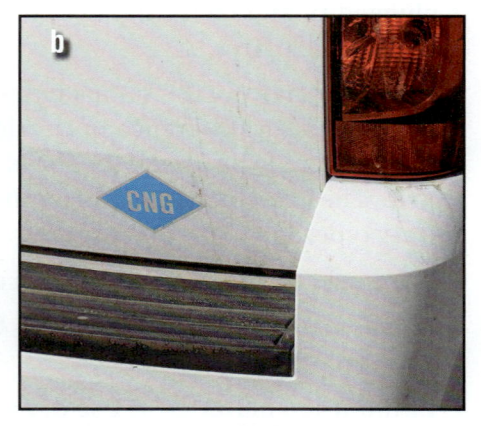

Figure 2.27 a. An SUV that stores alternative fuel in the trunk. **b.** A CNG logo on a passenger vehicle.

DOT Placard Parts

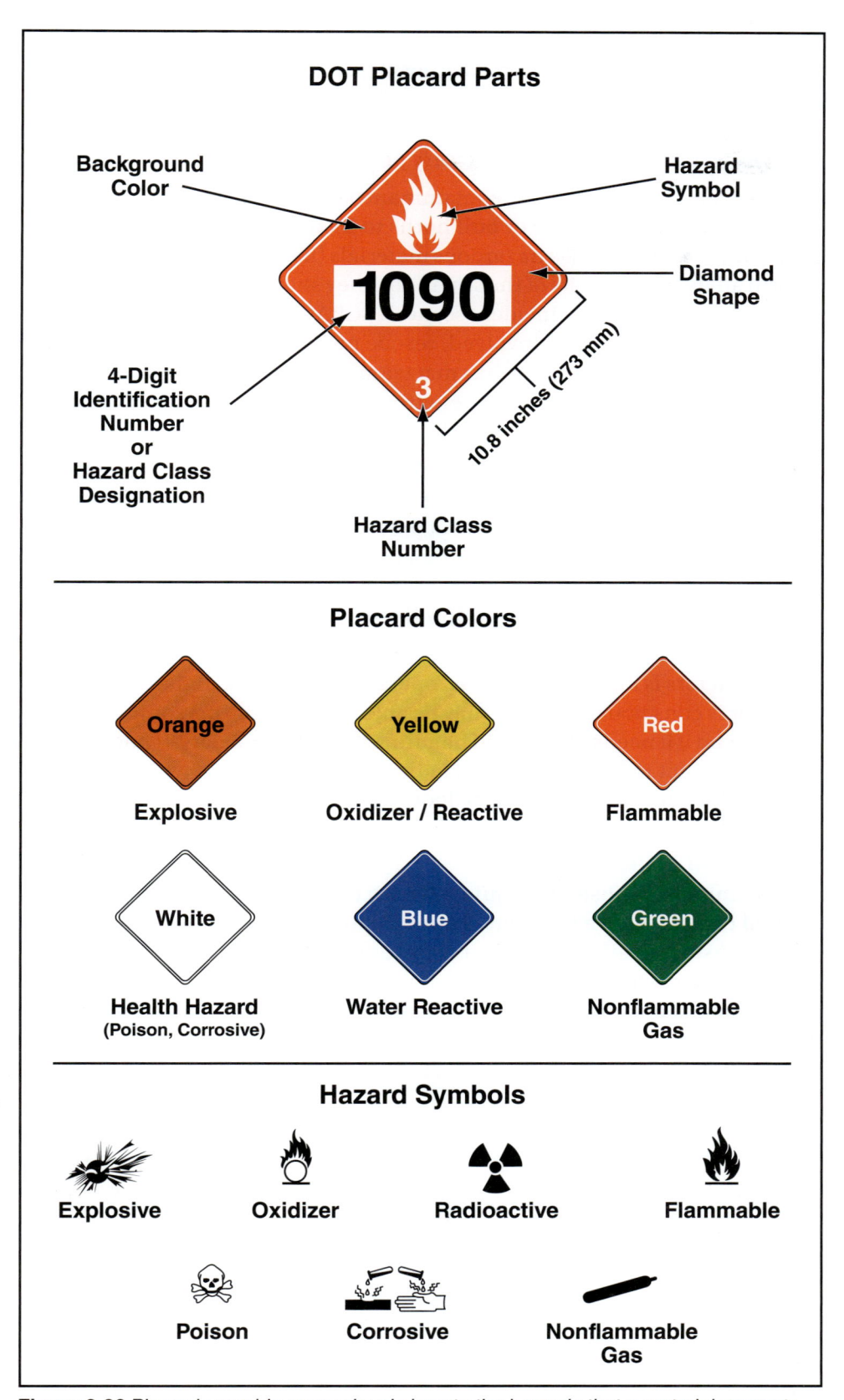

- Background Color
- Hazard Symbol
- Diamond Shape
- 4-Digit Identification Number or Hazard Class Designation
- Hazard Class Number
- 10.8 inches (273 mm)

(Example placard: 1090, Class 3)

Placard Colors

Color	Hazard
Orange	Explosive
Yellow	Oxidizer / Reactive
Red	Flammable
White	Health Hazard (Poison, Corrosive)
Blue	Water Reactive
Green	Nonflammable Gas

Hazard Symbols

- Explosive
- Oxidizer
- Radioactive
- Flammable
- Poison
- Corrosive
- Nonflammable Gas

Figure 2.28 Placards provide many visual clues to the hazards that a material presents.

Pedestrians fleeing the scene may be the first indication of the need to stop and assess the scene before approaching. If people are running from the scene with a look of panic on their faces or if pedestrians have collapsed in the area of the crashed vehicles, do not jeopardize rescue personnel by approaching the scene without taking the necessary precautions.

If it appears that an airborne contaminant has been released in the collision, use public address systems or bull horns to instruct those near the scene to vacate immediately. Call a hazardous materials (haz mat) response team, and inform all incoming units of the situation. They should be instructed to stage uphill and upwind of the incident scene. If SCBA and full PPE will protect the wearer from the chemical involved, rescue personnel should cordon off the scene and deny entry until the haz mat team arrives. If this level of protective equipment will not protect rescuers from the chemical involved, rescuers should stay out of the area.

Even if the cargo is labeled as hazardous, it may be contained and represent no immediate threat. Cordon off the cargo area until a hazardous materials specialist can assess the situation, but proceed with the extrication operation. Keep all nonessential personnel and spectators upwind of the scene in case of a subsequent release. Close the adjacent highway to all but emergency vehicle traffic. Stage emergency vehicles uphill and upwind.

When responding to a collision involving trucks, one of the most critical size-up factors is locating the driver/operator of the truck. If the truck driver/operator is conscious, he or she may be able to tell rescue personnel what the cargo is and if it needs any special handling to maintain safety. If not, rescuers should attempt to locate the bill of lading (cargo manifest), which is usually carried in a pocket on the driver's door.

Bus Haz Mat Incidents

Most commercial buses are equipped with overhead storage compartments located directly above the seats. These compartments are designed for passengers to stow small articles of carry-on luggage. Commercial buses also have large luggage compartments located below the seating area of the bus that open from the outside. While these compartments are primarily designed to carry large pieces of luggage, in many cases motor coaches also haul common freight. Regulations control the materials transported, however, regulations and laws are not always followed.

Chapter Review

1. What kinds of personal protective equipment should rescuers always wear at vehicle incidents?
2. What hazards related to conventional fuels, alternative fuels, and hybrid electric systems should rescuers be aware of?
3. How should hazards from conventional electrical systems be mitigated?
4. Which materials used to construct vehicle components can create hazards for rescuers and victims?
5. What are the "ABCs" of dealing with supplemental restraint systems during extrication operations?
6. What hazards do seat belt pretensioners pose to rescuers and victims?
7. What are the suggested minimum safety zone distances when working around airbags?
8. How can rescuers mitigate hazards related to passenger air bags?
9. What are three hazards related to vehicle suspension systems?
10. What substances could be a fire hazard or potential ignition source at a vehicle incident?
11. What potential explosion hazards may be present at a vehicle incident?
12. What should rescuers do in order to ensure that the scene is appropriately protected from fire and explosion hazards?
13. List the method(s) of extinguishment for vehicle fires involving each of the following alternative fuels: alcohol/gasoline blended fuel, natural gas, propane, hydrogen, biodiesel, hybrid or electric.
14. How should rescuers manage a vehicle incident when hazardous materials could be present?

Discussion Questions

1. You respond to a collision incident involving a biomedical waste truck and a transit bus. What types of hazards are likely to be present?
2. How common are hybrid/electric vehicles in your jurisdiction?

SKILL SHEETS

2-1
Access a vehicle to secure and disable hazards.

REMINDER: Not all agencies advocate the following practices. The following skill sheets present a snapshot of various procedures utilized during vehicle incident operations. Always follow manufacturer's recommendations and local SOPs. Rescuers must wear full PPE including hand, eye, and respiratory protection. It is recommended that rescuers maintain communication with victims and make them aware of pertinent rescue information.

WARNING: Rescuers must ensure that the vehicle is properly stabilized and the scene is safe.

CAUTION: Rescuers must take necessary precautions to protect themselves and victims from hazards including, but not limited to: glass fragments and dust, jagged metal, SRS gas cylinders, undeployed airbags, and fire hazards.

Step 1: Access the interior of the vehicle.

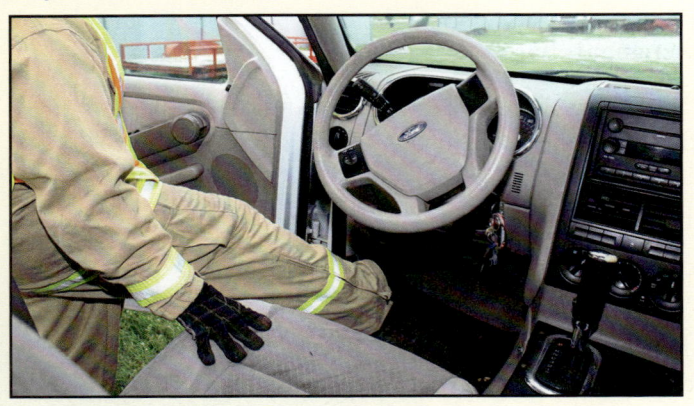

Step 2: Engage the emergency brake.
Step 3: Place the vehicle in park if it has an automatic transmission or into a low gear if it has a manual transmission.
Step 4: Turn the vehicle OFF using the key.
Step 5: Remove the key from the ignition.
NOTE: If a vehicle uses a smart key, the key must be placed out of range. Alternative fuel vehicles may have different power-down procedures than vehicles with internal combustion engines.
Step 6: Verify that the engine is not running.
Step 7: Identify and disable any secondary power sources, such as DVD players and laptops.

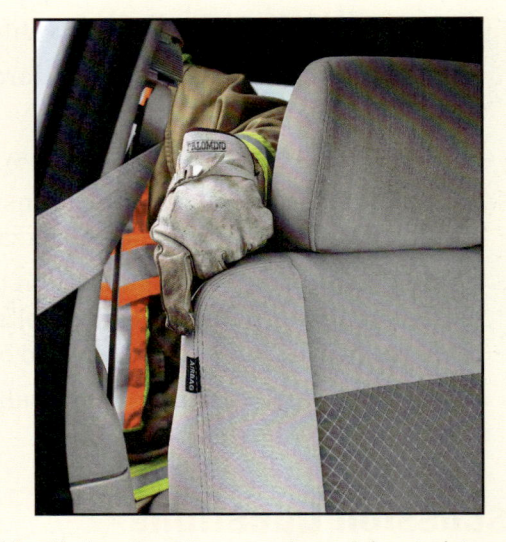

Step 8: Identify location of any supplemental restraint systems (airbags).
Step 9: Once the victim is properly supported, cut or release the seatbelt from the victim.

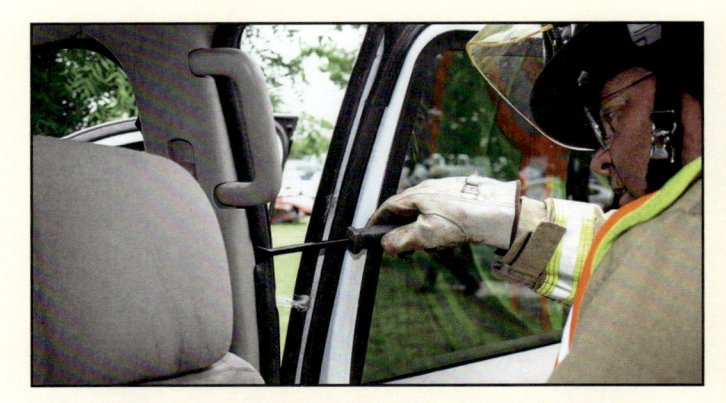

Step 10: If portions of the vehicle must be cut to access the victim, fully expose the area to be cut to identify any hazards.

Section B • Chapter 2 – Personal Protective Equipment, Hazards and Hazard Mitigation

2-2
Disconnect or disable a battery.

WARNING: Rescuers must ensure that the vehicle is properly stabilized and the scene is safe.

CAUTION: Rescuers must take necessary precautions to protect themselves and victims from hazards including, but not limited to: glass fragments and dust, jagged metal, SRS gas cylinders, undeployed airbags, and fire hazards.

Step 1: Locate and access the battery.

CAUTION: Disable the negative side first to reduce the chance of a short circuit while cutting the positive cable.

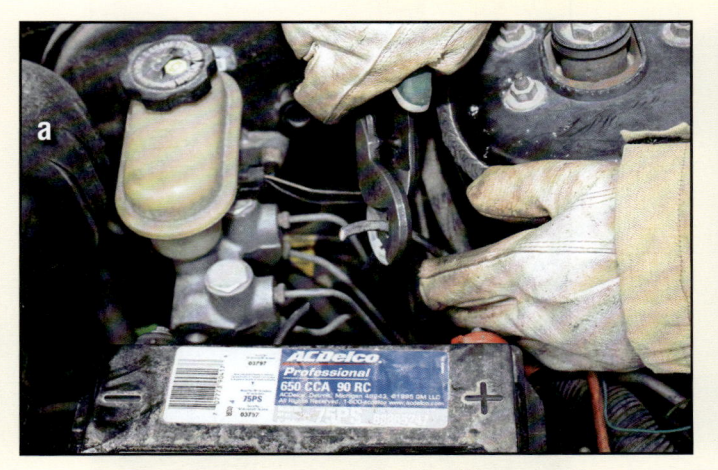

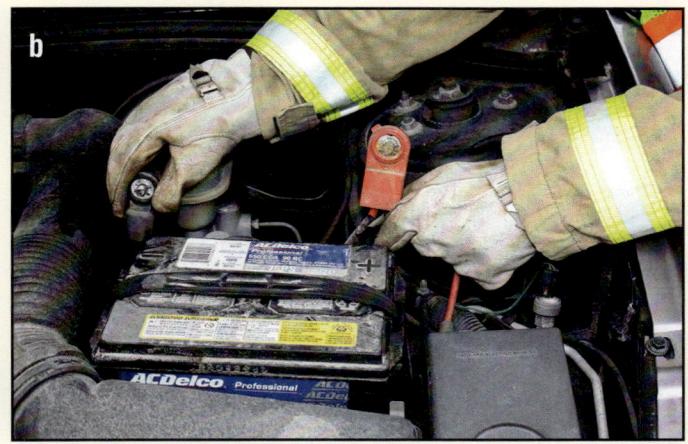

Step 2: Disconnect the power from the vehicle at the battery in accordance with local SOPs, such as by cutting the cable (method a) or by diconnecting the cables (method b)

Step 3: Verify power shutdown.

Section B • Chapter 2 – Personal Protective Equipment, Hazards and Hazard Mitigation

SKILL SHEETS

2-3
Secure suspension.

WARNING: Rescuers must ensure that the vehicle is properly stabilized and the scene is safe.

CAUTION: Rescuers must take necessary precautions to protect themselves and victims from hazards including, but not limited to: glass fragments and dust, jagged metal, SRS gas cylinders, undeployed airbags, and fire hazards.

Step 1: Identify support locations on the vehicle.
Step 2: Verify that the surface under these support locations will support the weight of the vehicle and equipment. If more support is needed, use alternative actions to provide base support (ratchet straps or pickets driven into the ground).
Step 3: Identify the location of the suspension system to be secured.

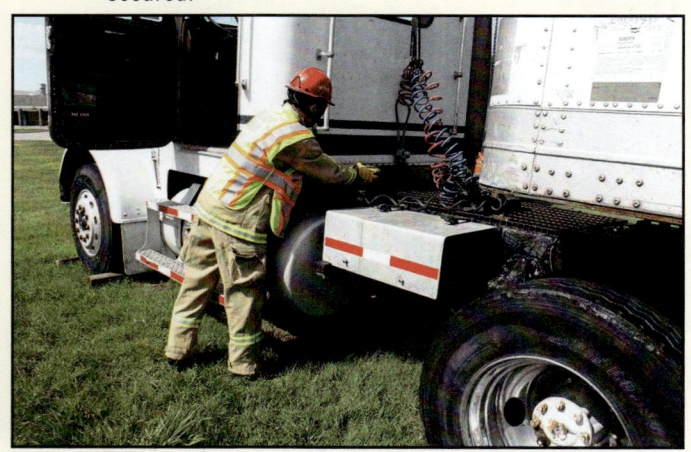

Step 4: Insert cribbing to capture the suspension between the vehicle frame and top of the rear spring.

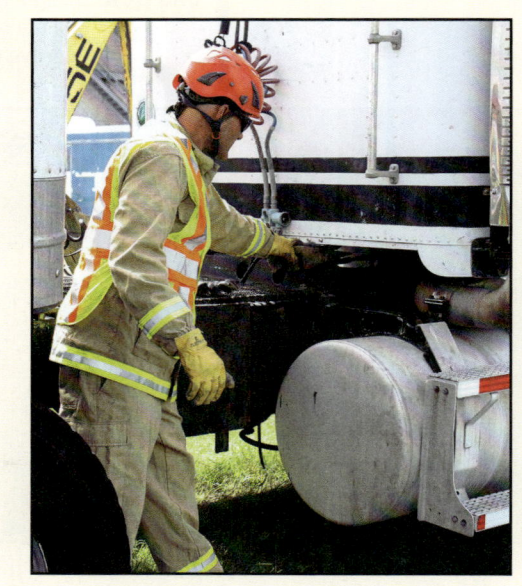

Step 5: Insert wedges between the frame and spring).

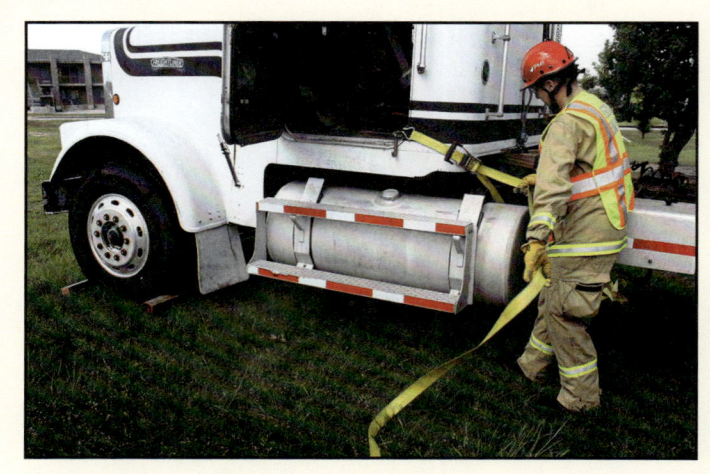

Step 6: Secure suspension to the frame.
Step 7: Inspect and maintain the integrity of the cribbing and wedges.

88 Section B • Chapter 2 – Personal Protective Equipment, Hazards and Hazard Mitigation

2-4 Secure an air-ride cab.

SKILL SHEETS

WARNING: Rescuers must ensure that the vehicle is properly stabilized and the scene is safe.

CAUTION: Rescuers must take necessary precautions to protect themselves and victims from hazards including, but not limited to: glass fragments and dust, jagged metal, SRS gas cylinders, undeployed airbags, and fire hazards.

Step 1: Identify support locations on the vehicle.

Step 2: Verify that the surface under these support locations will support the weight of the vehicle and equipment. If more support is needed, use alternative actions to provide base support (ratchet straps or pickets driven into the ground, etc.).

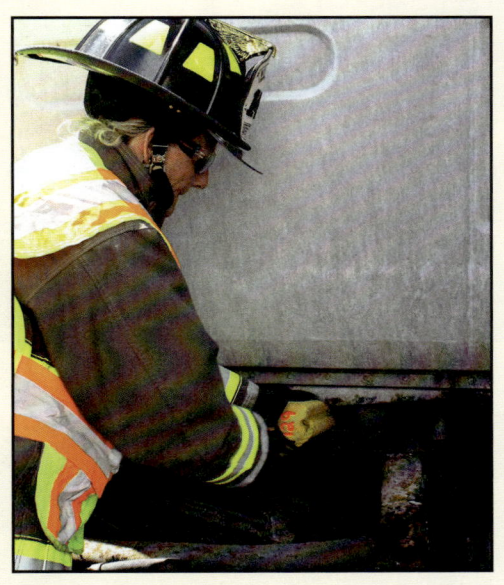

Step 3: Insert cribbing or wedges between the cab and frame rail.

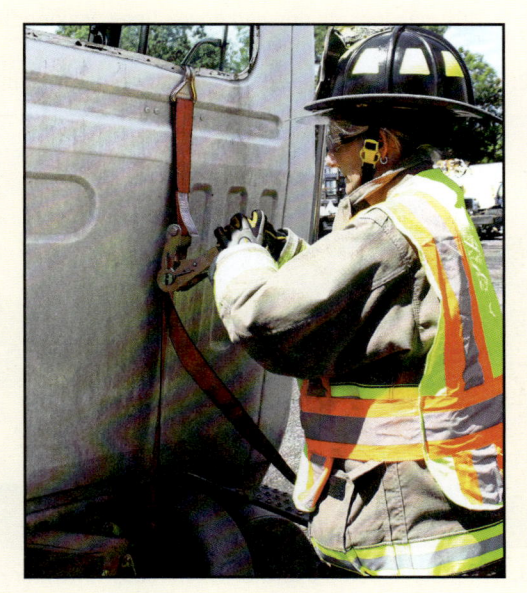

Step 4: Secure the cab to the frame.

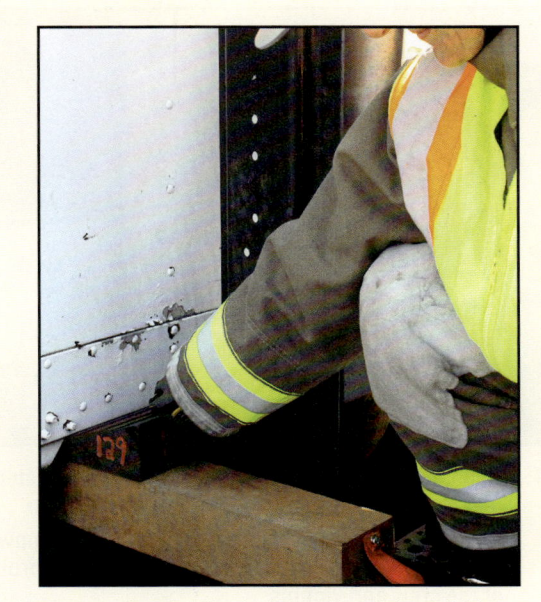

Step 5: Inspect and maintain the integrity of the cribbing and wedges.

Section B • Chapter 2 – Personal Protective Equipment, Hazards and Hazard Mitigation   89

SKILL SHEETS

2-5
Establish fire protection at a vehicle incident.

WARNING: Rescuers must ensure that the vehicle is properly stabilized and the scene is safe.

CAUTION: Rescuers must take necessary precautions to protect themselves and victims from hazards including, but not limited to: glass fragments and dust, jagged metal, SRS gas cylinders, undeployed airbags, and fire hazards.

Hoseline

Step 1: Verbalize the sequence for protection of the scene.
NOTE: This may include downed power lines, leaking fluids from the vehicle, etc.
Step 2: Deploy and advance an uncharged attack hoseline.

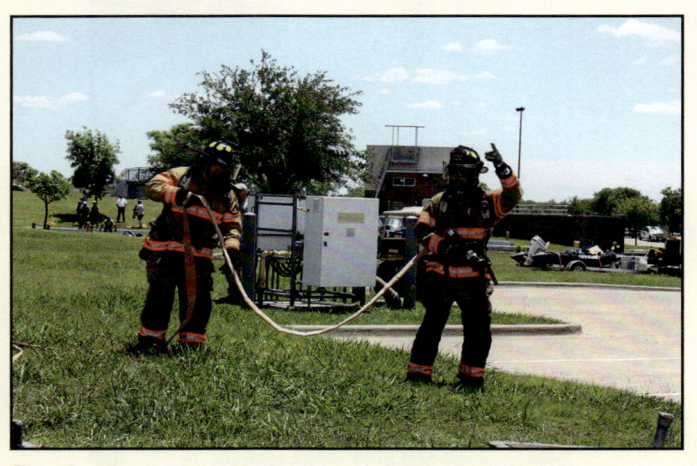

Step 3: Signal the pump operator when ready for water.

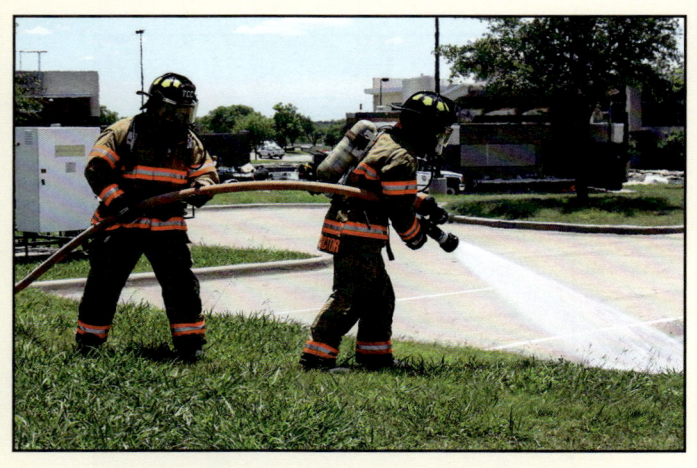

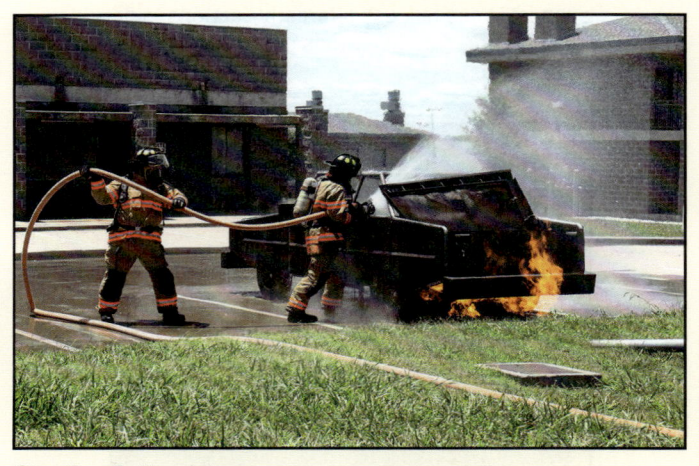

Step 6: Extinguish passenger compartment fire.

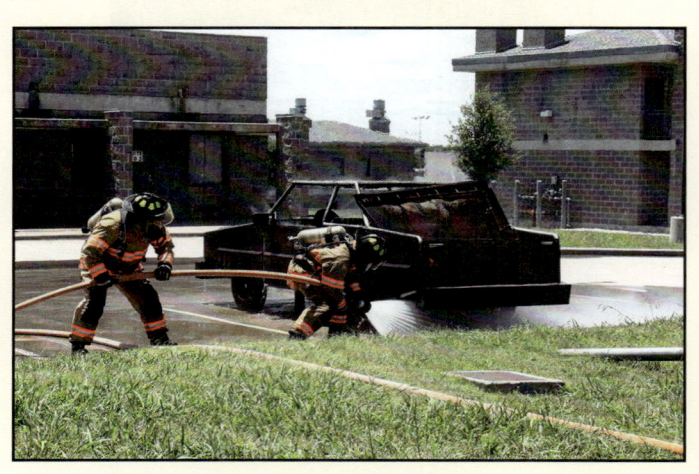

Step 7: Extinguish any other remaining fire.

Step 4: Open the nozzle to purge air and ensure that water has reached the nozzle.
NOTE: Approach the vehicle incident from uphill and upwind at a 45 degree angle whenever possible for best protection of the crew and victims.
Step 5: Extinguish any line of approach fires that would hinder advancement.

2-5
Establish fire protection at a vehicle incident.

Fire Extinguisher

Step 1: Verbalize the sequence for protection of the scene.

NOTE: This may include downed power lines, leaking fluids from the vehicle, etc.

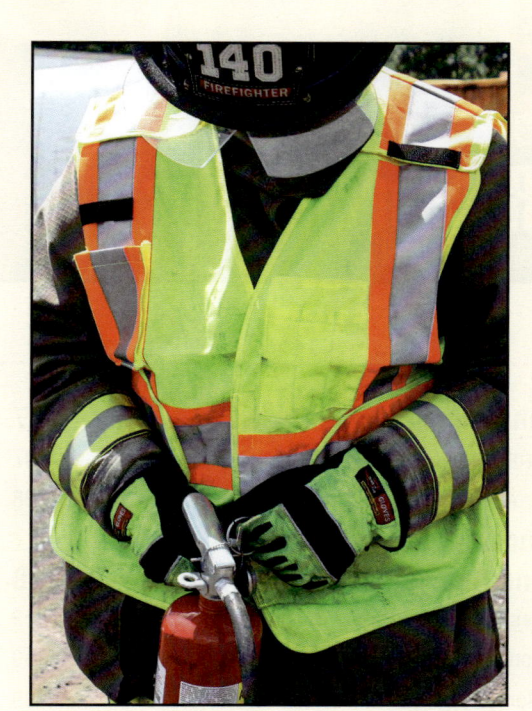

Step 2: Pull the pin at the top of the fire extinguisher to break the inspection band.

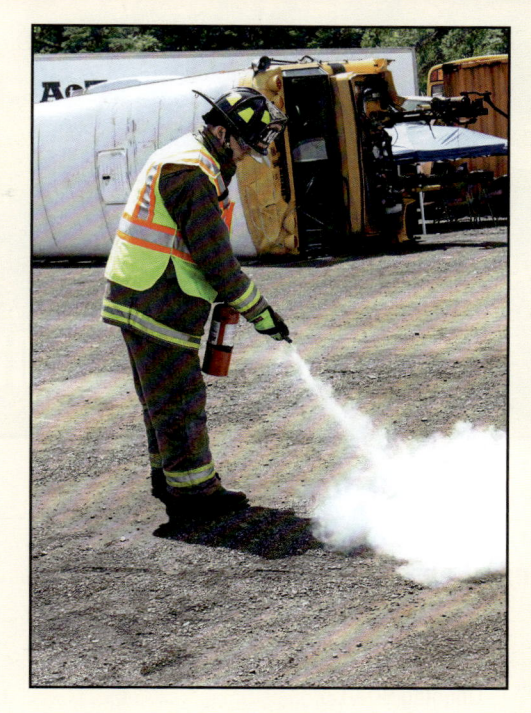

Step 3: Test the fire extinguisher to ensure it is in working order by briefly depressing the handle.

NOTE: Approach the vehicle incident from uphill and upwind at a 45 degree angle whenever possible for best protection of the crew and victims.

Step 4: Position the extinguisher nozzle to protect the incident.

Step 5: Extinguish any line of approach fires that would hinder advancement.

Step 6: Extinguish passenger compartment fire.

Step 7: Extinguish any other remaining fire.

Incident Management Responsibilities

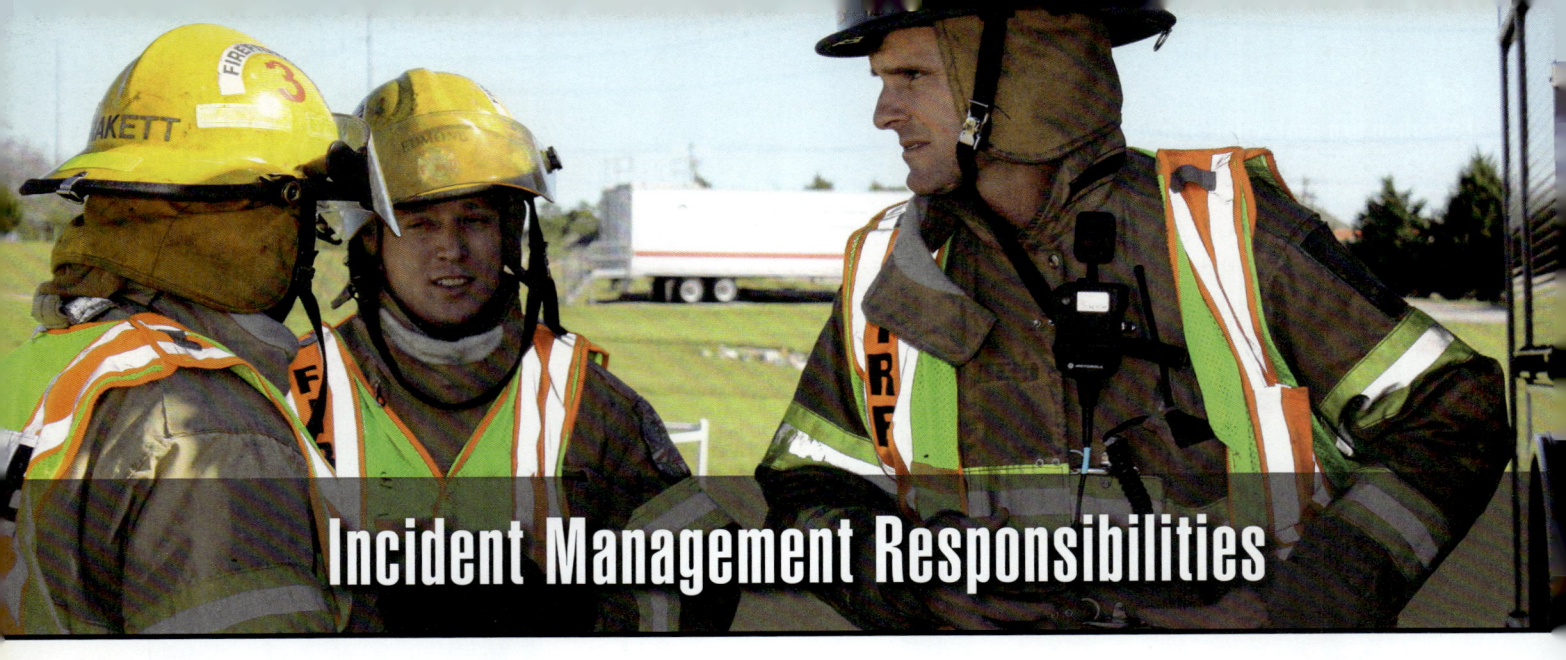

Chapter Contents

Initial and Ongoing Scene Size-up 95
    Initial Size-up 95
    Scene Assessment 96
    Ongoing Size-Up 99

Incident Command System 99
    ICS Standards of Performance 99
    Command and Control 100
    Incident Operation Groups 100
    Operating within the Incident Command System 103
    NIMS-ICS IAP Planning Process 104
    Situation Status Information 106
    Resource Status Information 106

Emergency Escape and Evacuation 106
    Escape and Evacuation Routes 107
    Emergency Evacuation and Safety Signals 107

Terminating an Incident 107
    Protecting Bystanders/Public 107
    Protecting Rescuers 108

Postincident Responsibilities and Analysis 108
    Restoring Operational Readiness 109
    Conducting an After Action Review (AAR) 109
    Monitoring Critical Incident Stress (CIS) 109
    Completing Documentation 110

Chapter Review 110
Skill Sheets 111

chapter 3

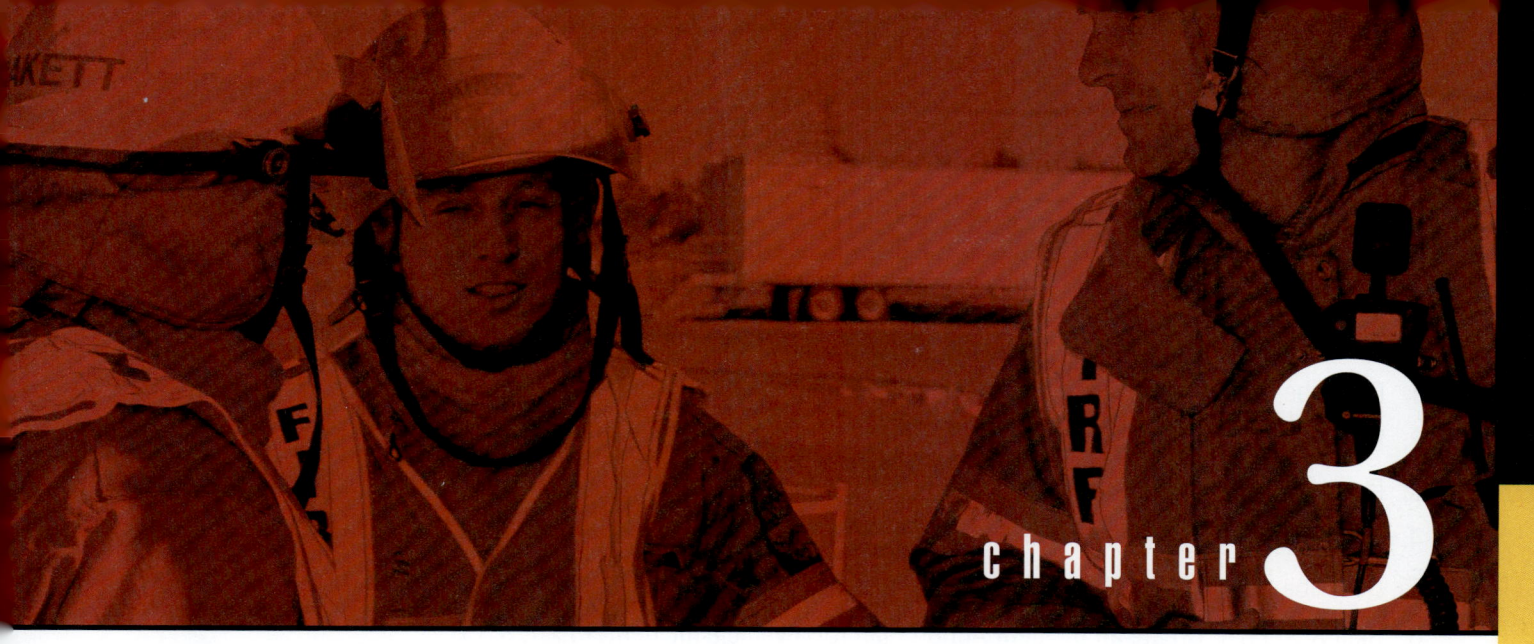

Key Terms

After Action Reviews (AAR)	109
Critical Incident Stress (CIS)	109
Extrication Group	101
Incident Command Post (ICP)	101
Incident Command System (ICS)	99
Operations Section Chief	100
Size-Up	95
Unified Command (UC)	104

JPRs addressed in this chapter

This chapter provides information that addresses the following job performance requirements of NFPA 1006, *Standard for Technical Rescuer Professional Qualifications (2017)*.

- 8.2.1
- 8.2.5
- 8.2.9
- 8.3.1
- 8.3.4

Incident Management Responsibilities

Learning Objectives

1. Describe the process of conducting initial size-up and ongoing size-up at a vehicle incident. [8.2.1, 8.3.1]
2. Explain the use of the Incident Command System (ICS) at vehicle incidents. [8.2.1, 8.3.1]
3. Describe emergency escape and evacuation considerations at a vehicle incident. [8.2.5, 8.3.4]
4. Identify the objectives of terminating a vehicle incident. [8.2.9]
5. Describe postincident responsibilities of emergency responders. [8.2.9]
6. Skill Sheet 3-1: Create an Incident Action Plan for a vehicle incident. [8.2.1, 8.3.1]
7. Skill Sheet 3-2: Terminate a vehicle incident. [8.2.9]

Chapter 3
Incident Management Responsibilities

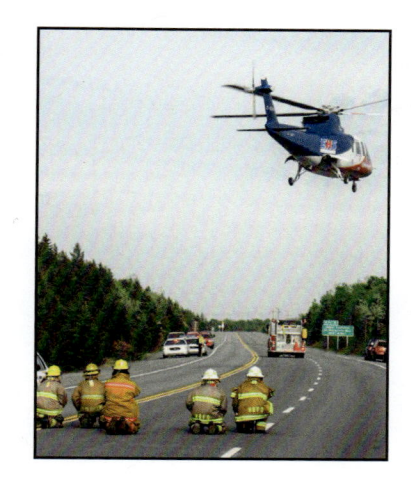

Operations and Technician level rescuers are responsible for not only participating in extrications, but for managing the scene as well. This chapter describes the responsibilities that these responders have at a scene. Operations and Technician level rescuers may also be assigned as crew leaders or be assigned direct actions to extricate victims. Chapter 1 of this manual provided a brief overview of vehicle incident safety. This chapter provides a more in-depth view of incident management as it pertains to Operations and Technician level rescuers.

Initial and Ongoing Scene Size-up

Before the first-due extrication team arrives at the scene, the officer in charge and every other member of the crew should **size-up** the incident to which they are responding. Before arrival, the crew(s) can analyze the information provided during the initial dispatch, as well as any available preincident planning information. In some cases, there may be a fully developed operational plan based on a preincident plan for the officer to reference. This plan may be available to the officer in hard copy or electronically. In any case, the more information that the responding rescue crew has available, the better prepared it will be to make the initial decisions upon arrival at the incident scene.

Size-Up — Ongoing evaluation of influential factors at the scene of an incident.

The sections that follow describe the process of completing a size-up of an incident. Responders need to be proactive in ordering resources based on the time/distance potential so that needed equipment arrives in a timely manner. For the purposes of this manual, the steps are drawn out and described in detail. At real incidents, experience and training make this process quick and decisive in most cases.

Initial Size-Up

Awareness level rescuers may complete the initial size-up at a scene. Awareness level rescuers should be able to identify hazards at the scene such as traffic, environmental, and incident related hazards. For a review of these details, please see Chapter 1, Vehicle Incident Safety. Building upon this fundamental knowledge, Operations and Technician level rescuers should expand size-up to include ongoing size-up during the operation.

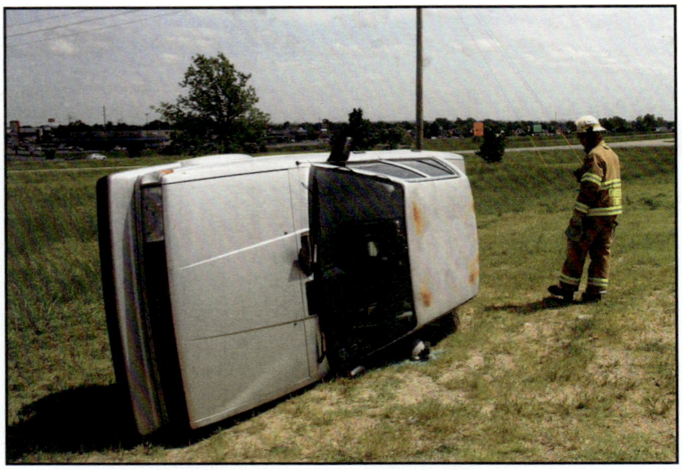

Figure 3.1 A rescuer making a general assessment of the situation.

Scene Assessment

At vehicle incidents, scene assessment involves observing a variety of variables and factoring them into the initial decision-making process. These variables include, but may not be limited to, the following:

- Weather
- Day of the week
- Time of day
- Vehicular traffic
- Pedestrians
- Vehicles involved
- Hazards

The first-arriving personnel must consider all these variables when attempting to see the big picture — to make a general assessment of the situation and to decide whether more resources will be needed **(Figure 3.1)**. On-scene personnel should be assigned to perform those tasks that relate to protecting everyone at the scene — themselves, pedestrians, and trapped victims.

Weather

Inclement weather may have the following effects on an incident:

- May have contributed to the incident occurring
- Hinders extrication operations
- Slows emergency vehicles response
- Obscures the vision of others approaching the scene
- May have an adverse effect on trapped victims
  — Cold weather can make trapped victims more susceptible to hypothermia.
  — Hot weather can put victims at risk of suffering heat-related conditions and dehydration.
- Temperature extremes may also have an adverse effect on rescue personnel

Day of the Week
Pedestrian and traffic patterns can vary significantly depending upon the day of the week. For example, during the week, many people are either at work or at school during the day, and relatively few are engaged in leisure and recreational activities. However, on the weekends, the reverse may be true. These variables can affect the volume of traffic to be expected in the vicinity of a particular crash scene.

Time of Day
The time of day can also have a significant effect on a vehicle incident. Incidents occurring during the morning or afternoon commute can be difficult for emergency responders to access. Traffic may be significantly affected during road construction projects and shift changes at industrial locations. Incidents occurring at night have the added problems associated with darkness and limited visibility.

At certain hours of the day, large numbers of school children might be walking to and from school. Likewise, heavy pedestrian traffic might be expected around shopping areas, theaters, hospitals, and sports arenas at particular times of the day or night.

Vehicular Traffic
The volume and speed of both emergency and nonemergency vehicular traffic approaching and already at the scene must also be considered as part of scene assessment. While it is important that emergency vehicles reach the scene as quickly as safely as possible, excessive speed and/or overly aggressive driving by emergency vehicle operators can cause additional collisions. Regardless of how well emergency vehicle operators drive, the greater the volume of traffic, the slower the response is likely to be. These possible delays must be factored into the initial size-up.

Pedestrians
Pedestrians at the scene of an incident may be curious spectators drawn to the scene or witnesses of the incident who can contribute valuable information during the extrication operations and/or the subsequent investigation. They may also be occupants of involved vehicles who were able to free themselves from the wreckage. In any case, they need to be protected, and their presence needs to be factored into the initial scene assessment.

Vehicles Involved
While a detailed assessment of each involved vehicle is part of a later step in the size-up process, a part of scene assessment is observing the number of vehicles involved **(Figure 3.2, p 98)**. The initial assessment will be different if the incident involves a single automobile or if it involves multiple vehicles and/or multiple victims.

Hazards
The following hazards could possibly place emergency responders and other personnel at the scene in danger:

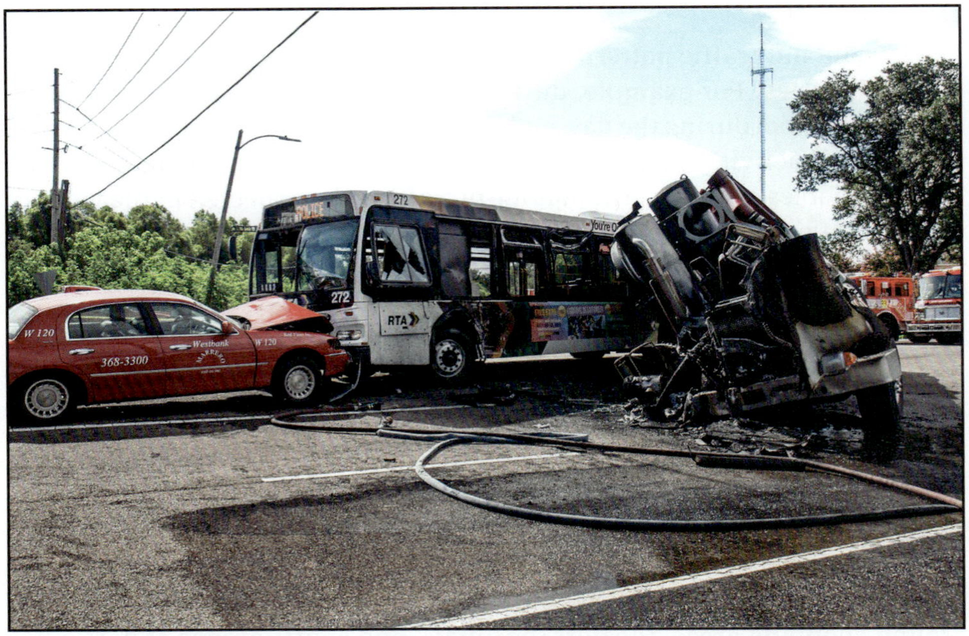

Figure 3.2 Part of scene assessment is determining the number of vehicles involved. *Courtesy of Chris Mickal.*

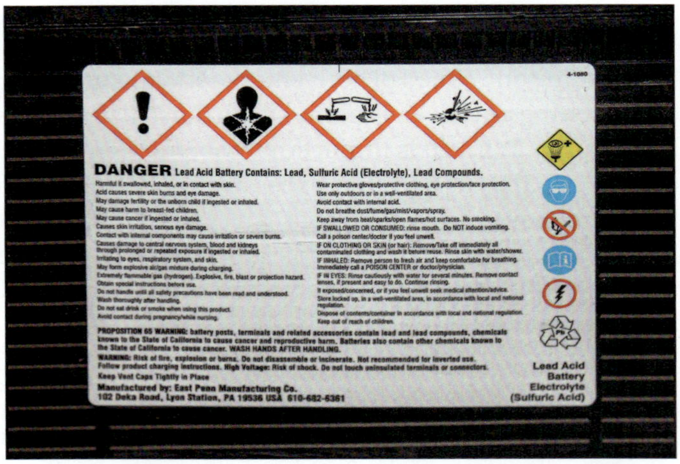

Figure 3.3 There are many hazardous chemicals in a vehicle, including battery acid.

- Leaking fuels and/or other flammable or combustible liquids **(Figure 3.3)**
- Traffic/crowd
- Downed power lines or broken power poles
- Hazardous materials spilled at the scene
- Terrain
- Slip, trip, and fall hazards

In some circumstances, rescuers may require specialized resources to help mitigate special hazards. For example, rescuers may request law enforcement's assistance with handling traffic/crowd control. Another example is the use of a hazardous materials team for incidents involving vehicles that are leaking hazardous materials.

Ongoing Size-Up

With the assistance of the assigned ISO at the scene, the officer in charge should monitor all hazards and other information discovered during the scene assessment. If there are changes to any of these conditions, especially changes that put responders' health at greater risk, the officer in charge should reassess the scene to account for the new risks. Rescuers should report their tactical status (accomplished tasks, progress, impediments to progress) and encountered hazards to the officer in charge so that operations can be adjusted as quickly as possible.

Incident Command System

Vehicle incidents can be as simple as a single-car accident with a trapped but uninjured victim to a multiple-car pileup with multiple trapped and injured victims. Depending on the nature and the scope of the incident, different levels of incident management will be needed. The entire **Incident Command System (ICS)** organization does not need to be implemented on every incident. Rescuers only need to use the parts of the system that are needed to handle that particular incident safely and efficiently.

> **Incident Command System (ICS)** — Standardized approach to Incident Management that facilitates interaction between cooperating agencies; adaptable to incidents of any size or type.

The more that rescuers practice using ICS on the simple day-to-day incidents, the more likely they are to use it effectively on a significant impact incident. The size and complexity of the incident organization should reflect the size and complexity of the incident. It is good practice for the officer in charge of the first (and perhaps only) apparatus at an incident to formally assume command as part of the initial report of conditions upon arrival. This keeps ICS in the forefront and makes for a smooth transition from a single apparatus incident to a much larger, more complex incident.

When a relatively small incident develops into a larger and more complex one, command may have to be transferred several times as the organization grows to meet the need. It is important that the transitions be made as smoothly and as efficiently as possible. The sections that follow introduce the reader to various components that make up the structure of the Incident Management System at a vehicle incident.

ICS Standards of Performance

The organization should train its members to implement appropriate components of local, state/provincial, or federal/national response plans. In the United States, for example, these plans would include the National Search and Rescue Plan, the Federal Response Plan, and the National Incident Management System (NIMS).

Rescue organizations should also conform to national standards of performance such as those created by the National Fire Protection Association (NFPA). NFPA 1006 and NFPA 1670 both identify a number of responsibilities the rescue organization or AHJ should meet in order to conduct rescue operations.

In the United States, the NIMS-ICS is a mandated command structure. NIMS-ICS is designed to be applicable to small, single-team incidents that may last only a few minutes as well as complex, large-scale incidents involving several agencies and many mutual aid responders that could possibly last much longer. IFSTA recommends this system for use in departments that respond to vehicle incidents in the United States. For vehicle incidents in Canada, personnel should follow a similar command structure as described by the Incident Command System Canada.

In order to safely and effectively operate at a vehicle incident, personnel should be familiar with the following:

- Operational protocols
- Communication
- Incident support operations and resources
- Transferring scene control

Command and Control

After an initial size-up, the Incident Commander (IC) must decide how to deploy the available resources and determine the need for additional resources. The IC should also continually reassess the needs of the incident. Under the rescue command and control category, there are several ways in which the IC can subdivide the resources into functional groups within the chain of command. These groups may vary from incident to incident or from agency to agency, but in general, those most commonly used are as follows:

- Scene control
- Vehicle stabilization
- Victim access and disentanglement
- Medical treatment
- Extrication
- Triage/treatment
- Transportation

The typical vehicle Incident Command chart looks similar to other Incident Command charts, except that the titles of some of the components are different. The system by which the functional groups and geographic divisions are organized should meet the specific needs of the particular extrication operation. The typical rescue scene organization may have to be modified to meet the demands of a specific incident. The involved agencies' needs, capabilities, and limitations will also factor into the rescue scene organization.

Within the limits of span-of-control, the IC is responsible for the actions and coordination of these groups **(Figure 3.4)**. On relatively small incidents, the IC can and should stay in constant contact with the supervisors of the groups and make certain that they are performing and interacting properly. On larger, more complex incidents, the IC should appoint an **Operations Section Chief** to coordinate the operations of the various functional groups.

> **Operations Section Chief** — Person responsible to the Incident Commander for managing all tactical operations directly applicable to accomplishing the incident objectives. Also known as Ops Chief or Ops Section Chief.

Incident Operation Groups

The Incident Command System is used when assigning functional groups at a vehicle incident. Each group should have one person in charge, a Group Supervisor, to see that all of its assigned responsibilities are completed. The Group Supervisor is also responsible for coordinating through the chain of command with the IC and with other groups. Personnel on the scene should be able to easily identify Group Supervisors, as well as the IC and all other

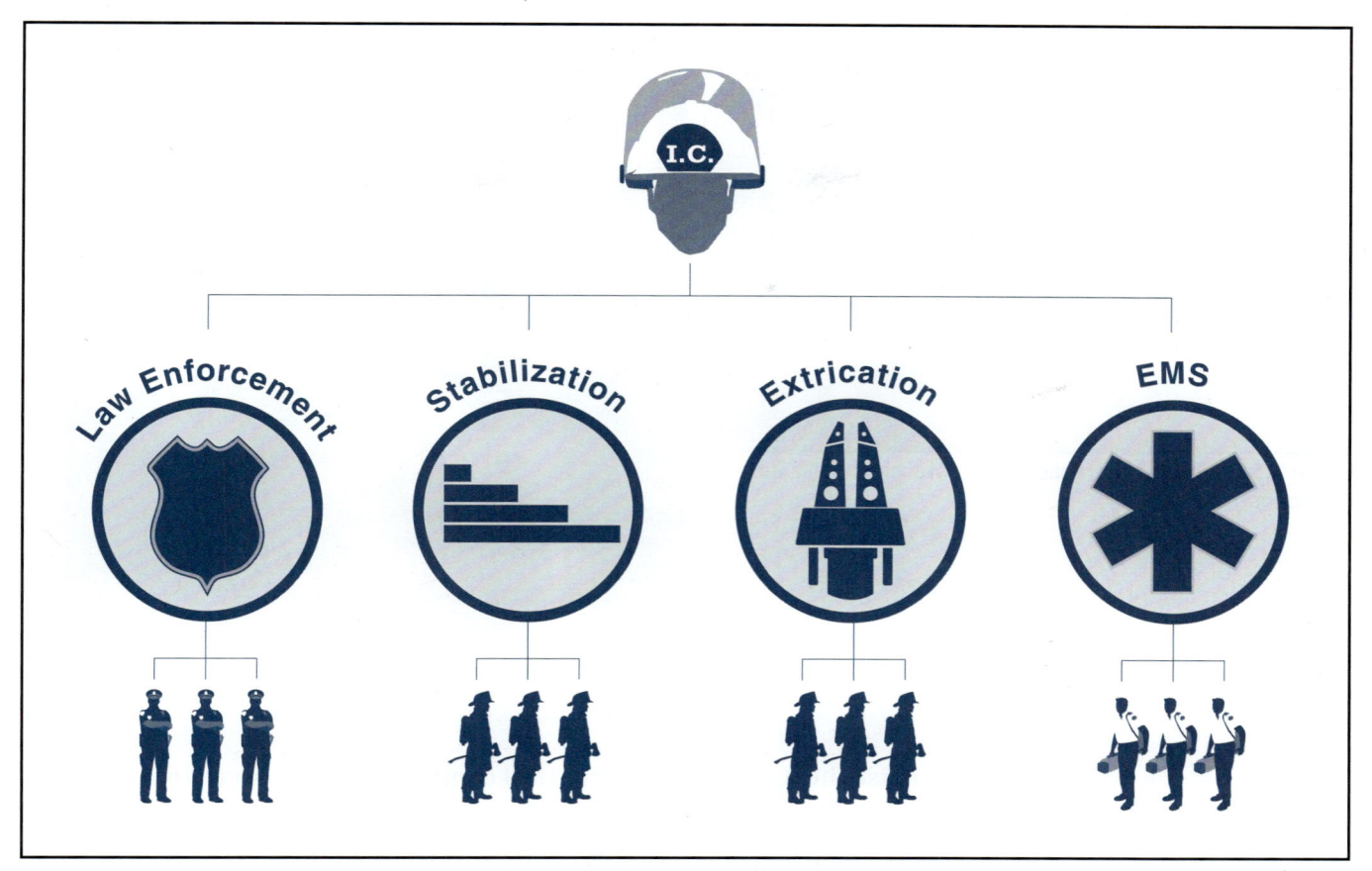

Figure 3.4 A diagram that demonstrates the groups involved in a vehicle incident.

position specialists. Wearing colored vests (labeled with the position titles) over protective clothing and marking a specific location or vehicle as the **Incident Command Post (ICP)** are the generally accepted ways of promoting easy identification.

Personnel should train and work within this system of organization regularly so that they can become and stay familiar with it. The sections that follow describe the activities associated with common functional groups that may be utilized at vehicle incidents.

Extrication Group

The responsibilities of the **Extrication Group** vary with the type, magnitude, and complexity of the situation. This group's activities can be conducted under the direction of an Extrication Group Supervisor. In general, its duties are as follows:

- Determine the number, location, and condition of the victim(s) that require extrication.
- Evaluate the resources required for the extrication of trapped victims and/or the recovery of bodies.
- Stabilize the vehicle(s) **(Figure 3.5, p. 102)**.
- Determine whether treatment is necessary and if it can be safely delivered on-site or if victims will have to be moved before treatment; if necessary, move victims to the triage/treatment area(s).

> **Incident Command Post (ICP)** — Location at which the Incident Commander and Command Staff direct, order, and control resources at an incident; may be co-located with the incident base.

> **Extrication Group** — Group within the Incident Management System that is responsible for extricating victims.

Section B • Chapter 3 – Incident Management Responsibilities

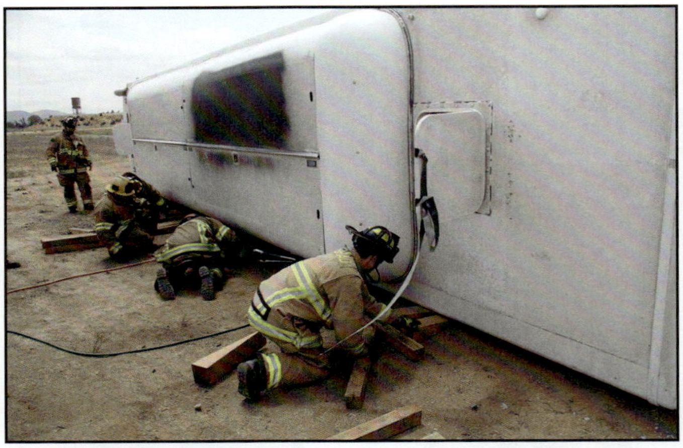

Figure 3.5 Responders practice heavy vehicle stabilization techniques.

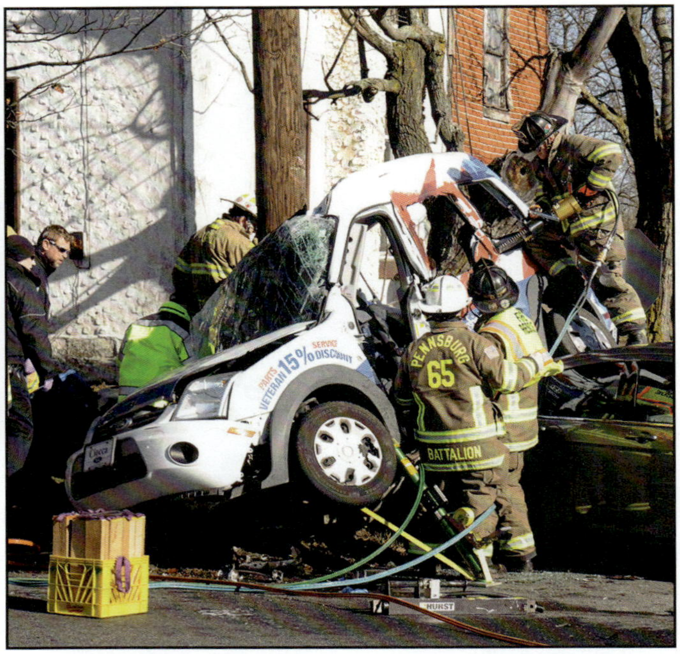

Figure 3.6 A crew of responders engaged in disentanglement procedures. *Courtesy of Bob Esposito.*

- Advise the IC (through the chain of command) of resource requirements.
- Allocate and supervise resources assigned to the extrication function.
- Perform disentanglement to extricate victims **(Figure 3.6)**.
- Report progress to the IC, and give an "all clear" signal when all of the victims have been removed.
- Coordinate with other groups through the chain of command.

Medical Group

The responsibilities of the Medical Group vary with the type, magnitude, and complexity of the situation. The activities of this group can be conducted under the direction of a Medical Group Supervisor. In general, the duties are as follows:

- **Triage** — Responsible for the assessment and categorizing of victims based upon the seriousness of their injuries
- **Treatment** — Provides on-scene, pre-hospital care
- **Transport** — Responsible for delivering victims from the scene to the appropriate medical facility whether by ground or air **(Figure 3.7)**

NOTE: The method in which these duties are carried out should follow the adopted protocols of the authority having jurisdiction. Personnel should follow local SOPs.

WARNING!
Operating near aircraft is inherently dangerous. Ensure that personnel are properly trained while operating around aircraft.

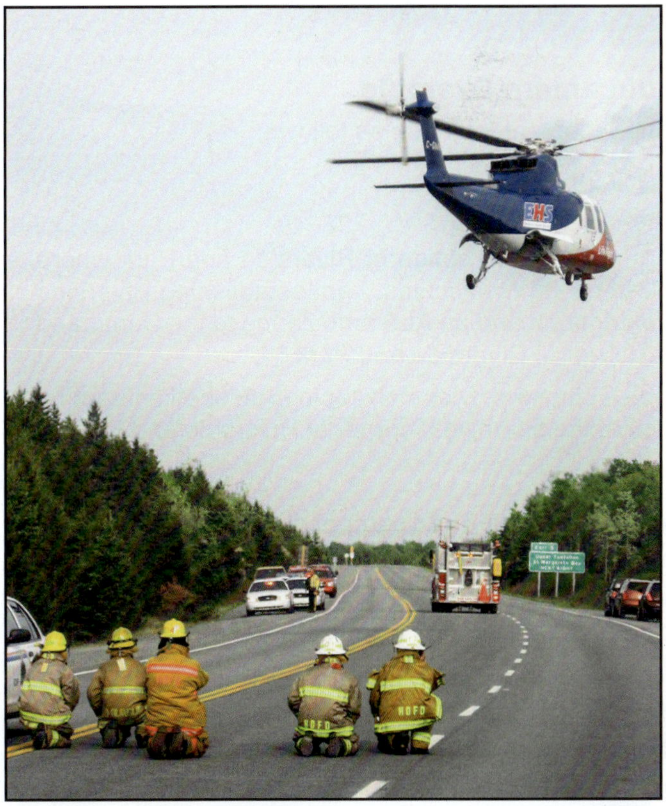

Figure 3.7 An EMS helicopter air lifting a patient to a local hospital after a vehicle accident. *Courtesy of Mike Wieder.*

Operating within the Incident Command System

The purpose of using any form of Incident Command System is to organize an emergency operation so that it can be conducted safely, efficiently, and effectively. The ICS should be established as part of the operational routine and used at every incident so that all department personnel will become familiar with it. Incident Command Systems are useful to large and small departments, but they can be especially beneficial to smaller departments that are not accustomed to working large-scale incidents. Staffing levels, equipment availability, and SOPs determine when and to what extent ICS will be implemented at any given incident.

Many extrication organizations have established ICS that specify who is in command at all times. ICS generally specify that the first member on the scene, such as a rescuer or a company officer, establishes command by advising the dispatcher that the individual is "establishing (name of incident) command." If more than one emergency vehicle arrives simultaneously, the senior person usually has this responsibility. The person establishing command has the full authority that goes with the position and remains in command until formally relieved or the incident is terminated.

The first rescuer or apparatus arriving on the scene of an emergency should initiate the ICS. If the size-up reveals that the Incident Management decisions required to make this a successful rescue are beyond the scope of this person's training, command should be transferred at the earliest opportunity to someone more qualified. In the meantime, the initial IC should do whatever the individual is qualified to do, such as initiating a command structure by naming the incident and announcing the location of the Command Post.

> **Incident Announcement Example**
>
> An actual incident announcement might be as follows:
>
> **Engine 31:** "Dispatch, Engine 31."
>
> **Dispatch:** "Go ahead, Engine 31."
>
> **Engine 31:** "We are at the intersection of Riverside and Park where there is a two-car collision with two victims. I am establishing Riverside Command. Dispatch extrication and an ALS ambulance to the Command Post at the southwest corner of Riverside and Park."
>
> **Dispatch:** "Riverside Command, Dispatch copies you need extrication and an ALS ambulance at the southwest corner of Riverside and Park."

If the company on scene is not trained and equipped to begin the extrication, members should begin to stabilize the incident to their level of qualification. This may be limited to cordoning off the area and identifying and isolating any witnesses to the accident.

Whenever the ICS is implemented, there should be only one Incident Commander, except in multijurisdictional incidents when a **Unified Command** is appropriate. Even when a Unified Command is used, the AHJ must clearly define the chain of command. To avoid confusion, one person should issue all orders through the chain of command.

If other agencies such as law enforcement are involved, each agency should be familiar with the type of system used by the host agency so that they can function properly within its structure. Agencies should offer regular (at least annually) joint-training exercises to achieve interagency cooperation and effectiveness.

The IC should assemble enough resources to handle the incident and organize them so that orders can be carried out promptly, safely, and efficiently. Having sufficient resources at the scene will help to ensure the safety of all involved. The organization must be structured so that all available resources can be utilized to achieve the goals of the IAP. If necessary, the IC can appoint a command staff to help gather, process, and disseminate information. Initially, establishing a formal ICP may not be necessary. However, it is recommended to at least designate the first-arriving emergency vehicle as the ICP until it is determined whether a formal ICP is needed. If the incident involves multiple emergency vehicles and it appears that it will be a prolonged operation, a formal, easily identified ICP should be established.

NIMS-ICS IAP Planning Process

Operations and Technician level rescuers may be responsible for taking command at a vehicle rescue incident. Creating an IAP is necessary at all incidents. As described in Chapter 1, Vehicle Incident Safety, an IAP can be either verbal or written. As the incident grows or has the potential for involving multiple units or agencies for an extended period, the IAP may need to be in written form. Operations and Technician level rescuers should be able to complete the necessary NIMS-ICS forms for an IAP.

Unified Command (UC) — In the Incident Command System, a shared command role in which all agencies with geographical or functional responsibility establish a common set of incident objectives and strategies. In unified command there is a single incident command post and a single operations chief at any given time.

The IC should formulate an IAP that reflects the following incident priorities:

1. Provide for extrication personnel safety and survival.
2. Prevent others from becoming victims.
3. Rescue those who can be saved.
4. Recover the remains of those beyond saving.

The IAP is based on information gathered during the incident size-up. The majority of emergency incident operations will be managed with a verbal IAP that is dynamic to the changing incident conditions. The IC may also use a tactical worksheet to track units and make field notes about the incident. The verbal IAP with the tactical worksheet may evolve into a written IAP as the incident grows in size and/or complexity.

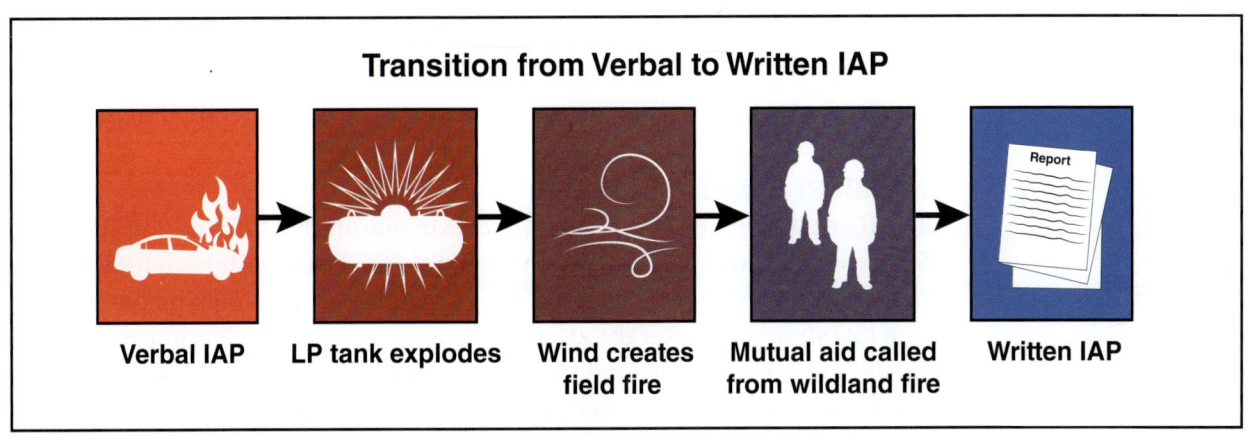

Transition from Verbal to Written IAP

Verbal IAP → LP tank explodes → Wind creates field fire → Mutual aid called from wildland fire → Written IAP

Figure 3.8 When an incident becomes more complex and more resources are deployed, it becomes more likely that a written IAP will be needed to document scene operations.

A written IAP should be forecasted early in the incident operations. By forecasting this need, the IC can expand the ICS structure to include a formalized planning process in which the written IAP is developed **(Figure 3.8)**. Following the NIMS *Planning "P"* form is an effective and standardized approach for developing the IAP and for all command and general staff personnel to understand their responsibilities in this process. Standardized ICS forms are available to record the various elements of the plan.

The IC develops and implements the initial written IAP with assistance from the Operations Section Chief when needed. As the incident grows in size and complexity, a formalized planning process will be needed. The *Planning "P"*, according to NIMS, takes the initial phases of Incident Command and develops a formal planning process with specific command and general staff responsibilities. In the *Planning "P"*, the ISO will develop a written general safety message and the *Incident Safety Analysis* (ICS form 215A). The ISO will be required to attend several meetings in the *Planning "P"* process and should ensure safety is addressed with a risk/benefit analysis in all aspects of the IAP planning process.

The following elements of IAPs were described in Chapter 1, Vehicle Incident Safety; the forms associated with these elements include:

- **Tactical worksheet** — May be created on the scene; the AHJ may develop its own form
- **Incident briefing** — ICS 201 Form

- **Incident objectives** — ICS 202 Form
- **Organization** — ICS 203 Form
- **Assignments** — ICS 204 Form
- **Support materials** — Site plans, access or traffic plans, and locations of support activities should be written down and remain part of the IAP
- **Safety message** — ICS 208 or 208H Form
- **Incident Safety Analysis** — ICS form 215A

The written IAP is maintained at the Incident Command Post and updated or revised as warranted or at the end of the specified time interval (NIMS *Planning "P"*). At the end of the incident, the plan is used as part of the postincident analysis and critique.

All incident personnel must function according to the IAP. Personnel should function according to the department's SOPs, but every action should be directed toward achieving the goals and objectives specified in the plan.

Situation Status Information

The IC, or if assigned, the planning section maintains the situation status information. Communication of situation status will generally be achieved from the tactical-level supervisors to the operations section chief and onto the IC. The ISO should monitor the effectiveness of this communication and ensure the operational strategy and tactics remain appropriate to the situation. It is the IC's responsibility to make changes to rescue tactics if status updates show little or no progress in affecting a rescue or extrication.

Resource Status Information

The IC or if assigned, the planning section – maintains the resource status information. After a briefing from the IC, the ISO should evaluate the resources assigned on scene, in staging, in rehab, and those that have been requested. The IC should ensure that all responders at the scene know where resources are located should they need them. If available resources are determined to be insufficient, the IC may need to call for additional resources. Communication for resource needs may start at the tactical level and proceed up the communication chain to the IC.

Skill Sheet 3-1 describes the process of creating an Incident Action Plan for a vehicle incident.

Emergency Escape and Evacuation

At some incidents, evacuation may be necessary. Depending on the number of people involved and their condition, evacuation can be a complex operation. Personnel accountability after an evacuation is paramount; therefore, crew integrity should always be kept intact. Upon exiting the unsafe area, all personnel should report to the predetermined area of refuge or safety. Immediately after the emergency evacuation, the IC will perform a Personnel Accountability Report (PAR) in an effort to ensure that all rescue personnel have reported to an area of refuge or safety.

Escape and Evacuation Routes

A contingency must be in place in the event that an operational area needs to be evacuated rapidly and without hesitation. The AHJ should establish procedures or guidelines that address rescue team evacuation and accountability measures that are to be followed in imminent danger situations. Procedures should exist for all types of emergency scenes, including vehicle incidents.

Every vehicle incident offers its own complications, and personnel should be aware of a potential evacuation route if the scene becomes too dangerous. An escape/evacuation route may be predetermined by the IC and announced to all personnel operating at an incident scene. This route may need to be protected by firefighters with a charged hoseline. In the event of an explosion or fire, the fire protection provided by the firefighters will help protect both victims and rescuers as they evacuate the scene.

Emergency Evacuation and Safety Signals

SOPs should address the methods used to notify rescue personnel of an evacuation. This notification can be a radio transmission or notification using visual and audible warning signals and devices. The IC or Safety Officer who receives information from on-scene personnel of a life hazard or potential for imminent danger to the rescue team members should announce an emergency traffic message over the radio, communicating the hazard to all personnel on the emergency scene. In addition to the radio transmission, a predetermined evacuation signal, such as air horn blasts, should also be performed. This signal means that all rescue operations are to be stopped and personnel are to retreat to an area of safe refuge.

Terminating an Incident

After all victims have been extricated, treated, and released or transported to a medical facility, all that remains is to terminate the incident. The objectives of terminating an incident include:

- Restoring the scene to as near normal as possible
- Making the scene safe for people to occupy
- Making the scene safe for vehicles to drive through

In some cases, after medical care is complete, emergency responders may have to maintain control of the scene to mitigate hazards or because of an ongoing investigation. During this time, personnel should be concerned with protecting any bystanders as well as the on-scene rescue personnel.

Protecting Bystanders/Public

Personnel must not overlook the need to provide protection to the public at an incident scene. Before terminating the incident, rescuers must ensure that a number of hazards are mitigated in order to make the scene safe for the public.

These duties include:

- Removing wrecked vehicles once law enforcement releases the scene **(Figure 3.9, p. 108)**
- Properly handling fuel spills or other hazardous materials that have contaminated the scene

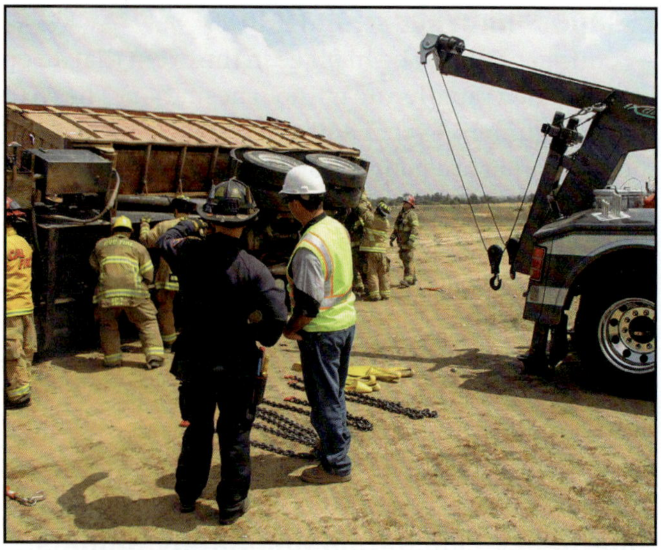

Figure 3.9 Emergency responders work with a tow truck to remove a heavy vehicle from a scene.

- Repairing power lines or removing broken or downed utility poles
- Barricading or closing roadways that have experienced damage from fire

Emergency responders may not be responsible for these duties; however, they should understand the importance of mitigating the hazards prior to terminating the incident. Until these hazards have been completely mitigated, the incident scene is not safe for the general public.

Protecting Rescuers

After all incident activity is complete, emergency responders must retrieve the tools and equipment they used during the incident. Personnel must inspect the tools and equipment and ensure their readiness for use at the next incident. Returning tools and equipment to the apparatus from which they came can be made much easier if all items are clearly marked.

First responders must maintain protection from traffic through proper control measures during this process. Traffic control should not be required once the incident is terminated and all debris, damaged vehicles, and emergency vehicles have been removed from the roadway. To restore normal traffic flow through the area, personnel should remove, in reverse order, all traffic control components, such as:

- Traffic-channeling devices.
- Flagger(s).
- Warning signs.

Skill Sheet 3-2 describes how to terminate a vehicle incident.

Postincident Responsibilities and Analysis

Once an incident has been terminated, responders still have the following responsibilities:

- Restoring operational readiness
- Conducting an After Action Review (AAR)
- Critical incident stress
- Documentation

Restoring Operational Readiness

Following an incident, all responding emergency vehicles must be restored to full operational readiness. This process should include the following:

- Re-servicing the apparatus' and equipment fuel and agent tanks
- Cleaning tools and equipment **(Figure 3.10)**
- Conducting postincident inspection, maintenance, and operational checks of tools and equipment
- Repairing or replacing damaged or expended tools and equipment
- Replacing expended extrication and medical materials

Conducting an After Action Review (AAR)

After an emergency, rescue personnel should review the incident from a technical standpoint to see whether future performance can be improved because of anything learned from this incident. Before leaving the scene of the incident, rescue personnel might conduct an **after action review** (AAR), also known as a postincident analysis (PIA). A more formal critique should be accomplished at the station.

AARs are learning tools used to evaluate a project or incident to identify and encourage organizational and operational strengths and to identify and correct weaknesses. Many organizations have successfully used the AAR process to improve their organizational operations and processes.

Monitoring Critical Incident Stress (CIS)

A critical incident is one that causes a person to have abnormal physiological and psychological reactions. **Critical incident stress (CIS)** can occur with a single incident or from cumulative events over time. Each responder will react to stress in an individualized manner. Adverse stress reactions can occur over a short- or long-term basis after a critical incident(s). Personnel must be able to function at a high level during operations; however, this ability to function can be diminished when stress remains unmanaged.

Stress has always been a part of the emergency responder's life due to the high level of uncertainty, limited control over the work environment, and the psychological effect of repeated emergency calls. They sometimes lack an effective way of acknowledging and dealing with the effects of CIS. Organizations should develop a program to assist members with CIS. This program should provide responders with access to professional help so that they can manage the CIS.

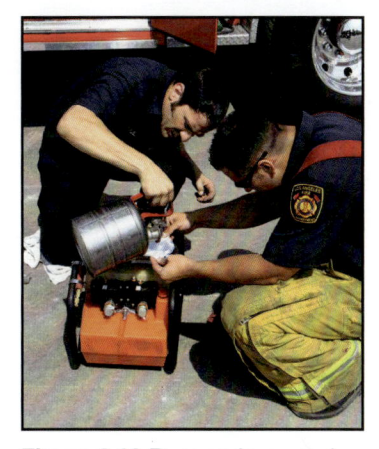

Figure 3.10 Responders need to clean tools and equipment regularly.

After Action Reviews (AAR) — Learning tools used to evaluate a project or incident to identify and encourage organizational and operational strengths and to identify and correct weaknesses.

Critical Incident Stress (CIS) — Physical, mental, or emotional tension caused when persons have been exposed to a traumatic event where they have experienced, witnessed, or been confronted with an event or events that involve actual death, threatened death, serious injury, or threat of physical integrity of self or others.

Changes to NFPA 1500 Regarding CIS

According to NFPA 1500, Chapter 12, recent research has challenged the benefit of what has been called Critical Incident Stress Management (CISM) or Critical Incident Stress Debriefing (CISD). In response to this research, NFPA 1500 has placed the emphasis on members utilizing professional services from "licensed and certified specialists [who may] include psychiatrists, psychologists, and clinical social workers." The current edition of the standard also excludes the terms CISD and CISM from the whole of the document.

If left untreated, the effects of critical incident stress can build up over time and lead to a serious condition known as post-traumatic stress disorder (PTSD). PTSD can produce some debilitating conditions that may be more than just career threatening; they may be life threatening.

NOTE: For more information on critical incident stress, refer to IFSTA's **Fire and Emergency Services Safety Officer** manual.

Completing Documentation

Documentation of incidents is critical to department and training records. All incidents require thorough, accurate, and factual documentation. These documents may be used in the court of law at a much later date.

Chapter Review

1. What variables must be considered when conducting an initial size-up?
2. How is ongoing size-up different from initial size-up?
3. How does the Incident Command System help vehicle incident response?
4. What type of incidents is NIMS-ICS designed to be applicable to as a command structure?
5. List five of the major duties of the Extrication Group.
6. What are the three major duties of the Medical Group?
7. How is Command established and transferred?
8. What priorities should be reflected in every Incident Action Plan?
9. How is situation and resource status information relayed at a vehicle incident?
10. What should take place if emergency evacuation becomes necessary at a vehicle incident?
11. List the objectives of terminating a vehicle incident.
12. What responsibilities do rescuers have after a vehicle incident has been terminated?

3-1
Create an Incident Action Plan for a vehicle incident.

NOTE: This skill sheet covers one method of terminating an incident. Always follow local SOPs. This skill assumes that incident operations have been underway and all incident objectives have been achieved.

Step 1: Conduct an initial size-up.

Step 2: Select the appropriate planning forms.

NOTE: Size up should be continued throughout the incident. The IAP should be modified to meet changing conditions as necessary.

Step 3: Identify hazards and create a plan for hazard mitigation.

Step 4: Determine scene safety zone placement and identify any additional scene security measures that are necessary.

Step 5: Identify the need for fire suppression.

Step 6: Identify type(s) of vehicles involved and stabilization needs.

Step 7: Identify victim location and develop a rescue plan or strategy.

Step 8: Assess the need for resources.

Step 9: Collect any other information required to develop an Incident Action Plan.

Step 10: Communicate the IAP information to other rescuers as necessary.

SKILL SHEETS

3-2
Terminate a vehicle incident.

NOTE: This skill sheet covers one method of terminating an incident. Always follow local SOPs. This skill assumes that incident operations have been underway and all incident objectives have been achieved.

Step 1: Ensure that the appropriate PPE is worn for the duration of the incident.

Step 2: Ensure that scene safety zones remain in place as necessary.

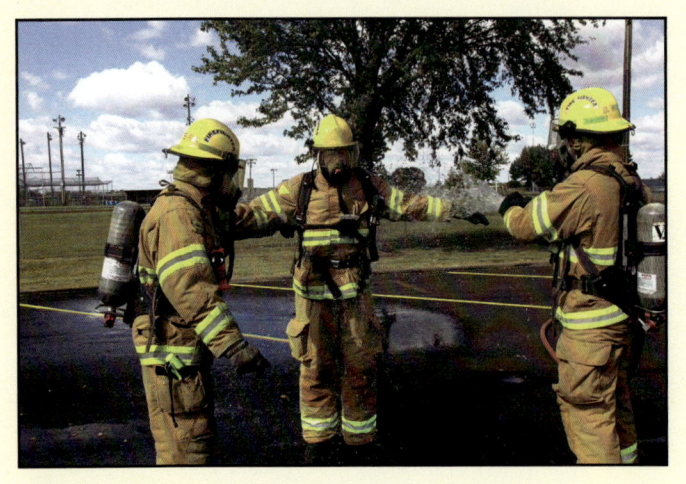

Step 3: Facilitate decontamination as necessary.

Step 4: Notify the party responsible for removal of the affected vehicle(s) and debris.

Step 5: Transfer scene control to the appropriate party.

Step 6: Communicate hazards and pertinent response information to the party responsible for assuming scene control.

Step 7: Terminate Command according to local SOPs.

Step 8: Collect information as needed for postincident analysis.

Step 9: Conduct postincident analysis activities.

Tools and Equipment

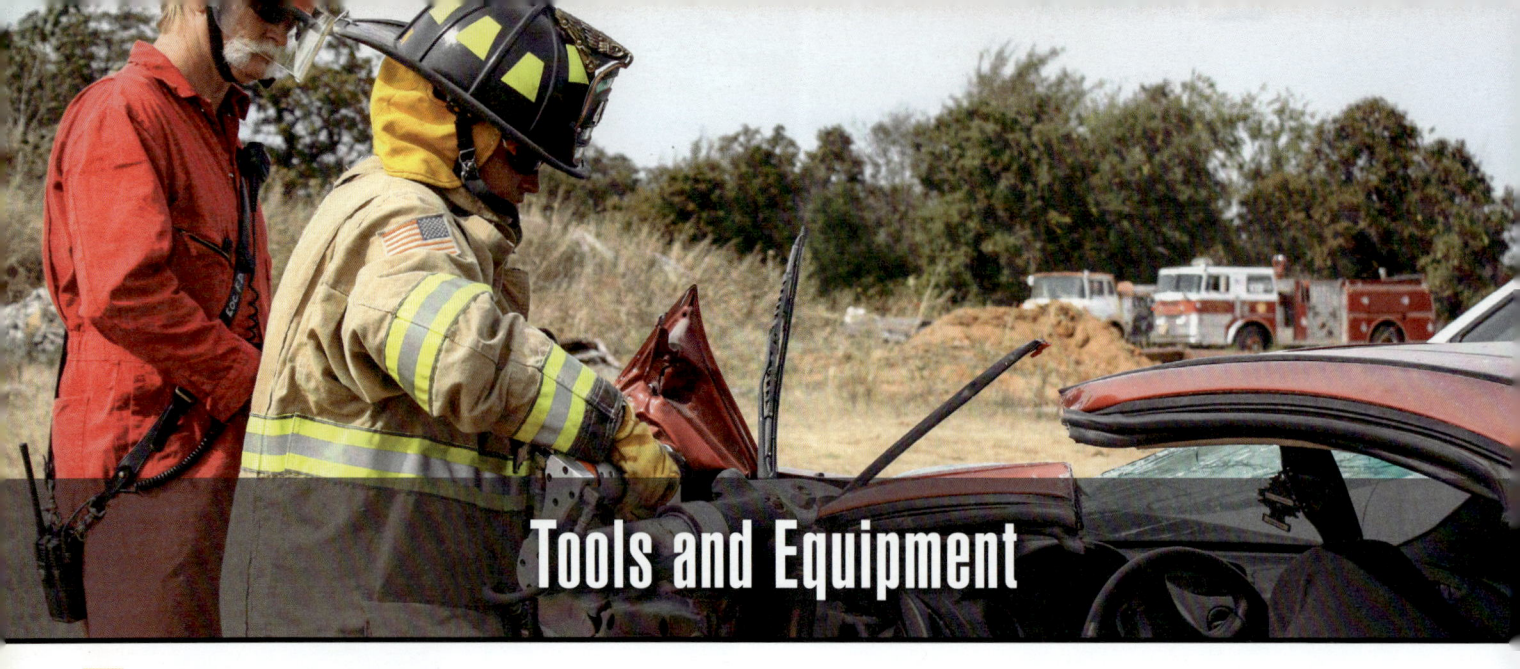

Chapter Contents

Rescue Vehicles, Vehicle Features, Equipment and Accessories 117
- Light Rescue Vehicles 117
- Medium Rescue Vehicles 118
- Heavy Rescue Vehicles 118
- Rescue Engines 119
- Standard Engines 120
- Ladder Trucks 120
- Rescue Vehicle Chassis 121
- Rescue Vehicle Compartmentation 121
- Rescue Vehicle Features and Equipment 122

Stabilization Tools and Equipment 127
- Cribbing 127
- Step Chocks 129
- Struts 130
- Rigging 130
- Ratchet Straps and Tie Downs 132

Extrication Tools and Equipment 133
- Hand Tools 133
- Electric Tools and Equipment 142
- Power Saws 145
- Hydraulic Tools and Equipment 148
- Pneumatic Tools and Equipment 152
- Lifting or Pulling Tools 156
- Come-Alongs 156
- Thermal Cutting Devices 158
- Routine Operational Checks and Maintenance 161

Chapter Review 162
Discussion Questions 162

chapter 4

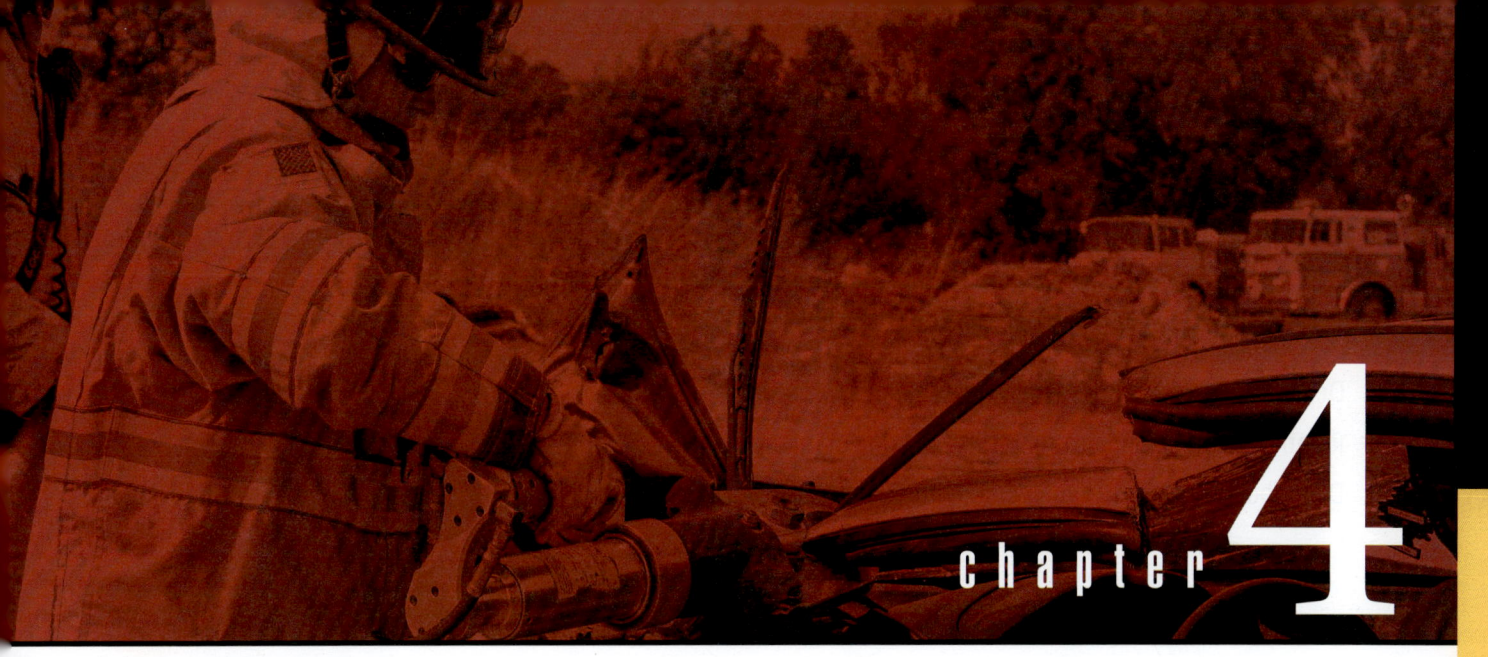

Key Terms

A-Frame 125	Ground Fault Circuit Interrupter (GFCI) 144
Apparatus Engine 123	Mechanical Advantage 136
Cascade System 126	Power Take-Off (PTO) System 143
Cribbing 127	
Gin Pole 125	

JPRs addressed in this chapter

This chapter provides information that addresses the following job performance requirements of NFPA 1006, *Standard for Technical Rescuer Professional Qualifications (2017)*.

8.2.3	8.3.2
8.2.6	8.3.4
8.2.7	8.3.5

Section B • Chapter 4 – Tools and Equipment   **115**

Tools and Equipment

Learning Objectives

1. Describe rescue vehicles used at vehicle incidents. [8.2.7, 8.3.5]
2. Identify types of stabilization devices and systems. [8.2.3, 8.2.7, 8.3.2, 8.3.5]
3. Describe types of tools and equipment used for vehicle extrication. [8.2.6, 8.2.7, 8.3.4, 8.3.5]

Chapter 4
Tools and Equipment

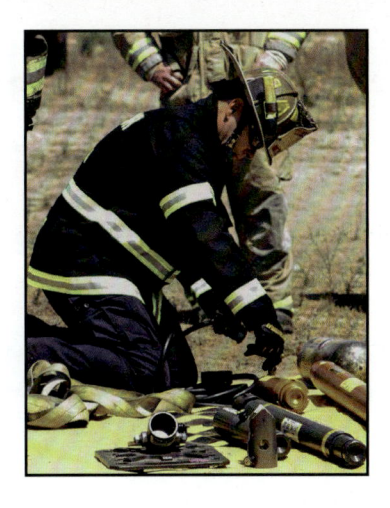

Some extrication tools and equipment have remained virtually unchanged since their introduction. Recently, however, a number of new traditional hand tools and power tools have been introduced, or existing equipment and tools have been greatly improved. In the past, auxiliary equipment such as generators, flood lights, and air compressors had to be added to rescue vehicles. These additions are now standard equipment on most new vehicles.

This chapter describes the tools and equipment that rescuers need in order to perform extrication safely. It also discusses various types of rescue vehicles and a variety of manually operated and power-driven tools used in extrication incidents. Finally, this chapter outlines routine operational and maintenance checks.

NOTE: Personnel should follow all manufacturer recommendations for all the tools and equipment that this chapter covers.

Rescue Vehicles, Vehicle Features, Equipment and Accessories

Fire departments and emergency response organizations use a wide variety of rescue vehicles and call them by a variety of names. For the purposes of clarity, rescue vehicles in this manual are referred to by the following classifications:

- Light rescue vehicles
- Medium rescue vehicles
- Heavy rescue vehicles
- Rescue engines
- Standard engines
- Ladder trucks

NOTE: This section will also discuss the rescue vehicle chassis and compartmentation.

Light Rescue Vehicles

Light rescue vehicles are designed to handle only basic extrication and life-support functions; they carry only basic hand tools and small equipment. Often, a light rescue unit functions as a first responder unit that attempts to stabilize the situation until more appropriate equipment arrives. The standard equipment carried by many ladder and engine companies gives them light rescue capabilities.

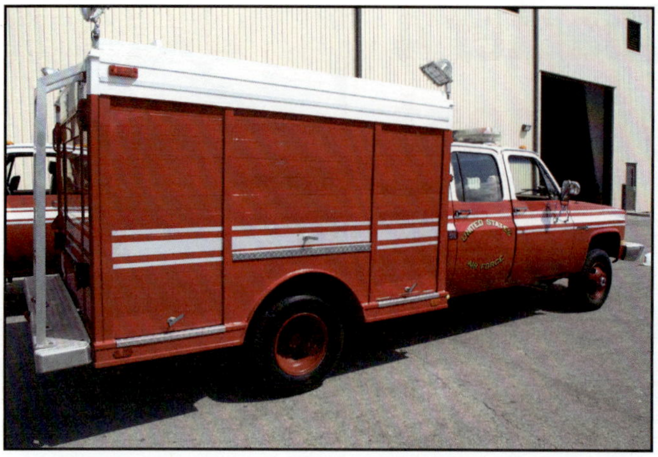

Figure 4.1 An example of a light rescue truck.

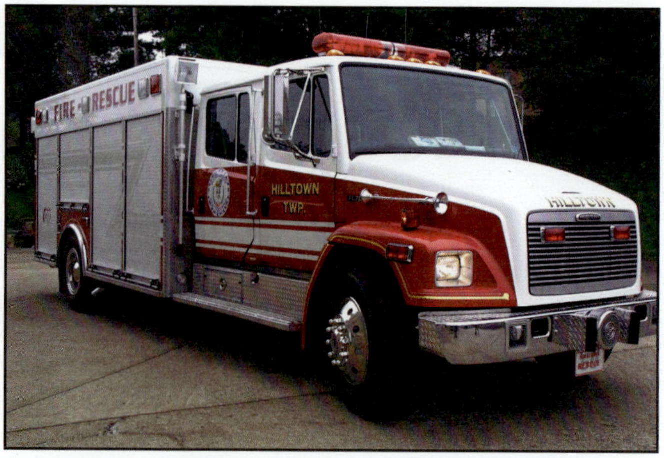

Figure 4.2 An example of a medium rescue truck.

Light rescue vehicles can be built on a 1-ton or 1 1/2-ton chassis. The rescue vehicle's body resembles a multiple compartment utility truck **(Figure 4.1)**. A light rescue vehicle can carry a variety of small hand tools such as saws, jacks, and pry bars, as well as smaller hydraulic rescue equipment and a small inventory of emergency medical supplies.

Medium Rescue Vehicles

Medium rescue vehicles have a wider range of capabilities than the light rescue vehicles. Medium rescue units are capable of handling the majority of vehicle rescue incidents **(Figure 4.2)**. They often carry a variety of fire fighting equipment, making them dual purpose units. In addition to basic hand tools, medium rescue vehicles may carry any of the following equipment:

- Hydraulic spreaders and cutters
- Pneumatic lifting bags and cushions
- Power saws
- Acetylene cutting equipment
- Ropes and rigging equipment

Specialized units may often be considered medium rescue vehicles. Specialized units have specific uses, but they may carry generalized equipment that can be used in other types of incidents. Some types of specialized units include:

- Hazardous materials units
- Water rescue and recovery units
- Bomb disposal units
- Mine rescue units
- Technical rescue units
- Lighting/power units

Heavy Rescue Vehicles

Heavy rescue units must be capable of providing the support necessary to extricate victims from almost any entrapment **(Figure 4.3)**. As their name

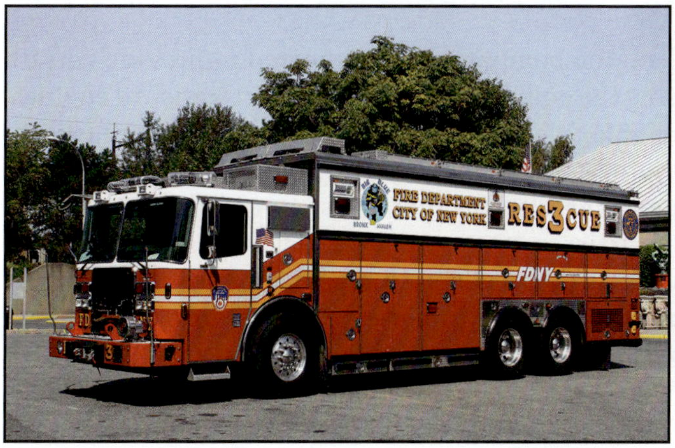

Figure 4.3 An example of a heavy rescue truck. *Courtesy of Ron Jeffers*

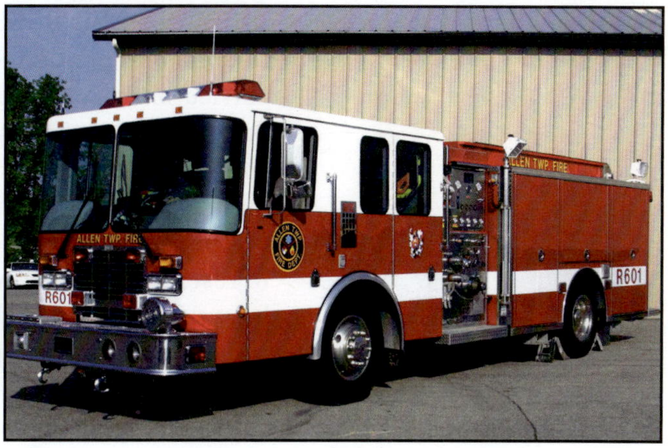

Figure 4.4 Some departments use rescue engines to respond to extrication incidents.

implies, heavy rescue vehicles carry more and heavier equipment than smaller vehicles. Equipment carried by the heavy rescue unit may include:

- A-frames or gin poles
- Cascade systems
- Larger capacity generators
- Trenching and shoring equipment
- Small pumps and foam equipment
- Large winches
- Hydraulic booms
- Large quantities of rope and rigging equipment
- Air compressors
- Ladders

Some modern heavy rescue vehicles have extendable light tower systems or hydraulic cranes mounted to the apparatus. Other specialized equipment may be carried according to the responsibilities of the rescue unit and the rescue exposures identified within the response district. Heavy rescue units are sometimes oriented more toward fire fighting than smaller units because they have more space available for fire fighting equipment.

Rescue Engines

A rescue engine can be a light, medium or heavy rescue vehicle that is specifically designed to serve as both a structural fire fighting pumper and a rescue vehicle **(Figure 4.4)**. As a result, this apparatus is useful at almost any type of incident and has sufficient rescue equipment to handle common extrication incidents. Because they are dual-purpose units, they generally cannot provide the same level of service in either fire fighting or rescue as can the same size unit dedicated to one discipline or the other.

Rescue engines vary in size. Some fire departments use mini-pumpers or midi-pumpers (initial-attack fire apparatus) with light rescue capabilities. Other departments use full-size engines that have been custom designed with extra-large compartments or other modifications for carrying rescue equipment. These larger apparatus are usually equipped with Class-A fire pumps and large water tanks.

Standard Engines

In some departments, engine companies are expected to provide certain extrication services. Using the equipment carried on most standard engines, company personnel are able to perform many vehicle extrication tasks. In some cases, the first-arriving engine company can perform extrication before other specialized equipment arrives. In other cases, the engine company can establish a perimeter, set up fire protection, and provide additional personnel to rescue companies working the incident. Pumping apparatus will usually have the ability to establish and maintain foam capabilities with the necessary proportioning and application systems needed.

Ladder Trucks

In many fire departments, ladder companies are better equipped than engine companies to perform extrication operations. Most ladder trucks carry a greater quantity and variety of equipment than engines **(Figure 4.5)**. Forcible entry tools and equipment carried on ladder trucks can often be used for vehicle extrication purposes. At large-scale incidents, ladder company personnel can supplement rescue personnel when additional help is needed but additional rescue companies are not readily available.

In departments whose fiscal constraints prevent the establishment of a dedicated rescue service, ladder companies normally carry a full complement of rescue equipment and routinely perform most of the extrication work. Ladder trucks typically have a large amount of compartment space to carry additional extrication equipment. Personnel who are already trained in ladder company operations are often cross-trained to perform extrication operations.

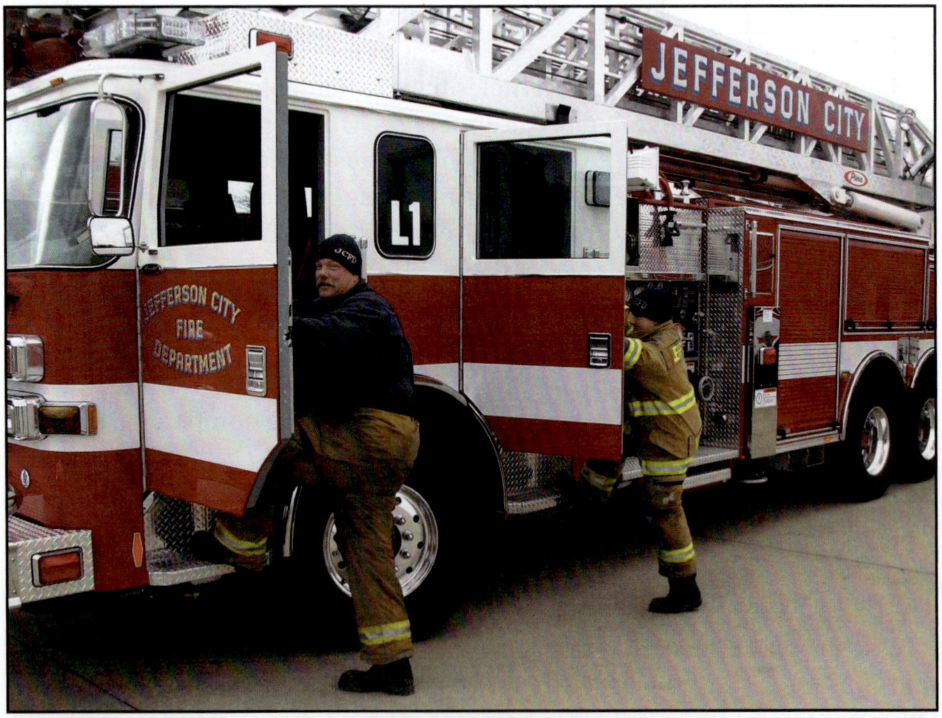

Figure 4.5 Some departments send response aerial apparatus (truck) companies to extrication incidents. *Courtesy of Alan Braun, University of Missouri Fire and Rescue Training Institute.*

Rescue Vehicle Chassis

The two primary types of rescue vehicle chassis are commercial and custom. Each is used for a specific purpose.

Commercial chassis are built by commercial truck manufacturers. These truck chassis are typically used for commercial vehicles, such as plumber's trucks, garbage trucks, dump trucks, and delivery trucks. Commercial chassis are the most commonly used chassis for rescue vehicles. All light and medium chassis units and a large percentage of heavy rescue chassis units are commercial chassis.

Custom chassis are built by manufacturers who specialize in fire apparatus chassis, so they are designed to withstand the heavy use of the emergency service. Custom chassis often incorporate special design features specified by the agency purchasing them.

Rescue Vehicle Compartmentation

Rescue vehicles are designed to transport rescuers, tools, and equipment to emergency scenes. The compartments for carrying the rescue tools and equipment vary from vehicle to vehicle but generally fit into the following three types:

- Exclusive exterior compartmentation
- Exclusive interior compartmentation
- Combination compartmentation

Exclusive Exterior Compartmentation

Exclusive exterior compartmentation is most commonly found in smaller rescue units. These vehicles offer no walk-in/walk-through area or interior storage. Tools and equipment are only accessible from outside the vehicle. Exterior compartmentation is advantageous because personnel do not have to enter the vehicle to access equipment **(Figure 4.6)**.

Exclusive Interior Compartmentation

Vehicles with exclusive interior compartmentation have all of their storage in an interior walk-in/walk-through area. This makes the entire inventory accessible from the inside of the vehicle and allows it to be stored out of the weather.

Vehicles designed with an interior walk-through area can sometimes transport more personnel inside the vehicle than vehicles with only exterior compartmentation. However, having to enter the vehicle for tools and equipment may slow procedures at an emergency scene. In addition, having to carry heavy tools and equipment from the walk-through level down to the ground level and back again can make extrication processes more difficult.

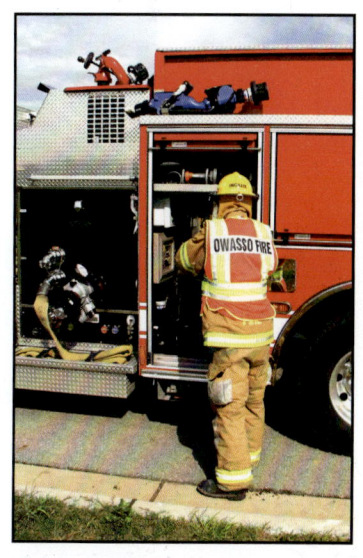

Figure 4.6 Equipment is carried in external compartments on this apparatus.

Combination Compartmentation

Another style of rescue vehicle body is one with a combination walk-in/walk-through area and both exterior and interior compartmentation **(Figure 4.7, p. 122)**. Vehicles with this type of body offer the advantages of each design. Having large compartments on the exterior promotes better ergonomics by allowing bulky and heavy pieces of equipment to be carried in a position where they are easily accessed. Likewise, protective clothing, medical supplies, and similar items can be carried inside and out of the weather.

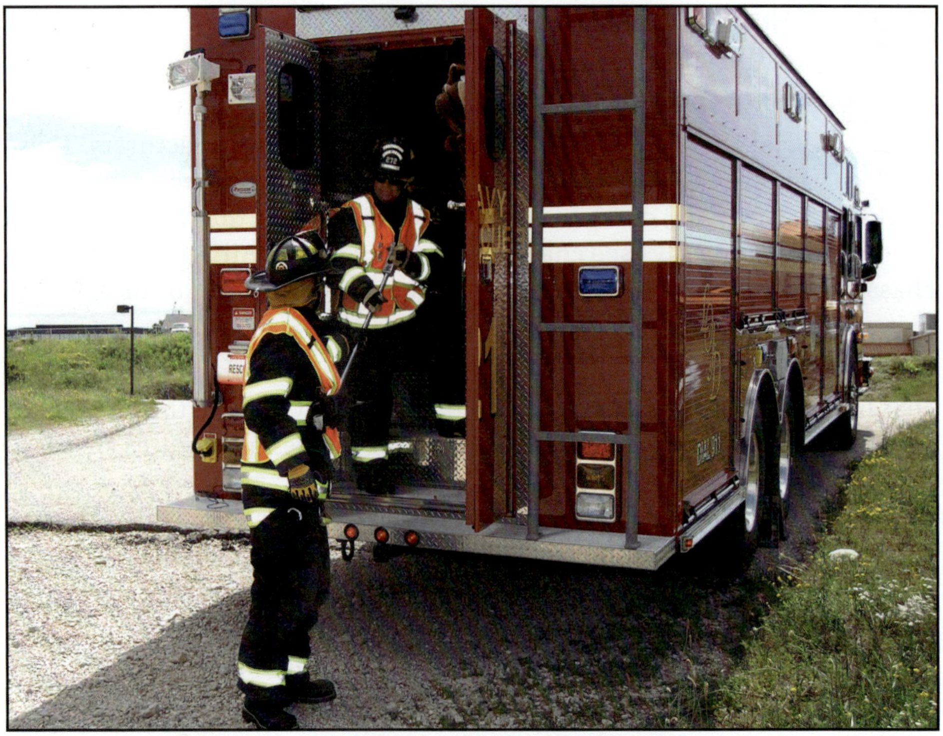

Figure 4.7 This rescue vehicle has both internal and external compartments in which equipment is stored. *Courtesy of Lake Ozark Fire District (MO).*

Rescue Vehicle Features and Equipment

Many emergency response organizations require special equipment and accessories to be incorporated into their rescue vehicles. Some of the most common of these special features include the following:

- All-wheel drive
- Rescue vehicle electrical equipment
- Vehicle mounted winches
- Gin poles and A-frames
- Hydraulic cranes
- Stabilizers
- Air supply systems

CAUTION
Wear appropriate PPE when using any of this equipment.

All-Wheel Drive

The nature of the response area will determine the need for this capability. Rough terrain within the district, or the likelihood of snow and ice in the winter, may necessitate that rescue vehicles be equipped with all-wheel drive. Districts containing mountainous areas and large areas under cultivation may require off road capability. All-wheel drive allows safer, more reliable vehicle operation during extreme conditions.

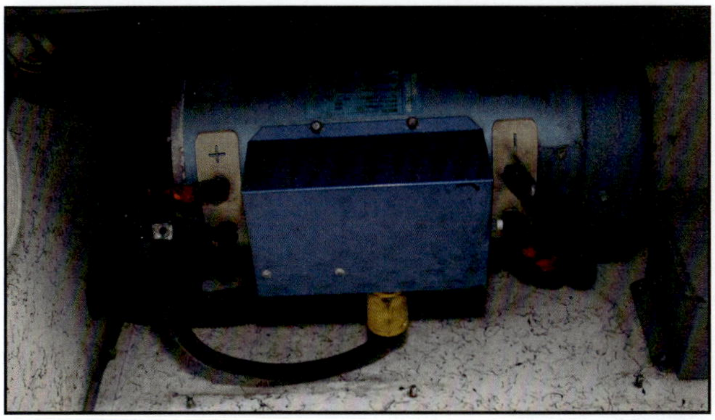

Figure 4.8 A power inverter built into a rescue vehicle.

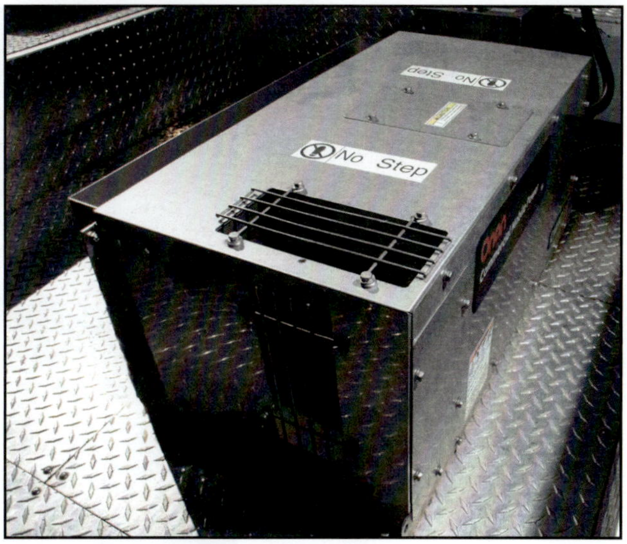

Figure 4.9 A vehicle-mounted electrical generator. *Courtesy of Pat McAuliff.*

Rescue Vehicle Electrical Equipment

Electrical equipment includes both power-generating equipment and the tools and equipment that use the power. Agencies should select power-generating equipment that will produce sufficient power for the tools and equipment that are to be used during extrication operations. This section will describe:

- Inverters
- Generators
- Stationary lights

Inverters. Rescue vehicles and ambulances use inverters, also called *alternators*, when large amounts of power are not necessary. Inverters convert the vehicle's DC into AC **(Figure 4.8)**. Inverters are fuel efficient and produce little or no noise during operation; however, they have limited power-generating capacities and limited range from the vehicle.

Generators. Generators are the most common power sources used on emergency vehicles. They can be either portable or permanently mounted on an apparatus. Portable generators are powered by small gasoline or diesel engines. Most portable generators are designed to be carried by one or two people. Portable generators provide electrical power to areas outside the reach of vehicle-mounted systems **(Figure 4.9)**.

Vehicle-mounted generators usually have a larger capacity than portable units. They provide power for portable tools and equipment and for the floodlighting system on the vehicle. Vehicle-mounted generators can be powered by gasoline, diesel, or propane engines or by hydraulic or **power take-off systems**. Switch-controlled floodlights are usually wired directly to the generators, and outlets are also provided for other equipment. These **apparatus engines**, also known as *power plants* generally have 110- and 220-volt capabilities with capacities up to 50 kilowatts and occasionally greater. Vehicle-mounted generators tend to be noisy during operation, making it difficult to communicate near them. Their exhaust fumes may contaminate the scene unless they are positioned downwind.

Power Take-Off (PTO) System — Mechanism that allows a vehicle engine to power equipment such as a pump, winch, or portable tool; it is typically attached to the transmission. Farm tractors are designed to operate the PTO shaft at either 540 or 1,000 revolutions per minute.

Apparatus Engine — Diesel or gasoline engine that powers the apparatus drive train and associated fire equipment. *Also known as* Power Plant.

Section B • Chapter 4 – Tools and Equipment **123**

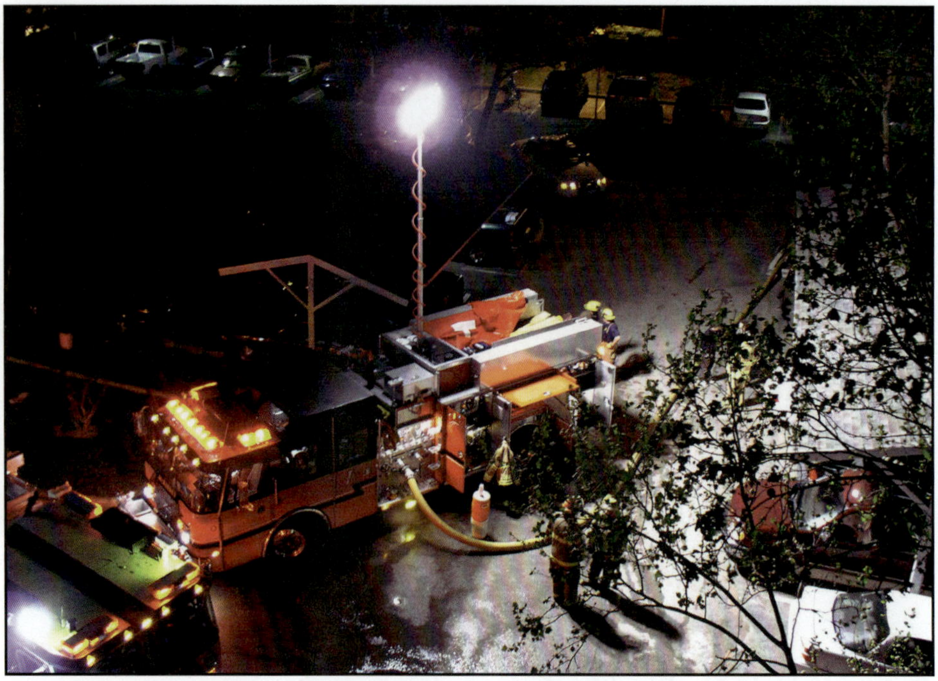

Figure 4.10 Apparatus-mounted lights provide lighting to an emergency scene. *Courtesy of Ron Moore and McKinney (TX) FD.*

Whether using a portable generator or a vehicle-mounted generator, do not exceed the rated capacity power of the generator. Overtaxing the power plant will provide poor lighting, may damage the power generating unit, and will cause electric tools to not function as designed.

Stationary Lights. Stationary lights are mounted on a vehicle using telescoping poles that allow them to provide overall lighting of the incident scene **(Figure 4.10)**. The telescoping poles can be raised, lowered, or rotated to provide the best possible lighting. Some dedicated lighting units have hydraulically operated booms with banks of lights and capacities ranging from 500 to 1,500 watts per light. Scene lighting should not exceed the rated capacity of the generator.

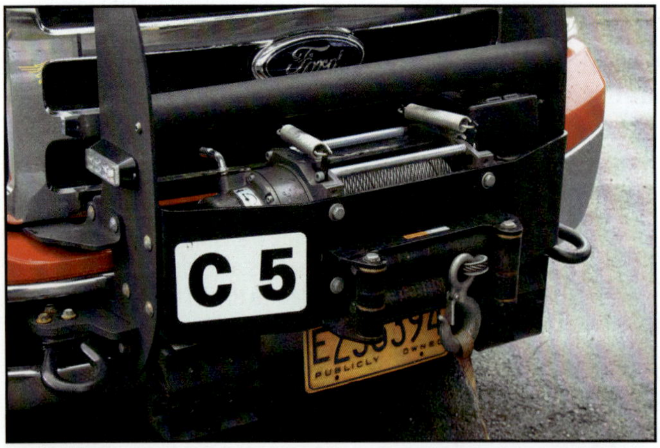

Vehicle-Mounted Winches

Many rescue vehicles, especially those designed as multipurpose vehicles, are equipped with winches. A winch uses either a wire rope cable or synthetic line. This rope or line is wound onto a rotating drum that is geared to give maximum pulling power. Winches may be powered by the apparatus engine or an electric motor. Most vehicle-mounted winches are operated with controls located adjacent to the winch, or remotely with controls attached to a long electrical cord **(Figure 4.11)**. Remote controls allow the operator to get a better view of the operation and, more importantly, allow the operator to remain outside of the winch danger zone.

Figure 4.11 Electric winches may be mounted on the front of the vehicle.

The rated capacity of winches varies. The winch is rated at its capacity when the first layer of cable is still on the drum. Never use a vehicle-mounted winch to move any object that is beyond the rated capacity of the winch. Winch and cable strength are strongest on the first wrap around the drum. As more cable is wrapped around the drum and the cable becomes layered, the strength decreases. As more cable is taken off the drum, the strength capacity increases. For safety reasons, the last layer of cable should not be removed from the drum.

When operating the winch, position it as close to the load as possible in order to limit the length of cable or chain between the winch and the load. This minimum distance reduces the size of the danger zone and reduces the chances of a broken chain or cable striking the operator or anyone else.

The winch danger zone is a circle around the winch with a radius equal to the length of cable or chain from the winch to the load **(Figure 4.12)**. Staying outside of this circle protects the winch operator and bystanders in case the cable or chain breaks.

Like all other extrication tools and equipment, periodically inspect winch components before and after each use to ensure that they are in proper working condition. Inspect the cable or chain for wear or damage and follow the manufacturer's recommended preventive maintenance schedule.

Gin Poles and A-Frames

Gin poles and **A-frames** are vertical lifting devices that may be attached to the front, rear, or side of an apparatus **(Figure 4.13, p. 126)**. Some of these devices have lifting capabilities in excess of three tons. Both gin poles and A-frames have a pulley at the working end that is used with a vehicle-mounted winch when lifting capability is needed. A gin pole consists of a single pole that is supported by guy wires to both sides of the vehicle. A-frames consist of two poles attached some distance apart on the apparatus roughly forming the letter A. Use stabilizers, when provided, to steady the rescue vehicle whenever A-frames are used.

Gin poles and A-frames are not designed to withstand lateral (sideways) stress. Guy wires or guide ropes may be used to increase lateral stability. When gin poles or A-frames are used, do not exceed the rated weight the apparatus chassis is designed to carry. Exceeding the gross vehicle weight limit may result in damage to the axles, chassis frame, or both. A gin pole system or A-frame should be engineered to work within the vehicle safety factors and working range.

Hydraulic Cranes

Cranes generate great power for lifting and pulling during extrication operations. Some rescue organizations have access to cranes through other agencies while a few others have added hydraulically operated cranes to their heavy rescue units. Hydraulic cranes assist in vehicle stabilization, removal of heavy vehicle components, and raising and lowering personnel and equipment. Some

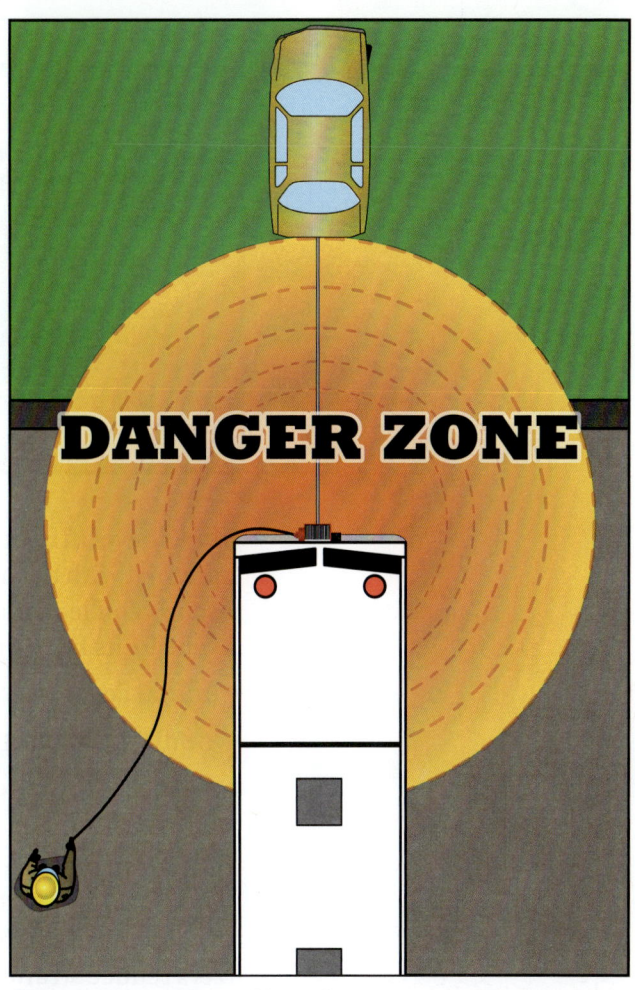

Figure 4.12 A winch cable under pressure can break at any point along its length, and if it does, it will whip back toward the winch box.

Gin Pole — Vertical lifting device that may be attached to the front or the rear of the apparatus; consists of a single pole that is attached to the apparatus at one end and has a working pulley at the other. Guy wires may also be used to stabilize the pole.

A-Frame — Vertical lifting device that can be attached to the front or rear of the apparatus; consists of two poles attached several feet (meters) apart on the apparatus and whose working ends are connected to form the letter A. A pulley or block and tackle through which a rope or cable is passed is attached to the end of the frame.

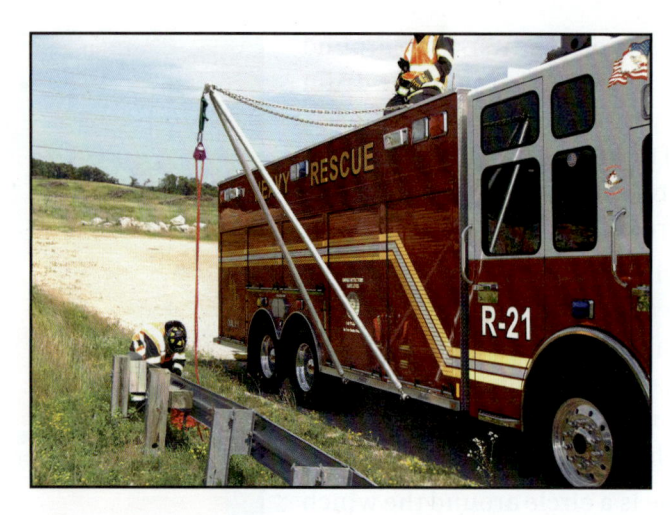

Figure 4.13 An A-frame rig attached to a rescue vehicle. *Courtesy of Lake Ozark Fire District (MO).*

cranes have lifting capabilities of up to eighteen tons or more. Rescue vehicles equipped with a crane must use stabilizers that are extended to stabilize the rescue vehicle while the crane is in use. Hydraulic cranes attached to heavy rescue units have three disadvantages:

- Initial cost of the crane
- Additional maintenance required
- Loss of space for other tools because of the crane's size

Stabilizers

Also known as stabilizing jacks or outriggers, stabilizers are used to steady the rescue vehicle when deploying a gin pole, A-frame, or hydraulic crane. Stabilizers reduce strain on the vehicle's suspension system when heavy loads are lifted and help prevent the vehicle from rolling over when parked on a slope. There are two types of stabilizer systems: hydraulic, which are set using lever controls, and manual, which resemble a screw-type jack and are set by hand.

Air Supply Systems

Rescue vehicles may be equipped with various systems to provide air for equipment and personnel. Air supply may come from tanks carried on the vehicle or be transferred from ambient air using air compressors. Three common air supply systems on rescue vehicles are:

- Cascade systems
- Breathing air compressors
- Non-breathing air compressors

Cascade Systems. Some rescue vehicles contain a bank of large capacity air cylinders called **cascade systems**. These systems refill SCBA cylinders during an emergency operation and refill cylinders used to operate pneumatic tools such as air chisels **(Figure 4.14)**.

Breathing Air Compressors. Some rescue vehicles contain air compressors that can generate breathing-quality compressed air. These units use generated air to fill cascade or SCBA cylinders, to supply airline equipment in confined spaces, or to purge areas of nonflammable, oxygen-depleting gases. Locate operating compressors in a clear atmosphere to avoid drawing contaminated

> **Cascade System** — Three or more large, interconnected air cylinders, from which smaller SCBA cylinders are recharged; the larger cylinders typically have a capacity of 300 cubic feet (8 500 L).

air into the units and supplying it to the users. Generally, place these units upwind of any emergency scene to avoid such contamination.

Non-Breathing Air Compressors. Non-breathing air compressors are used to operate pneumatic equipment. Because of the many styles and sizes, as well as their relatively low cost, non-breathing air compressors are found on many rescue vehicles. These compressors do not require a clear atmosphere for operation. They may be commercial construction style compressors or a use of the vehicle's engine compressor.

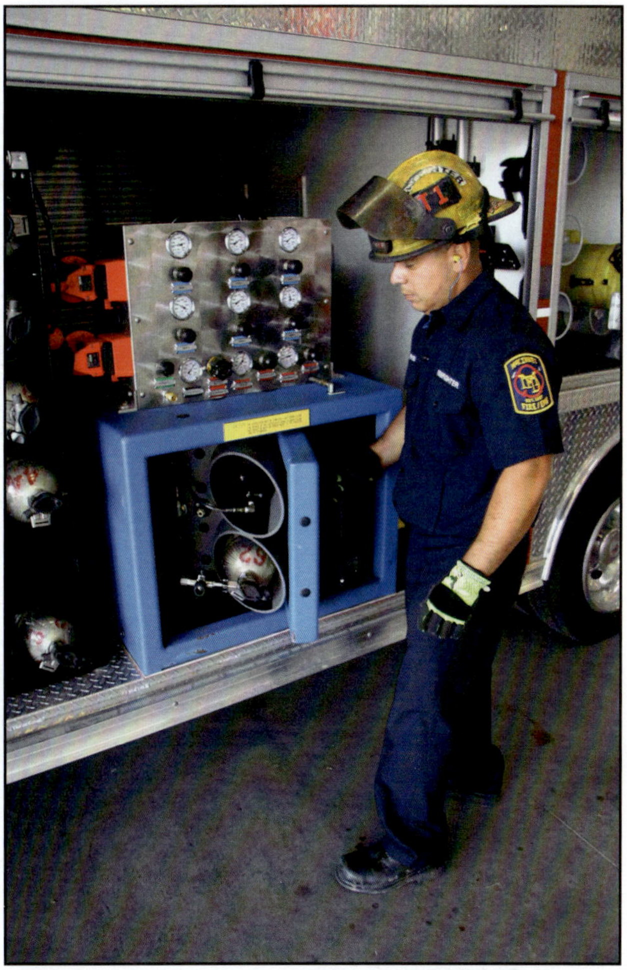

Stabilization Tools and Equipment

One of the first and most important steps in performing vehicle extrication safely — for the rescuers and victims — is stabilizing the vehicle. Any sudden and unexpected movement of the vehicle while rescuers and victims are inside can be dangerous, or even fatal. Therefore, rescuers must use the resources available at the scene to quickly and securely stabilize the vehicle. The means used to stabilize vehicles most often include the application of the following:

- Cribbing
- Step chocks
- Struts
- Rigging

Figure 4.14 Some rescue apparatus are equipped with air bottle reservicing cascade systems.

CAUTION
Wear appropriate PPE when using any stabilization equipment.

Cribbing

In addition to the wooden **cribbing** that has been used in extrication operations for many years, some cribbing available today is made of plastic. Each type of cribbing has certain advantages and disadvantages, as well as certain capabilities and limitations.

Wooden Cribbing

Much of the cribbing used in vehicle extrication is made of wood that is solid, straight, and free of major flaws such as large knots or splits. Various sizes of wood can be used, such as 2 x 2-inch (50 x 50-mm) and 6 x 6-inch (150 x 150-mm), but the most common is 4 x 4-inch (100 x 100-mm) wood timbers. Most pieces are 18 to 24 inches (450 to 600 mm) long. Some agencies paint the ends of the pieces different colors for easy identification by length. Other surfaces of the cribbing should be free of any paint or finish because the finish can make the wood slippery, especially when it is wet.

Cribbing — Wooden or plastic blocks used to stabilize a vehicle during vehicle extrication or debris following a structural collapse; typically 4 X 4 (100 x 100 mm) inches or larger and between 16 to 26 inches (400 to 650 mm) long.

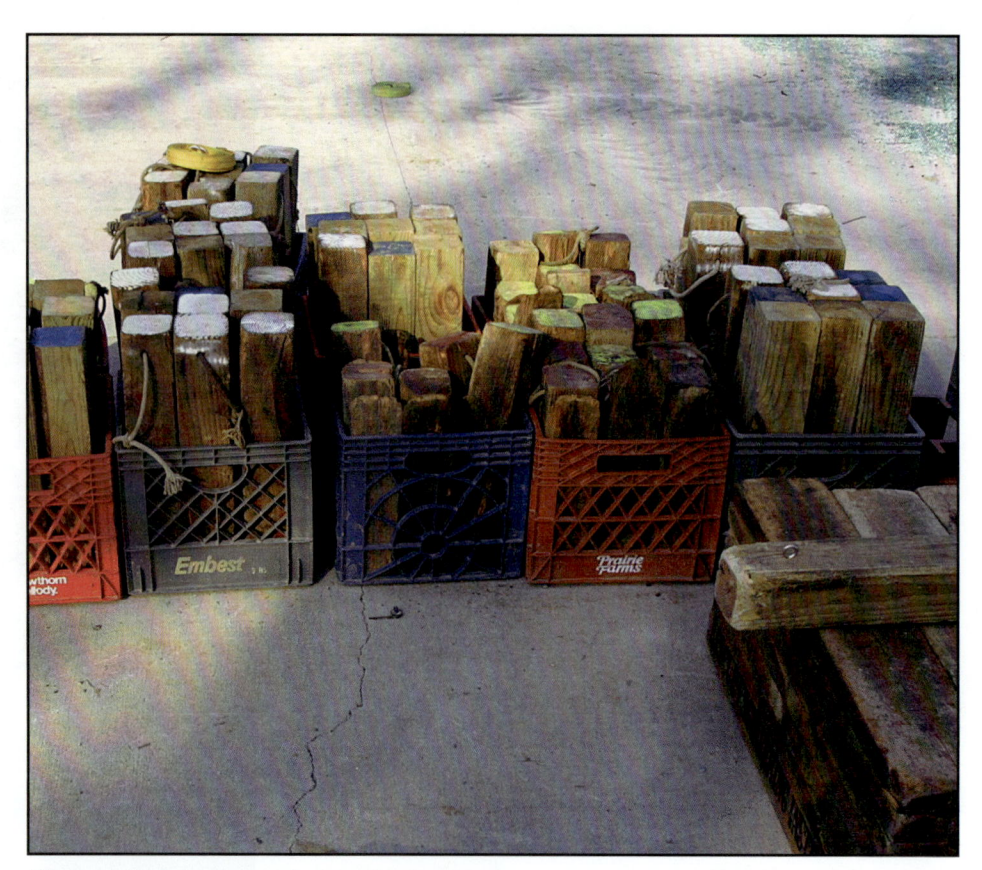

Figure 4.15 Cribbing stacked in plastic crates.

Cribbing pieces may have a hole through one end and a loop of rope or webbing tied through the hole to form a handle. Cribbing can be stacked in a compartment with the grab handles facing out for easy access, or it can be stored on end inside a plastic crate or box **(Figure 4.15)**.

Plastic Cribbing

A growing number of emergency response agencies use cribbing made of recycled plastic **(Figure 4.16)**. Plastic cribbing has the advantage of being twice as strong as wood. One disadvantage is that it provides no warning prior to failure, whereas wood cribbing will crack prior to failure. It is also impervious to oil, gasoline, and other substances that can soak into and contaminate wooden cribbing, however it may be slippery when wet. It also is more expensive and much harder to replace than wood cribbing.

Cribbing Applications

The most common application for cribbing in vehicle extrication is called a *box crib* **(Figure 4.17)**. This cribbing arrangement is named for the box formed when the pieces are set. A properly constructed box crib is a stable support.

One type of box crib, a 2-member x 2-member, is constructed by placing two pieces of cribbing parallel to each other on a flat, level surface. The distance between the two pieces is determined by the size of the cribbing, the intended height of the box crib, and local SOPs. A second layer of cribbing (two pieces) is placed perpendicular to and on top of the first layer. These two pieces should be spaced apart to provide a stable foundation. There should be a minimum

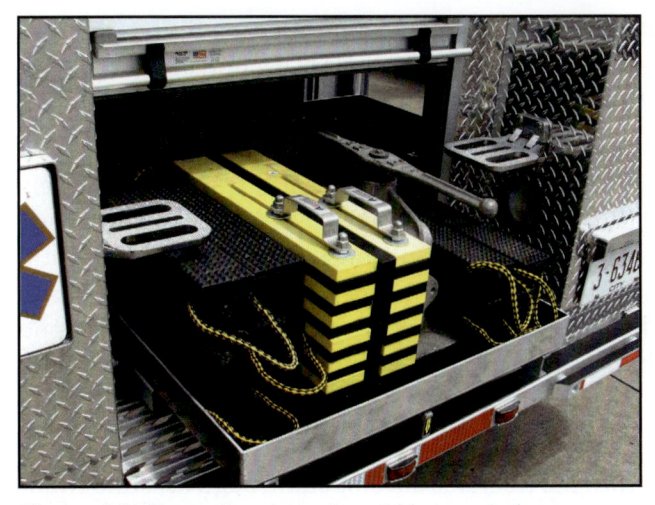

Figure 4.16 Examples of plastic cribbing made from recycled plastic.

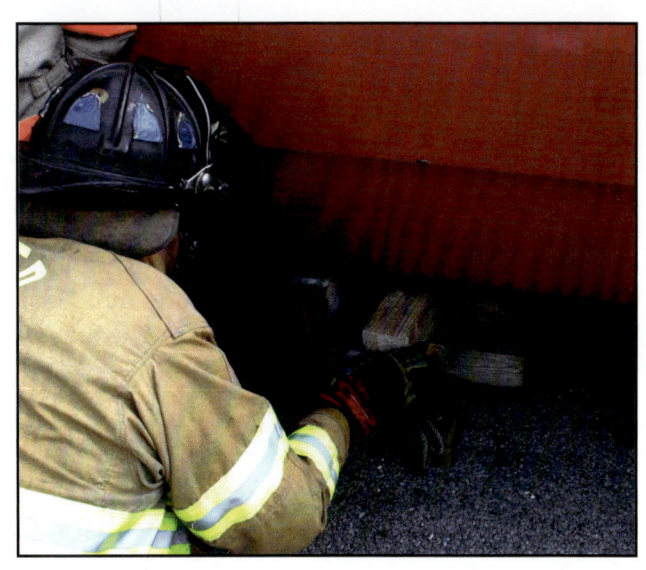

Figure 4.17 A rescuer building a box-crib using wooden cribbing.

of four inches of overlap on all four corners of the box crib, and cribbing ends should extend beyond the sides touching the layer. Continue this process in layers as necessary to reach a desired height. When constructing a box crib, follow departmental SOPs.

Other box crib configurations include the 3-member x 3-member, 4-member x 4-member, and solid. The more members used to construct individual layers will strengthen the box crib and increase its load-carrying capacity.

Box cribs have height limitations. According to the U.S. Army Corps of Engineers, the maximum height of a box crib is three times the shortest width of the box crib. They recommend maximum heights of four feet in 4 x 4 systems, and six feet in 6 x 6 systems. Be aware of these maximum heights when attempting to stabilize heavy vehicles that have higher ground clearances than passenger vehicles.

Use wedges and shims in conjunction with cribbing to stabilize vehicles. Wooden wedges are usually 4 x 4 x 18-inch or 2 x 4 x 12-inch (100 x 100 x 450 mm or 50 x 100 x 300 mm) material cut from corner to corner. Wedges are usually inserted in pairs, each wedge on opposite sides to tighten cribbing. Shims are the same shape as wedges but may be cut from smaller stock. Unlike wedges, shims are used singularly to take up space between cribbing and the object being supported.

A cribbing stack seldom completely fills the space between the base and the underside of the vehicle to be stabilized. For proper stabilization, the cribbing must fit that opening tightly to prevent any movement of the vehicle. Fill the gap between the top of the cribbing stack and the vehicle by setting a wooden shim into the gap atop each of the top cribbing pieces or by setting shims beneath the stack until the fit is tight.

Step Chocks

Step chocks are named for the series of steps that are formed when they are fabricated. Step chocks are made of recycled plastic or wood **(Figure 4.18)**. Some agencies purchase manufactured step chocks, others fabricate their own.

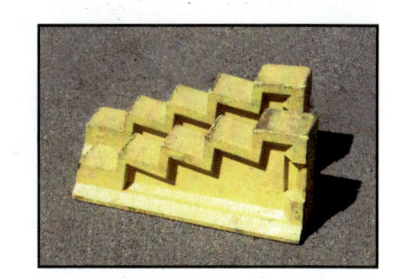

Figure 4.18 Examples of plastic step chocks.

Section B • Chapter 4 – Tools and Equipment **129**

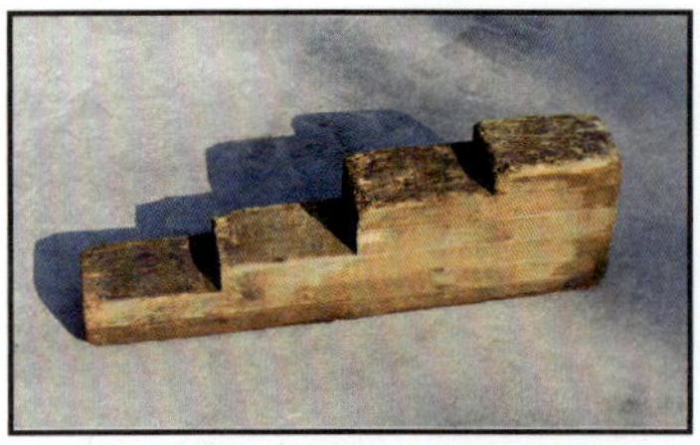

Figure 4.19 A wooden step chock made of varying lengths of 2- X 6-inch (50 x 150 mm) boards.

Either way, agencies should test materials under controlled conditions that will allow them to identify the capabilities and limitations of each. Testing will allow agencies to develop SOPs for the safe and effective application of these devices.

Wooden step chocks have a 2 x 6-inch (50 x 150-mm) base approximately 30 inches (750 mm) in length **(Figure 4.19)**. Centered on the base are progressively shorter lengths of 2 x 6-inch (50 x 150-mm) lumber stacked one upon the other. Each step is approximately 6 inches (150 mm) shorter than the one beneath. The total number of steps is limited by the length of the base. It is better to construct wooden step chocks by laminating the pieces together with wood glue and screws, rather than with nails.

Plastic step chocks have the advantage of being impervious to fuel, oil, and other liquids. Brand new or nearly new plastic step chocks and other shoring devices will be slippery until some wear has developed through use. Intentionally scratching and roughening new surfaces will provide better footing when the devices are in use.

Install a step chock by placing it on a firm, level surface and pushing the entire unit under the vehicle until the entire device is under the vehicle or one of the steps makes contact with the side of the vehicle. Do not install the step chock where it would interfere with the swing of the vehicle's doors. Eliminate any space between the highest step under the vehicle and the underside of the vehicle by setting a shim under the step chock or by letting the air out of inflated tires in a controlled manner to load the step chocks.

Struts

Adjustable struts that can be used in a variety of configurations. Some adjustable struts consist of a square tube attached to a base plate which spreads the load and provides more a secure footing. A series of holes along both sides allows a pin to be inserted to hold the tubes at the desired length **(Figure 4.20)**. Take up any space remaining between the top of the tube and the bottom of the vehicle with the screw jack in the end of the tube. Some innovative rescue agencies fabricate their own versions of these devices using wood and composite materials.

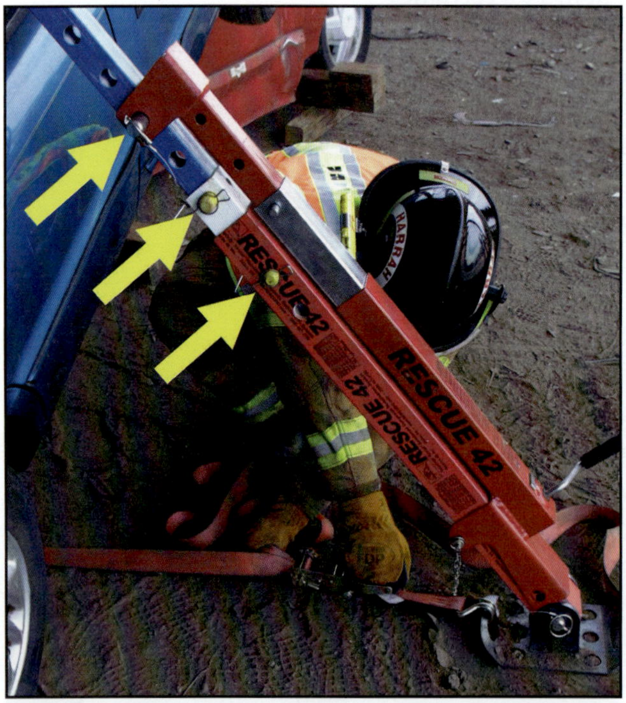

These devices can be extremely effective in certain situations. However, as with any other tool or device, there are conditions that do not lend themselves to their use and cribbing or step chocks may work better in these situations. Each individual extrication situation will dictate which stabilization device should be used.

Rigging

Rigging is a general term for some of the other tools and equipment that are used to stabilize vehicles. Rigging includes:

- Rope
- Chains
- Webbing

Figure 4.20 The arrows identify locking pin locations on a rescue strut.

Section B • Chapter 4 – Tools and Equipment

Rope

Rope is one of the most versatile and useful items carried on fire apparatus and rescue vehicles. It can be used for hoisting, lowering, securing and stabilizing vehicles, and for crowd control.

When used solely for securing and stabilizing vehicles, the rope used must be of high quality to withstand the stresses exerted on it, but it does not have to be life safety rope. Non-life safety rope is classified as *utility rope* and may be made of natural or synthetic fibers. Nylon rope is not ideal for vehicle stabilization because it stretches under load. If a nylon rope must remain in place for an extended period, it may have to be tightened periodically. If possible, use a different type of rope so that it will not have to be adjusted repeatedly during the operation.

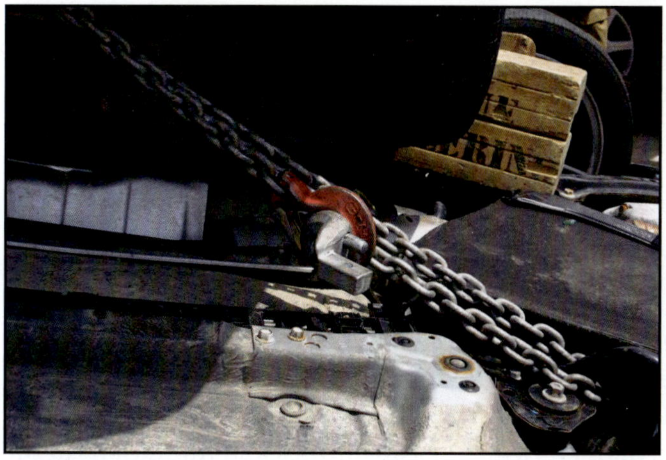

Figure 4.21 An alloy chain is the only approved type of chain in a rescue operation.

Chains

Use only alloy steel chains in vehicle extrication **(Figure 4.21)**. They are strong and highly resistant to abrasion and chemical degradation. Some special alloys are resistant to corrosive or hazardous atmospheres. The best chain for rescue work is Grade 80, also known as Grade 8 or Grade T. This chain can be identified by the 8 or T embossed on the links at regular intervals. The minimum chain size generally used for extrication operations is 3/8-inch (10-mm). Proof coil chain, also known as *common* or *hardware chain*, is not suitable for use in vehicle extrication operations.

For any operation, match the rated strength of the chain to the tools being used and the job being performed. All chains should have an attached tag that has the safe load weight stamped or printed on it.

Chain failures can occur when the chain is abused or neglected in use or storage. Improper treatment of chain components leads to metal fatigue and chain failure. Inspect chains link by link for signs of wear or damage on a regular schedule. Remove defective chains from service.

Observe the following safety rules when using chains:

- Do not drag a load with a chain under it.
- Do not cross, knot, or hammer a chain into position (for example, tying a knot in a chain to shorten it).
- Do not exceed the chain's listed safe working load.
- Do not use worn or damaged chains.

Section B • Chapter 4 – Tools and Equipment **131**

- Do not impact load a chain by lifting an object, dropping it, and then suddenly stopping its fall. This increases the strain on the chain.
- Do not connect chain hooks to anything but the chain itself.
- Do not weld links in alloy chain or otherwise expose them to excessive heat.
- Do not use chain appliances, such as hooks, pins, and links that are not of at least equal strength to the load being supported or controlled.
- Do not use hooks and attachments that are not made of the same alloy material as the rest of the chain.

CAUTION
While using hooks, orient the opening, or eye, towards the rescuer. If the hook fails and elongates, the hook will fail away from the rescuer.

- Do not attempt to splice a chain by placing a bolt through two links.
- Do not apply force to a kinked chain — make sure that all of the links are straight.
- Do not side load any of the chain attachments or components.

With few exceptions, chains and webbing of the appropriate size and strength may be used interchangeably. The choice between chains and webbing matters much less than knowing the capabilities and limitations of the chains and webbing available in a given situation. Using chains and webbing beyond their limitations can result in their failure - perhaps catastrophically.

Webbing

Conventional webbing is made from the same materials used in synthetic ropes, so similar precautions apply. There are two main types of webbing construction: flat and tubular. Both are similar in appearance except when viewed in a cross-section. Tubular webbing is woven in two ways: spiral and chain. Generally, the spiral weave is stronger and more resistant to abrasion than the chain weave.

The size of webbing varies with the intended use, but most webbing used for lifting and pulling operations starts at about 2 inches (50 mm) in width. The strength requirements for webbing are the same as for chain used in the same situation **(Figure 4.22)**.

Webbing is susceptible to ultraviolet light, abrasions, and chemical degradation. This makes it impractical for use in some extrication applications. If webbing must be used in a situation where it is exposed to abrasions, chemical contamination, or ultraviolet light for an extended period of time, protect it with edge protection or similar material.

Ratchet Straps and Tie Downs

Ratchet straps and tie downs typically consist of webbing straps, one to four inches (25 to 100 mm) in width with tie down hardware, including hooks, cam

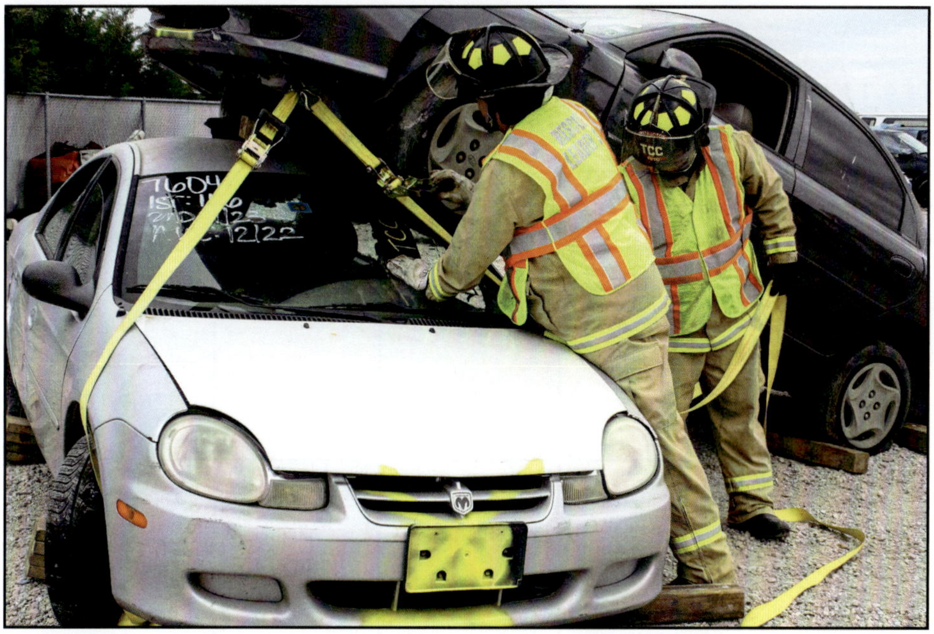

Figure 4.22 Rescuers practice marrying vehicles with a ratchet strap.

buckles, and ratchets. Uses straps in good condition (no frays or cuts in the webbing), with working ratchets and attached weight rating labels. Hooks can be flat safety hooks, wire hooks, and/or grade 80 grab hooks.

Rescuers use ratchet straps in numerous variations during stabilization operations, such as marrying a vehicle to an object or capturing a vehicle's suspensions. Rescuers also use ratchet straps to secure most rescue strut systems to vehicles. A ratchet strap may be the weak link in a tensioned buttress system.

NOTE: Rescuers must use appropriately rated straps for the situation.

Extrication Tools and Equipment

Acquiring the knowledge, skills, and abilities required to perform safe and effective vehicle extrication begins with learning the capabilities and limitations of the available tools and equipment. The tools and equipment procured by the response agency will depend upon the nature and extent of the rescue problems identified in the survey of the district required by NFPA 1670. The following sections that discuss the tools and equipment most commonly used in vehicle extrication incidents.

CAUTION
Wear appropriate PPE when using any extrication tools and equipment.

Hand Tools

A wide variety of hand tools are used in vehicle and machinery extrication. Most of these tools are the same tools used for structural fire fighting and other emergency work **(Table 4.1, p. 134)**. The following sections describe the hand tools that rescuers will use:

- Striking tools
- Prying tools

Section B • Chapter 4 – Tools and Equipment 133

Table 4.1
Table 4.1 Hand Tools Listed by Categorization

Striking	Prying	Cutting	Specialized	Lifting	Trench	Mechanic
Axes	Pry-axe	Chopping —Flat-head Axe —Pick-head Axe —Pry-Axe —Picks	Center Punch —Standard —Spring-Loaded	Screw Jacks —Bar Screw —Folding Screw	Short Handled Shovels	Sockets —Metric Set —Standard Set —Extensions —Large Ratchet —Small Ratchet
Battering Rams	Halligan	Snipping —Scissors —Shears —Tin Snips —Bolt Cutters —Wire Cutters	Glass Hammer	Rachet-Lever Jacks	Buckets —Collapsible —Canvas —Metal	Wrenches —Metric Set —Standard Set —Adjustable —Open-end —Closed-end
Ram Bars	Crowbar	Handsaws —Carpenter's Saw —Hacksaw —Coping Saw —Keyhole Saw —Windshield Cutters (Glass Saw)	Glass Saw			Pliers —Conventional —Channel-Lock® —Vise-Grip® —Wire Cutting
Punches	Claw Tool	Knives —Pocket —Linoleum —Utility —V-Blade				Screwdrivers —Metric Set —Standard Set —Phillips head —Flat Head —Various Sizes
Mallets	Pry Bar					Torx® Drivers (Star Drivers)
Sledge-hammers	Kelly Tool					
Mauls	Spanner Wrench					
Picks	Quic-Bar®					

- Cutting tools
- Mechanic's tools
- Specialized hand tools
- Lifting tools
- Trench tools

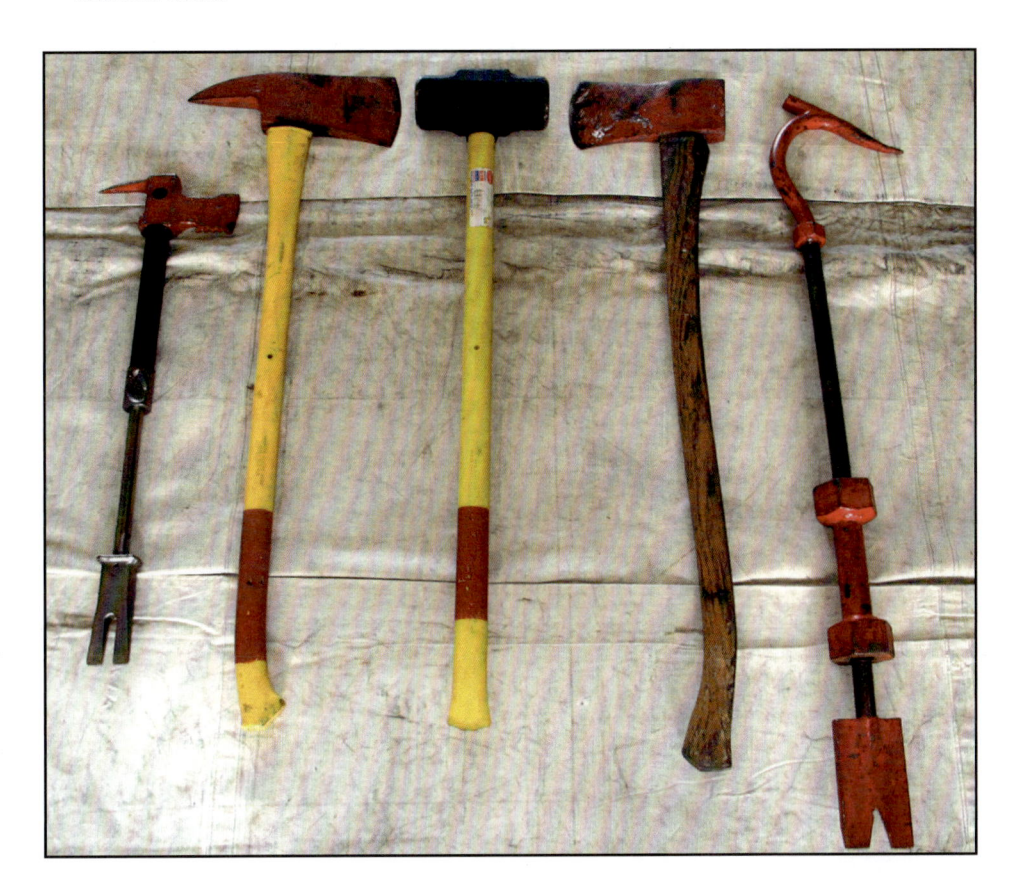

Figure 4.23 A selection of striking tools.

Striking Tools

The most common and basic hand tools are striking tools **(Figure 4.23)**. Most striking tools have a heavy metal head mounted on one end of a relatively long handle. This category includes:

- Axes
- Battering rams
- Ram bars
- Punches
- Mallets
- Hammers
- Sledgehammers or mauls
- Picks

Striking tools may cause serious crush or laceration injuries if used carelessly. Striking tools sometimes produce high-velocity chips and splinters capable of piercing skin and eyes. Take the following precautions to prevent injury:

- Wear proper protective clothing, helmet, and eyewear.
- Keep handles smooth.
- Ensure that all tool heads are well set.
- Keep the striking surface of the tool head free of chips and burrs.
- Keep axe blades clean and as sharp as their intended purpose and agency protocols dictate.
- Use striking tools with short, quick strokes. Long, sweeping strokes are more difficult to control and may strike anyone standing close by.

Prying Tools

Prying tools use leverage to provide a **mechanical advantage**. Using a prying tool properly can multiply the force applied. Prying tools may be used to pry open doors, windows, hoods, and trunk lids of vehicles **(Figure 4.24)**. These tools can even be used to lift vehicles or other heavy objects. Prying tools are excellent for widening a small opening for larger power tools to fit into. The following tools are examples of prying tools:

- Crowbar
- Pry bar
- Halligan (Hooligan) tool
- Claw tool
- Kelly tool
- Quic-Bar®

When used correctly, prying tools are safer than striking tools because of the absence of ballistic movement. However, prying tools can be just as dangerous as other types of tools if used incorrectly. For example, it is unsafe to strike the handle of a pry bar with another tool or to use a makeshift extension (sometimes called a cheater) on the tool handle. The most common type of cheater is a piece of pipe slipped over the end of a prying tool handle to lengthen it, thus providing additional leverage. Using a cheater can exert forces on the tool that are greater than the tool was designed to handle, which can destroy the tool and even cause serious injury to the operator or others. If a prying tool is inadequate for a particular application, an additional tool or a larger one should be used.

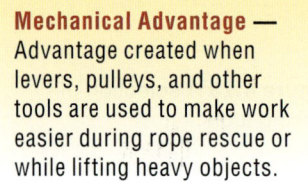

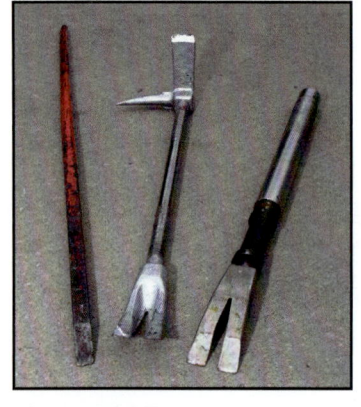

> **Mechanical Advantage** — Advantage created when levers, pulleys, and other tools are used to make work easier during rope rescue or while lifting heavy objects.

Figure 4.24 Three types of prying tools.

WARNING!
Do not use prying tools as striking tools unless designed for that purpose.

Cutting Tools

Cutting tools are the most diversified of the tool groups. Some cutting tools are designed to cut only specific types of materials **(Figure 4.25)**. Do not misuse a cutting tool by using it to cut a material it was not designed to cut or by using the tool in a way for which it was not designed. Misuse can destroy the tool and endanger the operator. This section addresses four distinct groups of manual cutting tools:

- Chopping tools
- Snipping tools
- Saws
- Knives

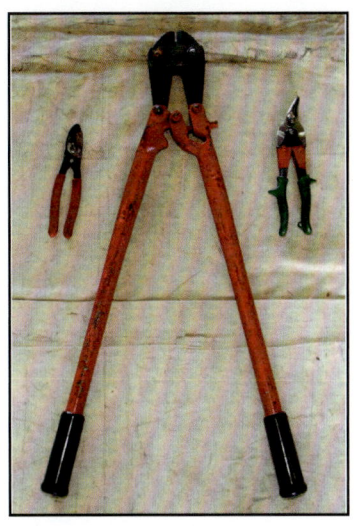

Figure 4.25 Three types of cutting tools.

Chopping tools. Chopping tools have a metal head with a cutting edge attached to one end of a relatively long handle. Chopping tools include the flat-head axe, pick-head axe, pry-axe, and various types of picks **(Figure 4.26)**. Take the following precautions to ensure maximum cutting efficiency of these tools while preventing corrosion:

- Keep the cutting edge free of paint and covered with a thin coating of light-grade machine oil.
- Keep the blade sharp, but not so sharp that the cutting edge chips when the tool is used.
- Check tool handles regularly for looseness, cracks, splinters, or warping.
- Maintain cutting tools according to agency protocols.

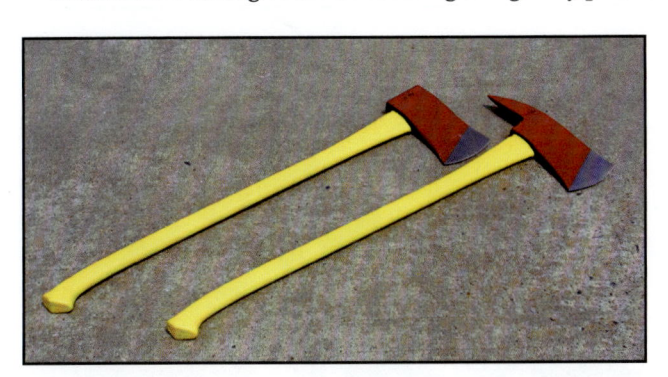

Figure 4.26 A flat head and a pick ax.

Snipping tools. Use snipping tools when the material must be cut in a controlled fashion or where space does not allow the use of larger tools. Snipping tools are generally safer than other types of cutting devices when working close to a victim. They are most effective on relatively thin material that can easily fit within the jaws of the tool. Snipping tools include various kinds of scissors or shears, tin snips, bolt cutters, and wire cutters.

The most common types of metal cutters are bolt cutters and insulated wire cutters, sometimes called *hot wire cutters*. These tools are similar in appearance, but they are not interchangeable. Using bolt cutters instead of insulated wire cutters when attempting to cut an electrical wire can result in electrocution. Only use cutting tools that are approved by a recognized agency, such as Underwriters Laboratories (UL), Underwriters' Laboratories of Canada (ULC), or FM Global, and maintained according to the manufacturer's recommendations to cut an energized electrical wire.

Section B • Chapter 4 – Tools and Equipment **137**

> **WARNING!**
> Do NOT use insulated wire cutters to cut downed power lines to facilitate a vehicle rescue.

Saws. Use handsaws on objects that require a controlled cut but do not fit into the jaws of a manual opposing-jaw cutter. Using handsaws takes more time than using powered saws or cutters; however, handsaws are safer to use when working close to a victim or when working in a hazardous atmosphere **(Figure 4.27)**. Handsaws commonly used for extrication include hacksaws and windshield cutters.

Keep all saw blades sharp, clean, and lightly oiled. Increase the cutting efficiency of any saw by periodically spraying the surface of the material being cut with bee's wax, a water-based cutting fluid, or soapy water to reduce friction between the material and the saw blade **(Figure 4.28)**.

The most specialized saws are the windshield cutter and the glass saw **(Figure 4.29)**. Windshield cutters have a short, heavy blade composed of coarse teeth. They are designed to quickly and efficiently remove a windshield from a vehicle. Glass saws consist of a glass cutting blade attached to a two-handed handle. They saw through laminated safety glass. Some glass saws have a built-in spike or spring-loaded punch. Protect any victims in the vehicle prior to removing glass with any device.

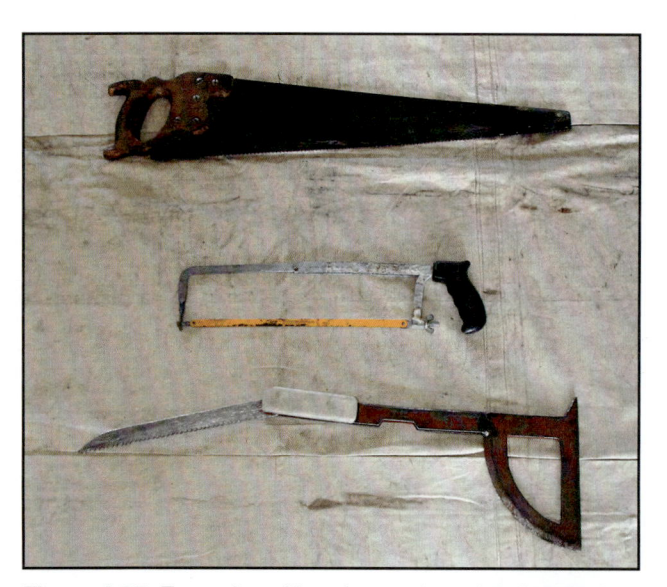

Figure 4.27 Examples of hand saws that might be used during an extrication operation.

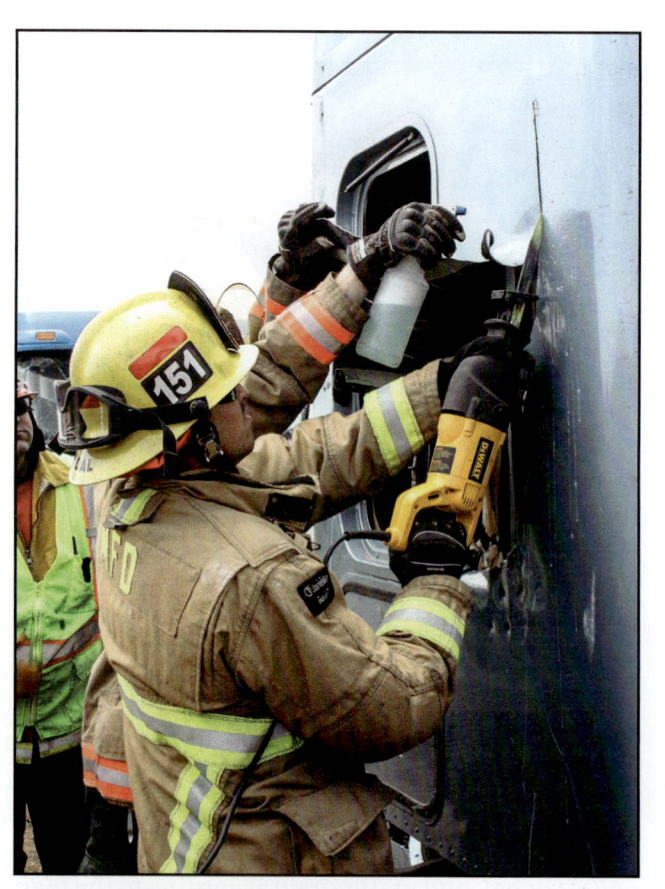

Figure 4.28 Soapy water reduces friction between metal and the saw blade.

138 Section B • Chapter 4 – Tools and Equipment

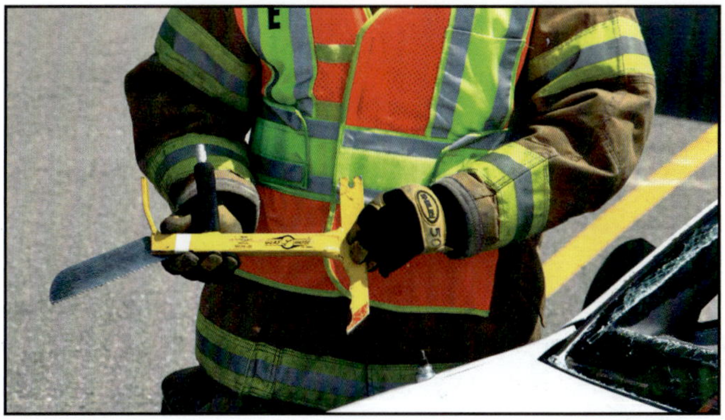

Figure 4.29 A glass saw is useful when cutting windshield glass.

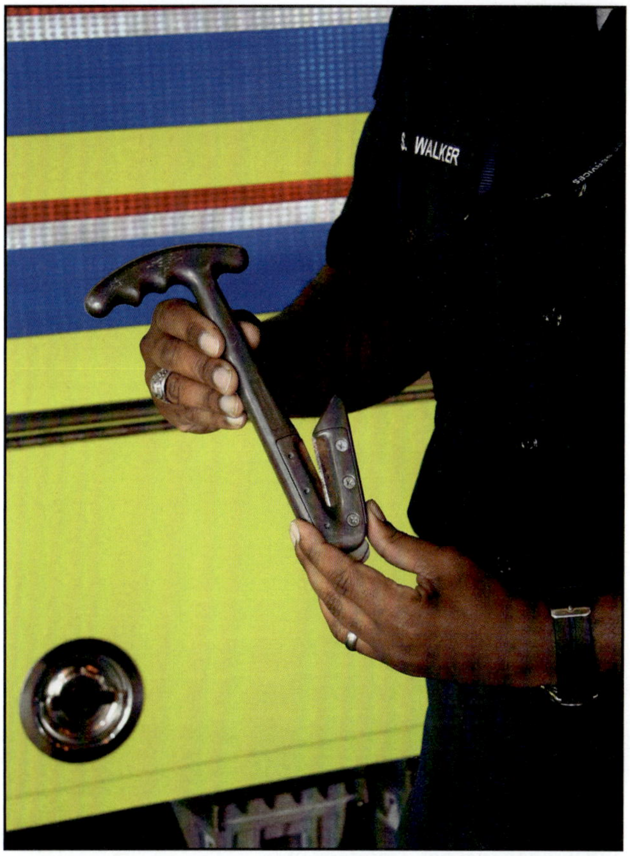

Knives. Various types of knives may be useful in vehicle extrications. While a sharp pocket knife may be adequate in some situations, knives specially designed for vehicle rescue are usually more efficient. Specially designed knives include V-blade (seat belt) knives, linoleum knives, and utility knives **(Figure 4.30)**. A locking-knife or fixed blade is preferred. Knife blades should be sharpened or replaced after each use to ensure that they are in optimum working condition for the next use.

Mechanic's Tools

In some cases, especially when working close to a trapped victim, it is better to disassemble a part of the vehicle rather than use a power tool to cut it. Disassembly eliminates the noise, vibration, and sparks that powered cutting tools produce. Rescue vehicles should carry a basic set of ordinary mechanic's tools — primarily sockets, wrenches, pliers, and drivers.

Figure 4.30 A V-blade can be used to cut seatbelts.

Sockets. Carry two sets of sockets — metric and standard — because vehicles manufactured outside the U.S. use nuts and bolts with metric dimensions, not standard (SAE) **(Figure 4.31, p. 140)**. Each set should include standard and deep-well sockets in a range of common sizes, extensions, and at least one ratchet wrench or socket handle. Having two socket wrenches — one large and one small — is recommended. In addition to allowing more options in their use, if more than one wrench is available, more than one disassembly operation can be performed at the same time.

Wrenches. Just as with socket sets, carry two sets of combination wrenches — metric and standard. Combination wrenches have an open head on one end and a closed head on the other end. Both sets of wrenches should include a range of common sizes. Also carry adjustable wrenches of various sizes.

Pliers. The tool inventory of any rescue vehicle should include a variety of types and sizes of pliers **(Figure 4.32, p. 140)**. Carry various sizes of the following types of pliers:

- Conventional pliers
- Channel-Lock type pliers
- Vise-Grip® pliers
- Wire cutting pliers

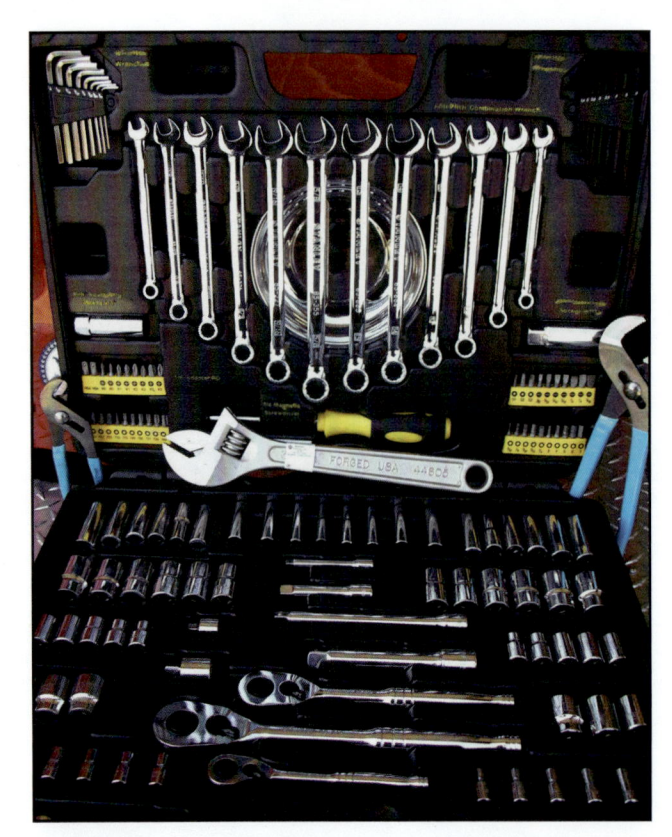

Figure 4.31 A mechanic's socket and wrench tool set. *Courtesy of Alan Braun, University of Missouri Fire and Rescue Training Institute.*

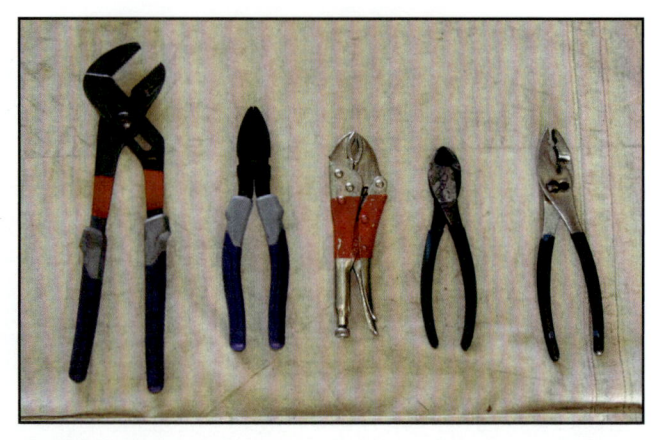

Figure 4.32 A variety of pliers that might be useful during extrication operations.

Drivers. The rescue vehicle's tool inventory should also include a variety of screw drivers and nut drivers. Include both Phillips- and slot-head screwdrivers in multiple sizes. Carry two sets of nut drivers — metric and standard — in a range of common sizes. Include other drivers, such as Torx® drivers (sometimes called star drivers).

Specialized Hand Tools

Some of the hand tools used in extrication are so specialized that they are almost never used for anything else. Examples of specialized hand tools are center punches and glass hammers.

Center punches. There are two basic types of center punches: standard and spring-loaded. A standard center punch is similar to a small chisel but with a pointed end. A standard center punch can be used to break tempered glass, but it must be struck with another tool to provide the breaking force. A spring-loaded center punch looks similar to a standard punch but provides its own breaking force when the tip is pressed against the glass.

Glass hammers. Glass hammers consist of a pointed metal head attached to a plastic handle. They are used to break tempered glass by striking the glass with the point of the metal head. Some have a built-in seat belt cutter in the handle (**Figure 4.33**).

Lifting Tools

With the exception of pneumatic lifting bags and cushions, which are discussed later in this chapter, the primary lifting tools used in vehicle extrication are various forms of non-hydraulic jacks. The jacks most often used are various screw jacks and ratchet-lever jacks. Although these tools are effective for their designed purposes, they do not have the same motive force as hydraulic jacks.

Screw jacks. Screw jacks are the easiest jacks to operate since they can be elevated or depressed simply by turning a threaded shaft. Check screw jacks for wear after each use and keep them clean and lightly lubricated, particularly the threaded shaft. Check the foot plates on which the jacks rest for wear or damage. The two most common types of screw jacks used in vehicle extrication are the bar screw jack and the folding screw jack.

Section B • Chapter 4 – Tools and Equipment

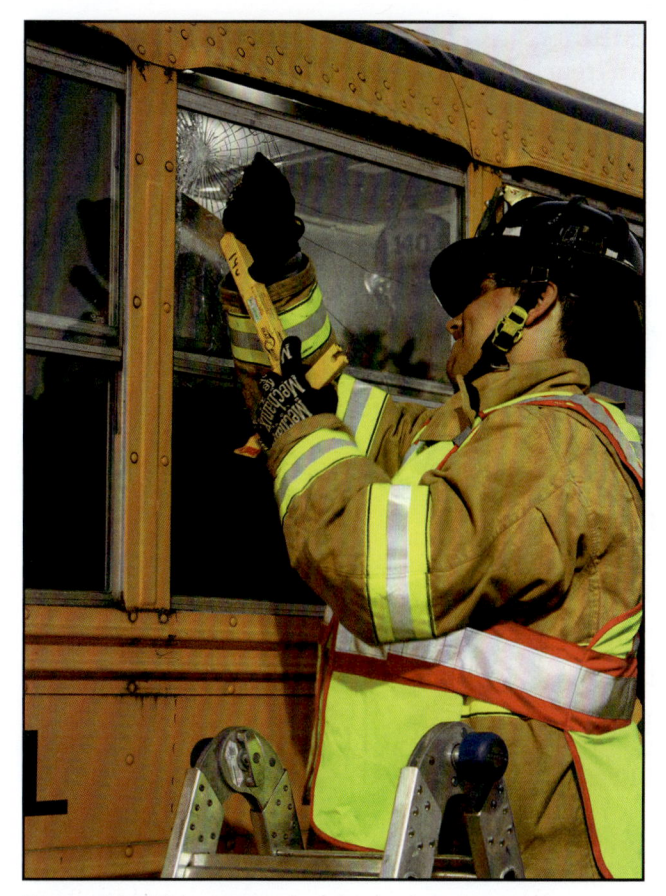

Figure 4.33 This rescuer is using a glass hammer.

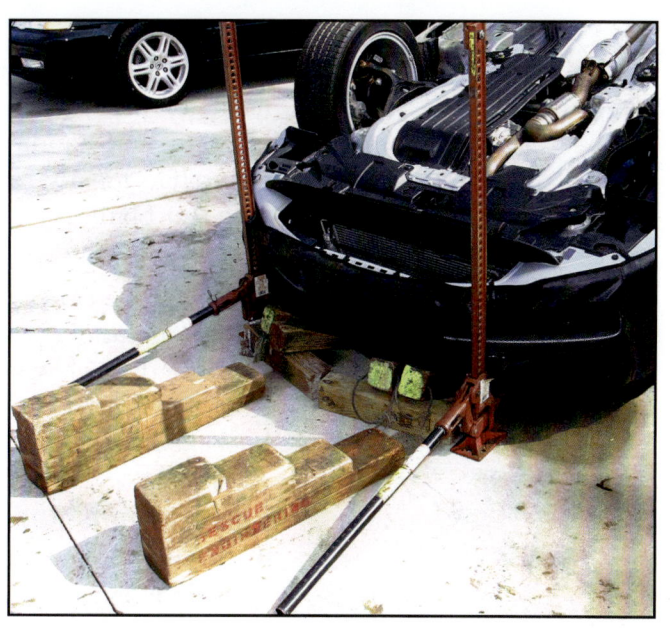

Figure 4.34 Ratchet jacks in use during an extrication training session.

The bar screw jack is an excellent tool for stabilizing loads but is considered impractical for lifting. The jack is extended or retracted by turning a threaded vertical shaft with a bar inserted into one of several holes in the jack's head.

The folding screw jack, also known as a scissor jack, consists of a top and bottom plate separated by levers that are drawn together or pushed apart by turning a threaded shaft. When fully collapsed, folding screw jacks fit into relatively small spaces (4 to 6 inch [100 to 150 mm] clearance). Folding jacks are not always stable under load and are therefore considered safe only for light loads.

Ratchet-lever jacks. Sometimes called Hi-Lift® jacks, these jacks consist of a vertical metal shaft, with notches or gear cogs along one side that fits into a metal base plate **(Figure 4.34)**. A movable jacking carriage fits around the shaft and has two ratchets on the notched side. One ratchet holds the carriage in position while the other works with a lever to move the carriage up or down. The ratchet jack is a good medium-duty jack but is the least stable under load. This type of jack can be used for limited spreading and pulling operations in the absence of hydraulic rams.

Hi-Lift® jacks carried on emergency apparatus should be dedicated to extrication tasks only and should be designed and purpose built specifically for extrication. Standard, factory issued and built components are not suitable for extrication operations.

Trench Tools

Due to space constraints in a trench, special scaled-down tools are sometimes needed to perform routine tasks such as removing dirt and debris. Trenching tools are short-handled shovels with a blade that can be swiveled 90 degrees to form a hoe. Ideally, rescue units should carry picks and other tools equipped with short handles for working in trenches; the working ends of these tools may be scaled down as well.

Collapsible canvas buckets are used to remove dirt from trenches during rescue operations. Conventional metal buckets can also be used, but they increase the risk of injury to rescuers in the trench if a bucket is dropped from above. Attach ropes to the bucket handles for hauling them up. Only use buckets with secure handles.

Electric Tools and Equipment

A variety of electrical tools and equipment are used in vehicle extrication. These tools may be DC battery powered, 110-volt AC, or both. Common electric tools and equipment include:

- Electric spreaders and cutters
- Electric impact wrenches
- Electric drills and drivers
- Portable lights
- Auxiliary electrical equipment

NOTE: Electrical saws are discussed along with other power saws later in this chapter.

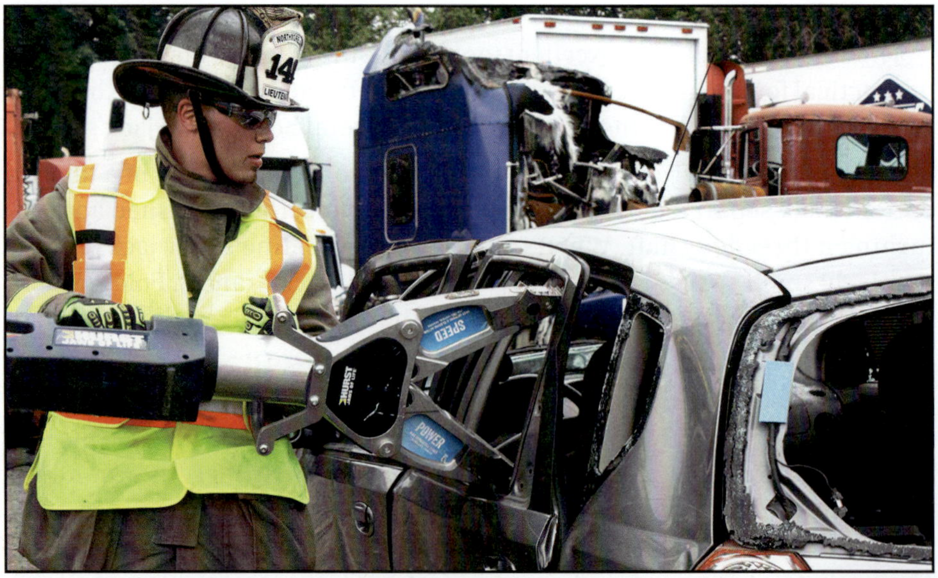

Figure 4.35 Powered electric spreaders serve many rescue functions.

Electric Spreaders and Cutters

Electrically powered spreaders and cutters are lighter and more portable than many hydraulic units. Electric spreaders can be equipped with conventional spreaders for pushing and pulling, with optional cutters, or with combination spreader/cutters **(Figure 4.35)**. These tools come in electric/gear-driven or electric/hydraulic-driven configurations.

142   Section B • Chapter 4 – Tools and Equipment

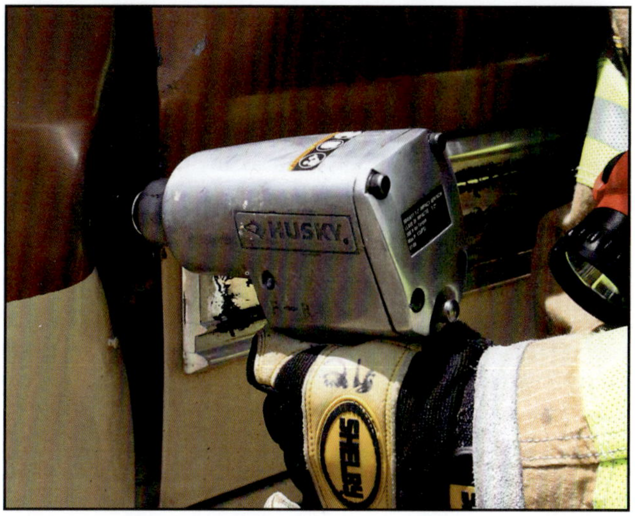

Figure 4.36 An electric impact wrench used to remove door hinge bolts. *Courtesy of Mark Stuckey, City of Owasso Fire Department.*

Electric Impact Wrenches

Electric wrenches are similar to the pneumatic impact wrenches discussed later in this chapter. They are used for the same purposes as the pneumatic versions **(Figure 4.36)**. Depending upon the brand and model, they may or may not be as powerful as the pneumatic wrenches.

Electric Drills and Drivers

Improvements in the batteries used to power electric drills and drivers have made these tools extremely useful at vehicle extrication incidents **(Figure 4.37)**. With replaceable battery packs and a variety of bits, these tools produce sufficient torque and rotational speed to be effective for use in dismantling vehicle components.

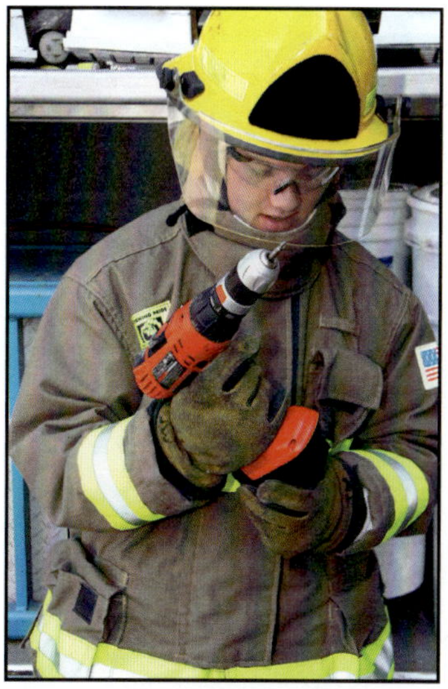

Portable Lights

Portable lights are used when the scene is beyond the effective reach of stationary lights or when additional scene lighting is necessary **(Figure 4.38)**. Portable lights generally range from 300 to 1,000 watts. They may be supplied by a cord from the power plant or may have an attached power unit. The Code of Federal Regulations requires that all such cords be equipped with **ground fault circuit interrupters**. The lights usually have handles for safe carrying and large bases for stability. Some portable lights are mounted on telescoping stands.

Figure 4.37 Rescuers now use a variety of battery powered tools such as this drill.

> **Ground Fault Circuit Interrupter (GFCI)** — Device designed to protect against electrical shock; when grounding occurs, the device opens a circuit to shut off the flow of electricity. *Also known as* Ground Fault Indicator (GFI) Receptacle.

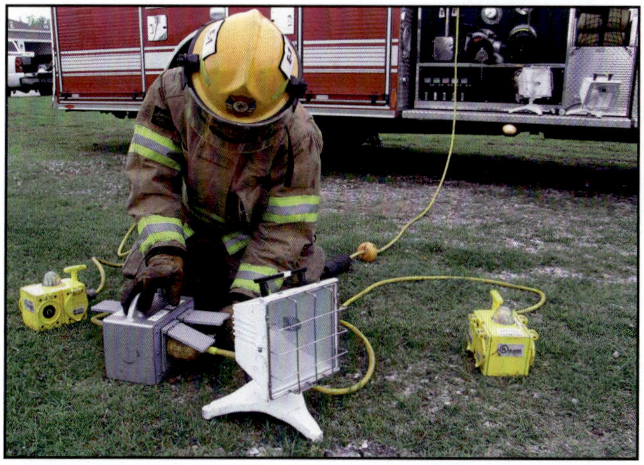

Figure 4.38 Portable lighting can be positioned on the ground.

Section B • Chapter 4 – Tools and Equipment 143

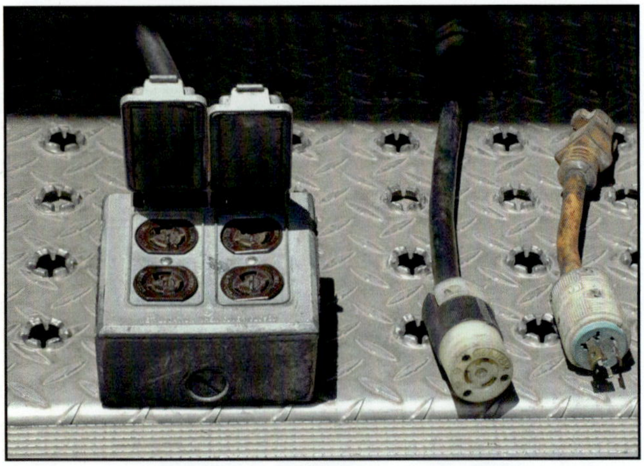

Figure 4.39 An electrical junction box and two types of adapters. Adapters allow equipment to be interchanged between different types of sizes of receptacles. *Courtesy of Ted Boothroyd.*

Auxiliary Electrical Equipment

A variety of other equipment may be used in conjunction with the previously described electric tools and equipment. Electrical cables or extension cords are necessary to conduct electric power to portable equipment. The most common size cable is a 12-gauge, 3-wire type. The cord may be stored in coils, on portable cord reels, or on vehicle-mounted automatic rewind reels. Twist-lock receptacles provide secure, safe connections. Electrical cable must be adequately insulated, waterproof, and have no exposed wires.

Junction boxes may be used when multiple connections are needed (**Figure 4.39**). The junction box is supplied by one inlet from the power plant and has several outlets. Many junction boxes have a small light on top that stays on as long as power is supplied to the unit.

In areas where automatic or mutual aid operations are common, some agencies may have different sizes or types of receptacles (for example, one has two prongs; the other three). Carry adapters so that equipment can be interconnected when necessary. Also carry adapters to allow rescuers to plug their equipment into conventional electrical outlets.

Signaling Devices

Signaling devices encompass a broad range of communication possibilities, not only to enhance scene safety and efficiency, but to assist in locating victims and improving rescue capabilities. From simple one-on-one communication about the extrication incident, to signaling approaching drivers through advanced warning and traffic channeling measures, most incidents use signals or indicators.

Signaling devices that are most commonly used at the scene of an incident are usually audio or visual in nature. Audio devices may include portable radios, cell phones, air horns, sirens, or even sonar victim location equipment. Visual devices can consist of simple hand gestures, flashlights, thermal imaging cameras, or chalk/paint/grease pencil marking kits for command boards or to warn of potential dangers. In addition, traffic cones, perimeter stakes, and boundary markers may warn the public or bystanders of potentially unsafe areas.

Voltage Detection Devices

When sizing-up an extrication incident, many potential hazards may exist that could harm personnel or the victim(s). Always anticipate, identify, and isolate electrical hazards prior to engaging in extrication activities. Electrical hazards may include downed power lines or a vehicle resting on a ground transformer. Every organization should have access to a power detection device for these situations. These devices usually detect AC electricity from frequencies between 20 to 100 Hz, and, in some cases, can alert the rescuers of an energy source from a safe distance. These detectors will not detect electricity in enclosed conduit nor will they detect DC electricity. Always contact the local utility company to verify power isolation and never assume that a power source is dead until verified by the power company.

Power Saws

Power saws are available in various designs, depending upon their intended purpose. Know the limitations of each type of power saw. Used improperly, power saws can be dangerous for both rescuers and trapped victims. Following a few simple safety rules will prevent most injuries from power saws:

- Match the saw to the task and the material to be cut. Never force a saw beyond its design limitations. Two things may occur: tool failure (including breakage) and/or injury to the operator.
- Use blankets or salvage covers to protect victims from the sparks, splinters, and debris chips created when using power saws.
- Wear appropriate protective equipment, including gloves, eye protection, and hearing protection.
- Do not use any power saw when working in a flammable atmosphere or near flammable liquids.
- Keep unprotected and nonessential people out of the work area.
- Follow manufacturer's guidelines for proper saw operation.
- Keep blades and chains well sharpened. A dull saw is more likely to malfunction than a sharp one.

The saws described in the following sections that follow may be powered by pressurized water, hydraulic pumps, gasoline, gas-oil mixtures, or electricity. Power saws can include the following types:

- Reciprocating saws
- Rotary saws
- Circular saws
- Chain saws
- Portable band saws

> ### Electric Saws
> Except for reciprocating saws, the electric saws used in vehicle extrication are electrically operated versions of the other power saws discussed in this section. Electrically operated saws include chain saws and circular saws. Like all other tools, electrically operated tools have advantages and disadvantages. They are often lighter in weight and quieter in operation than gasoline-driven tools. However, they must be tethered to a power supply by a power cord, and unless they are designed to be intrinsically safe, they cannot be operated in potentially flammable atmospheres.

CAUTION
The rotation of the blade of these saws creates significant torque that can cause the operator to lose control of the saw.

Reciprocating Saws

Reciprocating saws are easy to control and are well suited for cutting metal or wood. They produce far fewer sparks and airborne debris than rotary rescue saws. A reciprocating saw may be required when overhead cuts must be made or in areas with limited space **(Figure 4.40)**. Reciprocating saws have a short, straight blade that moves forward and backward in an action similar to a handsaw. Some have an optional orbital operation as well.

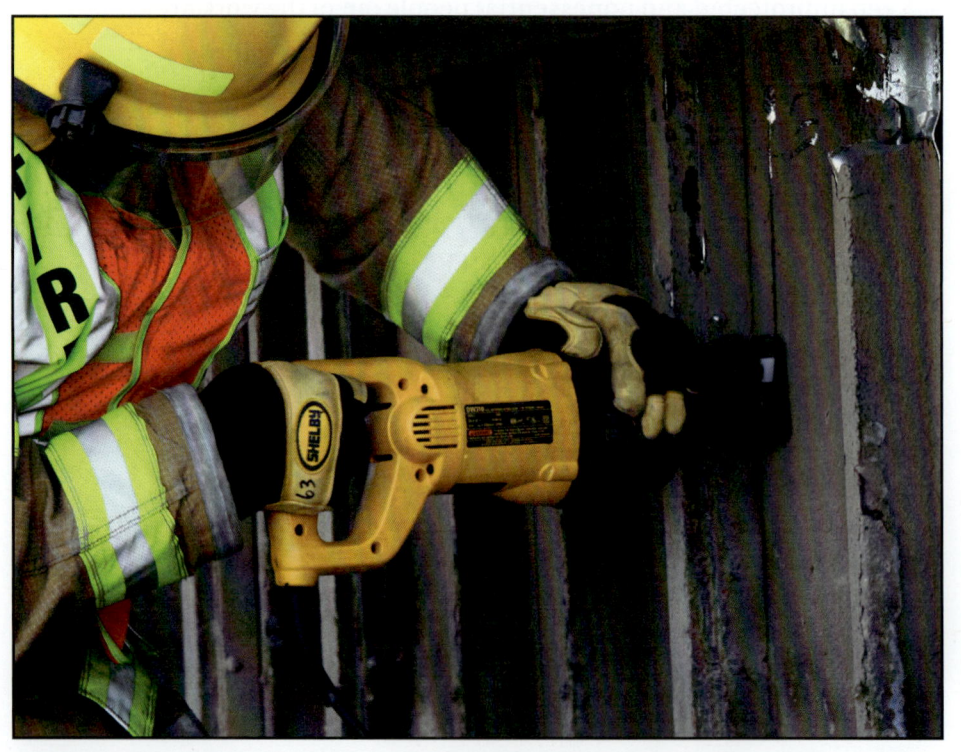

Figure 4.40 A reciprocating saw can cut straight lines in small spaces.

When equipped with metal cutting blades, reciprocating saws are extremely effective at bus and passenger vehicle extrication incidents. Other than the frame, these saws can easily cut almost any portion of a bus or passenger vehicle body.

Reciprocating saws can be powered by gasoline with the following disadvantages:

- Heavier and more awkward than the pneumatic and electric models
- May not be used in confined or oxygen deficient spaces
- Produce carbon monoxide

NOTE: Reciprocating saws are much easier to control and are safer to use than circular saws.

Rotary Saws

Also called rotary rescue saws, rotary saws will cut a variety of materials when equipped with the appropriate material-specific blade. Blade types include steel blades with carbide tips for cutting wood, Carborundum or other abrasive blades for cutting masonry and metals, and diamond-impregnated blades for cutting virtually anything. Because abrasive blades can degrade when exposed to hydrocarbon vapors, do not store them in the same compartment with fuel containers.

Use rescue saws with extreme care in order to avoid injury to operators and trapped victims. Protect victims and rescue personnel in close proximity to the cutting operation from sparks, chips, and splinters. Keep at least one charged hoseline standing by whenever cutting metal. In addition to providing fire protection, use water from the hoseline to cool the saw blade by applying a fine mist to the blade while it is in operation. Start the cooling water before cutting begins and continue it throughout the cutting operation. Putting cold water on a hot blade may cause it to shatter.

Circular Saws

Electrically or battery-operated circular saws used in vehicle extrication are usually the same as those used in construction. They are primarily designed for cutting wood and can be useful when cutting cribbing material on site. When equipped with a metal-cutting blade, circular saws can make straight-line cuts in metal **(Figure 4.41)**.

Chain Saws

Electric, gasoline, and hydraulically powered chain saws can be useful at some extrication incidents. They are often used for clearing brush and trees.

Chain saws with carbide-tipped chains can penetrate a large variety of materials, including light sheet metal. Although carbide-tipped chains cost almost four times as much as standard chains, they last considerably longer.

Chain saws often create more sparks, vibration and noise than other saws while cutting the sheet metal and plastic parts of most vehicles. These characteristics can frighten trapped victims in close proximity to the cutting operation. Additionally, victims are in danger of being struck by the cutting chain if it breaks during the cutting operation.

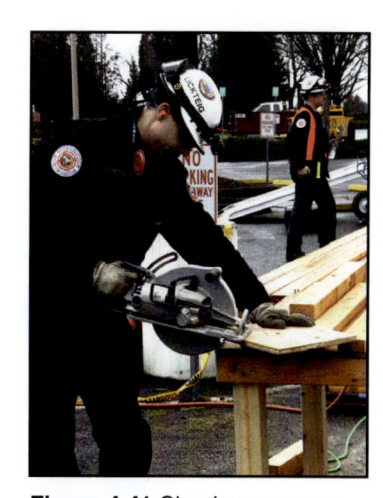

Figure 4.41 Circular saws are commonly available and easy to handle.

Portable Band Saws

Due to their superior cutting ability and lightweight design, portable band saws in certain circumstances, are the tool of choice for many rescuers. These saws are used extensively during impalement and industrial entrapment responses.

Portable band saws come in either cordless (battery-operated) or 110-volt corded configurations. The battery-type have smaller cutting capacity than the corded version, but corded saws require a power source.

Portable band saws are useful in cutting the ultra and advanced high strength metals found in new vehicle technology. They have the following advantages over reciprocating saws, grinders, and hydraulic cutters:

- They undergo minimal vibration since their blades spin in one direction (they do not reciprocate).
- They give off minimal heat.
- They rarely spark.
- They will not cause an object to fracture.

These advantages provide for better victim care and greater rescuer safety. They reduce hazards for victims and operators and allow for increased control and operation of the tool.

Hydraulic Tools and Equipment

There are two categories of hydraulic tools used for vehicle extrication: power-driven and manual. While most agencies that deliver vehicle extrication services use powered hydraulic tools and equipment on most extrication incidents, some situations require the use of manual hydraulic tools and equipment. The following sections describe both power-driven hydraulic tools and manual hydraulic tools.

CAUTION
Know the capabilities and limitations of the hydraulic tools and equipment available.

Power-Driven Hydraulic Tools

The development of power-driven hydraulic extrication tools has revolutionized the process of extricating victims. The versatility of uses, speed, and superior power of these tools has made them the primary tools for most extrication situations. These tools receive power from hydraulic fluid under pressure supplied through special hoses from a pump, commonly referred to as the *power unit*. The following means power hydraulic pumps:

- Compressed air
- Pressurized water
- Power-take-offs (PTOs)
- Electric motors
- Diesel or gasoline engines
- Battery

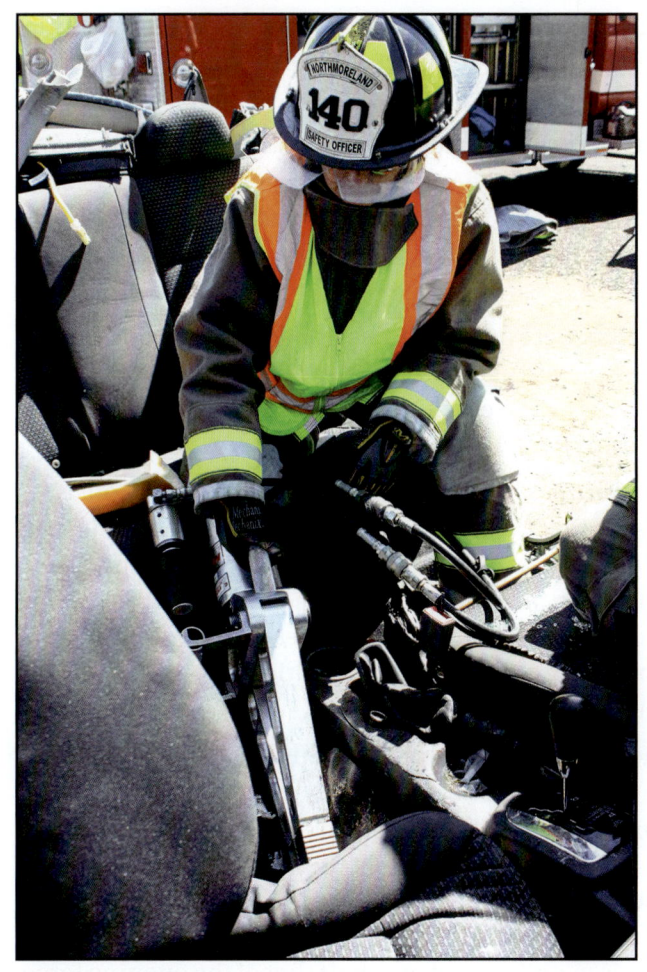

Figure 4.42 Hydraulic spreader being used to displace a seat during extrication training.

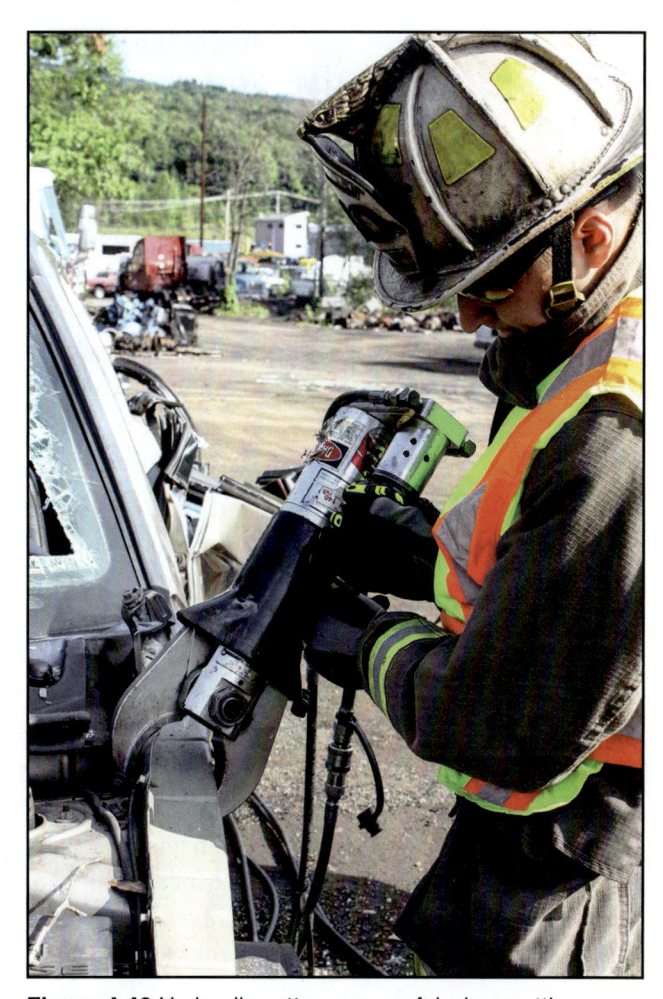

Figure 4.43 Hydraulic cutters are useful when cutting vehicle components.

Power units may be portable and carried with the tool, or may be permanently mounted on a vehicle and connected to a hose reel. The tools powered by these units may be powered by manually operated pumps if the power unit fails. Rescuers use the following power-driven hydraulic tools in vehicle extrication:

- Spreaders
- Cutters
- Combination spreader/cutters
- Pedal Cutters
- Rams

Spreaders. Powered hydraulic spreaders were the first powered hydraulic tools available for vehicle extrication **(Figure 4.42)**. They conduct a variety of different operations involving spreading, lifting, pulling, or displacing. Depending on the brand and model, some tools can produce more than 100,000 psi (700 000 kPa) of force. The tips of some large tools may spread more than 40 inches (1 000 mm), although rescuers use many smaller, lighter units.

Cutters. Hydraulic cutters can be used to cut roof support posts and other objects. These cutters can cut almost any object (metal, plastic, wood) that will fit between their blades **(Figure 4.43)**. However, some models cannot cut case-hardened steel or high-strength low-alloy (HSLA) steel. Cutters are limited because materials that they cannot cut are often located at potential impact points and at the corners of the compartment, prime cutting locations for vehicle extrication operations.

Cutters come in a variety of performance level ratings. NFPA 1936, *Standard on Powered Rescue Tools*, divides these ratings into five material categories based on the type of material: A, B, C, D, and E. It couples these categories with a numerical performance level rating (1-9) which indicates the size of the material category.

Pedal cutters. Pedal cutters were originally designed to cut reinforced steel bars in construction. These powerful devices easily cut through accelerator, brake, and clutch pedal arms. They can cut virtually anything that will fit between the blade and the anvil.

Combination spreader/cutters. Combination spreader/cutters consist of two arms equipped with spreader tips that can be used for pulling or pushing with cutters on the insides of the arms. These tools are excellent for use on small initial response vehicles or in areas where limited resources prevent the purchase of larger and more expensive individual spreader and cutting tools. The combination tool's spreading and cutting capabilities may be more or less than those of the individual units **(Figure 4.44)**.

Rams. Rams are designed primarily for straight pushing operations, although they are also effective at pulling **(Figure 4.45)**. They are especially valuable when it is necessary to push objects further apart than the maximum opening distance of the hydraulic spreaders. The largest of these rams can extend from a closed length of 36 inches (900 mm) to an extended length of more than 60 inches (1 500 mm). With extensions, these rams can extend up to 75 inches (1 900 mm). The closing force is usually about one-half that of the opening force.

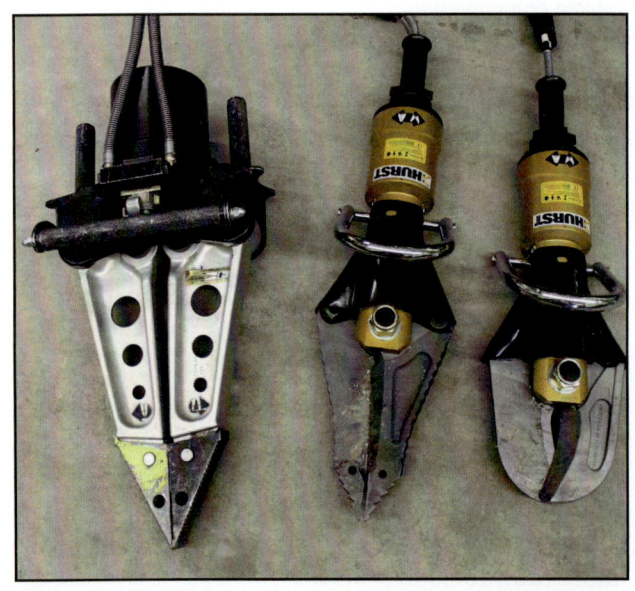

Figure 4.44 Spreaders, combination spreader/cutters and cutters are commonly used at an incident scene. *Courtesy of Shad Cooper/Wyoming State Fire Marshal's Office.*

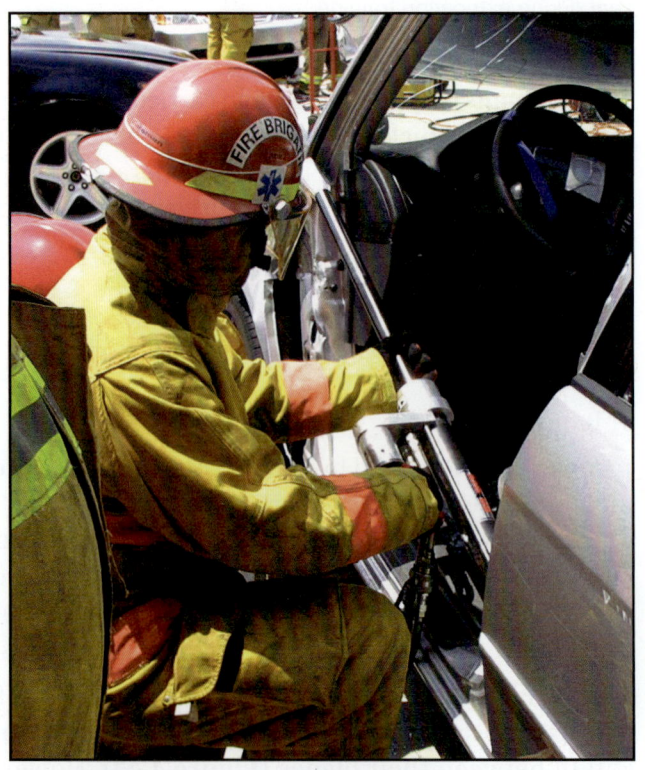

Figure 4.45 This rescuer is using a hydraulic ram to roll a dashboard.

Telescoping rams are also available. From a retracted length of as little as 12 inches (300 mm), some telescoping rams will extend to more than 60 inches (1 500 mm). Unlike conventional hydraulic rams, telescoping rams cannot be used for pulling. However, telescoping rams can have the same pushing force as conventional rams. They are available in two- and three-stage rams. After the first stage, the pushing force decreases by half for each additional stage.

Scratches or damage to a ram may render the tool inoperable. Do not side-load rams when using them during operation. Place rams in line with the desired load(s), and prevent any metal from contacting the piston section of the ram.

Manual Hydraulic Tools

Manual hydraulic tools operate on the same principles as powered hydraulic tools except that the hydraulic pump is powered by someone operating a pump lever. Manual hydraulic tools operate slower than powered hydraulic tools and with more limited range of operation. Two manual hydraulic tools are used most frequently in vehicle extrication: the hydraulic jack and the Porta-Power® system.

> **WARNING!**
> Never work under a load solely supported by a jack. Remember: lift an inch, crib an inch.

> **Jack Safety**
>
> When using any kind of jack, hydraulic or otherwise, ensure that the jack has a good, solid base and that the load is additionally supported by adequate blocking and cribbing. Block and crib the load as it is lifted to reduce the chances of it falling. The weight of the load being lifted is transmitted to the base of the jack. Therefore, to prevent the jack from sinking into the surface, place it on a weight-distributing base. This spreads the force placed on the jack. The base may be a wide board or steel plate; it should be solid, flat, and level. If it is not level, it should be shimmed level, while making sure enough room remains to place the jack. Only operate hydraulic jacks within the orientation for which they were manufactured.

Hydraulic jacks. Hydraulic jacks are excellent devices for many heavy lifting situations when used in conjunction with appropriate stabilization techniques **(Figure 4.46, p. 152)**. Hydraulic jacks are available in capacities up to 20 tons or larger.

Porta-Power®. The Porta-Power® tool system is an auto body shop tool used for vehicle extrication **(Figure 4.47, p. 152)**. It operates by transmitting hydraulic pressure from a hand-operated pump through a hose to a tool assembly. A number of different tool accessories give the Porta-Power® a variety of applications.

The Porta-Power® has accessories that allow it to be operated in narrow places in which the jack will not fit or cannot be operated. However, assembling complex combinations of accessories and the actual operation of the Porta-Power® is time consuming.

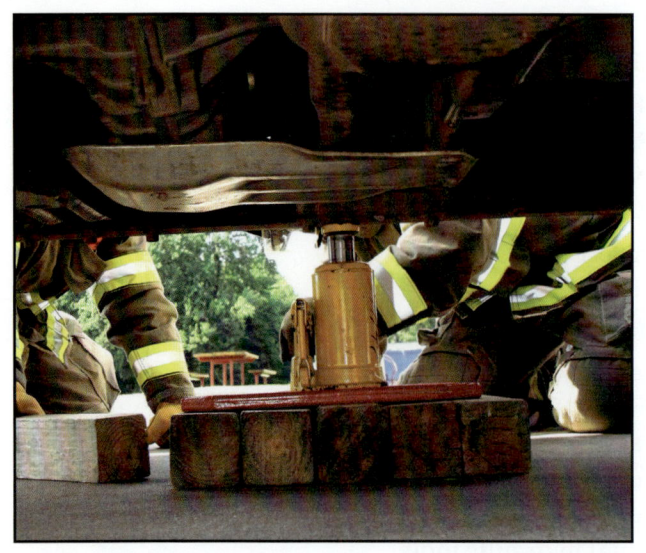

Figure 4.46 A hydraulic jack can be useful when lifting a vehicle.

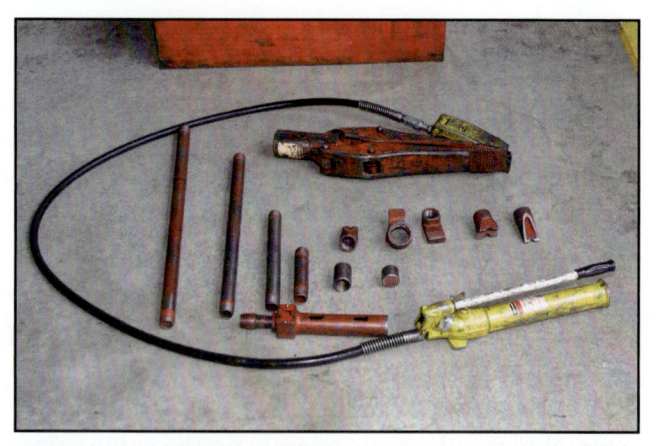

Figure 4.47 The Porta-Power® unit is largely replaced by other tools, but may still be used for extrication evolutions.

Pneumatic Tools and Equipment

Pneumatic tools use the energy of compressed air for power. Vehicle-mounted air compressors, apparatus brake system compressors, SCBA tanks, or cascade system cylinders can all provide air pressure. The most commonly used pneumatic tools in vehicle extrication include:

- Pneumatic chisels and hammers
- Pneumatic wrenches
- Pneumatic saws
- Pneumatic lifting bags and cushions

Pneumatic Chisels and Hammers

Most pneumatic-powered chisels (also called *air chisels*, *air hammers*, or *impact hammers*) are designed to operate at air pressures between 90 and 150 psi (630 and 1,050 kPa). Others operate up to 300 psi (2 100 kPa). Each tool should be operated at the manufacturer's recommended operating pressure.

Air chisels can be especially effective for cutting through the roof, roof support posts or doorjambs, seat bolts, and door lock assemblies. They are good for cutting medium to heavy-gauge sheet metal and for popping rivets and bolts. Cutting heavier gauge steel or other metals requires larger air supplies and higher pressures.

A variety of air chisel bits are available to fit many vehicle extrication situations. These include cutting bits and special bits for operations such as breaking locks or driving plugs. All bits should be kept sharpened and free of defects at all times.

> **WARNING!**
> Never use compressed oxygen to power pneumatic tools. Mixing pure oxygen with tool lubricants can result in fire or violent explosion.

> **CAUTION**
> Sparks produced when using air chisels in hazardous atmospheres may ignite flammable vapors.

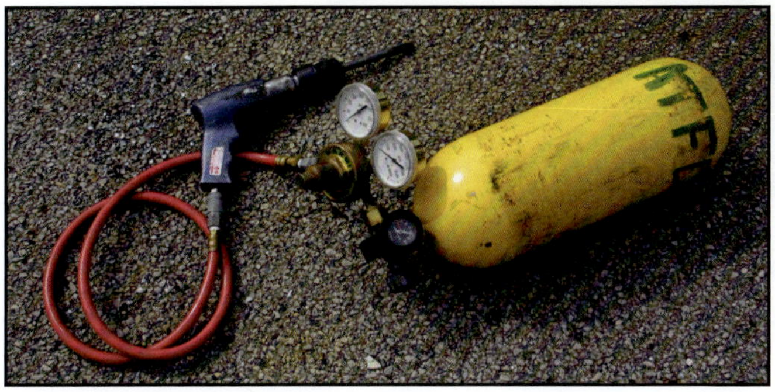

Figure 4.48 Pneumatic tools connected to SCBA cylinders use a high quantity of compressed air, but are very portable.

Pneumatic Wrenches

Air ratchets or impact wrenches are extremely useful for disassembling vehicle components **(Figure 4.48)**. With an adequate air supply and the right size socket, these tools can remove nuts and bolts rapidly. Their chief disadvantage is that they are quite noisy in operation.

Pneumatic Saws

Pneumatic saws include both rotary and reciprocating saws and are effective for cutting a variety of materials. They are noisy and can produce sparks.

The pneumatic whizzer saw is an air-driven cutting device with several advantages over other types of power saws **(Figure 4.49)**. At about 2 pounds (1 kg), the whizzer weighs about one-tenth as much as a circular saw, so it is much more maneuverable. Operating at 20,000 rpm, its 3-inch (75 mm) carborundum blade cuts case-hardened locks and steel up to 3/4-inch (19 mm) in thickness. The tool has a blade guard to protect the operator and the victim from flying debris. The whizzer operates much quieter than other power saws.

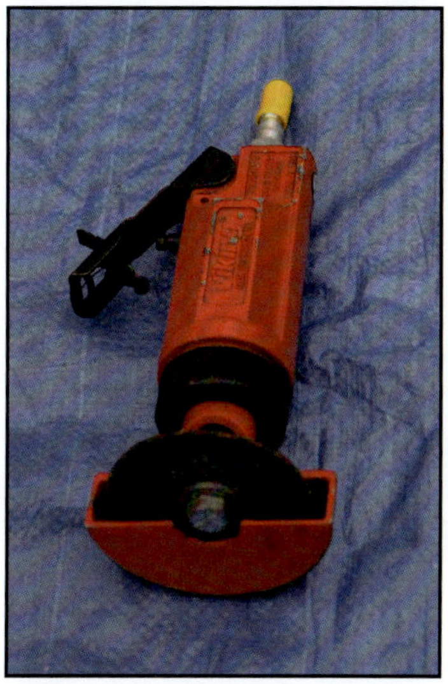

Pneumatic Lifting Bags and Cushions

Pneumatic lifting bags and cushions allow rescuers to lift or displace objects that cannot be lifted with standard extrication equipment **(Figure 4.50, p. 154)**. These tools have a wide variety of applications in extrication operations. They can be inserted into openings that are too small for other lifting equipment, and they are relatively quick and easy to use. However, their use is not without risks to safety. Operators should observe the following safety rules when using pneumatic lifting bags and cushions:

- Plan the operation before starting the work.
- Be thoroughly familiar with the equipment, its operating principles, capabilities, and limitations.
- Consult the appropriate operator's manuals and follow the recommendations for the specific system used.

Figure 4.49 A whizzer saw may run for 3 minutes on an SCBA cylinder.

Section B • Chapter 4 – Tools and Equipment 153

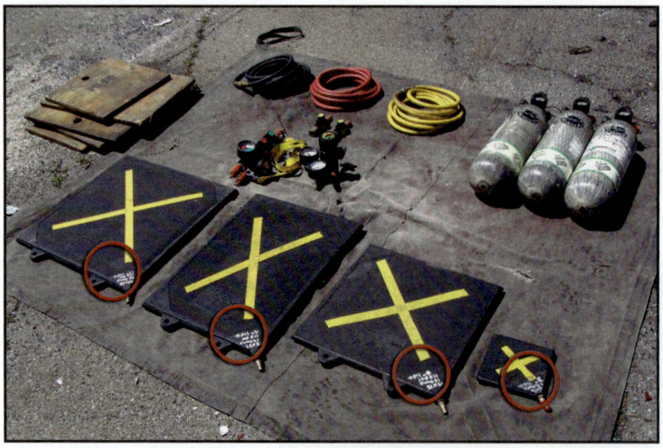

Figure 4.50 Pnuematic lifting capacities should be visibly marked on each bag.

- Keep all components in good operating condition and all safety seals in place.
- Have an adequate air supply and sufficient cribbing on hand before beginning operations.
- Position bag(s)/cushion(s) on or against a solid surface.
- Do not inflate bag(s)/cushion(s) against sharp objects — use a protective mat.
- Do not inflate bag(s)/cushion(s) fully unless they are under load.
- Inflate bag(s)/cushion(s) slowly and monitor them continuously for any shifting.
- Never work under a load supported only by lifting bags and cushions.
- Interrupt the process frequently to increase shoring or cribbing that will support the load in case of bag/cushion failure — lift an inch, crib an inch.
- Ensure that the top tier is solid when using box cribbing.
- Avoid exposing pneumatic bags and cushions to materials hotter than 220º F (105º C):
  — Insulate the bags with a nonflammable material.
  — Remove pneumatic bag(s)/cushion(s) from service if any evidence of heat damage is seen.
- Stack bags, as necessary, in accordance with manufacturer's recommendations.

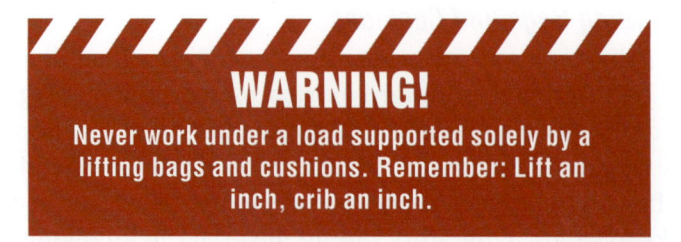

WARNING!
Never work under a load supported solely by a lifting bags and cushions. Remember: Lift an inch, crib an inch.

High-pressure lifting bags. High-pressure lifting bags are constructed of neoprene or butyl rubber reinforced with either steel wire or Kevlar® aramid fiber. These bags have a rough, pebble-grained surface to improve their grip.

They come in various sizes ranging from 6 x 6 inches (150 x 150 mm) to 36 x 36 inches (900 x 900 mm). Before inflation, the bags lie flat and are about ½ to 1 inch (13 to 25 mm) thick. The range of inflation pressure of the bags is about 116-150 psi (810-1 050 kPa).

The largest bags may inflate to a height of 20 inches (500 mm). The largest bags can lift approximately 90 tons (80 T). A lifting bag's weight-lifting capacity decreases as the height of the lift increases and its maximum lift capacity is generally rated at one inch (25 mm) of lift. The decrease in lifting capacity is due to the decrease in surface contact made by the bag as it is inflated. Rescuers cannot achieve maximum lift height and maximum lift weight on an operation simultaneously.

Use the following formula to determine the lift capacity of a high-pressure lifting bag: Length x Width x Operating Pressure (psi) = Lifting Capacity (lbs). Maximum lifting capacity is determined by the amount of surface area of the lifting bag that is in contact with the object being lifted multiplied by the pressure of the system. To ensure the maximum safe lift, use cribbing or another solid base as a foundation to position the bag as close as possible to the underside of the object to be lifted.

Low- and medium-pressure lifting cushions. Low- and medium-pressure lifting cushions (air cushions) are considerably larger than high-pressure lifting bags and are most commonly used to lift or temporarily stabilize large vehicles or objects. Low-pressure cushions generally operate on 7 to 10 psi (50 to 70 kPa), while medium-pressure lifting cushions use 12 to 15 psi (85 to 105 kPa).

Their primary advantage over high-pressure lifting bags is that they have a much greater lifting height range. Depending on the manufacturer and the model, these cushions may be able to lift an object upwards of 6 feet (2 m). Other advantages include:

- They maintain their entire lifting weight capacity throughout the entire lift.
- They are safer to use than stacking high-pressure lifting bags.
- They are easier to repair.

The disadvantages of low- and medium-pressure lifting cushions are:

- They are capable of lifting less weight than a high-pressure lifting bag.
- They require twice as much space for insertion between the base and the object being lifted.
- They are more vulnerable to puncture than high-pressure lifting bags.
- They do not operate the same as lifting bags and cannot lift a load straight up on their own; they must have a base or foundation point.
- They should never be stacked.

> **WARNING!**
> When lifting with low- and medium-pressure lifting cushions, the object being lifted may become unstable. An unstable object may shift or move, and cause harm to personnel.

Lifting or Pulling Tools

Rescue personnel often have to lift or pull a vehicle or some of its components away from a victim. The vehicle or components may weigh several tons, and the lift or pull may range from only 1 or 2 inches (25 to 50 mm) to several feet (meters). A variety of extrication tools exist to assist in this task. These include winches, cranes, come-alongs, Griphoists®, and mechanical advantage systems. Winches and cranes were discussed earlier in the chapter.

Wear durable leather or task-associated gloves when working with wire rope or cables. Broken strands will cut anyone who handles them carelessly. Use a hand-over-hand technique when handling a wire rope or cables.

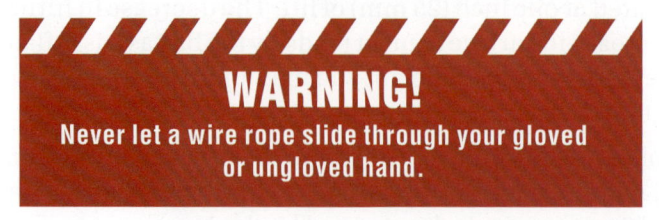

WARNING!
Never let a wire rope slide through your gloved or ungloved hand.

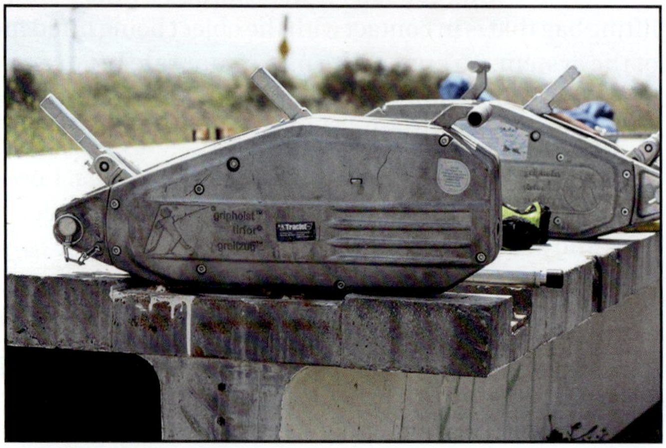

Figure 4.51 The Griphoist® is a diverse tool used for lifting, pulling, and securing objects.

Griphoists®

The Griphoist® is a portable manual hoist with traversing wire rope used for lifting, pulling, and securing objects **(Figure 4.51)**. These tools have many applications, such as removing vehicles from underride or override scenarios. There are multiple models of Griphoist® available. A common model used by rescue personnel is the TU-32, which is rated at 8,000 pounds (4 000 kg) for material-handling applications and 6,000 pounds (3 000 kg) for personnel-hoisting (man-riding) applications. The tool's capacity can be increased by two, three, or four times with the use of sheave blocks per manufacturer's recommendations. The 5/8-inch (15.5 mm) wire rope used with the TU-32 Griphoist® has a minimum breaking strength of 40,000 pounds (20 000 kg). Another common model, the TU-28 is rated at 4,000 pounds (2 000 kg) for material handling applications and 3,000 pounds (1 500 kg) for personnel hoisting (man-riding) applications. The TU-28 uses 7/16-inch (11 mm) wire rope that has a minimum breaking strength of 20,000 pounds (10 000 kg).

Come-Alongs

Come-alongs use leverage and a ratchet/pulley mechanism to increase pulling capacity. The come-along has a drum that is rotated by a lever handle directly or through gear action. A cable, chain, or webbing attached to the drum makes the effective pull of the come-along equal to the length of the cable. Anchor the come-along to a secure object, and attach the cable/chain to the load to be moved **(Figure 4.52)**. Once both ends are attached, operate the lever handle to pull the load toward the anchor point. The lever handles on some come-alongs are designed to bend before the chain or cable reaches the breaking point. The most common sizes or ratings of come-alongs are 1 to 10 tons (0.9 to 9.1 t).

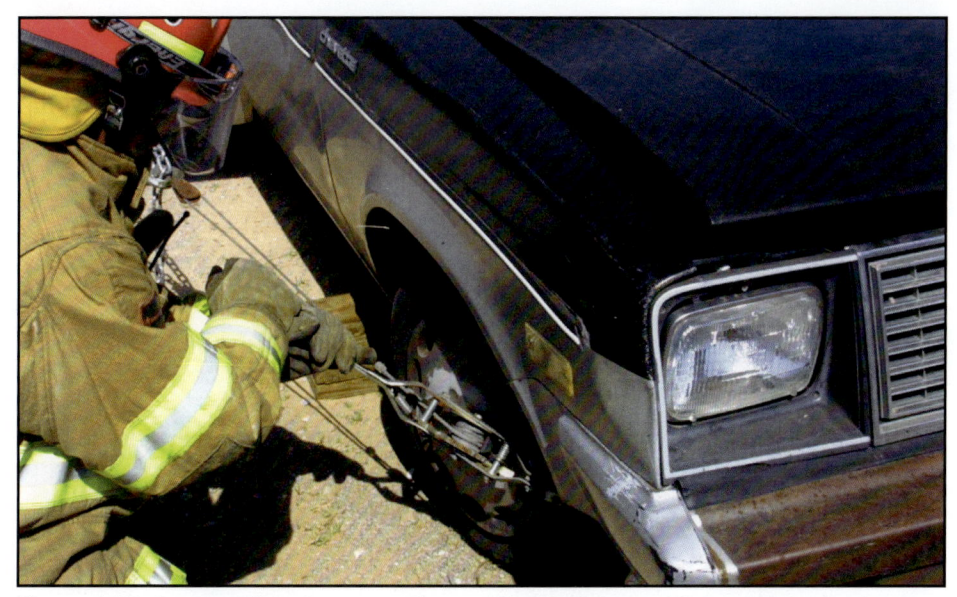

Figure 4.52 A come-along is operated manually to move an object toward a fixed anchor point.

> **CAUTION**
> Do not use an extension handle with come-alongs. Use only the calibrated handle that came with the device.

Mechanical Advantage Systems

Mechanical advantage systems lift or move light to heavy loads. They use leverage to reduce the amount of force required to move a certain amount of weight. These systems can be premade or constructed at the incident scene using pulleys, cables, chains, ropes, and other pieces of equipment. They help accomplish tasks such as lifting loads off of vehicles, victims or pulling a vehicle. One of the most commonly used in low-angle vehicle rescue is a three-to-one system used to deploy resources and equipment down a slight grade of 15-40 degrees and then bring victims and rescuers safely back up the slope.

When using a mechanical advantage system at vehicle extrication incidents, observe the following safety rules:

- Ensure the components of the mechanical advantage system are rated for the load to be moved.
- Pull in a direct line with the pulley or sheaves.
- Pull downhill whenever possible.
- Do not allow anyone to stand under or near the load in case the assembly fails. Block or crib all loads as they are moved.
- Lower suspended loads gradually, without jerking.
- "Mouse" a small rope on the hook to prevent slings or ropes from slipping off.

NOTE: Do not utilize life safety rope in mechanical advantage systems when a life is not involved.

Thermal Cutting Devices

Freeing trapped victims sometimes requires cutting through materials that are too dense to be cut with power saws. In these situations, a variety of thermal cutting tools can be used. Monitor safety at all times during any operation using thermal cutting devices. These operations are potentially dangerous. Observe the following safety rules to avoid most malfunctions and injuries:

- Do not use thermal cutting devices in any area in which the atmosphere may be flammable.
- Have charged handlines in place before beginning cutting torch operations.
- Handline personnel should wear appropriate PPE.
- Ensure that all cutting torch operators are experienced and efficient in using the tool in all situations.
- Train regularly in exercises that present a variety of cutting problems.
- Wear appropriate protective clothing and eye protection when operating thermal cutting devices.
- Store and use acetylene cylinders in an upright position to prevent loss of acetone. When an acetylene cylinder is considered empty of acetylene, it still contains acetone. Never place empty cylinders on their sides.

> **CAUTION**
> Thoroughly train rescue personnel in the safe operation of specific tools before they attempt to use them.

- Handle cylinders carefully to prevent damage to the cylinder or the filler. A dent in the cylinder indicates that the filler may be damaged. Damaged filler creates voids where free acetylene can pool and decompose, creating a potentially explosive condition.
- Dropping a cylinder may also cause the fuse plug to leak, creating a dangerous condition.
- Mark dented acetylene cylinders, and return them to the supplier.
- Avoid exposing cylinders to excessive heat. An ambient air temperature exceeding 130ºF (55ºC) is undesirable for storing or using acetylene cylinders.
- Do not store acetylene cylinders on wet or damp surfaces. Cylinders rust at the bottom as protective paint is worn away.
- Store acetylene cylinders in an area physically separated from oxygen cylinders and other oxidizing gas cylinders. Segregate full acetylene cylinders from empty or partially full cylinders.
- Design storage areas to prevent acetylene cylinders from falling over.
- Perform a soap test (applying a solution of soap and water on fittings) to detect leaks after making regulator, torch, hose, and cylinder connections. Slow leaks in confined areas could permit acetylene to accumulate in concentrations above the lower flammability limit, creating an explosive atmosphere. Acetylene has a wide flammability range: 2.5 to 81.0 percent by volume in air.

- Remove leaking cylinders to an open area immediately. Do not attempt to stop a fuse plug leak.
- Open acetylene cylinder valves no more than three-quarters of one turn. Do not use wrenches on cylinders that have handle valves. If the valve resists being turned, do not force it. Take the cylinder out of service immediately, and return it to the supplier for service.
- Do not use acetylene at pressures greater than 15 psi (105 kPa). Acetylene decomposes rapidly at high pressures and may explode as decomposition occurs.
- Do not exceed a withdrawal rate of one-seventh of the cylinder capacity per hour.
- Keep valves closed when not in use and when the cylinders are empty. After the valves are closed, bleed off the pressure in the regulator and in the torch assembly. Keep unconnected cylinders capped, whether they are full or empty, to prevent damage to fittings.
- Do not use grease or petroleum products on threads.

The following sections describe these varieties of thermal cutting tools:
- Exothermic cutting devices
- Cutting flares
- Plasma-arc cutters
- Oxyacetylene cutting torches
- Oxygasoline cutting torches

Exothermic Cutting Devices

Also known as *burning bars*, exothermic cutting devices are ultra-high temperature burning tools capable of cutting through virtually any metallic, nonmetallic, or composite material. They cut through materials such as concrete or brick that cannot be cut with an oxyacetylene torch. They also cut through heavy-gauge metals much faster than an oxyacetylene torch. Exothermic cutting devices can produce temperatures in excess of 8,000°F (4 400°C). The cutting bars or rods range in size from ¼ to ¾-inch (6 to 19 mm) in diameter and from 22 to 36 inches (550 to 900 mm) in length.

A type of exothermic cutting device is called an Arcair®. This tool uses a hollow magnesium rod fitted into a handle that allows oxygen to flow through the rod. The rod is ignited by an electric striker and burns as the oxygen is increased. This tool produces temperatures from 6,000°F to 10,000°F (3 300°C to 5 500°C). The rods last between 15 and 30 seconds.

Cutting Flares

Also available for cutting metal and concrete are exothermic cutting flares. Approximately the size and shape of highway flares, cutting flares are also ignited in the same ways as highway flares. Once ignited, these flares produce a 6,800°F (3 750°C) flame that lasts from 15 seconds to two minutes, depending upon the length and diameter of the flare. The obvious advantages of cutting flares compared to other exothermic cutters are the absence of a hose or power cord, and their light weight and portability.

Plasma-Arc Cutters

Plasma-arc cutters are ultra-high-temperature metal-cutting devices, generating temperatures of up to 50,000°F (28 000°C). Plasma cutters work by sending an electric arc through a gas that is passing through a constricted opening. This high speed gas cuts through the molten metal. In operation, they use up to 200 amperes of electrical power. They use many types of gases, including air, nitrogen, and argon. Air is the most common gas used for plasma cutters in the fire service. They work so fast that the heat travel through the material being cut is minimal compared to other cutting devices. These tools do not work well in wet conditions, or in poor conductive conditions.

Oxyacetylene Cutting Torches

The oxyacetylene cutting torch cuts by burning. It can cut heavy-gauge metal that is resistant to more conventional extrication equipment. The torch preheats the metal to its ignition temperature, and then burns a path in the metal with an extremely hot cone of flame caused by the introduction of pure oxygen into the flame.

Oxyacetylene cutting torches generate an extremely hot flame **(Figure 4.53)**. For preheating metal, the flame temperature in air is approximately 4,200°F (2 300°C). When pure oxygen is added through the torch handle assembly, a flame of over 5,700°F (3 150° C) is created. This is hot enough to burn through iron and steel with relative ease.

Like all other cutting devices that operate with a highly flammable gas and produce a flame, use oxyacetylene cutting torches with extreme caution. Oxyacetylene cutting torches use acetylene cylinders. Exercise extreme care in storing acetylene cylinders. Always keep acetylene cylinders in an upright position, whether they are in use or in storage. Acetylene is an unstable gas that is both pressure and shock sensitive. Acetylene storage cylinders are designed to keep the gas stable and safe to use. The cylinders contain a porous filler of calcium silicate, which prevents accumulations of free acetylene within the cylinder. They also contain liquid acetone in which the acetylene is dissolved and stored in liquid form. When an acetylene cylinder's valve is opened, the gas leaves the mixture as it travels through the torch hoseline assembly.

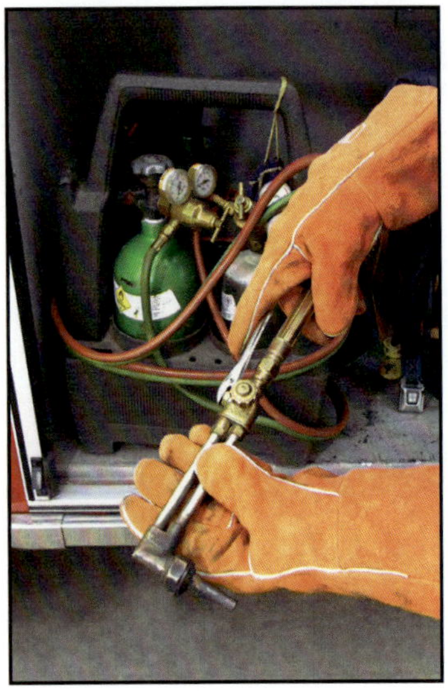

Figure 4.53 An example of an oxyacetylene cutting torch.

> **WARNING!**
> Keep acetylene cylinders in an upright position to prevent acetone, a flammable liquid, from flowing through the cylinder valve and pooling in the work area.

Oxygasoline Cutting Torches

Oxygasoline cutting torches, a relatively new cutting system, are fueled by a mixture of oxygen and gasoline. These systems use a conventional cutting torch and dual-hose configuration, but deliver the fuel (gasoline) to the torch in liquid form. These systems produce a cutting flame in the range of 2,800° F (1 500°C). With the help of special equipment, oxygasoline cutting systems may be used under water.

In addition to the ready availability of gasoline and its relatively low cost as compared to other fuels, the increased operational safety resulting from the fuel being delivered to the torch in liquid form is significant. Unlike systems that use gaseous fuels, in oxygasoline systems the flame cannot travel back through the supply hose **(Figure 4.54)**.

Routine Operational Checks and Maintenance

To ensure operability and extend their functional lifetime, all rescue vehicles, tools, and equipment must undergo operational checks and maintenance in accordance with manufacturer's recommendations. All personnel must be trained to perform these routine procedures for each type of apparatus, tool, and equipment the organization uses **(Figure 4.55).** Personnel must also be proficient in inspecting and maintaining their personal protective equipment.

The organization's SOPs should identify the frequencies and procedures to be followed for routine operational checks and maintenance on each type of equipment. Refer to the manufacturer's operations and maintenance manuals for more information on these topics.

A key part of any routine operational check and maintenance on equipment and vehicles is to ensure that the proper fuels and lubricants are used during re-servicing. The use of improper fuels and lubricants can severely damage emergency equipment and vehicles, causing them to fail.

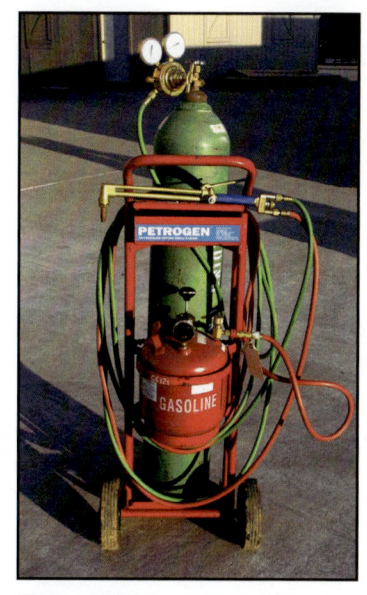

Figure 4.54 An oxygasoline cutting torch.

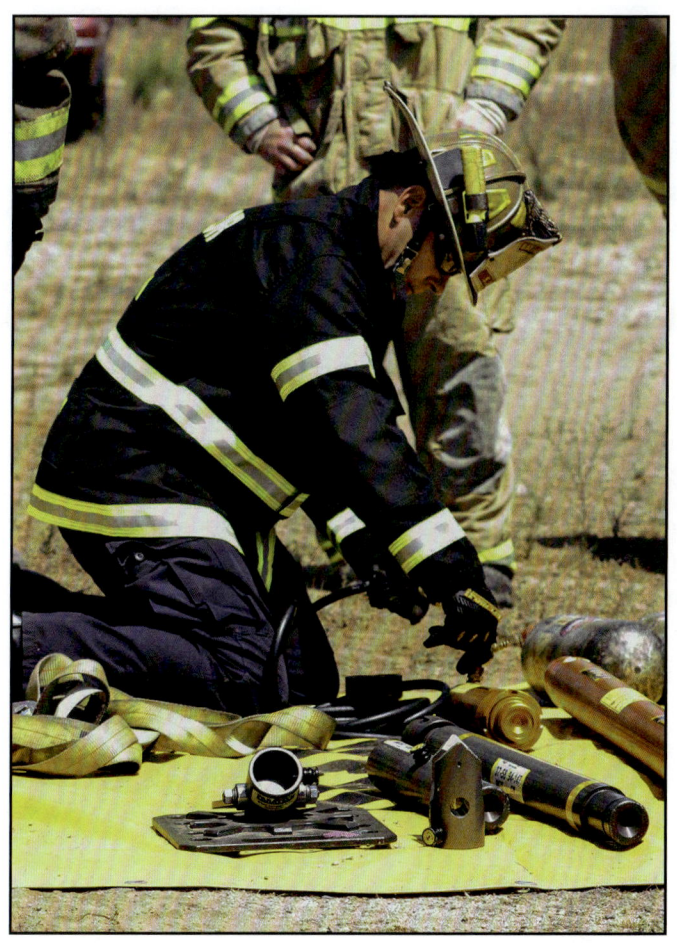

Figure 4.55 A rescuer performing routine maintenance on tools and equipment.

Section B • Chapter 4 – Tools and Equipment

Chapter Review

1. Compare and contrast the capabilities of light, medium, and heavy rescue vehicles.
2. How are ladder trucks often utilized for vehicle rescue?
3. Describe five types of specialized features or equipment that may be found on rescue vehicles.
4. What types of equipment are used to stabilize vehicles?
5. How is rope used at vehicle incidents?
6. What safety rules must be followed when using chain at a vehicle incident?
7. List five cutting, prying, or striking tools and tell how they would be used at a vehicle incident.
8. What types of electric tools and equipment are used at vehicle incidents?
9. What safety rules must be followed when using power saws?
10. Which types of hydraulic tools can be used to create access points for extrication?
11. For which extrication applications are pneumatic chisels, hammers, wrenches, and saws especially useful?
12. What safety rules should be observed when using pneumatic lifting bags and cushions?
13. How are Griphoists® and come-alongs used at vehicle incidents?
14. What safety rules must be followed when using mechanical advantage systems?
15. What safety rules must be followed when using thermal cutting devices?
16. Why is it necessary to routinely perform operational checks and maintenance on all tools and equipment?

Discussion Questions

1. Which type of rescue vehicles are used for vehicle incidents in your jurisdiction?
2. What types of specialized equipment is available for use at vehicle incidents in your jurisdiction?
3. You respond to an incident involving a car that has crashed into the guard rail near a steep drop-off and is resting on its side. Which stabilization and extrication tools are you likely to need?

Victim Management

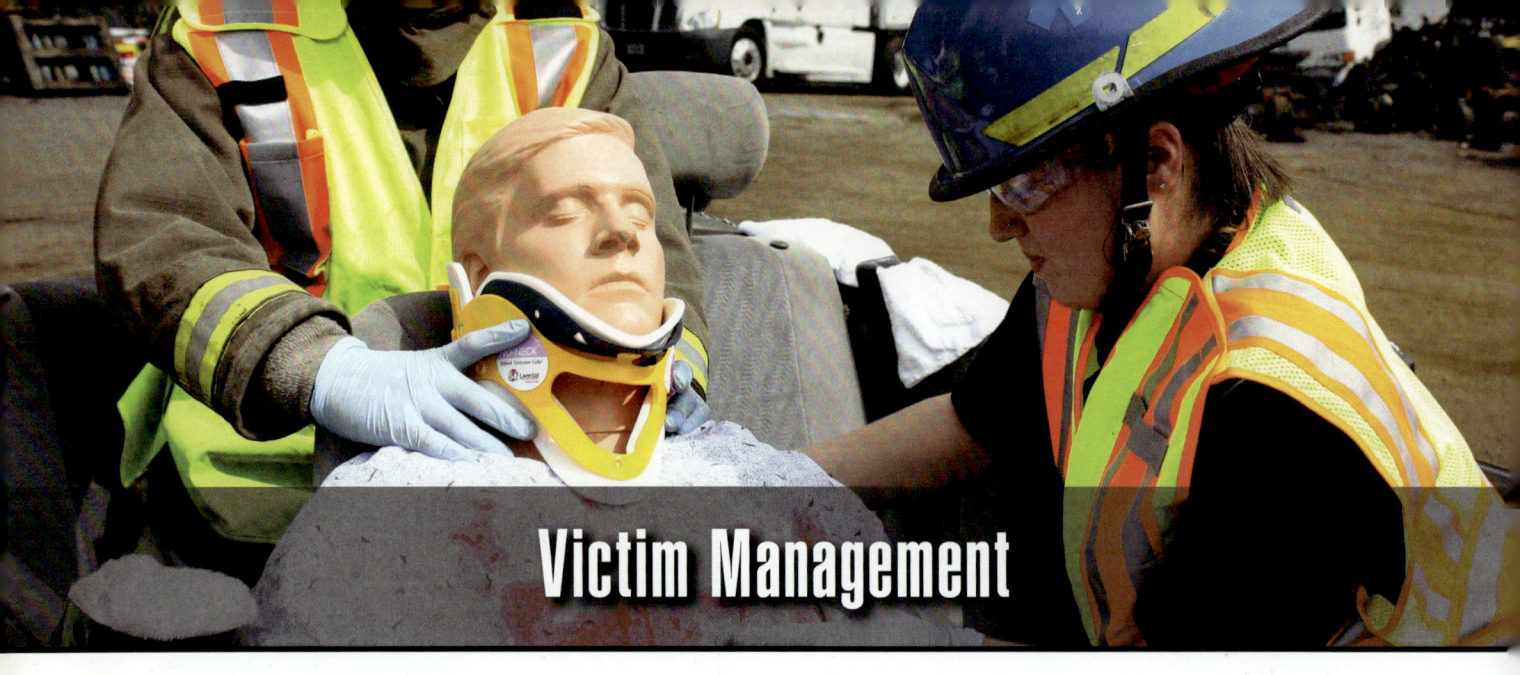

Chapter Contents

Administering Care 167
    Mechanisms of Injury 168
    Triage 173
    Preventing Further Injury 175
    Common Vehicle Incident Injuries 176
    Hazardous Materials Exposure 177
    Compartment/Crush Syndrome 177
    Field Amputations 178
    Internal Injuries 178

Immobilization, Packaging, and Transfer 178
    Types of Immobilization, Packaging, and Transfer Devices 179
    Immobilizing and Packaging a Patient 180
    Removing a Packaged Patient 181
    Transferring a Patient 182

Chapter Review 183
Discussion Questions 184
Skill Sheets 185

chapter 5

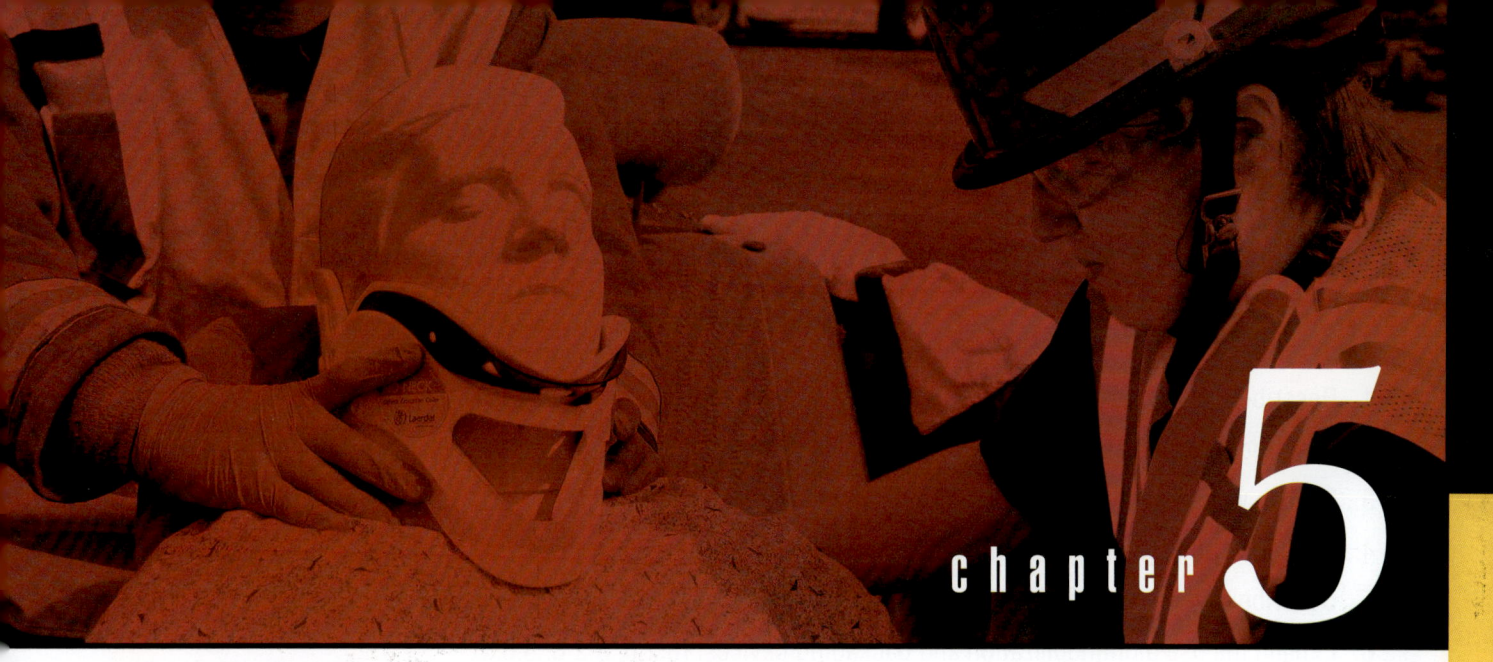

Key Terms

Advanced Life Support (ALS) 173
Aorta 171
Cervical Spine... 171
Compartment Syndrome 177
Crush Syndrome.. 177
Gross Decontamination........................... 177

Mass Casualty Incident (MCI)................. 174
Simple Triage and Rapid Treatment (START) 173
Triage 173

JPRs addressed in this chapter

This chapter provides information that addresses the following job performance requirements of NFPA 1006, *Standard for Technical Rescuer Professional Qualifications (2017)*.

- 8.2.6
- 8.2.7
- 8.2.8
- 8.3.4
- 8.3.5

Victim Management

Learning Objectives

1. Describe common mechanisms of injury in vehicle incidents.
2. Describe the process of assessing victim injury and exposure. [8.2.8]
3. Explain ways to prevent unnecessary victim injury. [8.2.8]
4. Describe common vehicle incident victim injuries. [8.2.8]
5. Describe different types of immobilization, packaging, and transfer devices. [8.2.6, 8.2.8, 8.3.4]
6. Explain the use of immobilization and packaging devices. [8.2.6, 8.2.8, 8.3.4]
7. Explain considerations for removing a packaged patient from the scene. [8.2.6, 8.2.8, 8.3.4]
8. Describe the process of transferring a patient to EMS care. [8.2.6, 8.2.8, 8.3.4]
9. Skill Sheet 5-1: Immobilize a patient using a cervical collar. [8.2.6, 8.2.8, 8.3.4]
10. Skill Sheet 5-2: Package a patient using a long board and remove the patient to a designated safe area. [8.2.6, 8.2.8, 8.3.4]
11. Skill Sheet 5-3: Package a patient using a seated spinal immobilization device and remove the patient to a designated safe area. [8.2.6, 8.2.8, 8.3.4]

Chapter 5
Victim Management

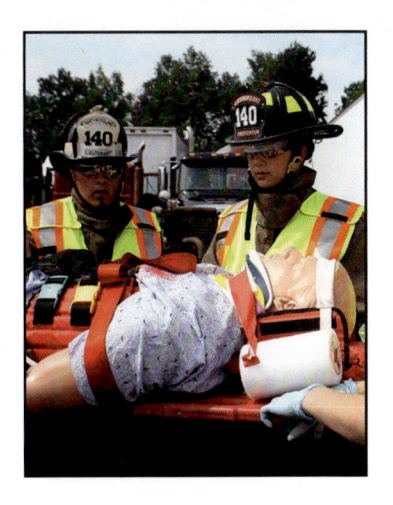

Victims' lives will often hinge on the rescuer's ability to combine their aptitude of incident management, safety, vehicle anatomy, tools, stabilization, and extrication techniques. In addition to these techniques, rescuers will need to provide patient care. This chapter will focus on the following:

- Administering care
- Immobilization, packaging, and transfer

NOTE: It is highly desirable for all rescuers to have at least some formal basic first aid or emergency medical technician (EMT) training.

The terms victim and patient have different meanings depending on one's location, jurisdiction, and/or experience level. For the purposes of this manual, the term *victim* will refer to persons who are involved with a vehicle incident and may have suffered injury or death, and the term *patient* will refer to persons who are receiving medical care.

This chapter provides general information. Each jurisdiction should have its own emergency medical service (EMS) protocols for operating at a vehicle incident. When providing care at a vehicle incident, rescue personnel should prioritize their safety and must wear full PPE at all times.

Administering Care

The types and severity of injuries that a victim of a vehicle accident may incur are almost limitless. Rescuers and medical personnel must prepare to provide a full array of care procedures to include:

- Protecting passengers from hazards, including extrication activities
- Immobilizing the cervical spine **(Figure 5.1)**
- Supporting the airway, breathing, and circulation (ABCs)
- Providing psychological support
- Providing oxygen therapy (usually high-flow oxygen by mask)
- Maintaining body temperature
- Monitoring cardiac activity
- Administering certain life support medications
- Immobilizing and packaging the patient for removal **(Figure 5.2, p. 168)**

Rescuers should also prepare to handle patients with physical and mental disabilities, as well as language barriers. These patients may require additional care considerations.

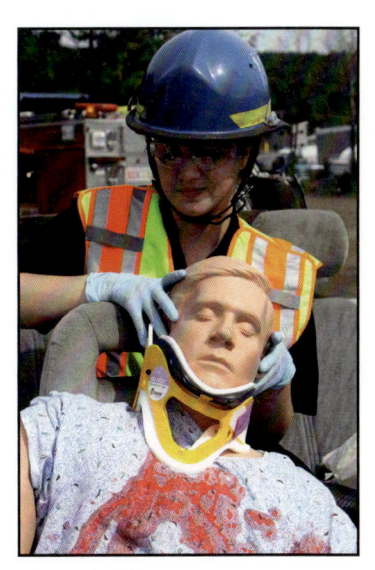

Figure 5.1 A rescuer practicing cervical spine immobilization.

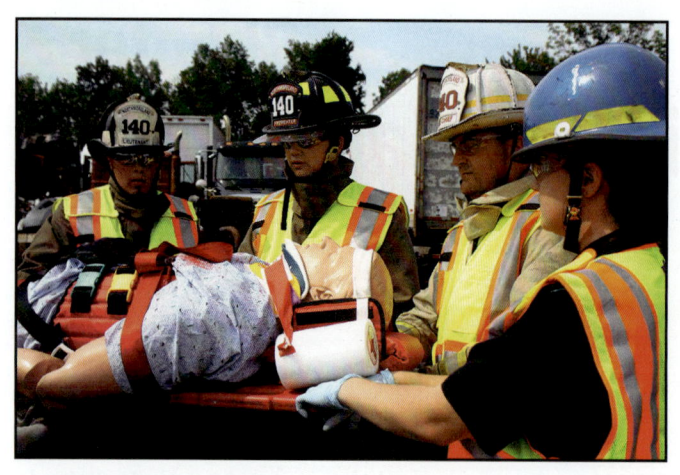

Figure 5.2 Responders practice immobilizing and packaging a patient for removal.

Monitoring a patient during rescue is just as important as conducting the initial evaluation. Patients' conditions can change dramatically during the rescue attempt and may require a change in care.

Victims of vehicle accidents, including entrapped victims may exhibit a number of common injuries. Those may include:

- Fractures and lacerations
- Hypovolemia (shock)
- Hypothermia and hyperthermia
- Hazardous materials exposure
- Compartment/crush syndrome
- Field amputations
- Internal injuries

According to the concept of the Golden Hour, a person suffering from internal bleeding should be treated, packaged, transported, and delivered to a surgeon in under an hour. The Golden Hour begins at the moment of crisis or impact **(Figure 5.3)**. EMS units also practice the concept of the Platinum Ten Minutes. The Platinum Ten Minutes is the maximum on-scene time goal that EMS units strive for when caring for patients.

At incidents of severe trauma, especially internal bleeding, no external treatment can replace the needed surgery. If the internal bleeding is not corrected early enough, the victim could suffer from, and potentially succumb to, shock. If a patient has injuries causing internal bleeding, rescuers should follow local protocols to arrange to transport the patient to a trauma center capable of handling the injuries.

The following section provides only general information on types of injuries and their treatment. Rescuers and emergency medical personnel should familiarize themselves with and follow local treatment protocols as established by the medical control within the AHJ.

Mechanisms of Injury

Vehicle incidents present some common causes and injury patterns. This section does not describe all types of injuries. Responders should always maintain attention when performing patient assessments.

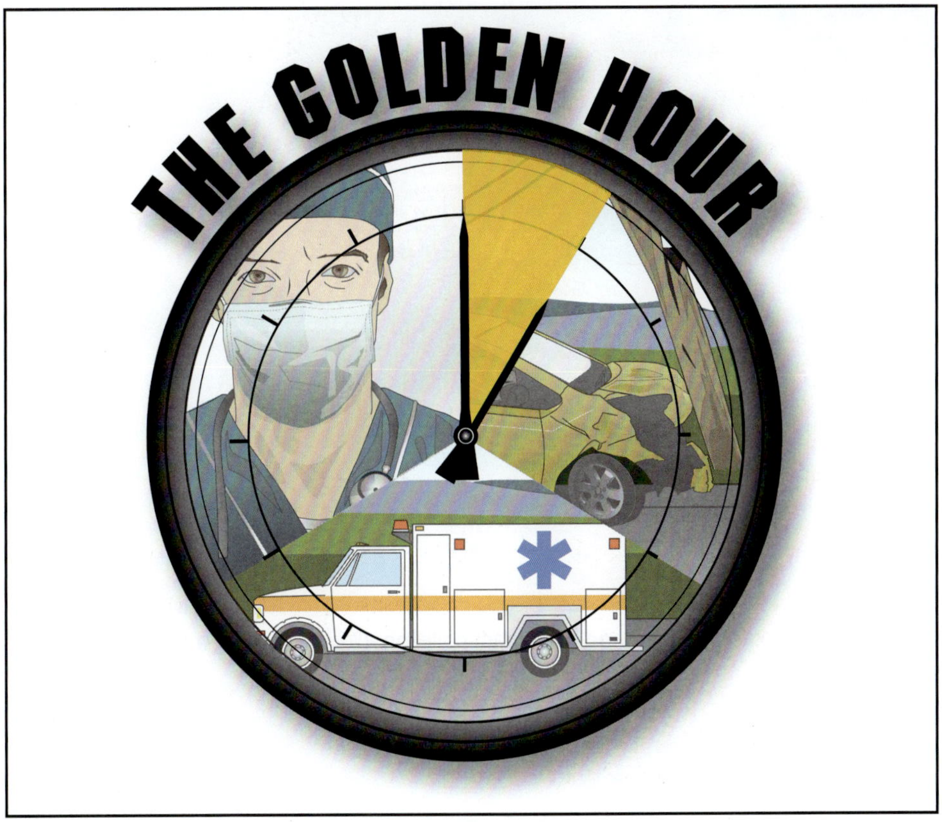

Figure 5.3 To increase their chances of survival, trauma patients should receive medical treatment at hospital facilities within the Golden Hour.

Fatality in the Same Vehicle
When assessing the mechanism of injury of victims, rescuers must consider factors such as fatality in the same vehicle. The forces applied to the bodies of the deceased were similarly applied to the surviving victim(s). In some cases rescuers may need to remove a deceased victim in order to best access another victim. When removing a deceased victim rescuers should treat the body with care and dignity. Rescuers should inform trauma center staff that the patient they are receiving was in the same vehicle as a deceased victim so that they too can understand the violent forces that may have been placed upon their patient during the collision.

Each type of collision has its own predictable pattern of injury. Awareness of the injuries associated with each type of collision will allow rescuers to provide care appropriately. The basic types of collisions include:

- Head-on impact collision
- Side impact collision
- Rear impact collision
- Rotational impact
- Rollover

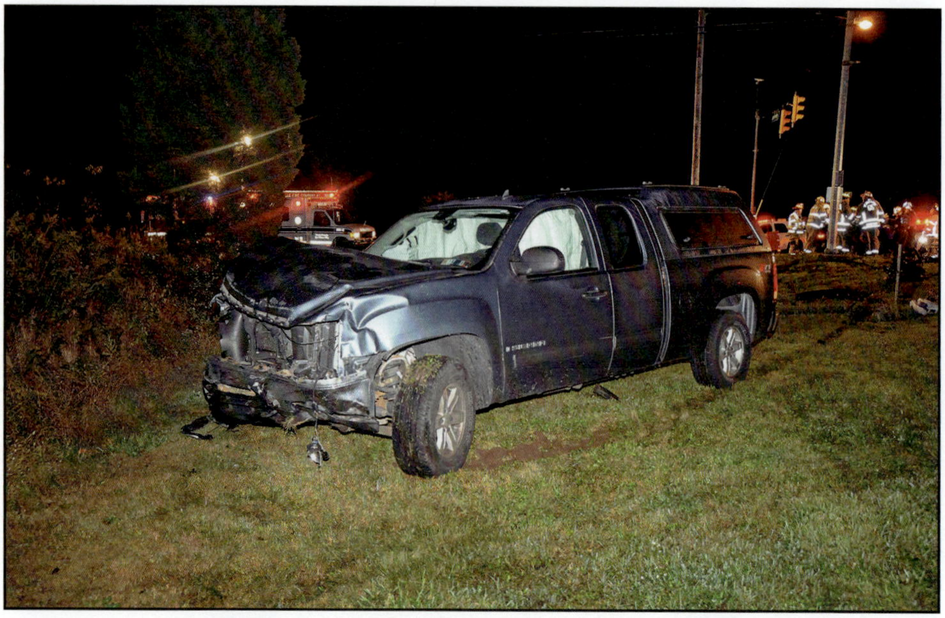

Figure 5.4 An example of a head-on impact collision. *Courtesy of Bob Esposito.*

Head-On Impact Collision

A head-on impact occurs when the front of a vehicle forcefully strikes another vehicle or object. When a vehicle's speed increases, the amount of energy increases, which increases the amount of damage the collision does to the vehicle and its occupants **(Figure 5.4)**.

When the car abruptly stops due to the impact, its occupants continue to travel forward. Victims take one of two possible pathways of motion and energy, either up and over the dashboard or down and under the dashboard. Each pathway has a distinctive pattern of injury. The use of a seat belt affects this pattern of injury.

Passengers that travel up and over the dashboard will sustain injuries to their chest and abdomen. They will commonly experience breaks and lacerations of the upper extremities. If the impact is severe enough, the passenger may crash into or through the windshield.

When passengers travel down and under the dashboard, the knees strike the dashboard and energy travels up the legs. The abdomen and then the chest strike the steering wheel. Common injuries include a dislocated hip and a broken patella (kneecap), femur (thigh bone), or pelvis. When an airbag deploys on an unrestrained passenger, the passenger tends to go under the bag (submarining), sustaining serious lower extremity injuries.

This section will address the following types of head-on impact injuries:

- Face, head, and neck injuries
- Chest injuries
- Abdominal injuries

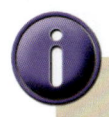

Injury Patterns: Blunt and Penetrating Trauma

Blunt trauma is caused by a blow or force that does not penetrate through the skin or other tissues in the body **(Figure 5.5)**. Penetrating trauma results when an object passes through body tissue. Sometimes the object may pass completely through the body, such as bullet, and other times the object may become impaled in the tissue.

Vehicle manufacturers have worked to engineer out objects that may penetrate a vehicle occupant during a collision. Many items along the roadside can cause penetrating trauma such as guardrails, sign posts, and fence posts. Items in a vehicle or its load such as rebar, pipe, or smaller dimension wood may all cause penetrating trauma. Rescuers must not remove an impaled object from the person's body. This needs to be done in surgery. Rescuers should stabilize impaled objects to prevent further internal injury. In some cases, rescuers may need to trim the impaled object in order to transport the patient. Rescuers should take care to not vibrate or move the object in the patient.

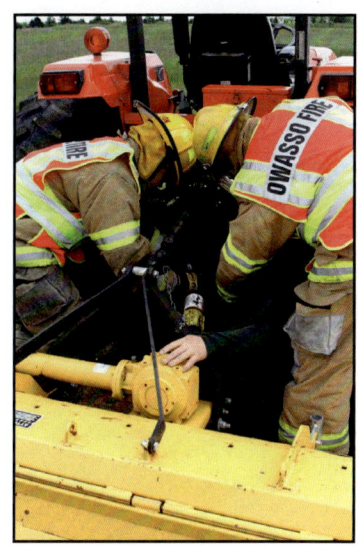

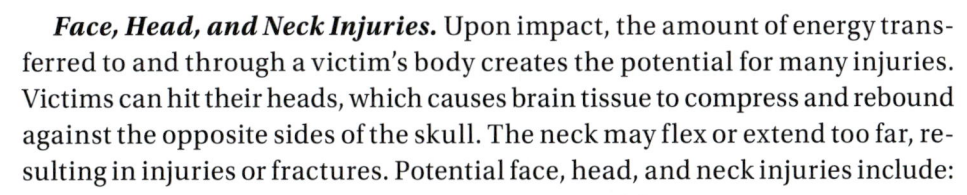

Figure 5.5 Rescuers disentangling a patient from a PTO shaft.

Face, Head, and Neck Injuries. Upon impact, the amount of energy transferred to and through a victim's body creates the potential for many injuries. Victims can hit their heads, which causes brain tissue to compress and rebound against the opposite sides of the skull. The neck may flex or extend too far, resulting in injuries or fractures. Potential face, head, and neck injuries include:

- Extensive soft tissue damage to the face
- Skull fractures
- Brain damage
- Fractures or injuries of the **cervical spine**
- Airway/breathing problems
  — May be present if there is bleeding from the mouth, nose, or face
  — Cartilage rings in the trachea (windpipe) may be separated or crushed

Cervical Spine — First seven bones of the vertebral column, located in the neck.

Chest Injuries. When the chest strikes the steering wheel, the ribs and sternum may break. Broken ribs may injure the lungs and heart. This may compress and bruise the heart, making it unable to pump blood effectively. The **aorta** may tear, resulting in life-threatening bleeding. As the lungs compress, they can bruise or rupture.

Aorta — Largest artery in the body; originates at the left ventricle of the heart.

Abdominal Injuries. When the abdomen strikes the steering wheel, the liver, spleen, and other organs may compress or lacerate. These injuries can cause internal bleeding. Abdominal pain and rigidity both indicate internal bleeding.

Side Impact Collision

The side impact is often called a T-bone collision. The occupant closest to impact absorbs more energy than the occupant on the opposite side **(Figure 5.6, p. 172)**. As the victim's body absorbs the energy of the impact, it pushes sideways and the head moves in the opposite direction. Upon impact, the

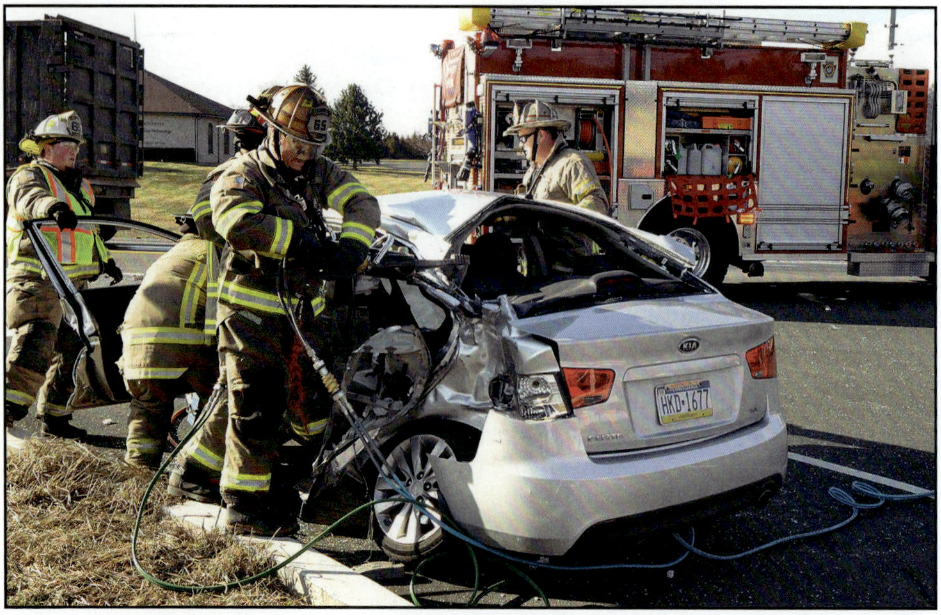

Figure 5.6 An example of a side-impact collision. *Courtesy of Bob Esposito.*

vehicle's components intrude into the passenger compartment and may cause additional significant injury to the victim. The following injuries commonly occur:

Face, Head, and Neck Injuries. The victim's head often impacts the door post. If there is more than one person sitting on a seat, heads can often collide. The impact/collision can result in skull and brain injuries, as well as injuries to the neck, such as cervical fractures.

Chest Injuries. If the vehicle door slams against the occupant's shoulder, the clavicle (collarbone) may fracture. If the arm is caught between the door and the chest, or if the door impacts against the chest directly, rescuers should suspect broken ribs and possible breathing problems. If victims are injured low in the rib cage or in the abdomen, they may suffer from an injured liver and/or spleen.

Abdominal/Pelvic Injuries. Lateral impact to the pelvis often causes fractures of the pelvis and femur. Damage to the iliac arteries and internal organs, such as the bladder, can also occur.

Rear Impact Collision

Rear impact occurs when a car is struck from behind by another vehicle traveling at a greater speed **(Figure 5.7)**. The car that is hit accelerates suddenly with the occupants' body(ies) slamming backward into the seat and then jerking forward. Rear impact may also occur if the vehicle loses control and strikes a stationary object, causing a sudden stop of the vehicle. This applies similar forces to the occupants. Rescue personnel should suspect the same kind of injuries as discussed for head-on collisions. If positioned properly, a headrest will prevent the head from whipping back. If the headrest is not in place or not properly fitted to the occupant, rescuers should suspect neck injuries.

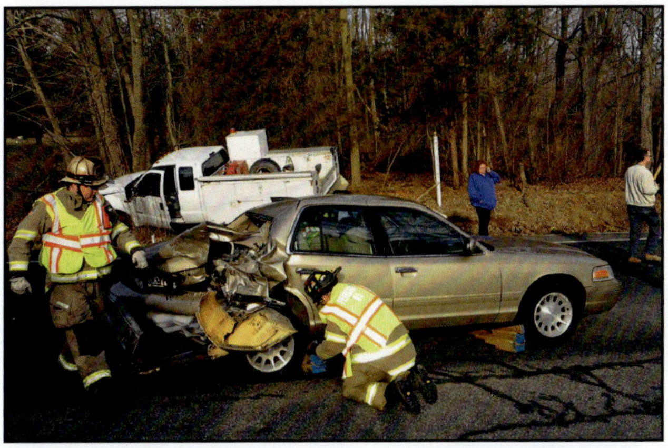

Figure 5.7 Responders stabilizing a passenger vehicle after a rear-end collision. *Courtesy of Bob Esposito.*

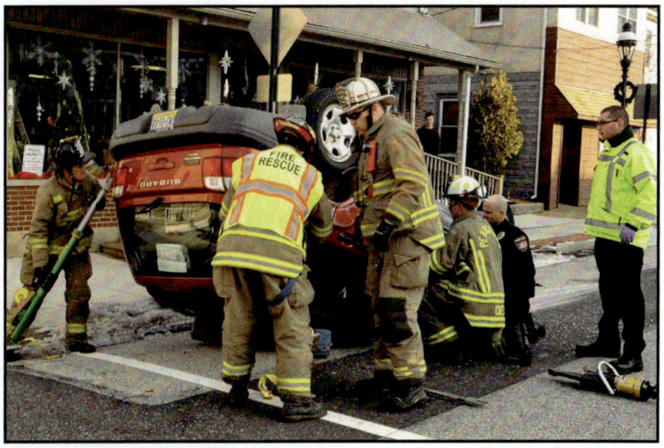

Figure 5.8 Responders stabilizing a passenger vehicle involved in a rollover collision. *Courtesy of Bob Esposito.*

Rotational Impact

A rotational impact occurs off center. The car strikes an object and rotates around it until the car either loses speed or strikes another object. Passengers are flung around the inside of the vehicle and often strike the steering wheel, dashboard, door posts, and windows, causing serious injuries. Rescuers should look for the same kind of injuries found in head-on and side impact collisions.

Rollover

During a rollover, car occupants change direction every time the car does. Every fixture inside the car becomes potentially lethal **(Figure 5.8)**. A specific pattern of injury is impossible to predict. Rescuers will often find occupants with severe soft tissue injuries, multiple broken bones, and crushing injuries (vehicle rolling over or settling on body parts).

Victims may eject from the vehicle during a rollover. These victims are subjected to unprotected collision with the vehicle they were in as they exit it, the ground, trees, buildings or even other vehicles. Ejected victims have a high chance of spine injury or death. Because of the many possibilities for blunt trauma to a victim during the collision event, rescuers should treat ejected victims as a high priority.

Emergency responders should use caution when approaching a scene to ensure they do not further injure an ejected victim. Rescuers should conduct searches of the area around a vehicle collision scene to account for victims that may have been ejected.

Triage

Triage is the process of identifying and prioritizing the most critically injured victims that have the highest chance of survival. One of the most knowledgeable EMS responders on the scene should conduct the triage **(Figure 5.9, p. 174)**. At times trained medical personnel may conduct triage, thus freeing up **advanced life support (ALS)** providers to work in the treatment area providing advanced life support skills to multiple patients.

The **simple triage and rapid treatment (START)** process allows responders to quickly identify life threatening conditions and to prioritize the allocation of medical resources and personnel. Rescuers may use information obtained

> **Triage** — System used for sorting and classifying accident casualties to determine the priority for medical treatment and transportation.

> **Advanced Life Support (ALS)** — Advanced medical skills performed by trained medical personnel, such as the administration of medications, or airway management procedures to save a patient's life.

> **Simple Triage and Rapid Treatment (START)** — Triage evaluation method for checking respiratory, circulatory, and neurological function, with the intention of categorizing patients in one of the four care categories: Minor, Delayed, Immediate, and Expectant. The START method is recommended for use by first-arriving responders for initial and secondary field triage.

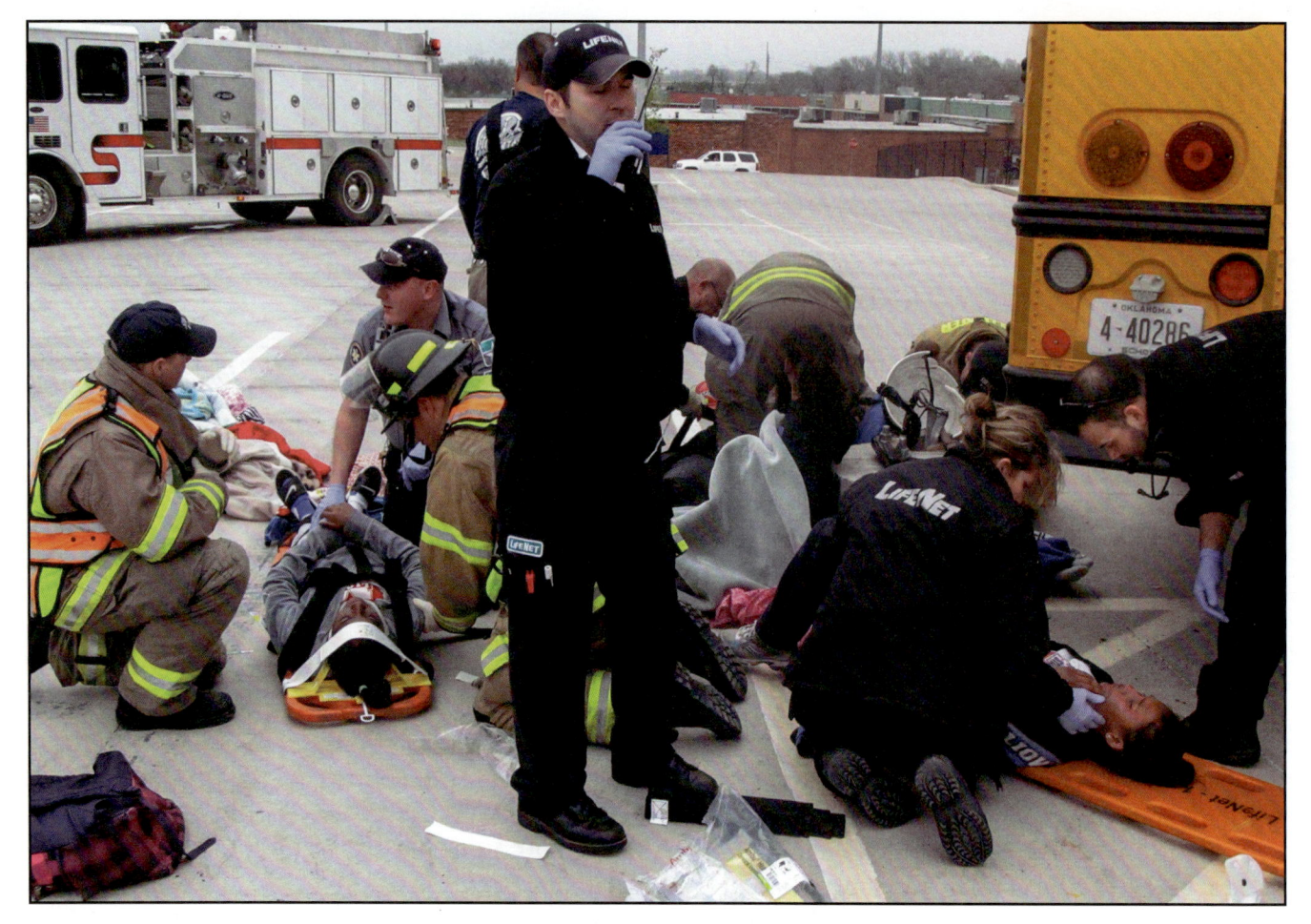

Figure 5.9 Responders conducting triage on an accident scene. *Courtesy of Mike Wieder.*

during triage to establish priorities for extrication or other incident activities. The START process is recommended for use by first-arriving responders for initial and secondary field triage. Initial triage takes precedence over any emergency treatment at the incident scene. Triage team members should limit any emergency care they provide to opening the victim's airway, controlling severe bleeding, and elevating victims' lower extremities. Personnel working in treatment areas shall perform secondary triage and annotate any additional injuries or conditions found on the victim's triage tag.

Many jurisdictions have varying definitions of what constitutes a **Mass Casualty Incident (MCI)** and when to employ field triage protocols. An MCI is any incident where the need for patient care overwhelms the available resources available. Incidents at which the responding resources can sufficiently address the incident are usually termed Multiple Patient Incidents (MPI). At an MPI, rescuers should follow normal treatment and transportation protocols of routine daily operations.

While many responders tend to think of MCI events as large-scale acts of terrorism, natural disasters, and crashed passenger jets, rescuers will more likely respond to MCI events of a smaller scale such as a multiple vehicle collision, bus accidents, and train derailments. Responders should familiarize themselves with MCI and triage protocols so they can rapidly employ these protocols when an MCI happens in their jurisdiction.

> **Mass Casualty Incident (MCI)** — Incident that results in a large number of casualties within a short time frame, as a result of an attack, natural disaster, aircraft crash, or other cause that is beyond the capabilities of local logistical support.

The first unit at an MCI should begin triage immediately, and they should report this action to the next arriving unit so that the arriving unit can set up Command. In addition to quickly establishing Command and implementing triage, rescuers should work to control the walking wounded. These people often wander off and self-transport to the closest hospital. They can easily overwhelm that medical facility, which takes staff away from providing care to patients arriving with more critical injuries.

Rescuers commonly use triage tags and checklists to identify and document the level of injuries a victim has sustained. The tags are color coded and remain with the victim to provide a visual indication to rescuers regarding treatment priority **(Figure 5.10)**. The triage process typically places victims into one of four categories:

- **Green: Minor** — Victims with minor injuries unlikely to require transportation from the scene for treatment. Frequently, EMS personnel treat such victims on the scene as resources become available.
- **Yellow: Delayed** — Victims whose injuries require transportation for evaluation and treatment but are not immediately life-threatening.
- **Red: Immediate** — Victims with life-threatening injuries who appear savable with immediate treatment and rapid transport. Immediate victims are priority for resources and, when accessible, should be the first transported.
- **Black: Expectant** — Victims who are dead or are expected to die regardless of treatment. In the case of limited on-scene resources, victims with a better probability of survival receive priority for treatment over expectant victims.

NOTE: Rescuers must triage victims in cardiac arrest as black when resources are limited. If resources become available, rescuers can re-triage these victims to a red level priority.

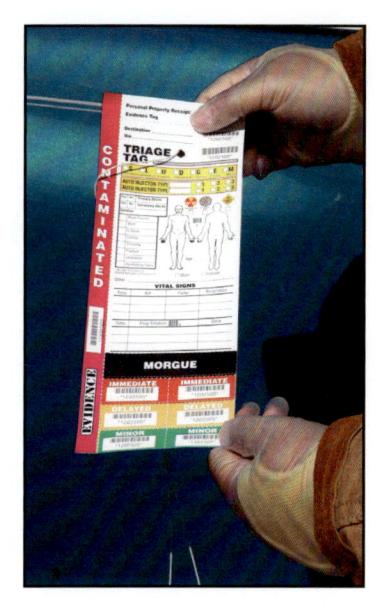

Figure 5.10 An example of a triage tag.

Preventing Further Injury

Rescuers should try to prevent further injury to victims. In some circumstances, such as when they have limited resources, rescuers may not be able to implement appropriate patient care. Rescuers will still have to perform other necessary operations, such as stabilization and extrication. Rescuers must ensure they do not cause any further and/or unnecessary injury to the victims.

Prior to any extrication activity, rescuers should make contact with patients, if possible **(Figure 5.11)**. Rescuers should communicate to the patients

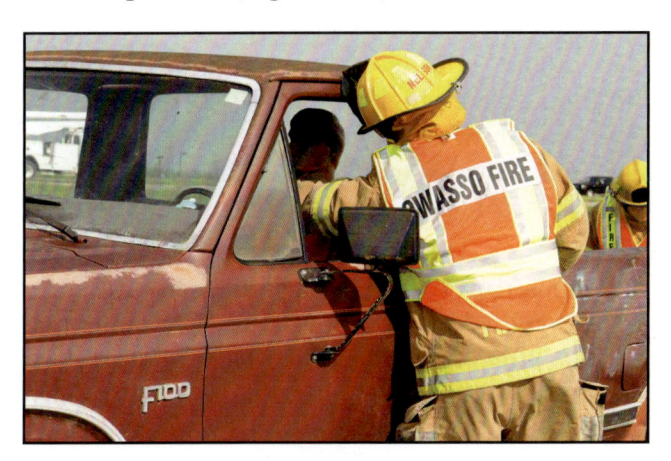

Figure 5.11 A rescuer assessing a victim.

what is happening and what is about to happen. Patients' anxiety levels may decrease if rescuers make them aware of the activities and sounds that are about to take place.

> **Psychological Concerns of the Victims**
> Victim assessment begins as soon as there rescuers establish voice contact with a victim. When rescuers establish contact with an entrapped victim they need to be sensitive to the fact that the person has been entrapped in the vehicle and is unable to get out. Once rescuers have established contact, an entrapped victim may be terrified of being alone. When possible, a rescuer should stay with the victim and explain what is happening. Rescuers must clearly communicate pertinent information with the victim.

A common way for rescuers to prevent further injury to victims is to protect them from glass hazards. Rescuers often cover victims with fire retardant protective coverings and, if possible, provide respiratory protection before breaking glass on the vehicle. Glass debris can cause serious harm to victims if rescuers do not take these measures. When possible, rescuers should break the glass furthest away from occupants to minimize occupant exposure to glass particles.

Whenever necessary, rescuers should make every effort to protect victims from inclement weather conditions. This may include using salvage covers or rapidly erected canopies to divert precipitation from the victims or to prevent direct contact by sunlight. Rescuers may use blankets and heating or cooling packs to control the temperature directly around the victim. In many circumstances, rescuers can leave windows and roofs intact and in place, which will provide victims with protection from inclement weather conditions.

Common Vehicle Incident Injuries

Rescuers are likely to find any of the following – or a combination of the following – injuries at vehicle incidents:

- Fractures and Lacerations
- Hypovolemia (blood loss)
- Hypothermia and Hyperthermia

Fractures and Lacerations

The force of a vehicle accident often results in orthopedic and soft-tissue injuries. In addition, these incidents create a high potential for cervical injury. Precautions such as cervical immobilization, use of cervical collars, and appropriate removal devices can have a positive effect on patient outcomes.

Hypovolemia (Blood Loss)

Hypovolemia, or loss of blood volume, can occur as a result of impact and injuries to the body. Shock as a result of hypovolemia is a life-threatening complication. Rescuers must stop the bleeding and provide oxygen and intravenous fluid replacement if possible. Bleeding or other complications may recur when objects that are compressing bleeding sites are removed during extrication.

Hypothermia and Hyperthermia

In addition to injuries from a vehicle accident, the victim may also develop hypothermia (decreased body temperature) or hyperthermia (increased body temperature) due to exposure to the environment. Wet clothing, lack of normal heating/cooling, weather, and duration of exposure during extrication all increase the possibility of body temperature-related emergencies. To lessen the effects of this problem, rescuers must protect the victim from the environment during rescue operations.

Victims who suffer from hypothermia or hyperthermia need aggressive basic techniques designed to raise or lower their core body temperature. To warm or cool a patient, rescuers can administer:

- Warm or chilled IV fluids
- Warm or chilled oxygen and blankets
- Warm air or cool air, through the use of a heater or air conditioner or blower that resembles ventilation equipment

Hazardous Materials Exposure

Many transportation related hazardous materials leaks result from vehicle collisions. Exposure to hazardous materials is a concern for all personnel. Ideally, rescuers should remove the victim from the source of any hazardous material, but this is not possible with an entrapped victim. In this situation, rescuers should remove the material from the victim. To do so, rescuers should cleanse the skin gently and, depending on the substance, flush with large amounts of water (**gross decontamination**). Cleansing, as well as the removal of contaminated clothing, should remove most of the contaminant. Rescuers should also provide respiratory protection if the material poses an inhalation danger and extrication will be delayed.

Compartment/Crush Syndrome

The body's muscle tissue is extremely vulnerable to sustained pressure. In a vehicle entrapment, structural components of the vehicle such as posts, steering wheel, and dash or the victim's own body weight may all cause compression. The amount of time before negative effects begin to develop depends upon the amount of pressure exerted at the time of the injury and other factors unique to each victim.

Compartment syndrome can occur when a victim's limb has experienced a traumatic injury. Muscle tissue, which is encapsulated in a sheath, swells as a result of a traumatic injury. As the muscle tissue swells to the limit of its sheath (or compartment), pressure in the compartment begins to build which reduces the body's ability to provide circulation to the muscle. Without access to advanced care and aggressive surgery to save the limb, permanent damage may occur.

Crush syndrome occurs as a result of external pressure that crushes part of the body and restricts blood flow to the injured area for an extended period of time. Without adequate blood flow, the injured tissue dies and releases toxins. When the victim is released from the entrapment, the toxins enter the bloodstream and spread throughout the body where they can impair critical organs and possibly cause death.

Gross Decontamination — Quickly removing the worst surface contamination, usually by rinsing with water from handheld hoselines, emergency showers, or other water sources.

Compartment Syndrome — Result of traumatic injury where the patient's muscle tissue becomes swollen and tightly encased. At four to six hours, crushed tissue begins to die and release toxins, which decreases the potential for saving the limb.

Crush Syndrome — Potentially fatal condition that occurs as a result of crushing pressure on a part of the body, typically the lower extremities. When blood flow to and from the injured area is absent for four to six hours, the injured tissue begins to die, giving off toxins; a sudden release of pressure may allow the toxins to flow into the bloodstream and to have an effect on other bodily organs.

To minimize the effects of crush syndrome, rescuers should recognize it as a possibility and provide treatment before victim extrication begins (as long as the entrapment does not compromise a vital function such as respiration). Prolonged entrapment times decrease the likelihood of a successful extrication. If available, advanced life support personnel familiar with compartment and crush syndrome should provide treatment for the victim.

Field Amputations

Victims of vehicle accidents may suffer partial or total amputation of one or more limbs. Rescuers and EMS personnel should treat the patient and handle the limb according to local protocols. On rare occasions, victims may require field surgical amputations of arms or legs. Such a drastic measure should be performed only after it has been determined that it is the only way a patient can be extricated and/or saved. Amputations create not only a psychological impact but also a biohazard. In these situations the rescuers should support medical personnel (surgeons) who perform the procedure at the scene. Jurisdictions should have protocols in place for this type of event.

Internal Injuries

Prior to advancements in vehicle safety technology, seriously injured occupants involved in vehicle accidents usually had such visible signs of injuries as facial lacerations, abrasions, bruises, and broken bones. Now, vehicle occupants protected by safety belts and supplemental restraint systems may not have as many visible injuries but may still need medical intervention for internal injuries. After an accident, serious internal injuries may be present but not apparent. To increase the chances that vehicle accident occupants receive timely and appropriate emergency care, medical personnel should always consider the possibility of internal injuries.

The impact of a motor vehicle accident can cause injuries to victim's internal organs such as kidneys, spleen, liver, lungs, heart, or aorta. Some vehicle occupants may suffer from a traumatic brain injury (TBI) if their heads get hit by or hit another object violently. TBI victims can suffer mild, moderate, or severe symptoms, depending on the speed, deceleration, and even the portion of the brain that is injured. Even when victims exhibit no visible sign of trauma, the force of impact may have injured the brain, causing bruising, bleeding and swelling. The initial trauma to the brain can be compounded when the deceleration event stops, causing the brain to collide with the inside of the skull, causing further injury to other portions of the brain. This type of injury is known as a coup contrecoup brain injury, which occurs at both the site of the impact, and the opposite side of the brain.

Immobilization, Packaging, and Transfer

Rescuers who perform vehicle extrication should know how to immobilize a patient. Even a rescuer who has no medical training may need to help immobilize, package, and transfer a patient. This section will cover the following:

- Types of immobilization, packaging, and transfer devices
- Immobilizing and packaging a patient
- Removing a packaged patient
- Transferring a patient

Types of Immobilization, Packaging, and Transfer Devices

Rescuers may use a number of different immobilization, packaging, and transfer devices. These devices include:

- Cervical collar
- Seated spinal immobilization device
- Long board
- Vacuum mattress

Cervical Collar

A cervical collar is typically a rigid or soft plastic or foam neck brace that secures and maintains the cervical vertebrae in their normal anatomical position. The term normal anatomical position, or neutral position, describes the position of the head, neck, and spine in the manner in which they appear with a human body lying supine with palms facing upward. Cervical collars prevent cervical flexion, extension, and rotation. Trained EMS personnel use them most often, especially in situations of trauma, falls, and vehicle accidents **(Figure 5.12)**.

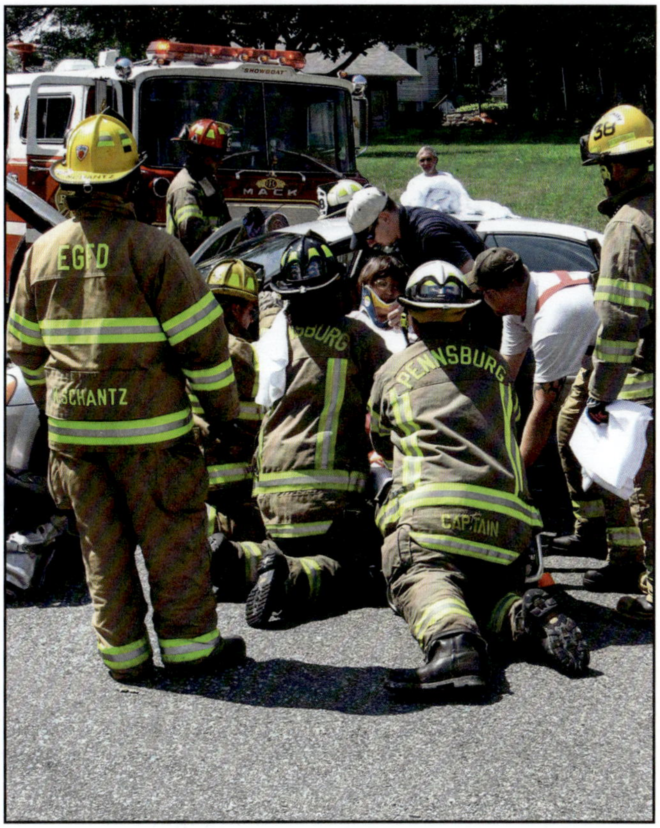

Figure 5.12 Rescuers stabilizing an accident victim with a cervical collar. *Courtesy of Mike Wieder.*

Seated Spinal Immobilization Device

Seated spinal immobilization devices, such as the Kendrick Extrication Device (KED®) or wooden short board, immobilize a suspected spinal injury on a seated patient. These devices allow immobilization of the head, neck, and torso. Rescuers should only use this device on a stable or non-critical patient.

Long Board

EMS personnel most often use a long board, also known as a spinal board, long spine board, backboard, or long backboard as a patient handling and transfer device in pre-hospital care at the scene of a vehicular incident **(Figure 5.13)**. It provides rigid support during movement of a patient with suspected or anticipated spinal injuries. The long board is most often constructed of rigid wood or composite material that will support the weight of the patient.

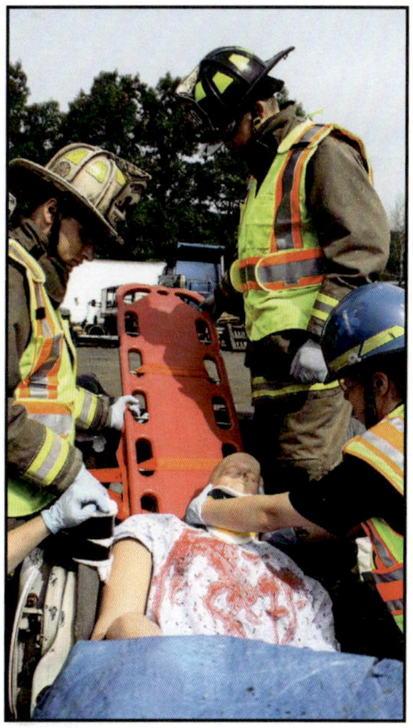

Vacuum Mattress

Vacuum mattresses are becoming more popular as studies indicate the discomfort of and challenge the effectiveness of long boards. Vacuum mattresses are most often filled with numerous polystyrene beads, encased in a flexible outer shell. This device is initially soft and malleable; however, when the air is removed (vacuumed), it becomes rigid, providing a form-fitting immobilization mattress. Similar to a long board, vacuum mattresses also have holes or handles to enable rescuers to carry the patient.

Figure 5.13 A long board provides rigid support for patients with suspected spinal injuries.

Immobilizing and Packaging a Patient

The guiding principle for immobilizing and packaging a patient is that personnel treat the spinal column as one bone that they need to immobilize from the base of the skull to the tailbone. Often, due to the nature of the collision, occupants are unable to move within the passenger compartment of the vehicle. Once extrication operations begin, the occupants gain more room to move within the vehicle, and their movements may aggravate their injuries. Rescuers must take precautions to limit patient movement as much as possible in order to minimize these injuries. Immobilization limits this movement.

Immobilizing the patient's cervical spine (c-spine) is the primary concern for rescuers. Rescuers should perform manual immobilization of the c-spine until total immobilization with a device is complete. To start this immobilization, rescuers use a rigid cervical collar to help hold the c-spine in a neutral position. Immobilizing the c-spine hinders the patient's ability to move his or her head and neck, which will lessen the chance of further injury. With a c-spine immobilization device in place, rescuers can then further immobilize and package the patient using other devices.

A cervical collar alone does not typically provide adequate immobilization. It should be used in conjunction with a long board, vacuum mattress, or possibly a seated spinal immobilization device.

NOTE: It is considered poor medical care to bend or twist an injured patient in order to remove them from the vehicle unless no other option exists.

If rescuers need to immobilize a child in child passenger safety seat for transport to a hospital, and the integrity of the seat is intact, rescuers can immobilize the child in the seat. Taking the seat as a single unit and securing it in the ambulance is considered the safest method for immobilization of children and infants. To properly immobilize a child in a car seat, the rescuer can use sheets, towels, or blankets to fill all void spaces between the seat and the child and then use tape to secure the child's head to the seat to prevent further movement.

Removing a Packaged Patient

Rescuers should be proficient in removing the packaged patient from the vehicle after the disentanglement process is complete. Rescuers should take care to limit further injury to the patient throughout the removal process. Rescuers will often remove the packaged patient from the vehicle to an awaiting ambulance, and transfer care to EMS personnel. Throughout this process, rescuers should practice proper lifting and carrying techniques. Confined work areas, vehicle position, and unstable terrain may complicate the rescuer's ability to remove a packaged patient, but rescuers should not compromise their own safety **(Figure 5.14)**.

NOTE: Rescuers should remove patients complaining of head, neck, or back pain from the vehicle in a manner that does not compromise spinal integrity. Ideally, rescuers accomplish this in a straight line with the direction of the patient's orientation.

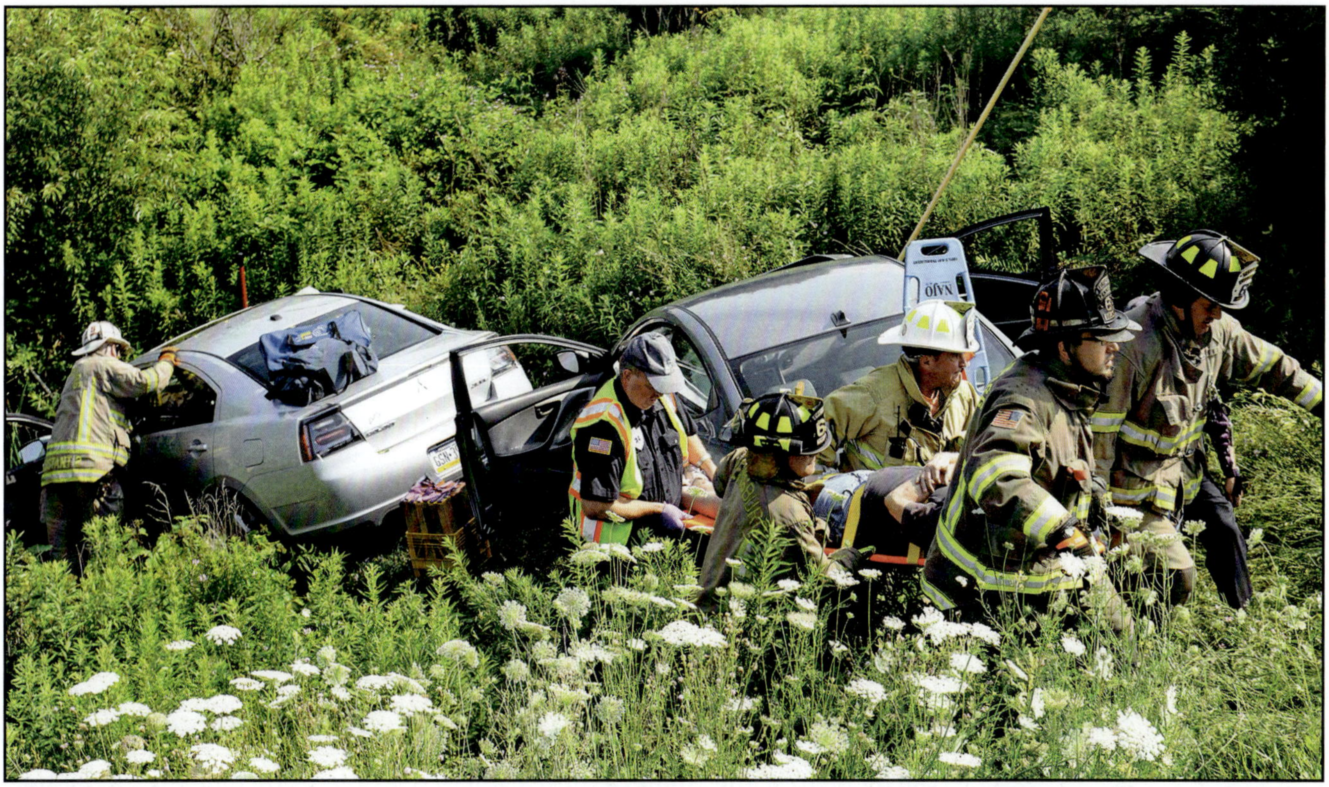

Figure 5.14 Uneven terrain creates more challenges and hazards for responders. *Courtesy of Bob Esposito.*

Rescuers should work as a team to safely remove the packaged patient from the vehicle, and all movement should be purposeful to complement the patient's care and removal. Rescuers can cause significant injury to the patient if they trip or slip on unstable terrain, or lose control of the patient.

Upon patient removal, rescuers should follow their pre-determined egress route to a safe area. They should keep this egress route free of vehicle debris, tools and equipment, and personnel. The safe area should be free of hazards. **Skill Sheets 5-1 through 5-3** list the steps for immobilizing and packaging a patient and removing a patient to a designated safe area.

Transferring a Patient

When transferring care of patients to EMS providers, rescuers should be effective and thorough in their communications **(Figure 5.15)**. Rescuers should relay patient information such as:

- Type of collision
- Known injuries
- Duration of incident
- Level of consciousness
- Vital signs
- Other pertinent information

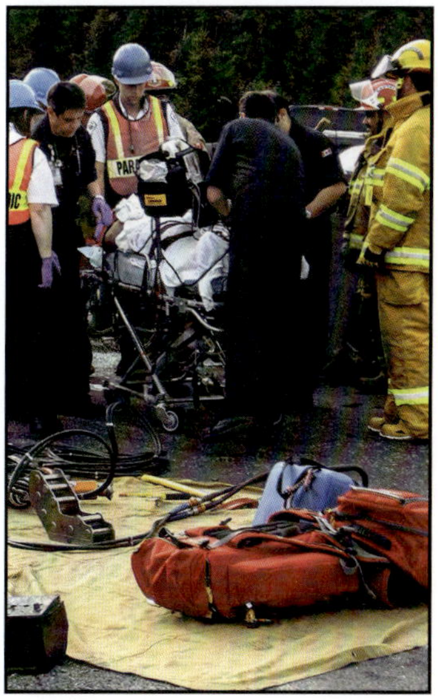

Figure 5.15 Responders must communicate effectively when stabilizing a patient for transfer. *Courtesy of Mike Wieder.*

> **Health Insurance Portability and Accountability Act (HIPAA)**
>
> The Health Insurance Portability and Accountability Act (HIPAA) was enacted by Congress in 1996 to set a national standard for electronic transfers of health data. U.S. Department of Health and Human Services establishes its administrative rules. Because of well-publicized changes, some emergency response units have questioned whether or not they could conduct Quality Assurance/Improvement AARs of incidents as previously done.
>
> It is allowable under HIPAA to conduct reviews for educational purposes, but all identifiable information (name, social security number, age, date, address) must be removed from the presentation before open discussion in a Quality Assurance/Improvement AAR occurs. The responders directly involved in patient care can discuss specifics of the call with other medical professionals who cared for that patient during the incident but all others are to be censored from the Protected Health Information.

Communications with EMS

Rescuers may need to communicate any problems with EMS that occur at the incident scene. Some of these principal problems include the following:

- Inherent delay in reaching trapped victims, so medical problems progress beyond normal pre-hospital trauma management
- Unusual medical problems, such as crush syndrome or hazmat exposure, which EMS personnel do not face on a regular basis
- Medical system chaos, such as overwhelmed/compromised EMS providers

While medical protocols vary, it is good practice to notify the receiving medical center of severely injured patients as early as possible after rescuers have made an accurate assessment of injuries. This information allows medical facility staff to prepare for the patient(s) and have specialty services ready upon arrival. In some cases, medical centers will have to call in medical providers such as surgeons or specialists, so providing advanced notification will minimize delayed care.

Patient Follow Up

Rescuers often follow up on patients to gain valuable feedback. Rescuers use this information to improve future patient care and extrication practices. The after-action review, or post-incident analysis, provides a process to gather information immediately following the incident, but patient follow up provides further information that allows rescuers to determine the effectiveness of the care delivered on-scene and other operations.

Chapter Review

1. What types of care should rescue personnel be prepared to administer at vehicle incidents?
2. What injuries are common to victims in a head-on collision?
3. How does the simple triage and rapid treatment (START) process help rescuers prioritize victims?
4. What can rescuers do to help ensure that victims are not injured further during extrication operations?
5. What should rescuers do for a victim who has lost enough blood to go into shock?
6. Which victim conditions result from exposure to the environment?
7. What actions must rescuers take if a victim is exposed to hazardous materials?
8. What are the effects of compartment/crush syndrome?
9. What types of internal injuries are victims of a vehicle incident likely to suffer?
10. Which type of device is used to maintain a patient's head, neck, and spine in neutral position?
11. What is the difference between a long board and a vacuum mattress?
12. How should rescuers treat the spinal column when immobilizing and packaging a patient?
13. What may complicate rescuers' efforts to remove a packaged patient to a safe area?
14. What patient information should be communicated to EMS providers when transferring patient care?

Discussion Questions

1. What medical training are vehicle rescuers required to have in your jurisdiction?
2. A victim has multiple lacerations and heavy blood loss. The victim is responsive, but is showing early signs of shock. Which triage category should be assigned to this victim?
3. Rescuers are often faced with difficult situations and decisions. One example of this is when a victim needs to be extricated quickly in order to provide medical care, but the scene requires a complicated stabilization process. As a rescuer, how do you prioritize these needs?
3. According to local SOPs, what responsibilities do rescuers in your jurisdiction have when transferring care of a patient to EMS personnel?

SKILL SHEETS

5-1
Immobilize a patient using a cervical collar.

REMINDER: Not all agencies advocate the following practices. The following skill sheets present a snapshot of various procedures utilized during vehicle incident operations. Always follow manufacturer's recommendations and local SOPs. Rescuers must wear full PPE including hand, eye, and respiratory protection. It is recommended that rescuers maintain communication with victims and make them aware of pertinent rescue information.

WARNING: Rescuers must ensure that the vehicle is properly stabilized and the scene is safe.

CAUTION: Rescuers must take necessary precautions to protect themselves and victims from hazards including, but not limited to glass fragments and dust, jagged metal, SRS gas cylinders, undeployed airbags, and fire hazards.

Step 1: Verbalize body substance isolation and scene safety.

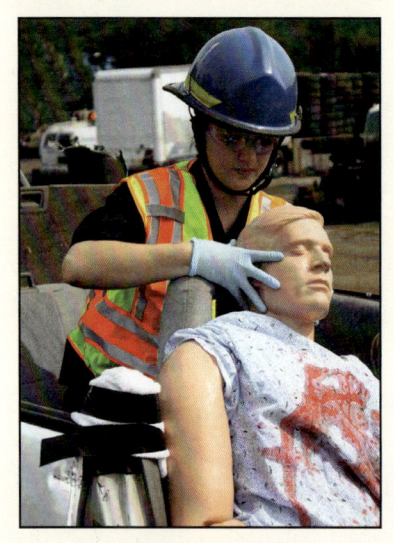

Step 2: Direct second rescuer to place and maintain head into a neutral in-line position providing manual support and immobilization.

Step 3: Assess pulse, motor, and sensory functions of the patient.

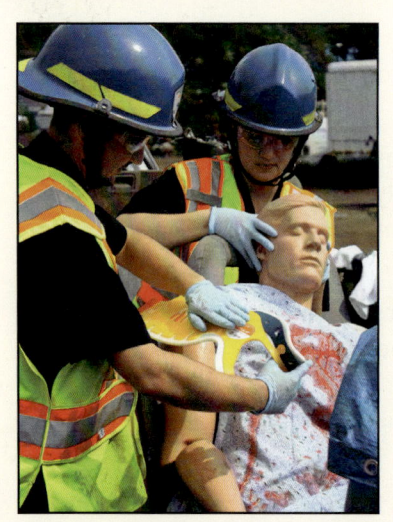

Step 4: Measure patient for appropriate cervical collar size.

Step 5: Appropriately size and apply the cervical collar.

Step 6: Ensure proper fit of the cervical collar. Remove articles of clothing or jewelry if they obstruct the proper fit of the cervical collar. Maintain neutral, in-line motion restriction until the patient is secured to an appropriate spinal immobilization device.

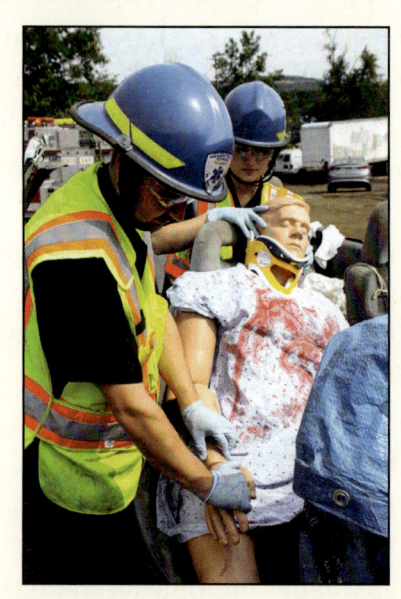

Step 7: Re-assess pulse, motor, and sensory functions of the patient.

184 Section B • Chapter 5 – Victim Management

5-2
Package a patient using a long board and remove the patient to a designated safe area.

SKILL SHEETS

WARNING: Rescuers must ensure that the vehicle is properly stabilized and the scene is safe.

CAUTION: Rescuers must take necessary precautions to protect themselves and victims from hazards including, but not limited to glass fragments and dust, jagged metal, SRS gas cylinders, undeployed airbags, and fire hazards.

Step 1: Verbalize body substance isolation and scene safety.

Step 2: Ensure that patient has a cervical collar applied and that the head is maintained in a neutral, in-line position while providing manual support and immobilization.

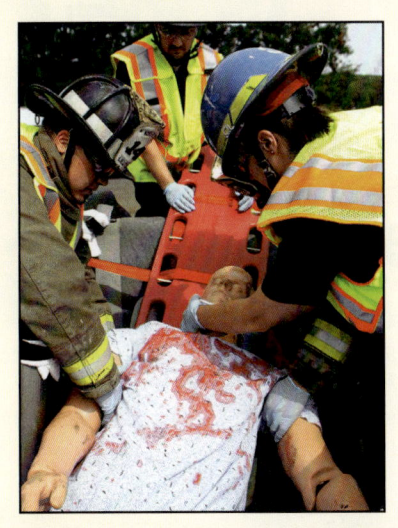

Step 3: Position the long board in an appropriate location for patient transfer.

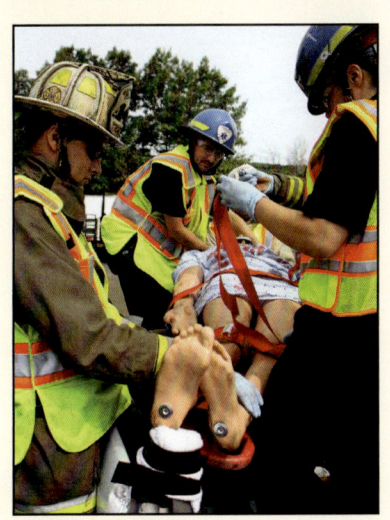

Step 4: Move the patient onto the long board without compromising the integrity of the spine.

Step 5: Center the patient on the long board without compromising the integrity of the spine.

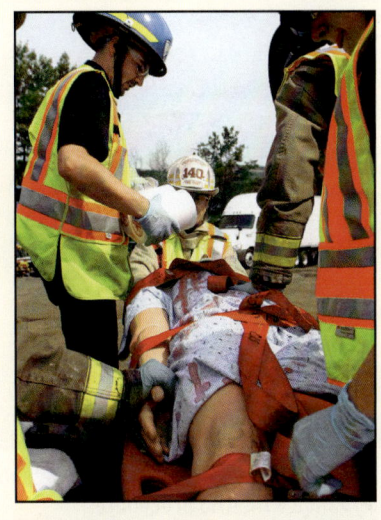

Step 6: Pad the voids between the patient and the long board as necessary in accordance with AHJ procedure.

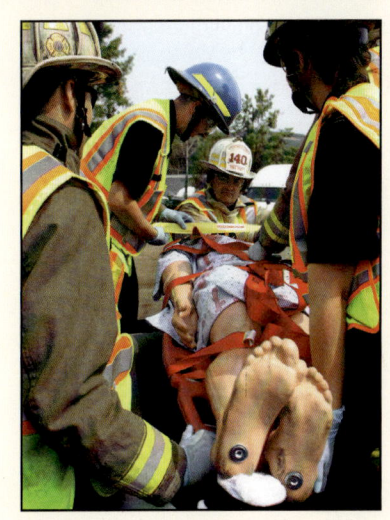

Step 7: Secure the patient to the long board in accordance with AHJ procedure.

Step 8: Assess pulse, motor, and sensory functions of the patient.

Section B • Chapter 5 – Victim Management

SKILL SHEETS

5-3
Package a patient using a seated spinal immobilization device and remove the patient to a designated safe area.

WARNING: Rescuers must ensure that the vehicle is properly stabilized and the scene is safe.

CAUTION: Rescuers must take necessary precautions to protect themselves and victims from hazards including, but not limited to glass fragments and dust, jagged metal, SRS gas cylinders, undeployed airbags, and fire hazards.

Step 1: Verbalize body substance isolation and scene safety.

Step 2: Ensure that patient has a cervical collar applied and that the head is maintained in a neutral, in-line position while providing manual support and immobilization.

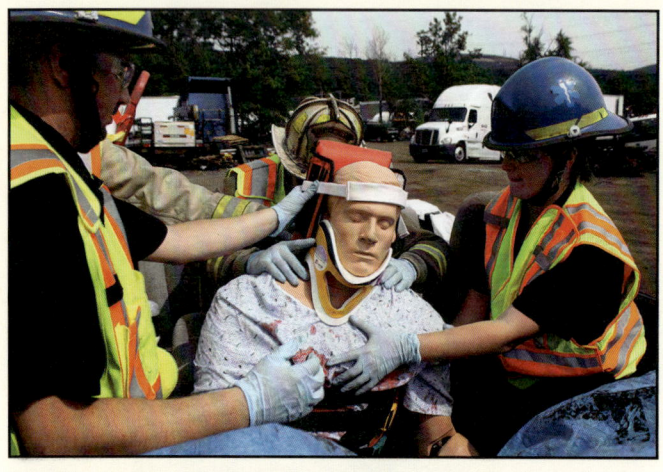

Step 3: Position the immobilization device behind the patient in accordance with AHJ procedure.

Step 4: Secure the patient to the immobilization device in accordance with AHJ procedure.

Step 5: Evaluate the fit and adjust as necessary.

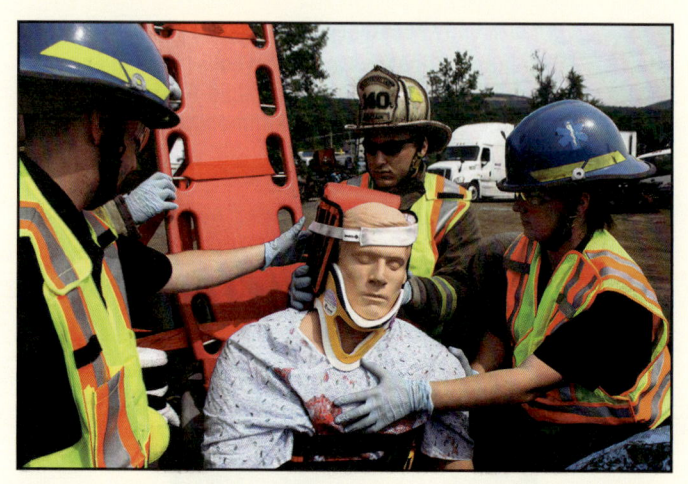

Step 6: Package the patient using a long board in accordance with AHJ procedure.

Step 7: Reassess pulse, motor, and sensory functions of the patient.

SECTION C: OPERATIONS LEVEL RESCUER — PASSENGER VEHICLE EXTRICATION

Passenger Vehicles

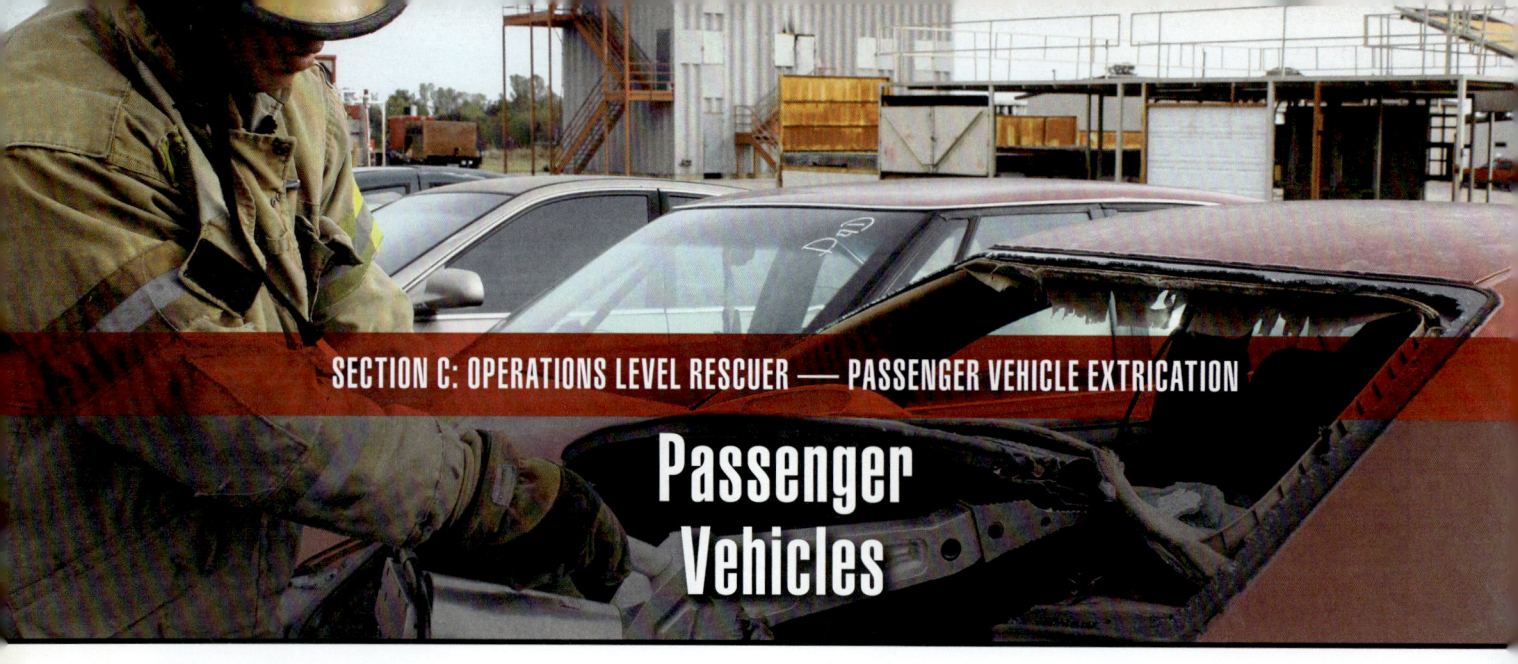

Chapter Contents

Types of Passenger Vehicles 191
    Passenger Cars 192
    Vans 197
    Sport Utility Vehicles (SUVs) 197
    Pickup Trucks 197

Passenger Vehicle Anatomy 198
    Common Vehicle Terminology 198
    Vehicle Frame 200
    Vehicle Windows 202

Passenger Vehicle Construction 204
    Passenger Vehicle Construction Materials 204
    Passenger Vehicle Fuel Systems 206
    Passenger Vehicle Electrical Systems 213
    Passenger Vehicle Exhaust Systems 216
    Passenger Vehicle Powertrain Systems 217
    Passenger Vehicle Suspension Systems 217

Passenger Vehicle Safety Features 219
    Collision Avoidance Systems 219
    Passenger Vehicle Supplemental Restraint
        Systems 220
    Energy-Absorbing Features 224
    Passenger Vehicle Rollover Protection Systems 229

Chapter Review 230

chapter 6

Key Terms

Chassis	200
Gross Vehicle Weight Rating (GVWR)	191
High-Strength-Low-Alloy Steel	228
Monocoque	200
Rollover Protection	229
Seat Belt Pretensioners	221

JPRs addressed in this chapter

This chapter provides information that addresses the following job performance requirements of NFPA 1006, *Standard for Technical Rescuer Professional Qualifications (2017)*.

- 8.2.1
- 8.2.5
- 8.2.6

Passenger Vehicles

Learning Objectives

1. Differentiate among types of passenger vehicles. [8.2.1, 8.2.6]
2. Describe elements of vehicle anatomy that are common to all passenger vehicles. [8.2.1, 8.2.5, 8.2.6]
3. Identify the types of materials used to construct passenger vehicles [8.2.5, 8.2.6]
4. Differentiate among passenger vehicle fuel systems. [8.2.5, 8.2.6]
5. Describe passenger vehicle electrical systems. [8.2.5, 8.2.6]
6. Describe passenger vehicle exhaust system components. [8.2.5, 8.2.6]
7. Describe passenger vehicle powertrain systems. [8.2.5, 8.2.6]
8. Identify components of passenger vehicle suspension systems. [8.2.5, 8.2.6]
9. Distinguish among types of collision avoidance systems. [8.2.5, 8.2.6]
10. Describe passenger vehicle supplemental restraint systems. [8.2.5, 8.2.6]
11. Identify energy-absorbing features of vehicles. [8.2.5, 8.2.6]
12. Explain the purpose of vehicle rollover protection. [8.2.5, 8.2.6]

Chapter 6
Passenger Vehicles

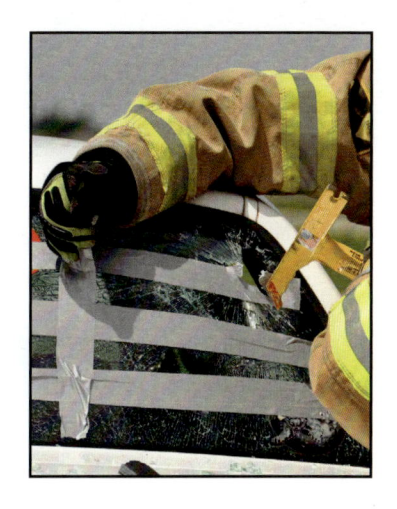

The majority of all vehicle incidents involve one or more passenger vehicles. Rescue personnel should be prepared to mitigate hazards, stabilize, and extricate a variety of types of passenger vehicles, ranging from compact cars to full-size vans. These vehicles contain multiple systems, such as fuel, electrical, and powertrain systems, and are constructed using many different materials and safety features. In order to perform vehicle extrication safely and effectively, rescuers should have a thorough understanding of passenger vehicles:

- Types of passenger vehicles
- General anatomy
- Passenger vehicle safety systems
- Passenger vehicle fuel systems
- Passenger vehicle electrical systems
- Passenger vehicle exhaust systems
- Passenger vehicle powertrain systems
- Passenger vehicle suspension systems

Types of Passenger Vehicles

Passenger vehicles are intended for one basic function — to transport people from one place to another in relative comfort and safety. Many designs exist and all vehicles will react differently in a collision, which may present unique challenges for rescue personnel.

In the United States (U.S.), the National Highway Traffic Safety Administration (NHTSA), under the direction of the Department of Transportation (DOT), classifies passenger vehicles according to the wheelbase and/or the **gross vehicle weight rating (GVWR)**. The wheelbase is the distance between the front and rear axles. The GVWR is the weight of the vehicle, including maximum cargo capacity. Additionally, some passenger vehicles are further defined by the total amount of passenger and cargo volume, measured in cubic feet (cubic meters), within the vehicle.

The NHTSA defines the most common types of passenger vehicles as the following:

- Passenger cars
- Vans
- Sport utility vehicles (SUVs)
- Pickup trucks **(Table 6.1, p. 192)**

Gross Vehicle Weight Rating (GVWR) — Maximum weight at which a vehicle can be safely operated on roadways; includes the weight of the vehicle itself plus fuel, passengers, cargo, and trailer tongue weight.

Table 6.1
Examples of Passenger Vehicles, Vans, and Light Trucks

Types	Example	Type	Example
Microcars shown: Smart Fortwo		**Station Wagons** shown: Dodge Magnum	
Subcompacts shown: Honda Fit		**Limousines** shown: Springfield Coach Body on a Mercury Lincoln Town Car Chassis	
Compacts shown: Toytota Corolla		**Sports** shown: Chevrolet Corvette	
Midsize shown: Honda Accord		**Convertibles** shown: Chrysler PT Cruiser	
Full size shown: Chevrolet Impala		**Roadsters** shown: Pontiac Solstice	

Continued on next page

Table 6.1 (Continued)
Examples of Passenger Vehicles, Vans, and Light Trucks

Types	Example	Type	Example
Kit Cars shown: Locust 7		**Crossover SUVs** shown: Toyota RAV4	
Pickup Trucks shown: Dodge Ram		**Utility Vehicles** shown: Mitsubishi Mini Truck	
Vans shown: Chevrolet Express (15-passenger)		**RV** shown: Four Winds RV Body on Ford E350 Chassis	
Minivans shown: Dodge Grand Caravan			
Sports Utility Vehicles (SUVs) shown: Suburban			

Section C • Chapter 6 – Passenger Vehicles

> **All-Terrain Vehicles**
>
> With the increased popularity of utility all-terrain vehicles (UATV) and all-terrain vehicles (ATV) in rural areas, the possibility of accidents involving these vehicles are continually increasing. In recent years, a continuing increase in size, weight, and carrying capabilities of these vehicles has progressed. Today, the common UATV/ATV is as large as most compact cars and trucks. Some are capable of carrying up to six people in fully encapsulated poly-carbon and steel-cab enclosures.
>
> Rescuers should be aware of the variety of challenges that UATVs/ATVs pose. These vehicles lack passenger protection and restraint systems, so there is a greater chance of passenger entrapment, ejection, and/or injury depending on the nature of the accident. Incidents involving UATVs/ATVs may occur at significant distances from main roadways, making it difficult for rescuers to access the site and transport necessary tools and equipment to the incident. Some other challenges include:
>
> - The terrain itself
> - Vehicle stabilization
> - Transferring victims

NOTE: For more specific information about passenger vehicles that are common within your geographical area, personnel should research the appropriate governmental regulations.

Passenger Cars

The NHTSA classifies passenger cars into separate categories according to wheelbase. Rescue personnel should know these categories and the types of cars included within each category. Types of passenger cars include the following:

- Minicompact cars
- Subcompact cars
- Compact cars
- Midsize cars
- Large (full size) cars
- Other cars

Minicompact Cars

Minicompact cars (also called station cars) are extremely small vehicles generally less than 10 feet (3 m) in length with interior volumes of less than 85 cubic feet (2.5 m^3) and a wheelbase of less than 86 inches (2 150 mm). Size restrictions limit the vehicles' occupant loads. Some minicompact cars have three wheels, while others have four. A wide variety of minitrucks based on minicompact designs has also been developed.

Subcompact Cars

The NHTSA classifies passenger vehicles with a wheelbase of less than 100 inches (2 500 mm) as subcompact. In general, subcompact cars are primarily economy cars. They are relatively smaller vehicles that typically have unibody construction, often do not have a trunk, and may have a third door or a hatchback in the rear. They may only have those safety features required by law.

Compact Cars
Compact cars, according to NHTSA, are those with a wheelbase between 100 and 104 inches (2 500 and 2 600 mm). They are typically slightly larger versions of those in the subcompact class and may have four doors, trunks, and even station wagon configurations. The majority of compact cars also have unibody construction.

Midsize Cars
According to NHTSA, midsize or intermediate class vehicles are those with a wheelbase of 105 to 109 inches (2 600 to 2 700 mm). They are some what larger than compacts, and many have unibody construction. This size class also includes midsize station wagons. A midsize car may have three to five doors and may or may not have a rigid frame.

Large Cars
Large cars have a wheelbase of 110 to 114 inches (2 750 to 2 850 mm). This class includes what some call luxury automobiles. Many large cars are built on rigid frames, while others have space frame or unibody construction. Their heavy construction can make extrication operations more difficult and time consuming.

Specialized Passenger Vehicles
There are several other types or variations of passenger cars than those previously mentioned, which include:

- Station wagons
- Limousines
- Sports cars/sports coupes
- Roadsters
- Convertibles
- Kit cars

Station wagons. Station wagons are generally modifications of sedan-type automobile bodies designed to carry two to nine passengers. The passenger compartment of a station wagon extends to the vehicle's rear window, replacing what would otherwise be a trunk. The rear space may be used for carrying loads or passengers and may be reached through a hatch or rear door(s).

Station wagons are distinguishable from hatchback vehicles, minivans, or SUVs in two ways. First, the height of the passenger compartment remains the same for its entire length. Second, the front body of the vehicle matches other vehicles in the manufacturer's production line. Station wagons can be categorized based on their total amount of passenger and cargo volume.

Limousines. Limousines are some of the largest passenger vehicles and have wheelbases of more than 114 inches (2 850 mm). The passenger compartment is usually divided between the front and rear seats by a movable glass partition. These vehicles may have extended chassis and multiple doors. In some instances, they may be armored. This category includes those vehicles that have been manufactured as or converted into limousines. They are all heavy vehicles built on rigid frames but are still vulnerable in side-impact (T-bone) collisions.

Although all vehicles have passengers that might not wear seat belts, limousine passengers are more than likely not to be wearing seat belts. In the event of a collision, passengers can be seriously injured by being thrown about inside the vehicle.

Sports cars/sports coupes. This category consists of two-seat roadsters, hatchback models, and muscle cars. Sports cars/sports coupes can be equipped with various types of rollover protection systems (ROPS). Many of these cars are involved in many high-speed collisions, perhaps rolling over numerous times before coming to rest. Manufacturers produce a variety of sports cars based on their various automobile production models.

Roadsters. Roadsters were conversions of popular older vehicles into two-seat open vehicles that offered limited protection from the weather and collisions because they lacked a roof, rear and side windows, and passenger protection systems. Modern roadsters are two-seat, convertible sports cars.

Convertibles. Many manufacturers offer a special variant of their more popular vehicle production lines. These vehicles are called convertibles and have a roof and rear window assembly that is removable or retractable. Many convertibles and sports cars have soft tops and may have ROPS installed in them. Some ROPS may be permanently deployed, while others may be deployed by crash or roll-activated sensors. Unlike roadsters, convertibles are equipped with roll-up side windows.

Kit cars. Kit cars are automobiles that may be purchased as a kit or set of parts that must be assembled. Major components, such as the transmission and engine, are normally taken from other donor vehicles. Kit cars often mirror the appearance of other factory production vehicles. Because these vehicles are often shop built, rescuers need to be aware of the potential presence of additional protection systems or the lack of typical passenger protection systems.

Vans

Vans are a functional type of passenger vehicle. They can be configured to hold up to ten passengers or be used to transport cargo. This category is further broken down into minivans and full-size vans.

Minivans

Minivans perform the same functions as both station wagons and sport utility vehicles and have a GVWR less than 8,500 pounds (4 250 kg) . Though minivans can be used to transport small cargo, their primary function is to transport people. Minivans can often transport an entire family or a children's sports team. When the rear seats are removed, they can accommodate large and bulky cargo that most other family vehicles cannot accommodate. Some minivans have only a driver's door on the left side and a passenger's door and a conventional or sliding door on the right side. Other minivans are built with a conventional or sliding door on the left side of the vehicle as well. They have either a single or double door in the rear of the vehicle. From a safety standpoint, their large profile makes them vulnerable to crosswinds, and their relatively high center of gravity makes them vulnerable to rollovers.

Full Size Vans

In North America, the term full size van refers to a full frame-based commercial vehicle with an integrated passenger/cargo compartment similar to that of a station wagon. Generally, the passenger version of this type of van has windows along the rear sides of the vehicle while the cargo version (called a panel van) does not. In some countries, the word van refers to a passenger-based wagon that has no rear side windows. Like minivans, their large profile makes them vulnerable to crosswinds, and their relatively high center of gravity makes them vulnerable to rollovers.

Sport Utility Vehicles (SUVs)

Sport utility vehicles (SUVs) evolved out of the truck-based station wagons of earlier decades. The older vehicles were basically designed as station wagons but were built on a truck chassis as opposed to a car chassis. SUVs with four-wheel drive capability are sometimes used for off-road recreational driving and they may be involved in off-highway incidents. The off-road environment can add considerably to the challenges for rescue personnel in these incidents.

Pickup Trucks

Pickup trucks are available in a wide range of sizes and styles. These vehicles are all constructed on full rigid frames, and many have four-wheel drive capability. Their carrying capacity ranges from ½ to 1 ton, and they can be equipped with a variety of suspension systems to support the rated carrying capacity.

NOTE: Like SUVs, pickup trucks with four-wheel drive capability are sometimes used for off-road recreational driving. Rescue personnel should be prepared to deal with off-highway incidents that involve pickup trucks.

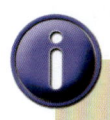

> **Sport Utility Trucks**
>
> Sport utility trucks are a combination of four-door passenger, vehicle interior luxury with the ability to haul payloads similar to that of a light pickup. The passenger compartment tends to be much larger than a standard truck, and the bed is typically much shorter.

Passenger Vehicle Anatomy

Most passenger vehicles consist of the same types of elements. These elements may vary in appearance across all different types of passenger vehicles, but serve the same purpose for every car. For example, the front of every vehicle varies dramatically; however, for vehicle extrication purposes, the front of the vehicle is consistent across all types of passenger vehicles. This section will introduce the areas that are common to all vehicles. These areas include the following:

- Common vehicle terminology
- Vehicle frame
- Vehicle windows

Common Vehicle Terminology

Common terminology is useful, particularly during emergency situations where confusion must be avoided. From an extrication standpoint, every vehicle can be considered to have eight sides with which rescuers must be concerned **(Figure 6.1)**. Regardless of the type or size of vehicle, rescuers must observe, evaluate, and deal with all aspects or sides. The following are common terms used to describe various areas of a vehicle:

- **Front**— End of the vehicle that the driver faces during normal operation, generally indicated by the headlights
- **Rear**—Opposite end of the vehicle from the front, generally indicated by the taillights
- **Interior** — Composed of the passenger compartment and may contain the storage compartment
- **Exterior** — Composed of the vehicle's body panels, windows, bumpers, and other components

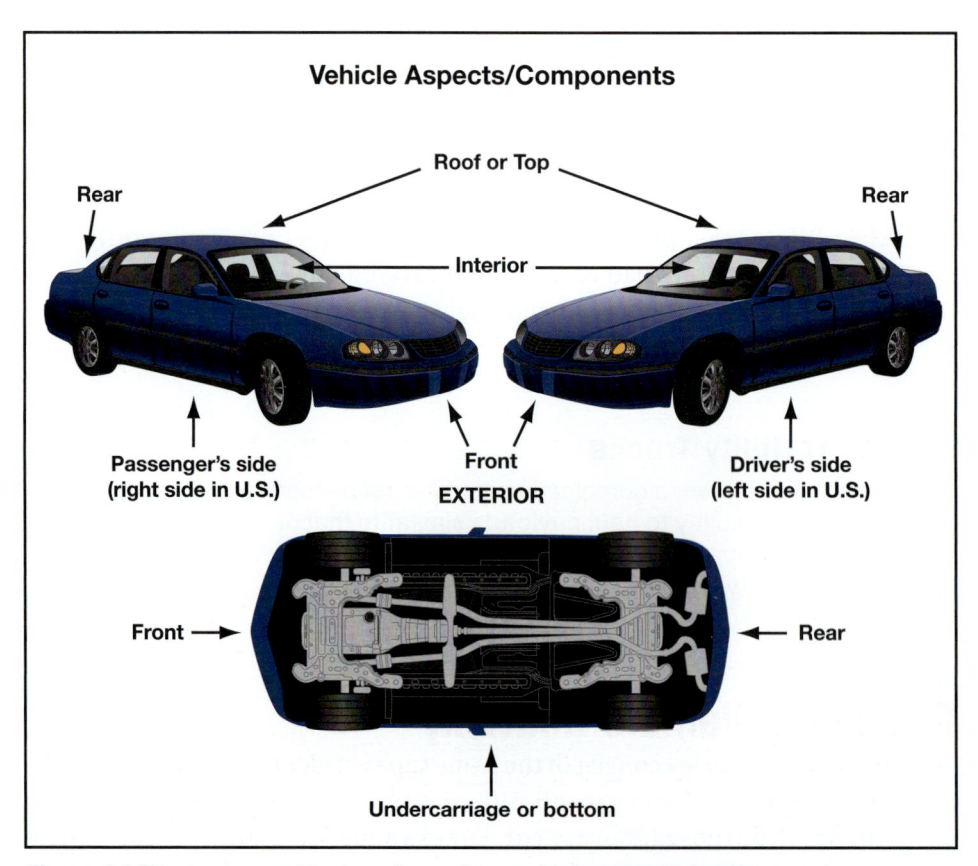

Figure 6.1 The terms used to describe various vehicle aspects or components.

198 Section C • Chapter 6 – Passenger Vehicles

- **Driver's side** — Side of the vehicle where the steering wheel is located
- **Passenger's side** — Side of the vehicle opposite the steering wheel
- **Undercarriage** — Underside of the vehicle, contains the chassis or frame, drivetrain, and the floor pan
- **Roof** — Top or cover of a vehicle

NOTE: The roof is always called the roof, no matter how the vehicle rests (wheel resting, side resting, or roof resting).

In addition, individual vehicle components are commonly described by specific terms. It is important that extrication personnel use the same terms for the door/roof posts and various other vehicle components. Terms for specific components are as follows:

- **Door/roof posts** — Structural members that surround the doors and support the roofs of vehicles:
  — Normally identified alphabetically from front to rear (A-post, B-post, C-post) **(Figure 6.2)**.
  — Also called pillars (A-pillar, B-pillar, C-pillar).
- **Hinges** — Allow vehicle doors to open and close:
  — Many sizes, shapes, and types of hinges
  — Bolted, glued, or welded to the vehicle
  — Focal point in many extrication scenarios
- **Latches and locks** — Mechanisms that capture the door when closed and lock it in place:
  — Focal point in various extrication techniques
  — Examples include the Nader bolt and the U-bolt.
- **Fenders** — Body material that surrounds the front tires. The fender, also called the front fender, starts at the front of the vehicle, proceeds around the front tire, and ends at the fire wall
- **Quarter panels** — Body material that surrounds the area of the rear tire
- **Firewall** — A partition between the engine compartment and the passenger compartment of a vehicle that is designed to protect vehicle occupants from the engine and its associated hazards

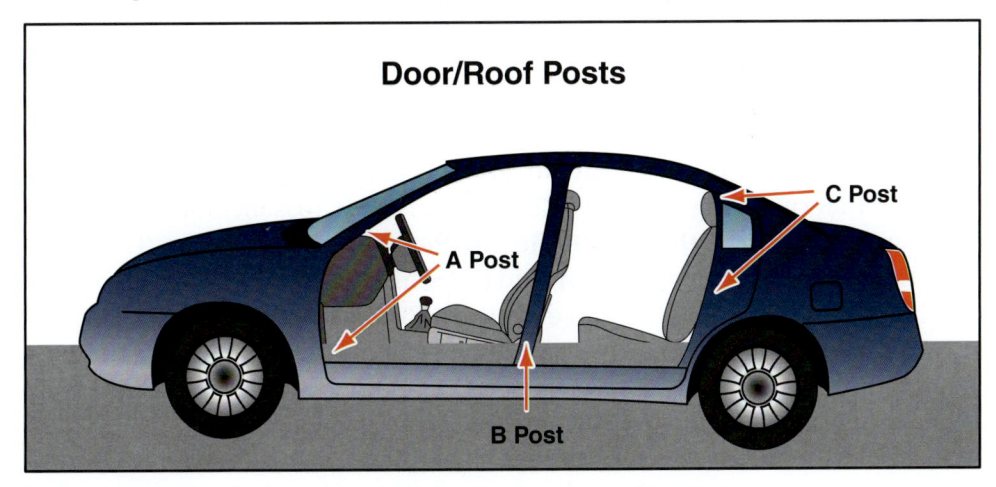

Figure 6.2 This illustration shows how door/roof posts are identified.

- **Kick panels** — Vertical panel wall in front of the A-post that is enclosed by several structural members
- **Rocker panels** — Rounded narrow body panels on each side of a vehicle below the doors and between the kick panel and the quarter panel. (Also known as *rocker channel*)

Vehicle Frame

A vehicle's frame provides the basic structural foundation or integrity of the vehicle. There are three basic frames used in modern vehicles: full or rigid frames, unibody, and space frames **(Figure 6.3)**. Additional specialty frames do exist, such as the **monocoque**.

A vehicle's structural integrity is determined by the remaining strength of the vehicle's **chassis** after a collision. The chassis may then be weakened further by rescuer's extrication efforts, such as removing the vehicle's roof or doors.

The type of vehicle frame may determine how a vehicle's structural integrity is affected by a collision and/or vehicle extrication. Full or rigid frame vehicles may be less affected by a collision than vehicles with a unibody or space frame. The structural integrity of vehicles with a full or rigid frame is also less affected by vehicle extrication, such as a door or roof removal, than vehicles with unibody frames. Rescuers should also be aware that older vehicles tend to retain more of their structural integrity because they contain more steel and less aluminum, magnesium, and plastic in their construction.

> **Monocoque** — Construction technique in which an object's external skin supports the structural load of the object.

> **Chassis** — Basic operating system of a motor vehicle consisting of the frame, suspension system, wheels, and steering mechanism but not the body.

CAUTION
When the chassis is weakened, the structural integrity is compromised, allowing unwanted and perhaps dangerous movement that must be prevented if rescuers and those trapped in the vehicle are to be protected.

Full or Rigid Frame

Full or rigid frames used in automobile construction have been around since the creation of vehicles. Early automobiles had frames made of wood, but steel has been the material of choice. Full or rigid frames are used in automobile body-on-frame construction. An advantage of body-on-frame construction is that it allows frequent changes to body styles without having to make changes to the chassis.

To form a chassis, a steel ladder frame is constructed using two parallel beams that run along the long axis of the vehicle. Cross members are bolted and welded between these beams to provide rigidity and support. This chassis then supports the powertrain, and the vehicle body is bolted to the frame. While smaller automobiles and even some SUVs have begun using unitized or unibody construction, manufacturers still use full or rigid frames on larger automobiles and trucks, particularly heavy-duty vehicles that carry or pull heavy loads.

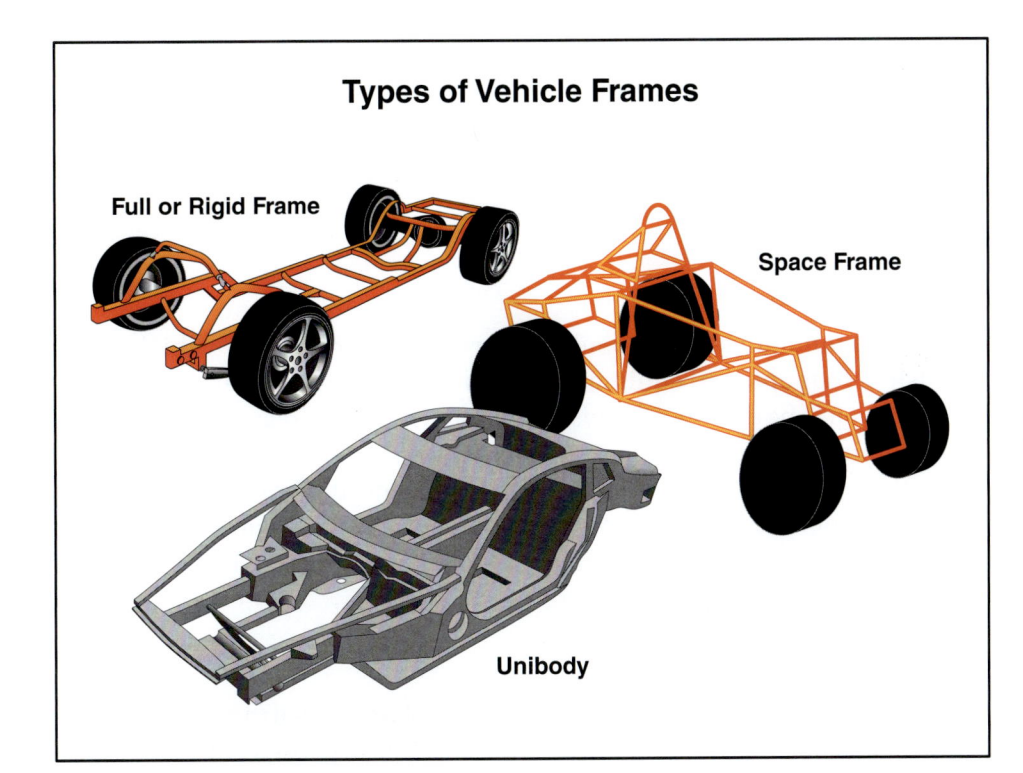

Figure 6.3 Examples of full (rigid), unibody, and space frames used in vehicle construction.

Unibody (Unitized Body)

As the price of aluminum dropped in the 1920s and 1930s, automobile manufacturers began to look at the use of unitized body (also called unibody or integral frame) construction that was becoming common in the aviation industry. In unibody construction, a vehicle's stress-bearing elements and sheet metal body parts are built together as one unit instead of attaching the vehicle's body to a frame as in body-on-frame construction. Unibody construction became more common following World War II, and today, spot-welded unibody construction is the dominant automobile construction technique.

Space Frame

Space frames are aluminum skeletons that are similar to aircraft frames upon which the aluminum, plastic, or composite skin of the vehicle's body is attached. The internal structure of these space frames provides the structural support for the vehicle while the skin provides aerodynamics, styling, and protection from the elements. Space frames are designed to support the entire load of the vehicle even if the skin of the vehicle is damaged. Because they are constructed of aluminum, these frames may weigh as much as 50 percent less than conventional steel or aluminum unibody frames.

Lighter vehicles built on space frames can be more fuel efficient and, in smaller production runs, less expensive to build than the more common steel or aluminum unibody vehicles.

Vehicle Windows

The windows of a vehicle are designed to do more than simply maintain the internal environment and to protect the occupants from being struck by insects or flying objects. Vehicle windows also serve to help keep the occupants inside the vehicle during accidents and can affect the vehicle's structural integrity. Vehicle windows can be made of the following:

- Glass
- Polycarbonates
- Laminated materials
- Tempered materials
- Transparent armor materials

Early automobiles were open-compartment, fair-weather vehicles with windshields as optional equipment. As time passed and passenger compartments began to be enclosed, windshields and windows of regular glass became more common. Regular glass was used in vehicles manufactured prior to 1927 when the laminated safety windshield was introduced. The trend toward safer glass for automobiles continued with the development of improved laminated safety glass, tempered glass, enhanced protective glass (EPG), and now polycarbonates and transparent armor.

Laminated Safety Glass

Laminated safety glass consists of two sheets of glass bonded to a sheet of plastic sandwiched between them **(Figure 6.4)**. This type of glass is most commonly used for windshields and some rear windows; however, with increasing safety standards, many vehicle manufacturers are starting to use laminated safety glass in all windows. Impact produces many long, pointed shards with sharp edges. The plastic laminate sheet holds most of these shards and fragments in place. When broken, the glass remains attached to the laminate and moves as a unit, which makes windshield removal easier.

Some manufacturers have laminated an additional layer of plastic to the passenger side of the windshield for added protection. Some laminated glass side windows are more than 1/3-inch (8 mm) thick. Many laminated wind-

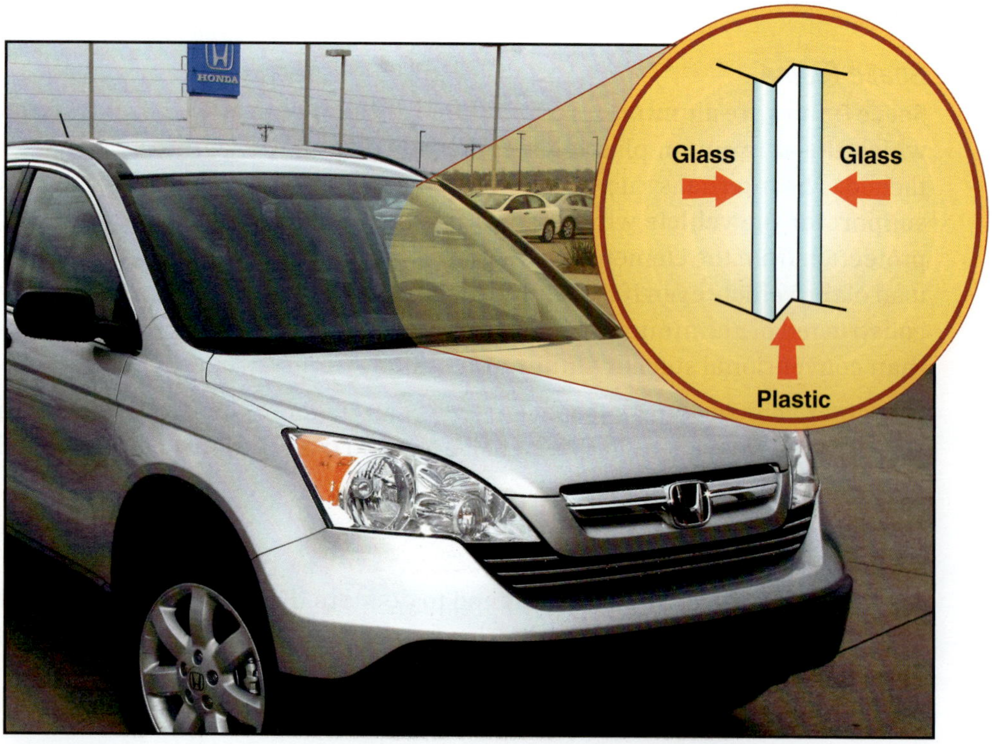

Figure 6.4 Laminated glass is required in passenger vehicle windshields.

shields and rear windows are now held in place with polyurethane glue. These windows can be identified by the black shading around the perimeter of the window, designed to protect the glue from sun damage.

Tempered Glass
Tempered glass is most commonly used in side windows and some rear windows. Tempered glass is designed to spread small fracture lines throughout the plate when struck. The glass then separates into many small pieces, decreasing the hazards of long, pointed pieces of glass. However, new problems are created such as small nuisance lacerations to unprotected body parts and the possible wounds to the eyes with tiny bits of glass **(Figure 6.5)**.

Enhanced Protective Glass (EPG)
Enhanced protective glass is usually used in side and rear-window locations. This glass is similar to laminate, but it is typically thinner, lighter, and stronger. EPG also has better soundproofing qualities than laminate. Current models that use EPG include Audi, Volvo, and Mercedes.

Polycarbonate
Advancements in the plastics industry have made the use of polycarbonate window glazing over glass for side and rear windows more common. These window systems provide greater scratch resistance, reduced weight, and a wider variety of window shapes. Some disadvantages of polycarbonate glass are its cost and the difficulty involved in penetrating it.

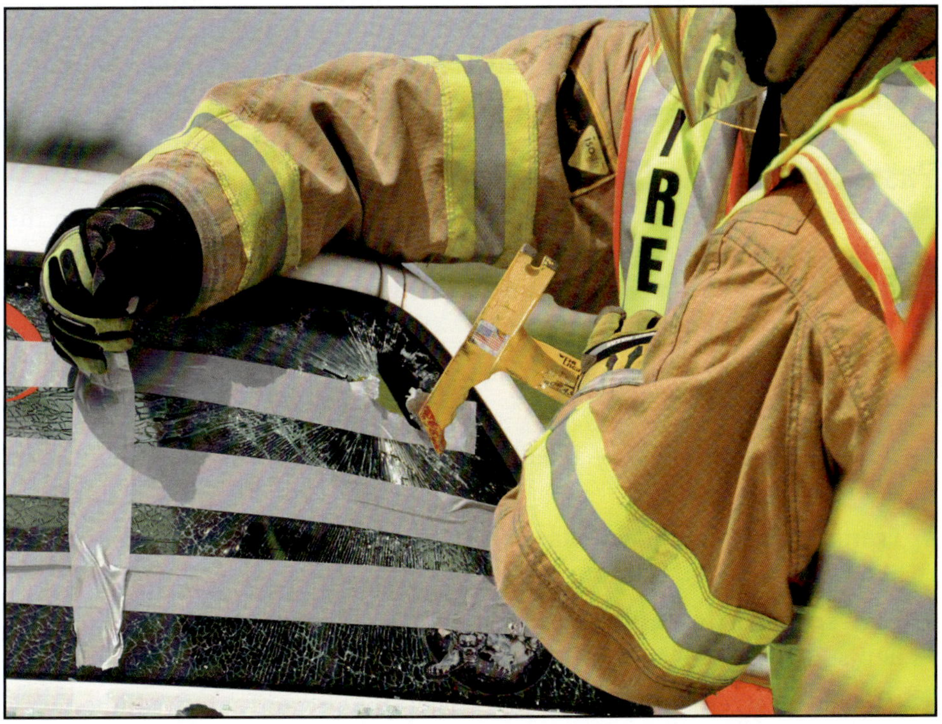

Figure 6.5 Rescue personnel preparing to break and remove tempered glass. *Courtesy of Sonrise Photography.*

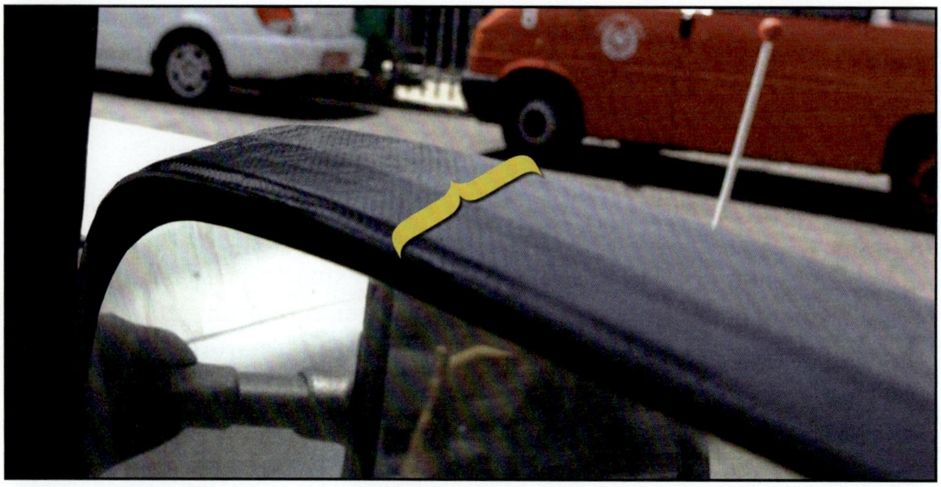

Figure 6.6 This photo shows the thickness of transparent armor or ballistic glass.

Transparent Armor
Transparent armor or ballistic glass and plastic are commonly made of sheets of polycarbonate material sandwiched between sheets of glass. Heat and pressure are used to laminate these materials together to form a ballistic glass capable of absorbing the impact of bullets or shrapnel and preventing them from piercing the glass **(Figure 6.6)**.

Passenger Vehicle Construction
Passenger vehicles are manufactured using a variety of construction materials and integral systems. Each type of passenger vehicle is unique, yet they all incorporate similar components such as fuel and electrical systems. The sections that follow describe the construction materials and integral systems common to most passenger vehicles.

Passenger Vehicle Construction Materials
A vehicle's construction materials and how those materials are used in the vehicle's construction can have an impact on vehicle extrication operations. Modern automobiles are constructed using many different materials in a variety of components such as:

- **Mild steel** — Used in vehicle frame, body components, and I-beam safety components
- **Dual phase (DP) steel** — Used in vehicle frame, body components, and safety components
- **Transformation induced plasticity (TRIP) steel** — Used in vehicle frame, body components, and safety components
- **High strength/low alloy (HSLA) steel** — Used in body and safety components. Includes DP and TRIP Steel
- **Ultra high strength steel (UHSS)** –Used in body and safety components. Includes boron and martensite
- **Aluminum** — Used in vehicle bodies, engines, and frames
- **Magnesium** — Used in tire rims, engine components, transmission housings, steering columns, frame support members, and dashboards

- **Copper** — Used in electrical system wiring
- **Plastics** — Used in light covers, body components, exterior/interior panels, dashboards, and seats
- **Composite materials** — Used in various vehicle components
- **Alloys** — Used in engines and vehicle body components
- **Glass** — Used in windshields, windows, lights, and light covers
- **Rubber** — Used in tires and electrical wiring insulation
- **Cast iron** — Used in agricultural and construction equipment bodies

> **WARNING!**
> Magnesium is highly reactive to water. If a magnesium component is on fire, use a Class D extinguisher. If one is not available, a large of volume of water can be effective and may minimize the magnesium/water reaction.

Due to changes in the Federal Motor Vehicle Safety Standards 214 and 216, ultra high strength steels, such as boron steel and martensite, are common in passenger vehicles manufactured since 2012. The standards state that manufacturers will decrease passenger vehicle injuries and fatalities in side-impact and rollover collisions; however, these standards give no direction as to how manufacturers will accomplish this goal. Manufacturers often choose to produce vehicles with more steel or stronger steel to reduce vehicle injuries and fatalities. Due to other limitations, such as fuel mileage restrictions, many manufacturers have also elected to use lighter steel.

> **CAUTION**
> Many construction materials present laceration and penetrating injury and inhalation hazards to rescuers and victims.

Passenger Vehicle Fuel Systems

Modern vehicles use a variety of different fuel systems which include the following:

- Conventional fuels
- Hybrid Electric Vehicles (HEV) **(Figure 6.7)**.
- Plug-In Hybrid Electric Vehicles (PHEV)
- Electric Vehicles (EV)
- Extended Range Electric Vehicles (EREV)
- Alternative fuels
- Fuel tanks

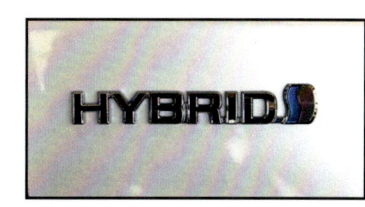

Figure 6.7 An example of a "Hybrid" label on an automobile.

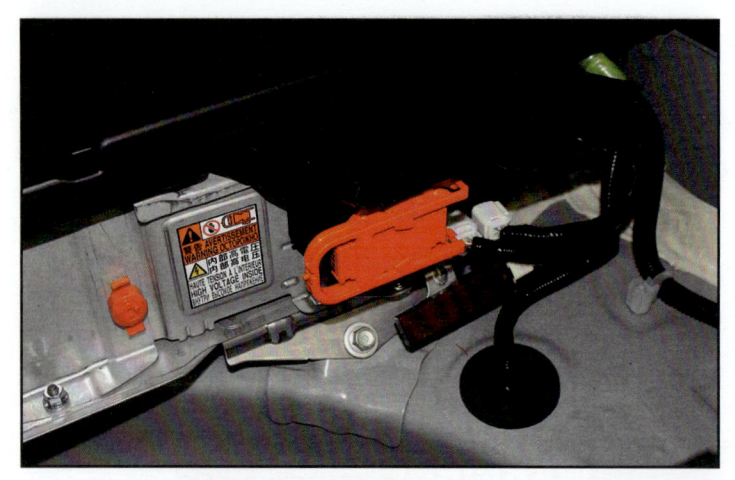

Figure 6.8 Batteries on some newer vehicles are found in the trunk.

Conventional Fuels

The two most common fuels used in automotive vehicles are gasoline and diesel, called petrol and petroldiesel in some countries. Gasoline and diesel are both hydrocarbon-based fuels, derived from petroleum , and can be ignited easily. During extrication operations, rescue personnel must ensure that gasoline or diesel leaks from vehicle tanks are controlled and ignition sources are isolated to prevent fires. If ignited, the fires should be extinguished rapidly.

Hybrid Electric Vehicles (HEV)

In the ongoing effort to minimize fuel consumption and to protect the environment, automobile manufacturers have been developing and constructing increasing numbers of hybrid vehicles. Conventional hybrid vehicles are powered by propulsion systems which have internal combustion engines and electric motors. HEVs cannot be plugged in and recharged. Instead, they utilize regenerative braking to collect kinetic energy and convert that energy into electricity, which is stored in the hybrid vehicle's batteries until needed. Most HEV batteries are housed in the trunk **(Figure 6.8)**.

The danger associated with hybrid vehicles is the high voltage stored within the batteries and running through wiring or cables connected to the vehicle's electric motor. These cables can carry as much as 650 volts of direct current. Rescue personnel may be exposed to the danger of electrical shock when attempting to isolate the electrical power system and batteries. Most manufacturers color code the cables orange, yellow, or blue to help rescuers and emergency responders recognize the power wires and cables for this system. However, there is no standard that mandates this. Several redundant safety measures are built into these systems to minimize accidental shock; however, rescue personnel should avoid the vehicle's electrical system as much as possible.

NOTE: HEVs also utilize a 12-volt (low voltage) battery similar to standard passenger vehicles.

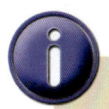

> **ℹ Vehicle Voltage**
>
> The automotive industry has adopted and implemented some standard terminology regarding voltage in vehicles. These voltage terms (high, medium, and low) are represented visually within the vehicle's electrical systems through color-coded wiring.
>
> - High Voltage (orange wiring) — Any voltage measurement greater than 60 volts
> - Medium Voltage (blue wiring) — Any voltage measurement between 30 and 60 volts
> - Low Voltage (any color wiring) — Any voltage measurement less than 30 volts

Currently, there is no standardized means to identify a hybrid vehicle by sight upon approach. Manufacturers use different symbols and different wording placed in different locations on the vehicles called badging to identify them as hybrids.

Rescue organization members are encouraged to monitor the development and production of hybrid cars by automobile manufacturers. Some manufacturers post information on their company websites for emergency responders to use when dealing with their vehicles during an emergency **(Table 6.2, p. 208)**.

NOTE: Personnel can access numerous information sources on HEVs, such as the NHTSA website, NFPA, *Hybrid and Electric Vehicle Emergency Field Guide*, manufacturer's emergency response guides, and various mobile applications.

Plug-In Hybrid Electric Vehicles (PHEV)

Plug-In Hybrid Electric Vehicles (PHEVs) are similar to the conventional hybrids in that they both are powered by conventional or alternative fuels as well as electric power stored in a battery. The PHEV battery can be charged by plugging it into an outside power source, by the internal combustion engine, or by regenerative braking. Unlike HEVs, which still depend on petroleum, it is possible for PHEVs to run on only electricity, up to 40 miles, when fully charged. However, because PHEVs can run off petroleum or electricity, they can be a good option for driving longer distances if recharging locations or options are unknown.

Electric Vehicles (EV)

Battery electric vehicles (EVs) run exclusively on electricity from onboard batteries. EVs are propelled by a battery-powered motor and are charged by plugging into an outlet at home or a public charging station. These vehicles have no gasoline engine; therefore, they produce no tailpipe emissions and have no exhaust systems. They have longer driving ranges as compared to PHEVs on the market today, and generally travel 60 to 80 miles (95 to 130 km) per charge, though a some models can travel over 200 miles (320 km) on a single charge. As emerging battery technology continues to improve, EV ranges will continue to extend, offering a greater number of drivers the option to drive exclusively on electricity.

Table 6.2
Examples of Hybrid Cars (by automobile manufacturer)

Manufacturer	Model Name	External Identification	HV Battery Locations	High Voltage (HV)	HV Cable Route	HV Isolation Methods
Ford/Mercury	Escape / Mariner	Ford Hybrid Green Leaf on fenders and tailgate	Cargo area under carpet	300+ volts Orange Cables	Under the vehicle from the right side near the rear axle to just off-center behind the front axle	Turn of ignition key, remove key from ignition, and place on dash. Disconnect negative cable on the 12 volt battery. Place high voltage service disconnect switch into service position, if possible.
General Motors	Chevrolet Silverado / GMC Sierra	"Hybrid" badge located on vehicle's doors and 120v outlets in bed	Under the rear seat	42 volts (intermediate voltage) Blue Cables	Under the vehicle from beneath the rear seat to the center behind the front axle	If 120 VAC APO indicator is on, depress the APO button, turn of ignition key, remove key from ignition, and place on dash. Disable the 42 volt battery pack using the service disconnect switch behind the lower right corner of the battery unit. Disconnect the 12 volt battery.
General Motors	Saturn VUE Green Line	"Vue" and "Hybrid" badges on lift gate and "Hybrid" badge on front doors	Under rear cargo floor	36 - 42 volts (intermediate voltage) Blue Cables	Under the vehicle from beneath the rear cargo floor to the center behind the front axle	Turn of ignition key, remove key from ignition, and place on dash. Disconnect both negative cables on the 12 volt battery. If ignition key can't be reached, remove the 30 amp ignition maxi fuse in engine compartment.
Honda	Accord / Civic	Word "Hydrid" on rear of vehicle	Behind the rear seat	144 volts Orange Cables	Under the vehicle from the right side near the rear axle to just off-center behind the front axle	**Best method:** Turn of ignition key, remove key from ignition, and place on dash. **Second best method:** Remove main fuse and disconnect both negative cables on the 12 volt battery.
Honda	Insight	Word "Hydrid" on rear of vehicle rear "wheel pants"	Behind the passenger seats and below the cargo area	144 volts Orange Cables	Under the vehicle from the left side near the rear axle to just off-center behind the front axle	**Best method:** Turn of ignition key, remove key from ignition, and place on dash. **Second best method:** Remove main fuse and disconnect both negative cables on the 12 volt battery.
Lexus	GS450h	Lexus GS450h logos on rear trunk and "Hybrid" logos on rear door moldings	In the trunk behind the rear seat.	288 volts Orange Cables	Under the vehicle from the center near the rear axle to the right side behind the front axle	**Procedure 1:** Turn of ignition key, remove key from ignition, and place on dash. If key cannot be removed, disconnect the 12 volt battery. **Procedure 2 (If ignition key can't be reached):** Disconnect the 12 volt battery and remove IGCT No. 4 fuse relay in engine compartment. **Power remains in the HV system for 5 minutes after disabling.**

Continued on next page

Table 6.2 (Continued)
Examples of Hybrid Cars (by automobile manufacturer)

Manufacturer	Model Name	External Identification	HV Battery Locations	High Voltage (HV)	HV Cable Route	HV Isolation Methods
Lexus (continued)	RX400h	Lexus RX400h logos on rear hatch	In the passenger compartment under the rear seat	288 boosted to 650 volts at engine. Orange Cables	Under the vehicle from the right side near the rear axle to just off-center behind the front axle	**Procedure 1** **(If READY indicator is on):** Push POWER button once. **(If READY indicator is not on):** Do NOT push POWER button. Keep SMART KEY at least 16 feet (5 m) from vehicle. If SMART KEY cannot be located, disconnect the 12 volt battery. **Procedure 2 (If POWER button can't be reached):** Disconnect the 12 volt battery and remove IGCT No. 1 fuse in engine compartment. Pull all fuses if unable to identify correct fuse. **Procedure 3 (If POWER button and engine compartment can't be reached):** Remove RH J/B-B fuse trunk. Pull all 3 fuses if unable to identify correct fuse. Then disconnect the 12 volt battery *Power remains in the HV system for 10 minutes after disabling.*
Toyota	Camry	Camry and "Hybrid Synergy Drive" logos on trunk lid. "Hybrid" logos on front fenders	In the trunk behind the rear seat	245 volts Orange Cables	Under the vehicle from the right side near the rear axle inboard to center line to just above center of the left front axle	**Procedure 1** **(If READY indicator is on):** Push POWER button once. **(If READY indicator is not on):** Do NOT push POWER button. Keep SMART KEY at least 3.3 feet (1 m) from vehicle. If SMART KEY cannot be located, disconnect the 12 volt battery. **Procedure 2 (If POWER button can't be reached):** Disconnect the 12 volt battery and remove IGCT No. 2 fuse in engine compartment. Pull all fuses if unable to identify correct fuse.
	FCHV (Hydrogen is stored in the vehicle's cylinder for at up to 5,000 psi [34 474 kpa])	FCHV Fuel Cell Hybrid Vehicle labels on the hood, both rear doors, and on right side of rear door	Cargo area under carpet	274 volts Orange Cables	Under the vehicle on the right side from just forward of rear axle inboard to just off-center right in the engine compartment	Turn of ignition key, remove key from ignition, and place on dash. Disconnect the 12 volt battery. *If unable to reach ignition key:* Disconnect the 12 volt battery and remove the IGCT and IGCTFC fuses in engine compartment. *Power remains in the HV system for 5 minutes after disabling.*

Continued on next page

Table 6.2 (Continued)
Examples of Hybrid Cars (by automobile manufacturer)

Manufacturer	Model Name	External Identification	HV Battery Locations	High Voltage (HV)	HV Cable Route	HV Isolation Methods
Toyota (continued)	Prius	Toyota Hybrid and Prius logos on trunk	In the trunk behind the rear seat	274 volts Orange Cables	Under the vehicle from the left side near the rear axle to just above the left front axle	Turn of ignition key, remove key from ignition, and place on dash. Disconnect the 12 volt battery. *If unable to reach ignition key:* Disconnect the 12 volt battery and remove the IGCT relay in engine compartment. **Power remains in the HV system for 5 minutes after disabling.**
	Highlander	Toyota Highlander "Hybrid Synergy Drive" logos on rear hatchback door	In passenger compartment under second row seat	288 volts Orange Cables	Under the center of the vehicle from under the second row seat to the engine compartment	Turn of ignition key, remove key from ignition, and place on dash. Disconnect the 12 volt battery. *If unable to reach ignition key:* Disconnect the 12 volt battery and remove the IGCT No. 4 fuse in engine compartment. If unable to identify the correct fuse, pull all 4 fuses. **Power remains in the HV system for 5 minutes after disabling.**

The information for this table was gathered from emergency response guides produced by the manufacturers for these vehicle models. The information was accurate at the time this manual was written.

The EV's high voltage battery system consists of a large, approximately 650 pound (325 kg), 400 volt lithium ion battery pack that is located on the exterior and underneath the vehicle. The battery pack is covered with a metal enclosure for protection and ease of mounting. These vehicles also have low voltage electrical systems that must be addressed during extrication events. Use caution with any high voltage and color-coded cables. Emergency response guides for first responders can be found on manufacturer websites.

CAUTION
Avoid electrical shock by using caution when working with high voltage and color-coded cables.

Extended Range Electric Vehicles (EREV)

An extended range electric vehicle (EREV) uses an internal combustion engine to power an electric generator that charges the battery system in a linear process — the engine powers a generator — which in turn charges the battery. Unlike dual-fuel hybrid and plug-in hybrids, only the electric motor powers the wheels of an extended range electric car. The internal combustion engine only charges the batteries. Each has an electric only range of about 40 miles (65 km). Both extend their range with a small internal combustion engine that charges the batteries and can also be recharged by plugging into a power source during periods of low power use.

Similar to the EV, the EREV's high-voltage battery system consists of a large, approximately 400 pound (200 kg), 350 volt lithium-ion battery pack that runs lengthwise on the exterior and underneath the vehicle, directly beneath the center console. This battery pack is also covered with a metal enclosure for protection and ease of mounting. As with all other hybrid vehicles, use caution when working with any high voltage and color-coded cables.

Alternative Fuels

For fuel economy and environmental protection, a variety of alternative fuels can be used to power modern vehicles. Rescuers need to be aware that at an extrication operation they may encounter these alternative fuels and the hazards associated with them. Alternative fuels include but are not limited to:

- Propane and Liquefied Natural Gas (LNG)
- Auxiliary fuel cells
- Alcohol/gasoline blended mixtures
- Hydrogen
- Biodiesel
- JP-8

Propane and Liquefied Natural Gas (LNG). Some passenger vehicles are equipped with a fuel selector that allows the engine to run on either gasoline or propane. Propane is a by-product of petroleum refining and natural gas production. Also known as liquefied petroleum gas (LPG or LP-Gas) in the U.S., propane is often used to power buses, forklifts, and taxis. Propane can also be used as a fuel for heating and cooking in campers and recreational vehicles. When used as a vehicle fuel in other countries, propane is called autogas.

Liquefied natural gas is produced from oil and natural gas fields around the world. Because LNG burns cleaner and produces fewer greenhouse gases than petroleum fuels, it is viewed as an environmentally friendly fuel **(Figure 6.9)**.

Should a propane or LNG tank leak or rupture during an accident, the fuel released will vaporize and could be ignited by an ignition source. Fire department personnel need to be standing by to provide fire protection during extrication operations.

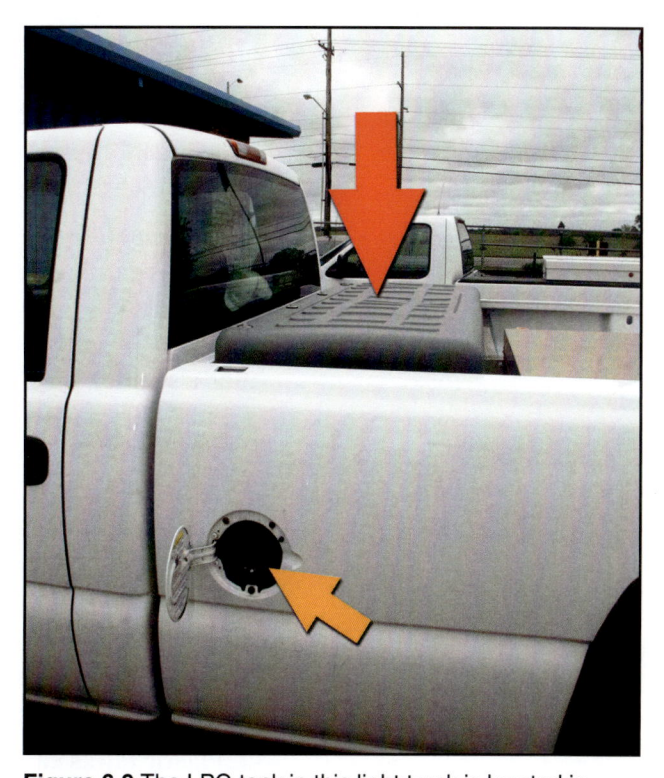

Figure 6.9 The LPG tank in this light truck is located in the plastic box in the bed of the truck while the fill point is located near the gasoline tank fill point.

Auxiliary Fuel Cells. In essence, fuel cells are electrochemical energy conversion devices that produce electricity while converting hydrogen and oxygen into water. Because the electrical output of a single fuel cell is quite limited, a bank or stack of fuel cells is used to generate sufficient DC current to power electrical motors in vehicles.

The production of hydrogen does result in a net loss of energy. Currently hydrogen is not readily available for automotive use and the storing of hydrogen for fuel cell usage is difficult. Because of hydrogen's very low density storage, storing it in cryogenic storage tanks or as a liquid in pressurized tanks simply does not store enough energy for extended driving. Some fuel cells use reformers to draw the hydrogen for the cells to use from gasoline, methane, or ethanol. Because hydrogen is highly flammable, use caution around hydrogen storage tanks during extrication operations to prevent the release and ignition of this fuel.

Alcohol/Gasoline Blended Mixtures. Alcohol/gasoline blended mixtures, such as E85 (85 percent ethanol and 15 percent gasoline), are becoming more commonplace in the United States and in other countries. E85 is less costly to purchase than gasoline but in vehicles manufactured in 2002 and before, they are less fuel efficient. In newer, flexible fuel engines, E85 runs more efficiently.

Hydrogen. Hydrogen can also be burned in internal combustion engines to produce motive power for vehicles. Again, the problems associated with using hydrogen as a fuel include:

- Limitations in hydrogen production and storage
- Flammability
- High pressure compressed gas storage

Biodiesel. Biodiesel is a fuel similar to diesel and derived from animal fats or vegetable oils such as corn and soy. It is nontoxic, biodegradable, and produces fewer emissions than petroleum-based diesels during the combustion process. Biodiesel is classified as a nonflammable liquid with a flash point of 320° F (160° C).

Jet Propellant-8 (JP-8). Since the 1990s, the U.S. military and North Atlantic Treaty Organization (NATO) have been using JP-8, a kerosene derivative, as a single fuel to power diesel and turbine engines in land-based vehicles. While JP-8 is primarily used as an aircraft fuel, military forces have begun using it as a fuel for land-based vehicles such as Humvees, heavy military trucks, military fire apparatus, and other tactical military vehicles.

Fuel Tanks

Historically, vehicle fuel tanks were constructed of aluminum or terne coated steel. Older tanks tend to corrode, weigh more than plastic tanks, and are more expensive to produce than modern plastic fuel tanks. One hazard that plastic tank manufacturers have had to overcome was the flammability of the tank materials themselves when the tank became involved in fire. Recent advances in the plastics industry have led to the development of less flammable materials.

Plastic tanks can be punctured easily during an accident or rapidly fail in the event of a fire. Rescue personnel should maintain situational awareness of a vehicle incident regarding the potential failure of the fuel tank.

> **CAUTION**
> Fuel that is released from a failed reservoir can pose a serious risk to rescue members, victims, and the environment.

Passenger Vehicle Electrical Systems

Vehicle electrical systems are a likely ignition source. These include battery systems, window defoggers, and other systems. Battery systems can impart heat energy to various parts of a wrecked vehicle which increases the risk of spark and ignition of spilled fuels and/or hydraulic fluids. Defoggers can produce sparks or shock a person during window removal.

Some modern passenger vehicles may have onboard power inverters that provide electricity to remote power outlet (RPO) sites. These allow the use of AC power for the operation of electrically powered equipment such as drills, saws, or other devices at various locations on or in the vehicle **(Figure 6.10)**. Many work/service vehicles have higher capacity power inverters that are capable of high energy output.

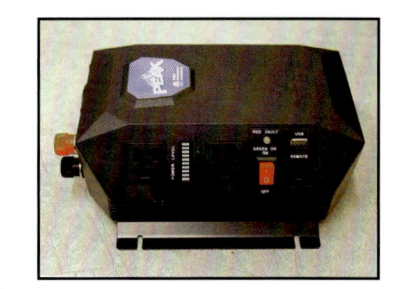

Figure 6.10 A remote power outlet found in some vehicles.

Isolating and managing these electrical systems eliminates a potential source of ignition, deactivates the vehicle's supplemental restraint system, and de-energizes any additional accessories or power equipment that may still be running. Isolating the electrical system may require disconnecting or cutting the battery cables, or can be as simple as flipping a master disconnect switch.

Rescuers should verify that the battery system has been isolated by observing systems that normally operate on battery power. Some jurisdictions perform this by activating the hazard lights and verifying their inoperability.

> **WARNING!**
> When isolating the vehicle's electrical system, rescuers should ensure that all electrical cables have been disconnected or cut.

The electrical system of a vehicle is designed to store and deliver the electricity needed to start the engine and to power and operate the various electrical components of the vehicle. A typical vehicle electrical system is composed of the following:

- Battery (stores electricity)
- Alternator (produces electricity)
- Wiring
- Fuses (protect electrical system)
- Ancillary equipment:
  — Lights
  — Fans
  — Air conditioning
  — Stereo
  — Power windows and seats

At extrication operations, rescue personnel must isolate electrical power to the vehicle(s) or piece(s) of equipment involved. Most vehicle electrical systems are low-voltage systems. Passenger vehicles and light trucks are usually 12-volt systems while larger trucks, recreational vehicles, and military vehicles operate on 24-volt systems. Passenger vehicles can also have auxiliary systems that operate at higher voltages.

Vehicle electrical systems include any of the systems and subsystems that comprise the automobile wiring harnesses. These electrical systems include the starting and charging systems, as well as the following:

- Keyless entry and smart key ignitions
- Headlights
- Battery systems
- Electric engine cooling fans
- Electronic front and rear defoggers

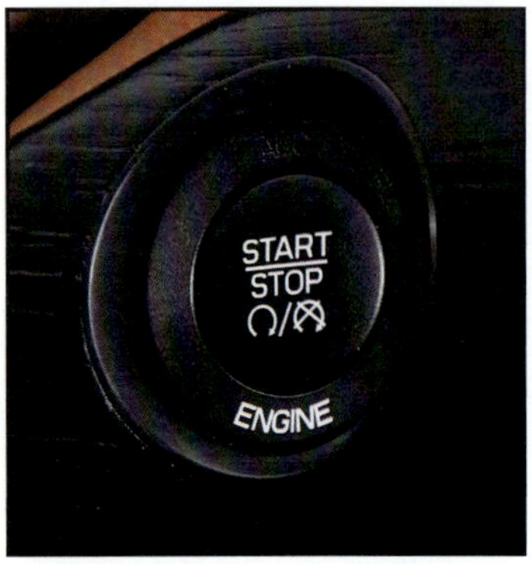

Keyless Entry and Smart Key Ignitions

Keyless ignition systems are becoming more common in passenger vehicles. In the early stages of a vehicle incident, it is critical to locate the keyless ignition button or switch and then know how to shut down the keyless ignition system **(Figure 6.11)**. These systems are becoming more common, with more than 150 different makes and models offering keyless ignition systems.

Rescuers should be aware that the vehicle is still capable of being operated, although the vehicle's key may not be in the ignition. If rescuers locate a smart key(s) during vehicle extrication operations, they should remove it a safe distance from the vehicle to keep the vehicle from being activated. Responders should power down the vehicle, activate the emergency brake, and locate and disconnect the battery.

Figure 6.11 A keyless ignition switch found in newer vehicles.

Headlights

A vehicle's headlight systems can incorporate conventional headlights or high-intensity discharge (HID) headlights. Conventional headlight systems are similar to standard residential lightbulbs in that the lightbulbs contain a filament and are rated in watts. When voltage is applied, light is produced in a yellowish hue.

HID headlights use an inert and highly pressurized xenon gas to produce a slightly bluish-looking light. Xenon is an odorless, colorless, nontoxic, and chemically inert gas. It is contained inside a small, sealed bulb deep inside the HID assembly. HID headlights are up to three times brighter than the more common halogen headlights.

HID headlights operate on high voltage; however, the amperage is low. An electric ballast, similar to that found in a fluorescent lamp, converts the car's 12-volt DC to up to 25,000 volts of AC when the headlight is first turned on. This high voltage creates an arc that jumps across the small gap inside the electrodes of the sealed lamp unit. This energizes the xenon gas, causing the gas to produce the bright light. Once the arc is formed and the headlight warms up, the voltage drops to approximately 80 volts AC.

Battery Systems

An automobile battery serves as the storage device for the electrical energy needed to start the vehicle or may serve as the power supply for electrical vehicles. Automobile batteries used in ignition systems are generally of the lead-acid type. Battery packs used to power electrical or hybrid vehicles include **(Figure 6.12)**:

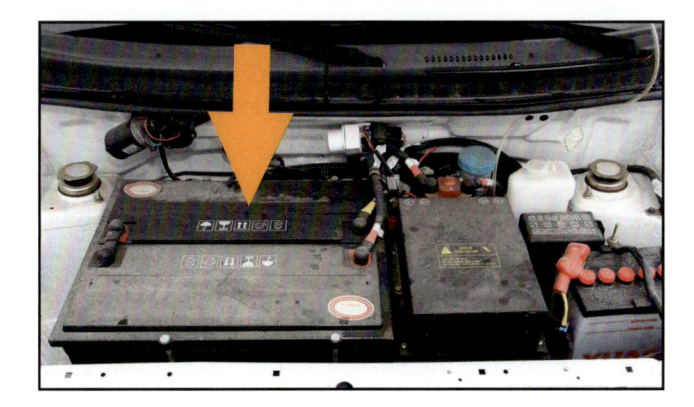

Figure 6.12 A battery pack for an electric car.

- Lead-acid
- Absorbed glass mat
- Nickel cadmium (NiCad)
- Nickel metal hydride (NiMH)
- Zinc-air
- Lithium ion (Li-ion)
- Lithium ion polymer (Li-poly)

CAUTION
Avoid touching battery systems unless absolutely necessary. Battery systems can impart heat energy to various part of a wrecked vehicle which increases the risk of shock, spark, and ignition of spilled fuels and/or hydraulic fluids.

The battery/batteries in passenger vehicles and light trucks may be found in the engine compartment, passenger compartment, fender wells, or in the trunk. In some vehicles, batteries may be covered by a retaining bar, a cover made of plastic or some other material, or the windshield washer fluid reservoir. In larger vehicles, the battery or batteries are usually in a special compartment separate from the engine compartment.

Diesel trucks, diesel passenger vehicles, and hybrid vehicles most always have more than one battery. Due to additional technology power requirements, some standard passenger vehicles now in production also have more than one battery. In select Mercedes C and E class vehicles, which are non-hybrid and non-diesel, the main battery is located in the trunk and the auxiliary battery is located in the engine compartment. The main battery starts the vehicle while the auxiliary battery powers active and passive restraint systems and other items such as the global positioning system (GPS) and lighting system.

Electric Engine Cooling Fans

Most vehicles have an engine cooling fan run by the electrical system that provides additional cooling for the engine during vehicle operation. Some vehicles have an auxiliary or supplemental electric engine cooling fan that is used to assist in maintaining the engine coolant temperature. These cooling

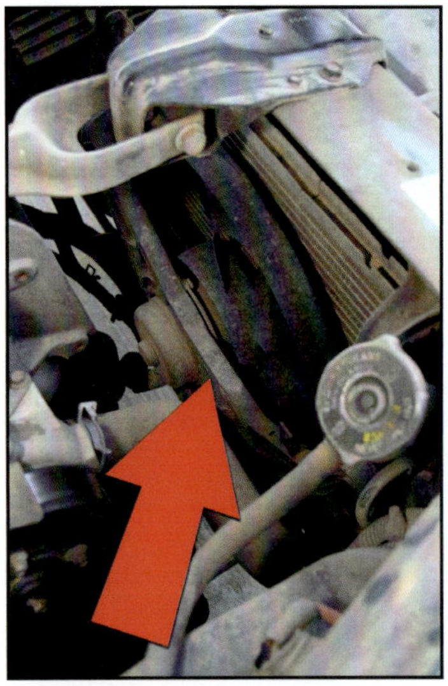

Figure 6.13 An example of an engine cooling fan.

fans are controlled by the engine's computer or by a thermostat that turns them on and off based upon the coolant temperature. Because these fans are electrically driven, rescue personnel should exercise caution while working near them **(Figure 6.13)**.

Electronic Front and Rear Defoggers

Some vehicles are equipped with electronic defoggers in the front windshield or rear windows. When removing the windshield, rear window, or displacing the dashboard, rescuers should ensure the electrical power to the vehicle has been isolated to prevent shock or the production of sparks due to the amperage carried by these devices.

Passenger Vehicle Exhaust Systems

Modern automobile exhaust systems are designed to carry the exhaust gases away from the vehicle and its occupants. These systems also help improve vehicle performance and fuel consumption, as well as reduce engine noise. Exhaust systems consist of the following components:

- **Exhaust piping** — Generally constructed of stainless steel or zinc-plated steel. This piping channels the exhaust gases from the engine exhaust manifolds to the catalytic converter (if so equipped), from the catalytic converter to the muffler, and from the muffler to the outside air.

- **Catalytic converters** — Catalytic converters, sometimes called a catalyst, are stainless-steel canisters that are integrated into a vehicle's exhaust system that convert vehicle exhaust emissions into less harmful materials. Each catalytic converter is composed of a thin layer of catalytic material, platinum, rhodium, and palladium, arranged over inert supports. Highly efficient three-way catalysts are available in vehicles that employ a feedback fuel-air ratio control system to produce a precise combustion control.

- **Mufflers** — Mufflers reduce the volume of noise that the engine produces and the exhaust gases carry.

Exhaust gases are hot when they leave the engine; therefore, exhaust system piping and components tend to be hot as well. The heated piping and components can be dangerous for rescuers to touch because of the risk of getting burned.

> **CAUTION**
> Do not touch hot vehicle exhaust systems. Wear appropriate personal protective clothing and equipment when working near these systems.

Passenger Vehicle Powertrain Systems

A vehicle's powertrain, sometimes called the drivetrain, includes all of the parts that create and transfer power to the road **(Figure 6.14)**. Powertrain components include the following:

- Engine/motor
- Transmission
- Drive shafts

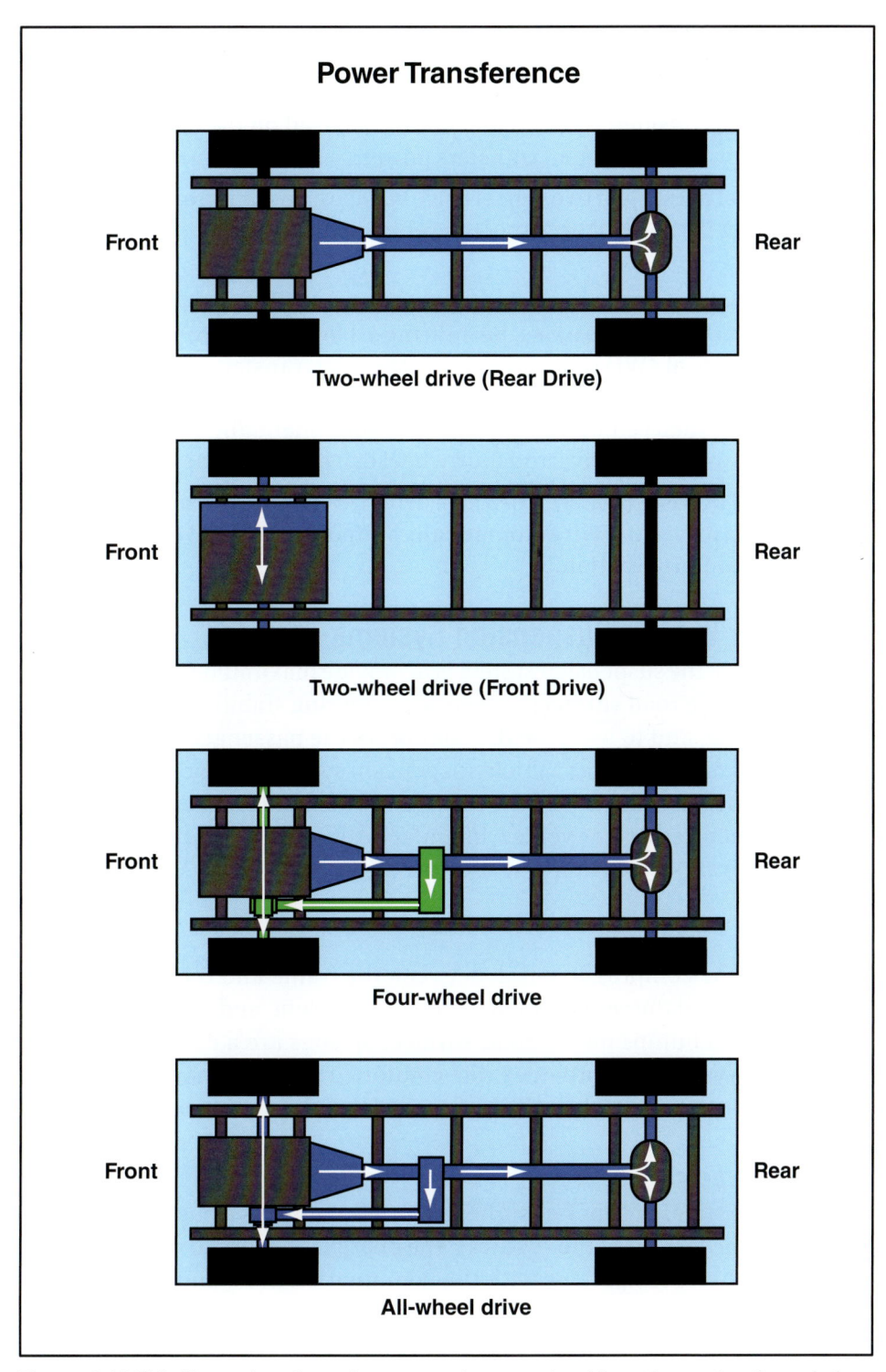

Figure 6.14 This illustration shows how power is transmitted from the engine through the power train for two, four, and all-wheel drive.

- Differentials
- Drive wheels or tracks

A vehicle is considered one of the following based on the configuration in which the powertrain system transfers power:

- **Two-wheel drive** — In two-wheel drive vehicles, power is transferred to one axle, either in the front or rear of the vehicle, which then transfers power to the surface.
- **Four-wheel drive** — Four-wheel drive (also called 4x4 or 4WD) vehicles have power sent to two axles, permitting all four wheels to receive power. An advantage of 4WD is the greater traction and transfer of power when the vehicle is operating in areas of low traction such as gravel, mud, ice, and snow. Many such vehicles are equipped to shift (manually or automatically) between two-wheel drive and four-wheel drive as necessary.
- **All-wheel drive** — Modern all-wheel drive (AWD) vehicles normally run in two-wheel drive and will automatically shift into all-wheel drive as necessary to maintain traction.

Passenger Vehicle Suspension Systems

The purpose of the suspension system is to provide maximum friction between the tires and the road surface, to help with steering stability, to improve vehicle handling, and to increase the comfort of the passengers. The foremost components of a passenger vehicle suspension system are springs, shock absorbers, suspension struts, and the tires. As the demand for passenger comfort and safety increases, some vehicle manufacturers are now equipping modern vehicles with air suspension systems as well.

Springs
Springs are the compressible link between the frame and the body. Springs bear the weight of the vehicle, maintain the ride height, and absorb the energy resulting from bumps on the road surface. Springs are a component of the suspension system that provides ride comfort. Three commonly used types of springs are the coil spring, the leaf spring, and the torsion bar.

Shock Absorbers
As the name states, a shock absorber absorbs energy. As a passenger vehicle negotiates the terrain of the roadway, the energy is absorbed into the shock. The shock absorber operates with the combination of oil and a series of internal valves. As the vehicle negotiates the bumps in the roadway, the oil can only flow through the internal valves of the shock absorber at a certain rate; therefore, the suspension movement becomes slower, smoother, and considerably more predictable.

Suspension Struts
Struts are similar to shocks internally with oil and valves, but they are constructed differently on the exterior. Struts are mounted to the chassis of the vehicle, usually attached to a coil spring, and designed to be an integral and structural part of the suspension system. Unlike shocks, if the struts were not attached, the car would not be supported and would be totally immobile.

Tires
Tires are often not included as a part of the suspension system. However, tires support the total weight of the vehicle and are the point of contact of the vehicle with the road surface, absorbing the initial energy. Tires have a direct impact on the safe handling and ride quality of the vehicle based on tire size, construction, and inflation pressures.

Passenger Air-Suspension Systems
Some modern passenger vehicles are now being equipped with air-suspension systems. Air ride suspension systems give the vehicle self-leveling capability, increasing the stability, handling, and comfort. These systems have sensors that inform the computer of the height of the vehicle and any need for center of gravity modification. If the vehicle height is too low, an onboard compressor pumps up the air suspension until the car is leveled out. If the vehicle height is too high, the air-ride computer releases the pressure, reducing the profile of the vehicle. The computer can control the adjustment of the individual air-ride components in milliseconds, depending on the driving situation.

Passenger Vehicle Safety Features
Passenger vehicles are manufactured to include a variety of safety features. Each type of passenger vehicle is unique, yet they all incorporate similar components. For example, the seat belt is a universally common feature that is included in the manufacture of vehicles. This section will explain the following topics:

- Collision avoidance systems
- Passenger vehicle supplemental restraint systems
- Energy-absorbing features
- Passenger vehicle rollover protection systems

Collision Avoidance Systems
Improvements in vehicle technology have improved passenger vehicle safety systems. While these systems may not have a specific impact on vehicle extrication, they do play a role in the avoidance and detection of collision potential through emerging technology. These systems ultimately achieve a reduction in fatalities and injuries.

Collision avoidance systems can use radar, laser, infrared or other sensors to detect objects, nearby vehicles, and potential roadway hazards in the path of the vehicle. Drivers are alerted audibly and/or visually so that they can take corrective action. To avoid or mitigate the severity of a collision, some systems also take proactive measures such as providing automated braking assistance and engaging vehicle stability control systems.

Forward-Looking Collision-Avoidance Systems
These systems typically use radar or laser sensors to detect and warn the driver of potential danger (approaching or stationary) in front of the vehicle. The typical system scans a distance of 330 feet (100 m) or more forward of the vehicle. As stated previously, some systems take automatic control of the braking system if the driver does not respond.

Side-Sensing Collision-Avoidance Systems

These systems are sometimes called active blind-spot assistance. By using cameras, radar, or lasers, they generally sense objects from 6.5 to 30 feet (2 to 10 m) from the side of the vehicle in the blind spot area. They warn the driver of potential danger through audible and/or visual alarms.

Rear-Looking Collision-Avoidance Systems

This system operates and senses distances of 20 feet (6 m) or less by using a camera, radar, or laser. When driving forward, the system senses objects that are approaching from the rear, such as a vehicle approaching at a high rate of speed. When driving in reverse, the system can sense pedestrians and fixed objects toward the rear of the vehicle.

Adaptive Cruise Control

When the cruise control is activated, a radar or laser senses the distance between vehicles. This system measures, monitors, and maintains a safe distance between the vehicles by controlling the speed of the host vehicle through either throttle control or braking.

Infrared Night Vision Systems

This technology uses and operates infrared sensors to detect people, animals, objects, or vehicles and warns the driver well before the headlights can illuminate them. These systems are similar in technology to the thermal imaging cameras utilized in the fire service today.

Passenger Vehicle Supplemental Restraint Systems

Passenger vehicle restraint system technology is rapidly evolving. Rescue personnel are encouraged to stay current on vehicle restraint systems. Increased collision protection for vehicle occupants is provided by a variety of supplemental restraint systems (SRS) such as:

- Seat belts, seat belt pretensioners, and load limiters
- Airbags
- Child safety restraint devices

Although the supplemental restraint systems have saved many lives, they have also added a potential safety hazard for both rescuers and vehicle occupants. This hazard is the accidental activation of one or more of these systems during extrication operations. Some modern vehicles have multiple systems whose locations may not be readily identified.

Seat Belts, Seat Belt Pretensioners, and Load Limiters

Since 1968, all passenger vehicles manufactured in the U.S. have had to be equipped with seat belts. These systems consist of a belt that attaches across the wearer's lap and extends across the upper torso **(Figure 6.15)**. They are intended to restrain the wearer in an upright position in the seat and keep the wearer from bolting forward in a frontal impact collision. More importantly, they are designed to keep the wearer inside the vehicle if the doors come open.

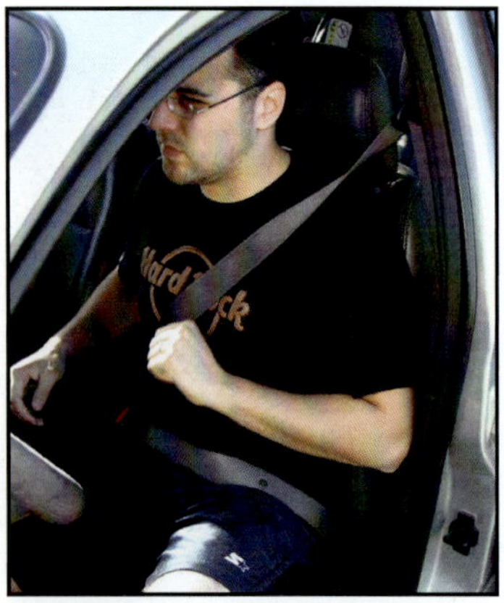

Figure 6.15 A driver wearing a standard seat belt.

Both testing and experience have made it clear that seat belts are most effective when they are pulled tightly across the wearer's body. Because this can be rather uncomfortable, few vehicle occupants tighten their belts as snugly as they should. Therefore, some manufacturers have added **seat belt pretensioners** to their vehicles. When the front-impact airbags activate, they instantly tighten (pretension) the seat belts so that the wearer receives maximum benefit of the seat belt. Pretensioners prevent the occupant from sliding forward and underneath the dashboard during a collision. They also reduce the amount of movement in which an occupant would move forward then backward during a frontal impact, possibly reducing occupant injury.

In some cases, the belts may be tightened to the point that they cause injury or may restrict the wearer's ability to breathe normally. In an effort to decrease this injury potential from crash force, some vehicles now have load limiters that work in harmony with the pretensioners. Load limiters are designed to release belt tension in a controlled manner so that the passenger is introduced into the airbag more gently **(Figure 6.16)**.

Seat Belt Pretensioners — Protective devices designed to tighten the belts as the front-impact airbags deploy.

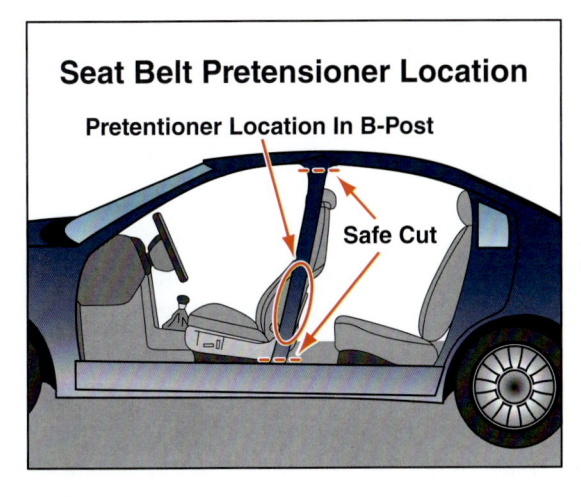

Figure 6.16 The appropriate location of a seat belt pretensioner in a vehicle's B-post.

Airbags

Airbags are a form of restraint that is intended to help reduce passenger injuries. Airbags prevent passengers from striking the following:

- Other passengers
- Steering wheel
- Dashboard
- Windshield
- Side windows
- Door frames

Airbags are automatically activated in the event of a collision **(Figure 6.17)**. Electronic or mechanical means deploy the airbags. Chemical or stored gas inflators fill the airbags. Chemical inflators, currently used in all driver frontal restraint systems and many passenger frontal restraint systems use sodium azide (enhanced with potassium nitrate) to create nitrogen gas, which inflates the airbag. Most side impact Airbags, curtains, tubes, and some passenger frontal airbags use stored gas inflators, usually filled with inert gas, to inflate the airbags.

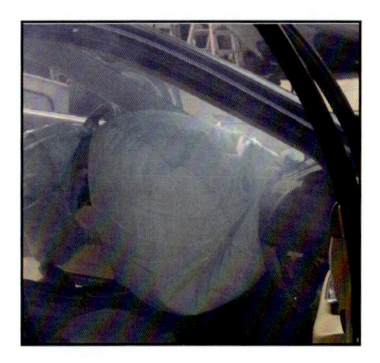

Figure 6.17 Front air bags immediately following deployment.

Section C • Chapter 6 – Passenger Vehicles **221**

> **WARNING!**
> Airbags can deploy at speeds of up to 200 mph (320 km/h) exerting a potentially lethal force. Rescue personnel must know where these Airbags may be located and the possible procedures to avoid and mitigate them.

A variety of Airbags exist in today's passenger vehicles, including the following:

- Frontal impact airbags
- Side-impact protection systems (SIPS)
- Head protection systems (HPS)
- Neck protection systems (whiplash protection systems)
- Seat belt airbags
- Center mounted airbags
- Knee bolsters

Frontal Impact Airbags. Frontal impact airbags are considered SRS because they are intended to supplement seat belts, not replace them. Children under the age of twelve should not ride in the front seat of vehicles with an armed passenger frontal airbag.

Electronically operated restraint systems receive their energy from the vehicle's battery. They are designed to activate through a system of mechanical or inertia switches located forward of the passenger compartment and by microelectronic controls that may be located under the front seats or in the console between the front seats.

These systems have a reserve energy supply that is capable of deploying an airbag even if the battery is disconnected or destroyed in a collision. When the battery is disconnected, the reserve energy supply will eventually drain away, disarming the restraint system. Vehicle manufacturers list different time estimates on how long it takes for the reserve energy to deplete entirely. These estimates range from as little as one second to as much as thirty minutes. Many pickup trucks have features that allow the passenger air bag to be disarmed.

Side-Impact Protection Systems (SIPS). Some side-impact protection systems can be electronically or mechanically operated and may or may not require power from the vehicle's electrical system to activate. Therefore, some SIPS bags may deploy even if the battery has been disconnected. In mechanical systems, isolating or preventing airbag deployment may require that the connection between the sensor and the airbag inflation unit be cut. Electronically activated SIPS will need to be isolated by isolating the battery. The procedures for cutting the airbag connection and isolating the battery will vary from vehicle to vehicle. Rescue personnel should refer to manufacturer's instructions for clarification on these procedures.

Head Protection Systems (HPS). A growing number of vehicles have HPS installed. On vehicles equipped with side-impact collision, these airbags deploy from a narrow opening between the headliner and the top of the door frame. The two types of HPS are:

- **Window curtains** — Upon activation, a high-pressure cylinder instantly inflates window curtains. These HPS automatically deflate shortly after deployment.
- **Inflatable tubes** — Inflatable tubes instantly inflate upon activation. Inflation will shorten the tubes and snap them down into place across the side window. Unlike other airbags, inflatable tubes remain inflated after deployment. Rescue personnel can easily remove this HPS by cutting their nylon straps or can deflate them by puncturing the tube with a sharp object.

One danger with both of these systems is that if a rescuer is working through the window opening, he or she is likely in the deployment path of the airbag. This danger can be mitigated by a complete roof removal. However, when cutting the posts for roof removal, rescuers must be careful not to cut into high-pressure cylinders.

> **CAUTION**
> Do not cut high-pressure cylinders. Peel and peek prior to performing cutting operations.

Neck Protection Systems (Whiplash Protection Systems). Neck protection systems, commonly called whiplash protection systems or active restraint systems, are a type of passive restraint device. When a vehicle is involved in a rear-end collision, sensors will immediately recognize the type and severity of the impact and trigger a gas generator, which inflates a small bladder within the headrest. This action moves the headrest up and forward, reducing the space between the neck, head, and headrest, minimizing backward movement and injury potential. The process, from recognition to deployment, takes only .03 to .04 seconds and significantly reduces the risk of neck and spinal injuries to those involved in the collision. Although this type of system is usually utilized for front-seat passengers, developing technology suggests that rear-seat passenger neck protection will be developed in the near future.

Seat Belt Airbags. Some newer vehicles are equipped with seat belt Airbags. Although they can be located in the front or rear seats, most are located in the rear seats due to the presence of frontal and side impact protection systems in the forward passenger compartment. Inflatable seat belts help reduce head, neck and chest injuries for passengers who may be more vulnerable to such injuries, such as children and the elderly. Once the belt has been deployed, each of the tubular, accordion-folded Airbags inflate and expand up to three times its normal size to cover the wearer's torso and shoulder, providing better protection for a larger area of the body as well as a tighter hold due to the increased size. The speed at which the seat belt Airbags inflate is slower than in regular Airbags. It is already pressed against the wearer's body through the seat belt and does not need to be prevented from hitting anything. The whole process, from detection to inflation, lasts only 40 milliseconds.

Center-Mounted Airbags. Center-mounted Airbags deploy from the right side of the driver's seat and position themselves between the front row seats near the center of the vehicle. As with other SRS, it is designed to be used in conjunction with the seat belt. The Airbag is designed to provide restraint during passenger-side crashes when the driver is alone and also acts as an

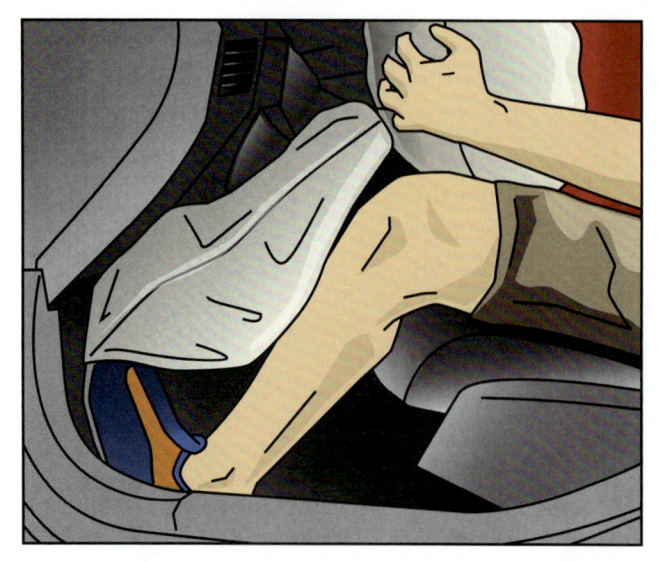

Figure 6.18 This illustration shows how a knee bolster deploys to protect a driver's legs.

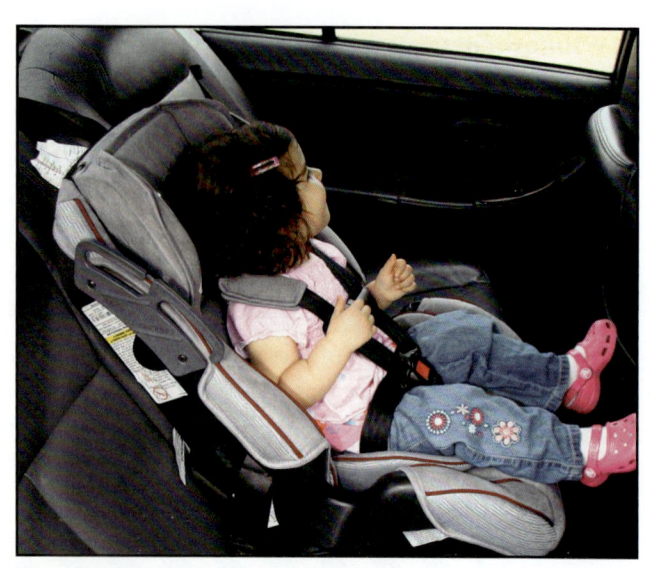

Figure 6.19 Child safety seats like this one save many lives.

energy-absorbing cushion between driver and front passenger in both driver and passenger side-impact crashes. The Airbag can also help minimize injury in rollover accidents.

Knee Bolsters. Some vehicles are equipped with restraint devices that are intended to protect the lower legs of the driver. They are also intended as "antisubmarine" devices — that is, they are intended to help prevent the driver from sliding forward and becoming wedged under the dashboard. The same precautions apply as with other front-impact restraints **(Figure 6.18)**.

Child Safety Restraint Devices

For years, child safety seats had to be purchased separately and fastened securely into the backseat of most automobiles. Because of the wide range of child seat sizes and securing mechanisms, as well as the equally wide range of rear seat belt configurations, some installations were not as safe as intended.

Many automobiles are being manufactured with child safety restraint devices and integrated child safety seats as original factory equipment **(Figure 6.19)**. An integrated child safety seat is normally located at the center of the rear seat and folds down to form a child seat complete with seat belts. Rescuers may need to extricate an infant or toddler from one of these devices at an emergency scene. Knowledge of these systems will assist rescuers with maintaining the safety of the young victim.

Energy-Absorbing Features

Many automobiles are equipped with energy-absorbing features designed to absorb the force of side, front, and rear collisions. These features are intended to reduce the monetary and human costs of vehicle collisions. However, they also add some potentially lethal hazards for emergency response personnel, and they can increase the difficulty of performing vehicle extrication. These energy-absorbing features include:

- Crushable bumpers
- Bumper struts
- Steering column

224 Section C • Chapter 6 – Passenger Vehicles

- Collision beams
- Crumple zones

Crushable Bumpers

Vehicle manufacturers used a number of different energy-absorbing feature designs to meet federal standards to reduce the monetary costs of low-speed collisions — those at 5 mph (10 km/h) or less. The low-speed collisions were later reduced to 2.5 mph (4 km/h). The first most prevalent design for energy-absorbing features was crushable bumpers.

Crushable bumpers are designed to absorb energy by flexing when struck. Some bumpers are made of polystyrene foam molded into an egg crate structure, covered by a flexible rubber shell, while others are made of synthetic rubber molded into a honeycomb structure covered with a flexible shell **(Figure 6.20)**.

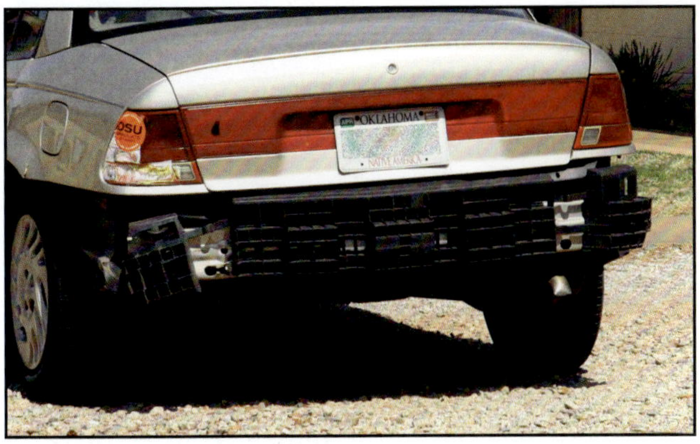

Figure 6.20 A crushable bumper system minus the flexible rubber shell.

Crushable bumpers are not a hazard in a fire until the fire is out. As these bumpers cool after being exposed to the heat of a fire, beads of a clear liquid form on the surface of the bumper. This liquid may appear to be water, but it is actually concentrated hydrofluoric acid (HF), which is a highly corrosive substance. Rescue personnel should flush these bumpers with copious amounts of water to minimize the presence of HF.

> **WARNING!**
> Avoid skin contact with the hydrofluoric acid (HF) that forms on the surface of crushable bumpers after a fire. Hydrofluoric acid is absorbed through the skin, and contact could be fatal.

Bumper Struts

In addition to crushable bumpers, many automobiles are equipped with energy-absorbing bumper struts. These struts make the vehicle less vulnerable to damage in low-speed collisions. Two struts are mounted between the front bumper and the vehicle frame or chassis, and two more are mounted in the rear of the vehicle. Similar to conventional shock absorbers, these sealed units contain hydraulic fluid and compressed gas.

When these struts are exposed to the heat of a fire, they can explode with tremendous force. If both struts attached to a bumper explode simultaneously, they can launch the bumper and/or the struts 100 feet (30 m) or more from

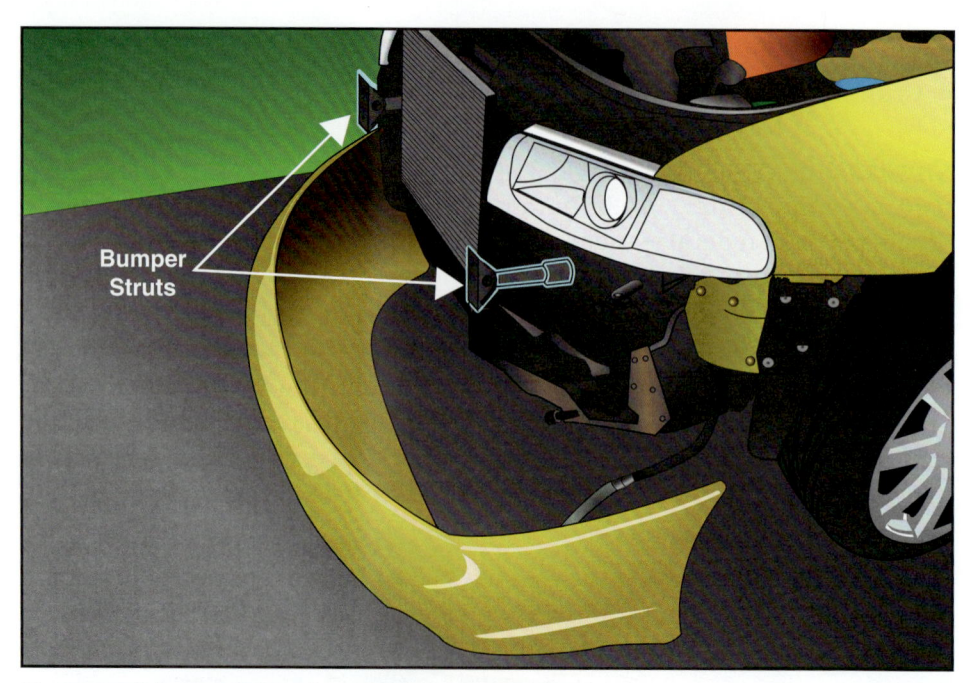

Figure 6.21 An illustration of a bumper strut system.

the vehicle. If only one strut explodes, the other acts as a pivot point and the bumper can swing in an arc across the front or rear of the vehicle. Anyone in the path of a bumper attached to an exploding strut is in jeopardy. Therefore, when the front or rear bumper of an automobile is exposed to heavy flame impingement, all personnel should stay out of the danger zone — directly in front of the bumper and to each side a distance equal to the length of the bumper **(Figure 6.21)**.

> **WARNING!**
> Do not approach a vehicle's bumper from directly in front or within the length of the bumper on each side of the vehicle when the bumpers are exposed to direct flame impingement or when they have been impacted.

Rescuers should also be aware of the hazards associated with gas-filled struts used to support the hoods and hatchbacks (when open) on some vehicles. When exposed to the heat of a fire, these struts can explode and launch parts many feet (meters) from the vehicle at speeds sufficient to cause fatal injuries. Rescuers have been impaled when these struts have exploded and forcibly ejected strut components from the vehicle.

Another strut system on vehicles is the suspension system. Some front suspensions are equipped with a shock absorber that is mounted directly below the coil spring. Struts are also used in some independent, rear-suspension systems that have a shock-absorber strut assembly on each side. Piston rods are composed of a plated rod that is attached to the piston of the shock-absorber and usually extend up to the top of the shock to attach to the vehicle.

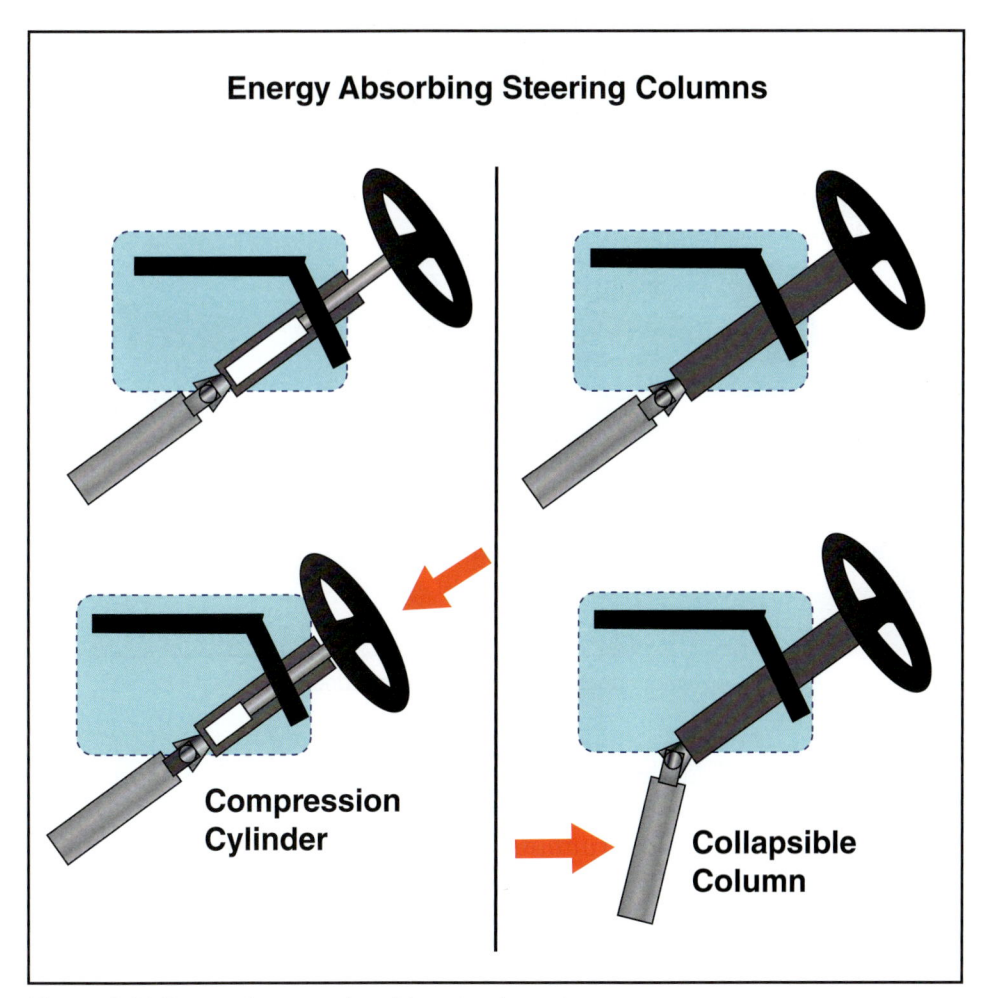

Figure 6.22 Types of energy absorbing steering columns.

Steering Column
Introduced in the late 1960s, the energy-absorbing steering column has proven effective in saving lives and limiting injuries during front-end crashes. These devices, along with driver-side airbags, protect the driver by absorbing the force of the driver's forward movement during a collision. With the introduction of tilt, collapsible, and tilt-steering columns, use extreme caution if the steering column is pulled or relocated **(Figure 6.22)**.

Collision Beams
Used since the late 1960s, collision beams have helped to reinforce vehicles' resistance to side-impact collisions. Early designs consisted of several layers of ordinary mild steel formed into a corrugated beam about 7 inches (175 mm) wide and about 2 inches (50 mm) thick, installed across each side door. Because mild steel has a tensile strength of about 20,000 to 23,000 psi (140 000 to 160 000 kPa), these beams were relatively easy to cut with hydraulic shears. However, newer designs have made two major changes — the construction of the door beams and the addition of a dashboard support beam **(Figure 6.23, p. 228)**.

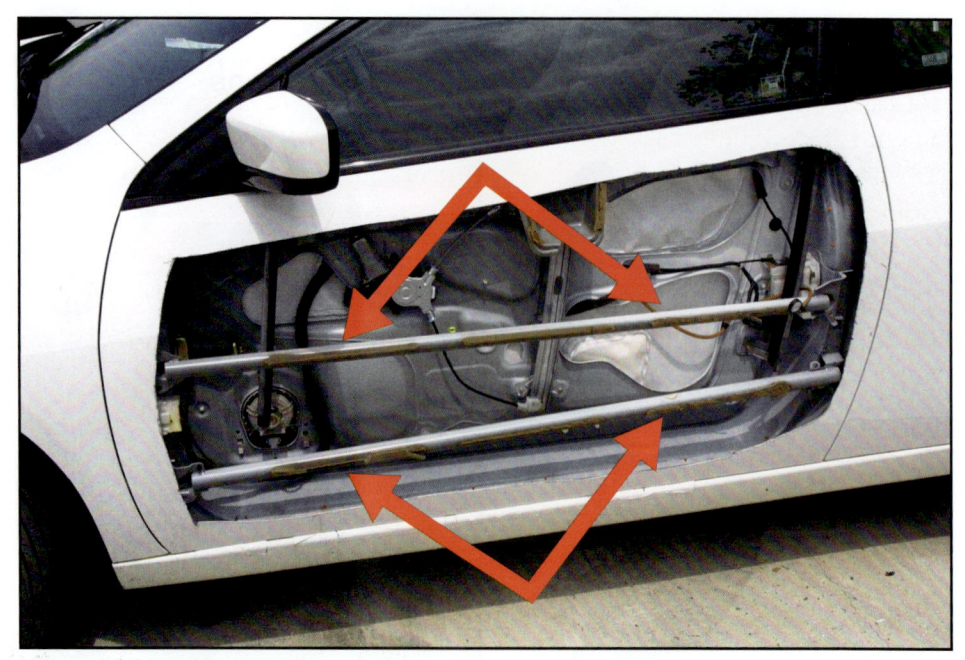

Figure 6.23 Example of side impact bars inside a vehicle door.

> **High-Strength Low-Alloy (HSLA) Steel** — Alloy steel developed to provide better mechanical properties or greater resistance to corrosion than carbon steel; different from other varieties of steels in that it is designed to possess specific mechanical properties.

Newer designs of side-impact protection incorporate stronger materials such as **High-Strength-Low-Alloy steel**, micro-alloy (MA) steel, and UHSS. The materials make up long bars running horizontally or diagonally within a door.

- HSLA steel has a tensile strength of 40,000 to 70,000 psi (280 000 to 490 000 kPa).
- MA steel has a tensile strength of 110,000 to 215,000 psi (770 000 to 1 500 000 kPa).
- UHSS has a tensile strength of up to 442,000 psi (3 100 000 kPa).

These new materials may be too hard for the blades of available power cutters. If this is the case, rescuers may have to make relief cuts above and below the bar and use spreaders to move the end of the bar. These bars may embed themselves into the A, B, or C posts when the vehicle is compressed front to back creating a "deadbolt lock."

These new alloys add significantly to the structural integrity of any vehicle and reduce the likelihood of the vehicle folding in the middle when struck from the side. They are also used in the construction of some dashboard support beams. These collision beams span the width of the vehicle from A-post to A-post.

Crumple Zones

Another energy-absorbing mechanism utilized on modern vehicles is the crumple zone. Certain body and frame components at the front and rear of a vehicle provide adequate structural support for normal vehicle operations and usage but are designed to give way or compress in a calculated manner during a collision. Crumple zones lengthen the time a vehicle takes to come to a complete stop during an accident, thus reducing the force of deceleration upon the vehicle's passengers.

Passenger Vehicle Rollover Protection Systems

Many convertible automobiles and open body vehicles that lack the C-post of hardtop vehicles are equipped with roll bars, a form of **rollover protection** systems (ROPS). Roll bars are made of hardened, tubular-steel stock, that is anchored to the vehicle body or frame, and extended up behind the passenger cabin. Roll bars are intended to protect the vehicle occupants in rollover crashes.

Currently, all other passenger vehicles are now required to have roof supports, commonly called roll cages, that will withstand a force equal to 2.5 times the weight of the vehicle. In the near future, the roof and support structure will be required to support three times the weight of the vehicle in a rollover crash situation. Even though roll bars and cages are designed to withstand significant impact without collapsing, they are not indestructible and can collapse onto the occupants, pinning them in their seats. Roll bars and cages can add to the challenge for rescuers in extrication situations.

Some manufacturers provide an extendable roll bar system on some of their newer models **(Figure 6.24)**. This pop-up-style roll bar system activates and rapidly extends up behind the passengers when the vehicle exceeds 23 degrees from the horizontal, a lateral angle limit of 62 degrees, or a longitudinal angle of 72 degrees. Additionally, these systems can deploy if the vehicle experiences a 3G acceleration force or becomes weightless for at least 80 milliseconds. While these devices allow better visibility to the rear of the vehicle and a more aesthetic appearance while maintaining rollover protection, they pose a significant safety hazard to rescuers when they deploy.

NOTE: Roll bars should not be confused with anti-roll bars, which are stabilizer bars that are designed to prevent a vehicle from rolling over.

> **Rollover Protection** — Roll bars and roll cages within automobiles that protect passengers in the event of a rollover.

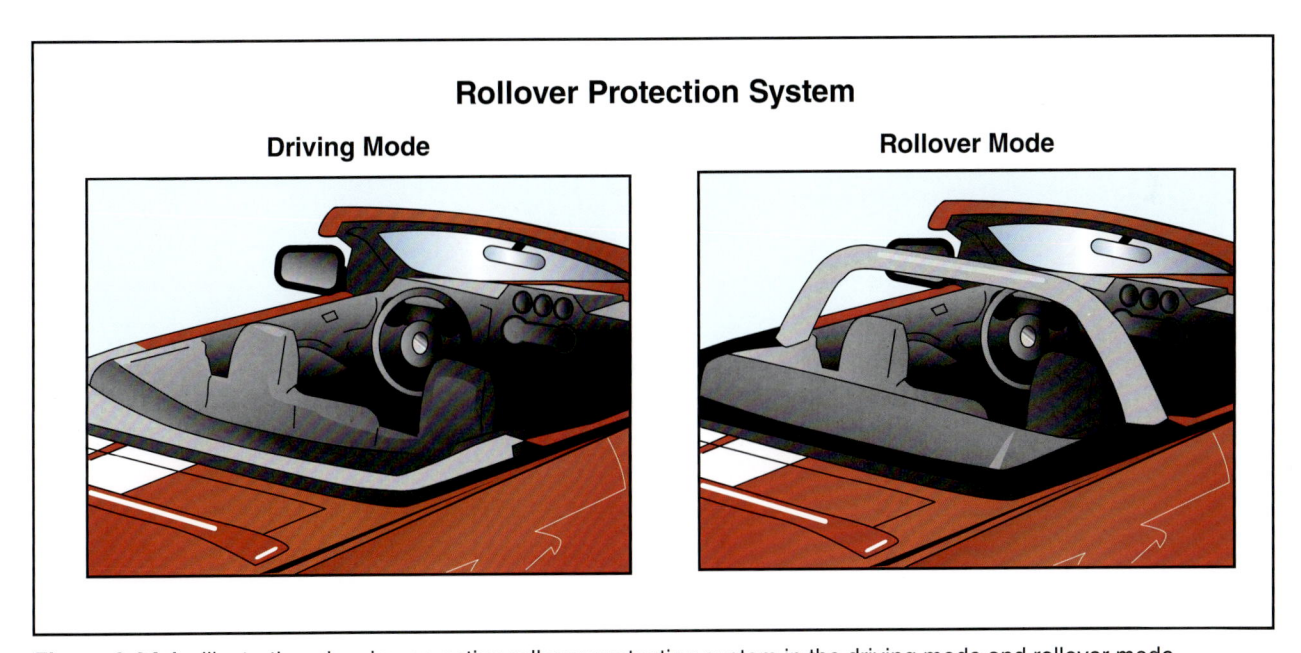

Figure 6.24 An illustration showing an active rollover protection system in the driving mode and rollover mode.

Chapter Review

1. What are four types of passenger vehicles?
2. Define the eight common terms used to describe the areas of a passenger vehicle.
3. What is the difference between full frame, unibody, and space frame vehicle construction?
4. What types of windows may rescuers encounter in passenger vehicles?
5. What materials are used in passenger vehicle construction?
6. What are the different types of fuel systems used by modern passenger vehicles?
7. List the components of a passenger vehicle electrical system.
8. What is the function of passenger vehicle exhaust systems?
9. What is the difference between two-wheel drive, four-wheel drive, and all-wheel drive?
10. List the components of passenger vehicle suspension systems.
11. What types of collision avoidance systems may be included in a passenger vehicle?
12. What is the purpose of seat belts and seat belt pretensioners?
13. What types of airbags may be found in modern passenger vehicles?
14. Why must rescuers take precautions when working around crushable bumpers and bumper struts?
15. What is the purpose of a roll cage?

Passenger Vehicle Stabilization Operations

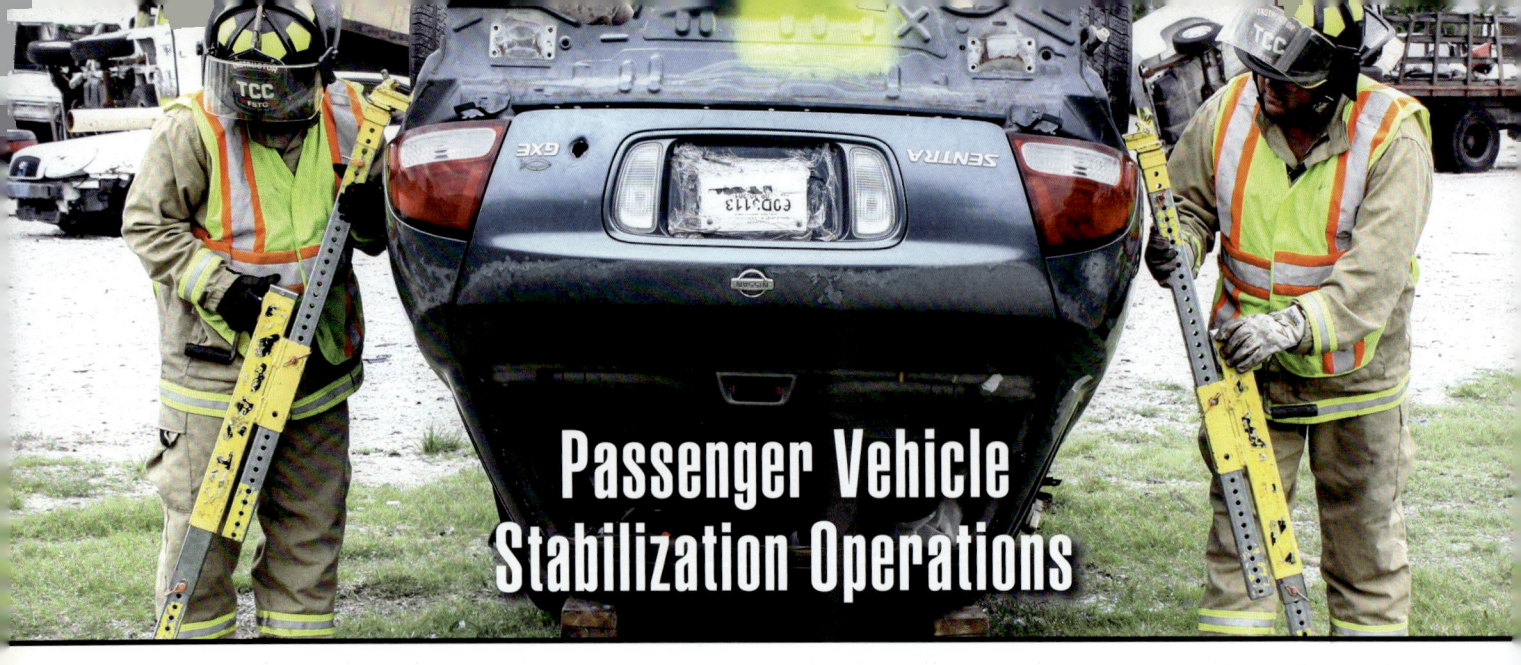

Chapter Contents

Introduction to Vehicle Stabilization 235
    Mechanism of Movement 236
    Stabilization Points and Surfaces/Terrain 238
    Lifting 239

Application of Stabilization Tools and Equipment 242
    Wheel Chocks 242
    Cribbing Materials 242
    Pneumatic Lifting Bags and Cushions 243
    Jacks 245
    Levers 246
    Hitches 247
    Chains 249
    Wire Rope 250
    Synthetic Slings 251
    Rigging 253
    Struts 255
    Recovery Vehicles 255

Passenger Vehicle Stabilization Operations 255
    Passenger Vehicle Structural and Damage Characteristics 256
    Maintaining Vehicle Stability 257
    Wheel-Resting Passenger Vehicle Stabilization 257
    Side-Resting Passenger Vehicle Stabilization 259
    Roof-Resting Passenger Vehicle Stabilization 261
    Passenger Vehicles in Other Positions Stabilization 261

Chapter Review 263
Discussion Questions 263
Skill Sheets 264

Chapter 7

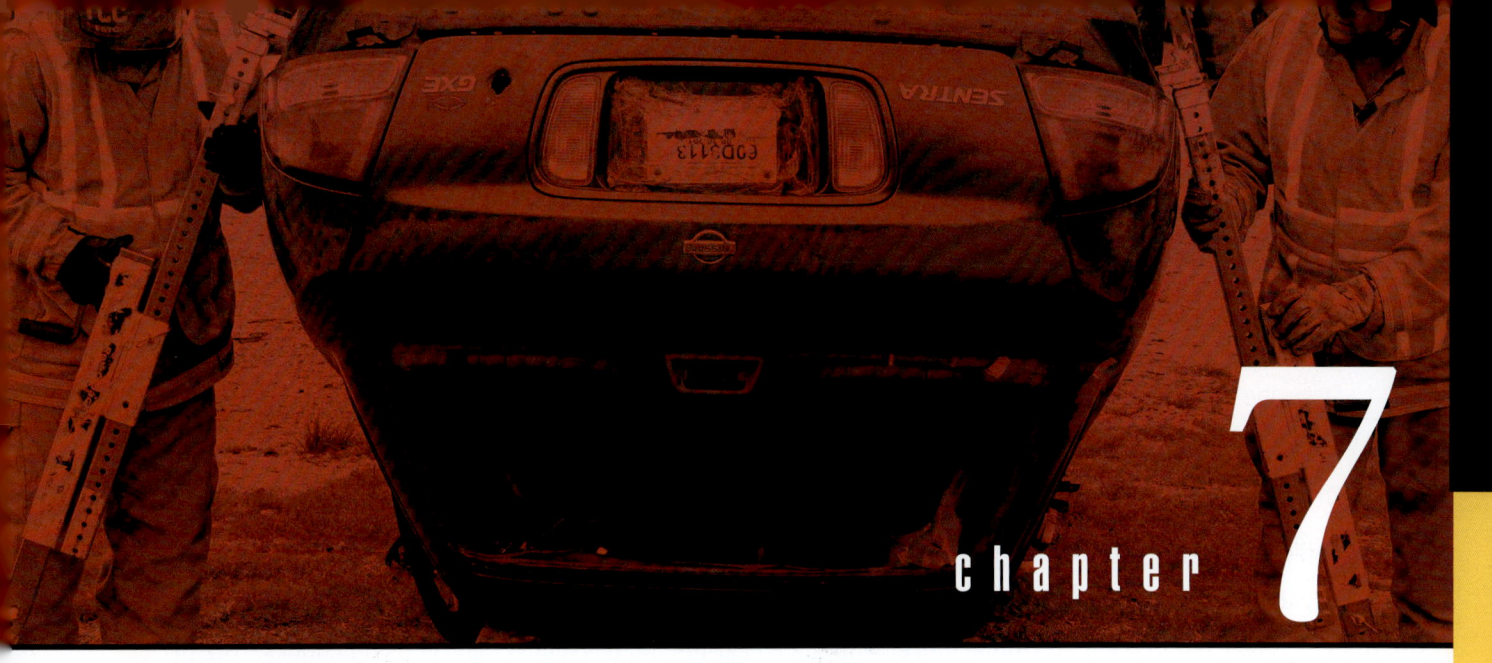

Key Terms

Center of Gravity 236
Fulcrum..246
Lever..246
Rigging..253
Sling..247
Vehicle Stabilization............................235

JPRs addressed in this chapter

This chapter provides information that addresses the following job performance requirements of NFPA 1006, *Standard for Technical Rescuer Professional Qualifications (2017)*.

8.2.3

8.2.7

Passenger Vehicle Stabilization Operations

Learning Objectives

1. Describe the mechanism of vehicle movement. [8.2.3]
2. Identify vehicle stabilization points and surfaces. [8.2.3]
3. Describe situations that may require vehicles or objects to be lifted at a vehicle incident. [8.2.3]
4. Explain considerations for the application of stabilization tools and equipment. [8.2.3, 8.2.7]
5. Explain ways to maintain vehicle stability during rescue operations. [8.2.7]
6. Skill Sheet 7-1: Prevent horizontal movement of a wheel-resting passenger vehicle using chocks. [8.2.3]
7. Skill Sheet 7-2: Lift a wheel-resting passenger vehicle using pneumatic lifting bags. [8.2.3]
8. Skill Sheet 7-3: Lift a wheel-resting passenger vehicle using a jack. [8.2.3]
9. Skill Sheet 7-4: Lift a wheel-resting passenger vehicle using a Class I lever. [8.2.3]
10. Skill Sheet 7-5: Stabilize a wheel-resting passenger vehicle using step chocks. [8.2.3]
11. Skill Sheet 7-6: Stabilize a wheel-resting passenger vehicle using cribbing. [8.2.3]
12. Skill Sheet 7-7: Deflate the tires of a wheel-resting passenger vehicle. [8.2.3]
13. Skill Sheet 7-8: Stabilize a side-resting passenger vehicle using struts (same-side opposing force system). [8.2.3]
14. Skill Sheet 7-9: Stabilize a side-resting passenger vehicle using struts (tensioned buttress system). [8.2.3]
15. Skill Sheet 7-10: Stabilize a roof-resting passenger vehicle using struts (tensioned buttress system). [8.2.3]
16. Skill Sheet 7-11: Attach or "marry" a vehicle to another vehicle or object. [8.2.3]

Chapter 7
Passenger Vehicle Stabilization Operations

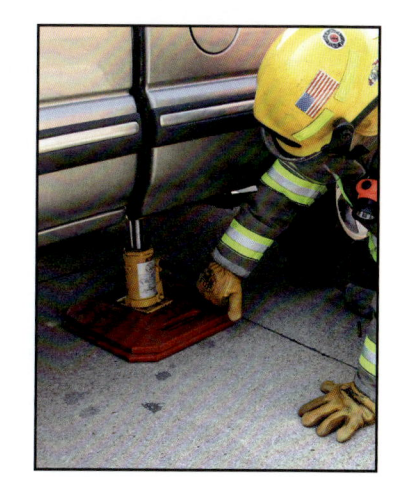

Adequate vehicle stabilization establishes sufficient points of contact between the vehicle and a stable surface to prevent the vehicle from moving in any direction. Vehicle stabilization requires rescuers to continuously evaluate numerous factors while performing the operation. Every vehicle stabilization incident is unique. This chapter will cover the following topics:

- Introduction to vehicle stabilization
- Application of stabilization tools and equipment
- Passenger vehicle stabilization operations
- Maintaining vehicle stability

Introduction to Vehicle Stabilization

Rescue personnel must stabilize each vehicle involved in a collision. This prevents further injury to the vehicle's occupants, prevents possible injuries to rescue personnel, and prevents further degradation of the vehicle's structural integrity. **Vehicle stabilization** refers to the process of providing additional support at key points between the vehicle and the ground or other solid surface. Good stabilization maximizes the area of contact between the vehicle and the ground to prevent any sudden or unexpected movement of the vehicle. Rescuers use a variety of tools, equipment, and techniques to stabilize vehicles **(Figure 7.1, p. 236)**.

Rescuers practice stabilization in phases. The initial phase of stabilization happens quickly and includes using wedges, wheel chocks, and step chocks **(Figure 7.2, p. 236)**. The secondary phase of stabilization includes using struts, chains, straps, and cribbing. The ongoing phase of stabilization includes the reassessment of current stabilization and the application of new stabilization as necessary.

Rescuers should not test vehicle stability prior to stabilization operations. They should not push, pull or shake a vehicle, regardless of its orientation. The slightest push, pull, or accidental contact in the wrong place may move a vehicle significantly, perhaps compounding the occupants' injuries and potentially injuring rescue personnel. Rescuers should add wheel chocks to a wheel-resting vehicle to prevent horizontal movement of the vehicle.

Prior to attempting to stabilize any vehicles, rescuers should have working knowledge of a vehicle's mechanism of movement, the vehicle's stabilization

> **Vehicle Stabilization** — Providing additional support to key places between a vehicle and the ground or other solid anchor points to prevent unwanted movement.

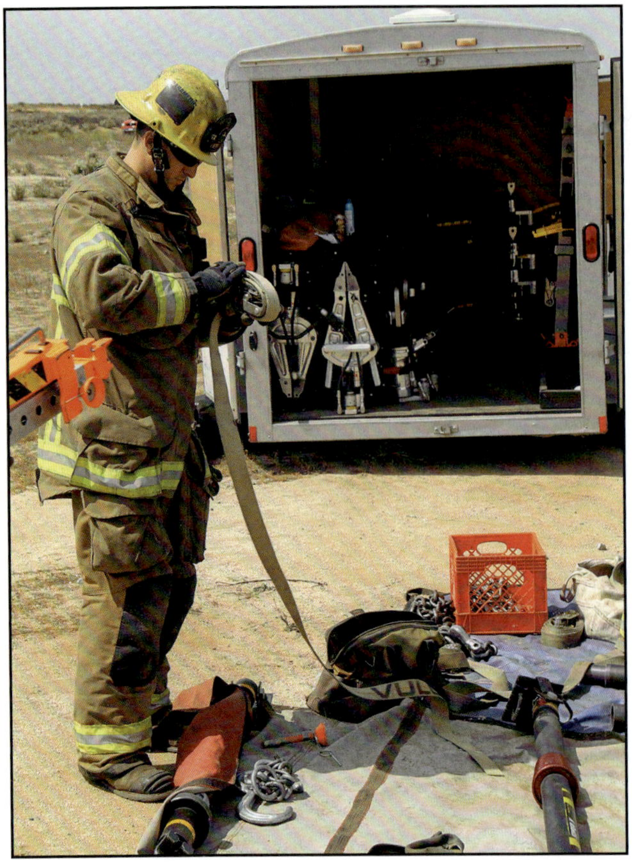

Figure 7.1 A variety of tools and equipment are used for vehicle stabilization operation.

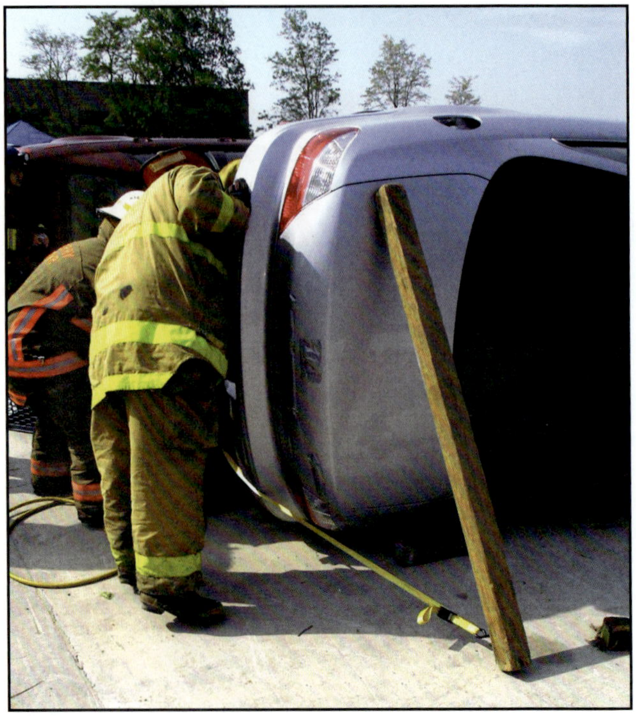

Figure 7.2 Extrication personnel often used a combination of cribbing, rigging, and struts to stabilize passenger vehicles resting on their sides.

points, various stabilization surfaces, and basic vehicle anatomy. Also, rescuers will have to understand how lifting vehicles and objects may factor into vehicle stabilization operations.

NOTE: Chapter 6, Passenger Vehicles, describes vehicle anatomy.

Mechanism of Movement

In order to properly stabilize a vehicle, rescuers should have knowledge of the directions that unstable vehicles might move **(Figure 7.3)**. An understanding of the mechanism of movement will help rescuers make decisions on their approach to stabilizing vehicles. This section discusses a vehicle's center of gravity and the various directions an unstable vehicle might move.

Center of Gravity

A vehicle's **center of gravity** will significantly affect its stability. Half the total weight of a vehicle is on each side of its center of gravity. A vehicle's center of gravity acts as a pivot point around which the vehicle will move unless prevented from doing so. The higher a vehicle's center of gravity, the more susceptible the vehicle is to rolling over. Proper vehicle stabilization supports the vehicle on all sides of its center of gravity to prevent any movement.

When most passenger vehicles are empty, the center of gravity is slightly forward of the front door in the center of the vehicle. However, filling the fuel tank, placing objects in the trunk, or adding occupants to the car will all change the weight distribution in the vehicle and, thus, the vehicle's center

> **Center of Gravity** — Point through which all the weight of a vessel and its contents may be considered as concentrated, so that if supported at this point, the vessel would remain in equilibrium in any position.

236 Section C • Chapter 7 – Passenger Vehicle Stabilization Operations

of gravity. Rescuers may encounter particular difficulty when attempting to determine the center of gravity of a collision-deformed vehicle. Because the center of gravity may change dramatically with weight distribution, vehicles that appear stable may actually be unstable. Rescuers should stabilize any vehicle containing injured and/or trapped occupants to prevent any further movement.

The mass and weight of a vehicle also affect its stability after a collision. The heavier the vehicle, the greater its tendency to settle toward the stability of the ground. When a vehicle rests on a slope, its mass makes it susceptible to sliding or rolling down that slope. Rescue personnel should identify this potential movement and take action to safely and effectively counteract it.

NOTE: The center of gravity on vehicles varies greatly based on the type of vehicle, the vehicle's load, fuel supply, and many other factors. Rescuers should become familiar with the vehicles common to their jurisdiction to gain a better understanding of the center of gravity of those vehicles.

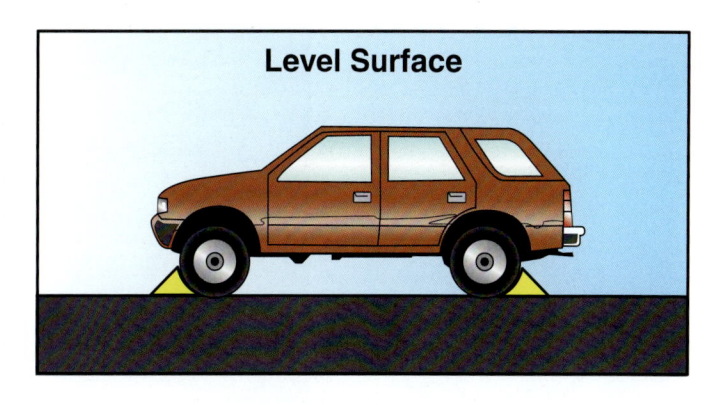

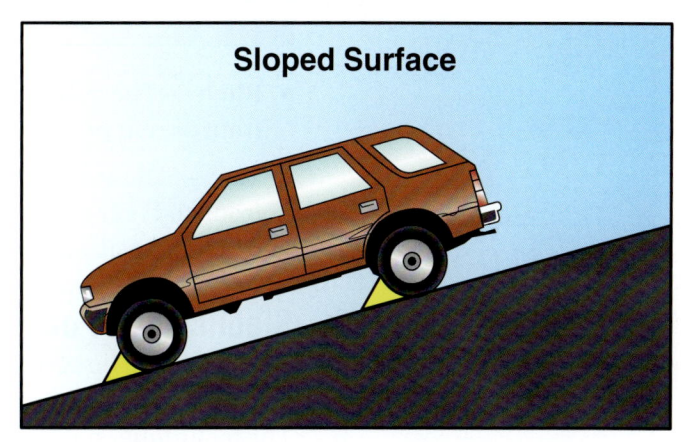

Figure 7.3 Methods for chocking a vehicle on a flat surface and on a slope.

Directional Movement

In order to understand the potential movements of an object, envision three imaginary lines drawn through the vehicle. Each line represents a different axis: longitudinal (horizontal), vertical, and lateral.

- **Longitudinal (horizontal) axis** — Imaginary horizontal line that extends lengthwise from the front to the rear of the vehicle and passes through the center of the passenger compartment.

- **Vertical axis** — Imaginary vertical line that extends from the top of the vehicle to the bottom of the vehicle, stops at the ground, and passes through the center of the passenger compartment.

- **Lateral axis** — Imaginary horizontal line that extends from the outside of the passenger side of the vehicle to the outside of the driver side of the vehicle, and passes through the imaginary center point of the passenger compartment.

Stabilizing a vehicle means preventing sudden and unexpected movement of the vehicle in any direction along any of these axes **(Figure 7.4, p. 238)**. An unstable vehicle will move in one or more of the following directions:

- **Horizontal** — The vehicle can move forward or rearward on the longitudinal axis or can move horizontally along the lateral axis.

- **Vertical** — The vehicle can move up or down in relation to the ground while moving along the vertical axis.

- **Roll** — The vehicle can move side to side while rotating along the longitudinal axis but remain horizontal in orientation.

Section C • Chapter 7 – Passenger Vehicle Stabilization Operations 237

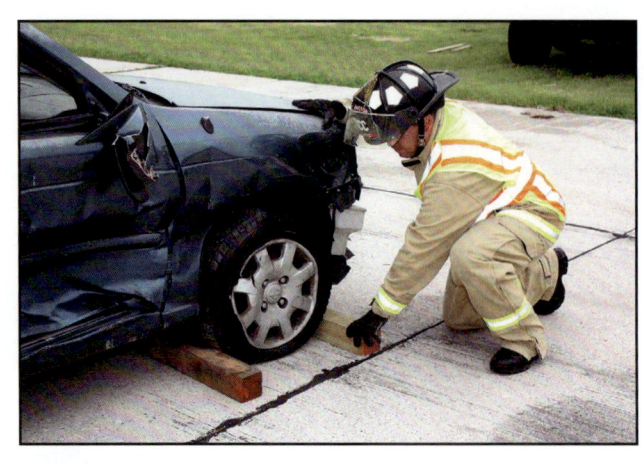

Figure 7.4 This vehicle has been chocked to prevent movement.

- **Pitch** — The vehicle can move up or down on the lateral axis causing the front or rear of the vehicle to rise or fall.
- **Yaw** — The vehicle can twist or turn on the vertical axis and causes the front and rear portions to move in a left or right direction in relation to their original position.

Stabilization Points and Surfaces/Terrain

The structural integrity, balance point, shape, and resting position as related to slope and grade determine the stability of any movable and untouched object. The technique, stabilization points, and stabilization surfaces applied during stabilization efforts determine the final stability of an object. Stabilization points and surfaces can vary greatly and are determined by many factors. For the purpose of this text, stabilization points will refer to the specific physical areas of the vehicle, machinery, or object to be stabilized. Stabilization surfaces/terrain will refer to the locations situated away from these stabilization points, such as the ground or other surfaces. In most cases, responders should attempt to obtain four-point or six-point stabilization; however, some situations may require more points of contact to effectively achieve the desired level of stabilization **(Figure 7.5)**.

Stabilizing a Vehicle Resting on its Roof

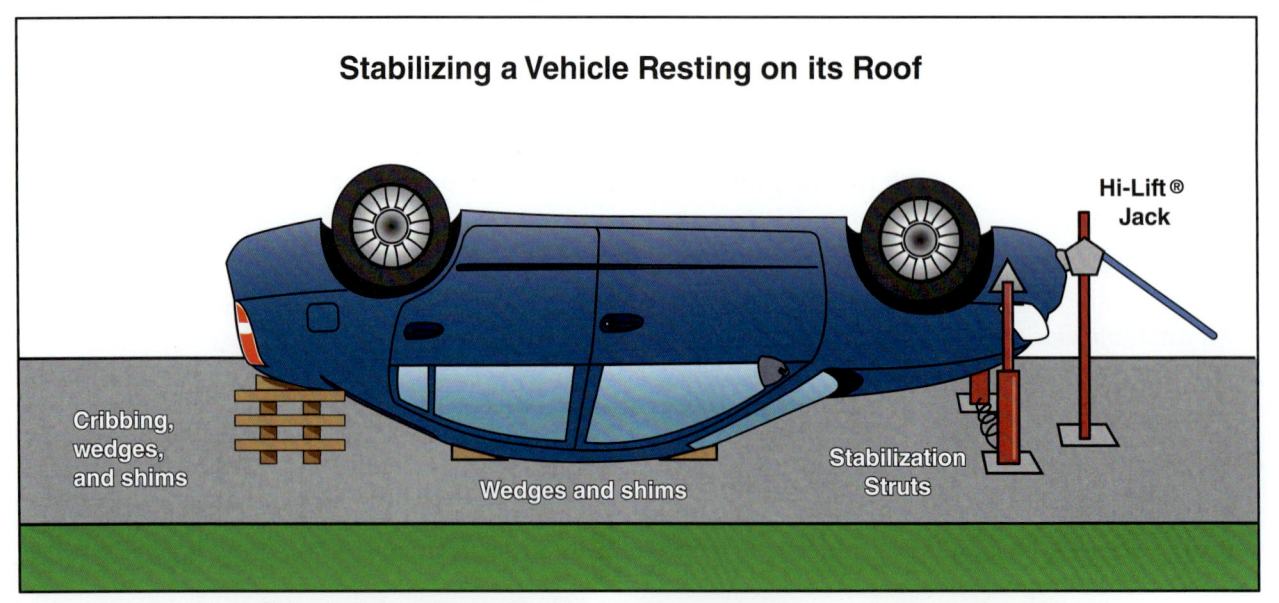

Cribbing, wedges, and shims | Wedges and shims | Stabilization Struts | Hi-Lift® Jack

Figure 7.5 The rounded shape of a vehicle's hood, roof, and trunk can present a challenge when stabilizing an upside down vehicle.

238 Section C • Chapter 7 – Passenger Vehicle Stabilization Operations

Stabilization Points

Dependent upon the type of vehicle and the position of that vehicle (wheel resting, side resting, roof resting), the rescuer will face varying shapes, sizes, and points of contact to utilize for stabilization **(Figure 7.6, p. 240)**. Rescuers must make an effort to ensure that any stabilization point does not impede or block potential victim access, egress, or extrication operations.

Using cribbing or step-chocks strategically located at the strongest or most structurally sound points of the vehicle will appropriate stabilize most wheel resting vehicles. These points may include the frame components where the pillars or posts meet the frame on passenger vehicles.

Side- and roof-resting vehicles present challenges because the roofs of most vehicles are rounded above the door openings, and their surfaces have a smooth, painted finish. This provides less purchase for cribbing or step chocks. Because of the rounded contours of vehicle roofs, rescuers may need to support the vehicle front and rear with cribbing, struts, or other suitable means **(Figure 7.7, p. 241)**. The contours of the side of the vehicle are usually more rounded and offer fewer positive purchase points than a wheel-resting vehicle. The sheet metal or plastic fenders and side panels are not as strong as other structural members; they tend to bend when used as stabilization points.

Rescuers should strive to use fixed components of the vehicle as stabilization points, such as the vehicle's frame. However, rescuers may use intact and undamaged dynamic components, such as the suspension system. Rescuers should not use other vehicle components, such as exhaust systems and the drivetrain, for stabilization.

NOTE: Avoid any component of the exhaust system due to the extreme heat associated with these systems.

Stabilization Surfaces/Terrain

Surfaces, also known as terrain, may include concrete, asphalt, dirt, sand, or sod. The weather conditions at the time of the event affect the terrain. Place a solid base of cribbing, a flat board, or a steel plate under the equipment to prevent it from sinking into soft, wet, or muddy surface/terrain. Additionally, many manufacturers offer additional accessory equipment such as ratchet straps or pickets to secure and/or displace weight on specific stabilization equipment.

Lifting

Rescuers sometimes need to remove other objects involved in the incident away from or off of the vehicle in order to stabilize the vehicle. For example, if the vehicle struck a tree, power pole, or a building, the struck object may have collapsed onto the vehicle, trapping the occupants inside **(Figure 7.8, p. 241)**. Rescue personnel then face the challenge of lifting the collapsed object from the vehicle while limiting the amount of vehicle movement. Prior to lifting an object off the vehicle, rescuers should first capture the vehicle's suspension.

Types of Accidents

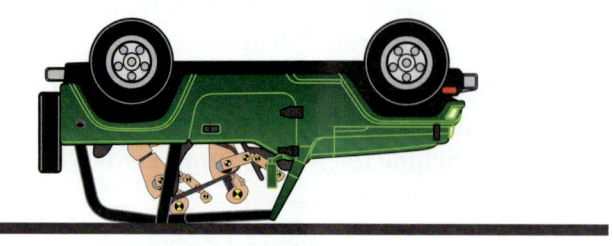

Roof Resting

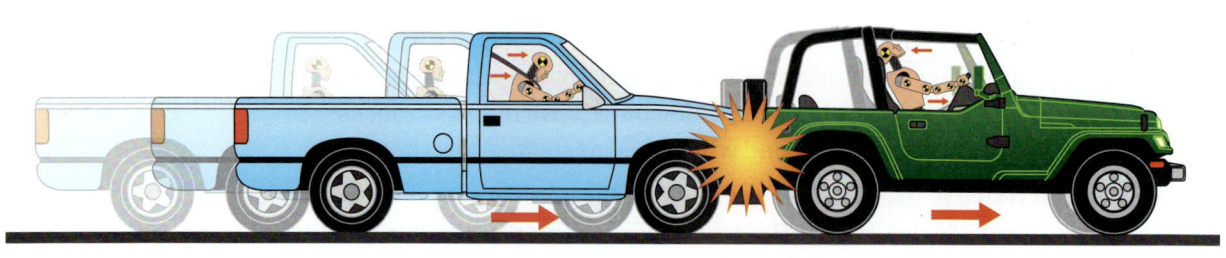

Front/Rear Impact-Wheel Resting

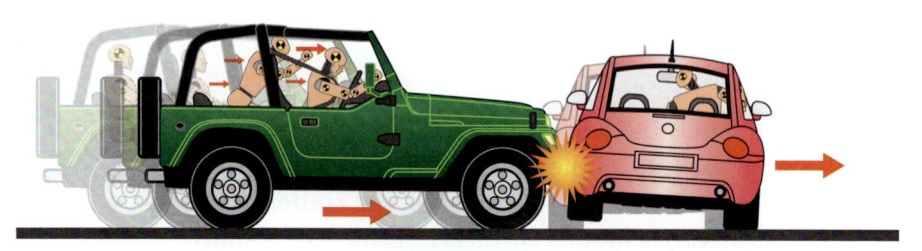

Wheel Resting

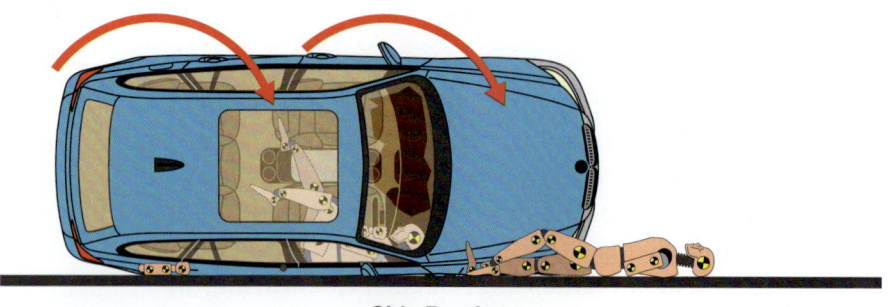

Side Resting

Figure 7.6 Knowledge of common types of vehicle impact injuries helps emergency responders to determine the correct response.

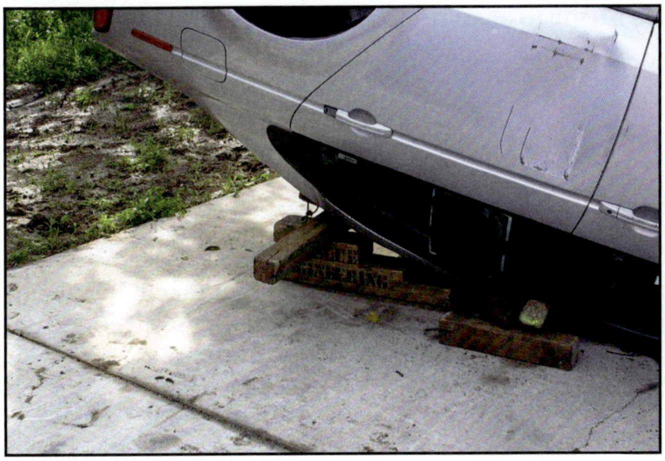

Figure 7.7 This roof-resting vehicle is being stabilized by cribbing and chocks placed underneath the roof.

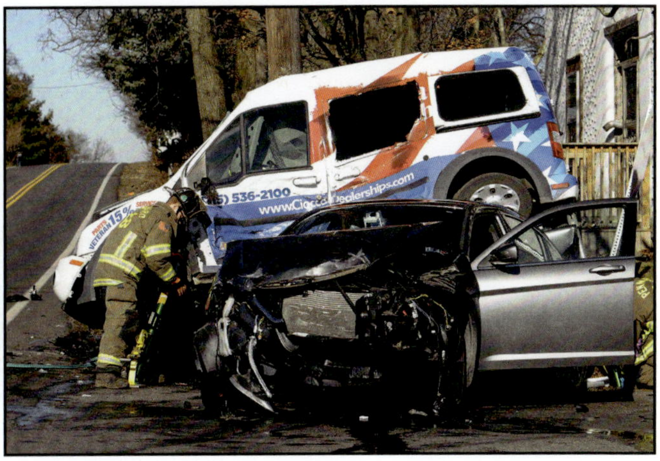

Figure 7.8 A responder stabilizing a vehicle with struts. *Courtesy of Bob Esposito.*

> **WARNING!**
> When dealing with an incident that involves a power pole, collapsed building, or other significant hazard, rescuers may need to consult other agencies before starting rescue operations.

Depending upon the situation and the resources available on scene, lifting objects from crashed vehicles may involve the use of pneumatic lifting bags/cushions, jacks, levers, or even booms or cranes. Successful lifting operations require rescuers to establish a reliable contact point between the mechanism and the object being lifted. As rescuers lift the object, they need to capture it with cribbing or some other resource in order to prevent the object from falling back into its original position (lift an inch, crib an inch).

In some cases, the object resting on the vehicle may be too massive to lift intact. Before removing any object, rescuers must capture the crushed vehicle's suspension to reduce the amount of reactionary movement when they lift the overlying load. Removing larger objects may require dividing them into liftable pieces. Rescuers may use a chain saw to cut objects like trees or wooden power poles into smaller, more manageable pieces. Rescuers should attempt to free the underlying vehicle while making as few cuts as possible. If the overlying object is made of metal, rescuers may cut it with a power saw, oxyacetylene cutting torch, or other thermal cutting device. Rescuers may cut a wood frame wall into sections with a chain saw or rotary saw. Rescuers can lift, cut, or break a masonry wall to create access to the victim.

Another option involves supporting the overlying object or load so it will not move in any direction and pulling the vehicle from under it. To remove the vehicle, rescuers must lower the vehicle until it no longer contacts any portion of the object or load. Rescuers should first capture the suspension of the vehicle, then either remove air from the vehicle's tires or dig underneath the tires to lower the vehicle. After separating the object or load and vehicle, rescuers can use a winch, come-a-long, or Griphoist® to slowly pull the vehicle from underneath the object or load as smoothly as possible.

Section C • Chapter 7 – Passenger Vehicle Stabilization Operations

Rescuers may also use lifting to accomplish the following:
- Help position the vehicle for better stabilization (common)
- Lift one vehicle off another to gain access into the lower vehicle
- Lift a vehicle off of a trapped victim

Application of Stabilization Tools and Equipment

Rescuers will likely encounter numerous variations of vehicle accidents. Each variation will require the rescuer to utilize different applications of stabilization tools and equipment. Rescuers should familiarize themselves with the application of the following tools and equipment:

- Wheel chocks
- Cribbing materials
- Pneumatic lifting bags and cushions
- Jacks
- Levers
- Hitches
- Chains
- Wire rope
- Synthetic slings
- Rigging
- Struts
- Recovery vehicles

Wheel Chocks

The first step in the stabilization process may require application of wheel chocks **(Figure 7.9)**. General wheel chock guidelines include placing and centering the chocks on both sides of the tire, applying the vehicle's parking brake, and re-assessing the vehicle throughout the operation. **Skill Sheet 7-1** describes the steps for preventing horizontal movement of a vehicle using chocks.

> **CAUTION**
> Never rely on the vehicle's mechanical systems as the only means of stabilization. Use them only in conjunction with other methods.

Cribbing Materials

Responders normally use cribbing in a box formation and typically push the pieces into position with a mallet or with another piece of cribbing. Wedges may ensure solid contact between the cribbing and the vehicle. Cribbing placed under the sides of a vehicle prevents lateral movement **(Figure 7.10)**.

The box crib commonly provides a base for a pneumatic lifting device. This application requires a solid top tier of cribbing, with several pieces laid side by side with no opening in the middle. Leaving an opening in the middle would allow the lifting bag to bulge into the opening, reducing its lifting ef-

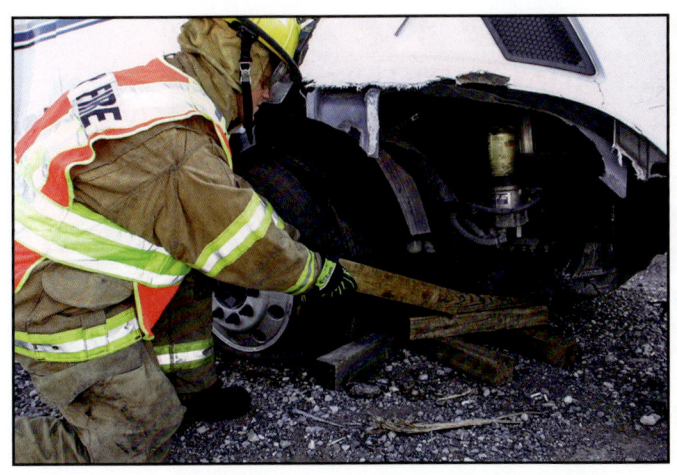

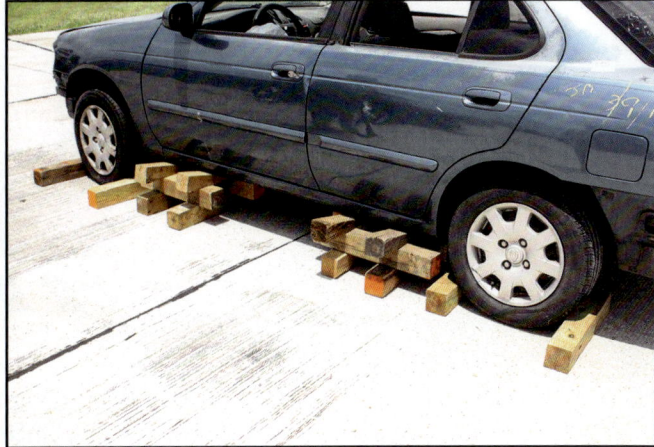

Figure 7.9 Chocking is a non-damaging method of stabilizing and maintaining a vehicle's wheels. *Courtesy of Jennifer Ayers/Sonrise Photography.*

Figure 7.10 A box crib provides a base for lifting.

ficiency and perhaps damaging the bag. The inflating bag might also push the top pieces off the side of the stack. To reduce the possibility of the pneumatic bag shifting atop the cribbing stack, some agencies place a mat made of foam rubber or belting material on top of the cribbing and under the lifting bag.

NOTE: When lifting a vehicle, rescuers need to maintain a stable platform and stabilize the vehicle as the load rises (lift an inch, crib an inch).

Pneumatic Lifting Bags and Cushions

Pneumatic lifting bags or cushions, designed for lifting heavy objects, may be used to lift vehicles **(Figure 7.11)**. **Skill Sheet 7-2** describes the procedures for using pneumatic lifting bags to lift a vehicle.

When using pneumatic lifting bags or cushions to lift a vehicle, rescuers should use solid pieces of plywood or heavy-duty mat material at least as large as the bags/cushions to protect the bags/cushions from damage. Place one piece of the plywood, mat, or industrial belt material as needed to prevent undue damage to the bag/cushion. This will protect the pneumatic lifting device from glass and sharp edges.

NOTE: Although it is common practice to place a protective mat or a piece of material between the bag and the object to be lifted, most manufacturers do not recommend this practice because it potentially reduces the gripping surface of the bag.

When using any form of pneumatic lifting device, rescuers should perform the following:

- Control hazards (if possible).
- Determine victim location and provide care (if possible).
- Crib the vehicle and insert the bag under the vehicle in a way that allows maximum surface contact.
- Maintain vehicle stabilization.
- Protect the bag from punctures.
- Lift an inch, crib an inch.

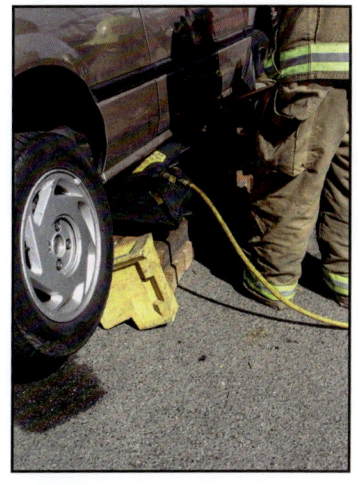

Figure 7.11 Pnuematic lifting bags should be used in pairs at opposing sides of an unstable vehicle.

Section C • Chapter 7 – Passenger Vehicle Stabilization Operations   **243**

> **WARNING!**
> Improper use of bags or cushions can cause the bag/cushion to violently eject from under the load to be lifted. Always follow manufacturer's recommendations.

> **CAUTION**
> Do not place pneumatic lifting devices near the vehicle exhaust system's catalytic converter(s).

Throughout the lifting operation, the officer in charge monitors the lifting evolution and gives commands to the controls operator. These commands should be simple, such as "up on red," "hold on red," or "down on red." The lifting bag or cushion operator should be in position to see that the equipment is functioning correctly, determine how much to lift or lower a load, and take corrective action if necessary. Successful application of lifting bags or cushions requires communication between all personnel.

High-Pressure Lifting Bags
Rescuers should perform the following actions when using high-pressure lifting bags during extrication operations:

- Assess the load to be lifted.
- Calculate the load to be lifted.
- Use the proper lifting bag for the load to be lifted.
- Insert the bag under the object to provide a straight upward lift.
- Ensure appropriate load capture throughout the lifting operation.
- Inflate the bag.
- Adjust the lifting platform higher.
- Repeat the above steps until meeting desired lift.

Some manufacturers' recommendations allow high-pressure lifting bags to be stacked for lifting operations. While manufacturer's recommendations allow this, stability decreases with each additional lifting bag. Rescuers need special training and experience when performing these operations.

NOTE: Stacked bags can only lift the capacity of the lowest rated device.

> **WARNING!**
> Stacking high-pressure lifting bags may cause instability.
> An unstable object may shift or move causing harm to personnel.

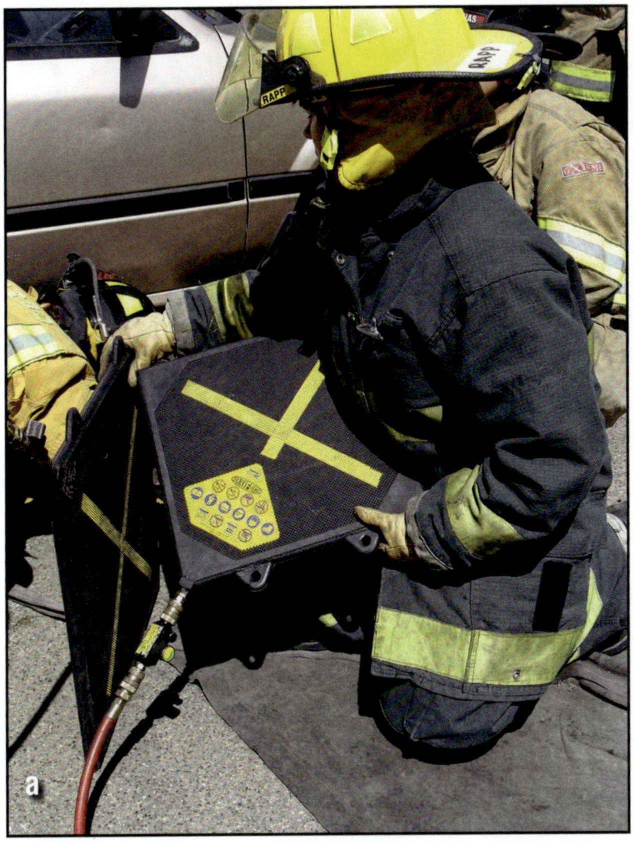

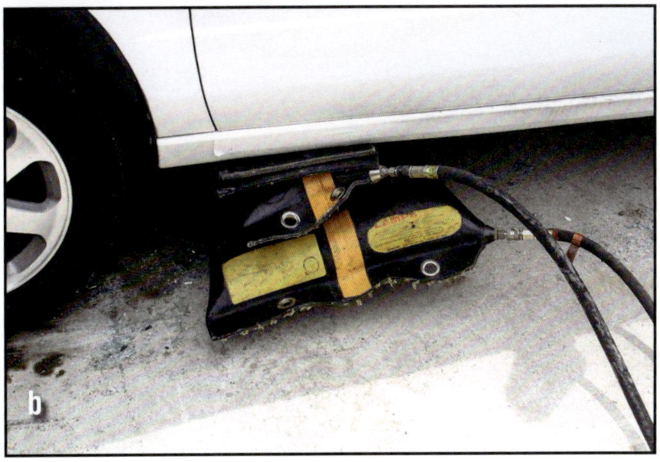

Figure 7.12 a. An example of a high-pressure lifting bag. **b.** A low-pressure lifting cushion is used temporarily to stabilize the vehicle.

Low- and Medium-Pressure Lifting Cushions

When using low- and medium-pressure lifting cushions, rescuers should only lift the object enough to remove the victim(s). They must crib the pivot side (opposite of the lift side) of the object, to avoid crushing the victim(s) **(Figure 7.12 a and b)**.

Jacks

Rescuers should follow these guidelines when using jacks during extrication operations:

- Crib the vehicle specifically for the type of jack and/or lift.
- Establish a firm base to set the tool against so that the tool will not push into the ground when lifting **(Figure 7.13, 246)**. Use cribbing or a platform to provide a good base.
- Capture the load throughout the lifting operation.
- Move only the material the amount needed to extricate the victim.

NOTE: Skill Sheet 7-3 describes the procedures for lifting a wheel-resting passenger vehicle using a jack.

CAUTION
Never allow the object that is being moved to come back into the area it is being moved away from. This will help prevent re-impingement of the object onto the victim.

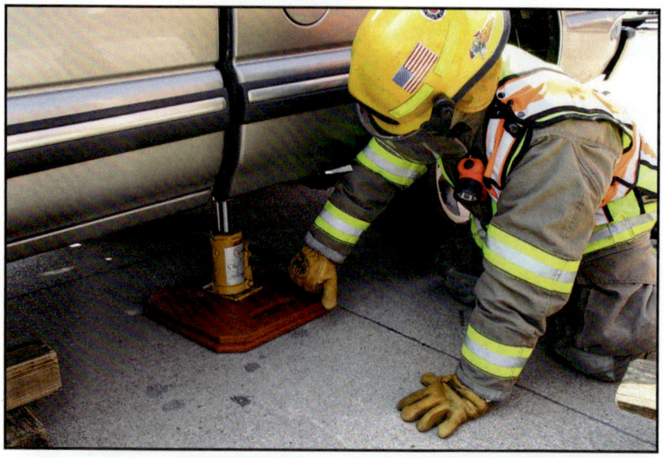

Figure 7.13 A jack must be placed on a solid level surface.

Lever — Device consisting of a bar pivoting on a fixed point (fulcrum), using power or force applied at a second point to lift or sustain an object at a third point.

Fulcrum — Support or point of support on which a lever turns in raising or moving a load.

Levers

A **lever** is a rigid bar, either straight or bent, that freely moves on a fixed point called a **fulcrum**. The lever transfers a force from one place to another while at the same time changing the direction of the force.

To calculate the potential mechanical advantage of a lever, measure the distance between:

1. The load and the fulcrum (load side)
2. The fulcrum and the point of applied force (force side)

If the length of the lever is three times as long on the force side of the fulcrum as on the load side, the lever has a 3-to-1 mechanical advantage. For example, if you have a 300-pound (150 kg) load to lift and a 3:1 lever, it will take 100 pounds (50 kg) of force to lift the load. The three lever classifications vary based on the location of the fulcrum as it relates to both the load and the force.

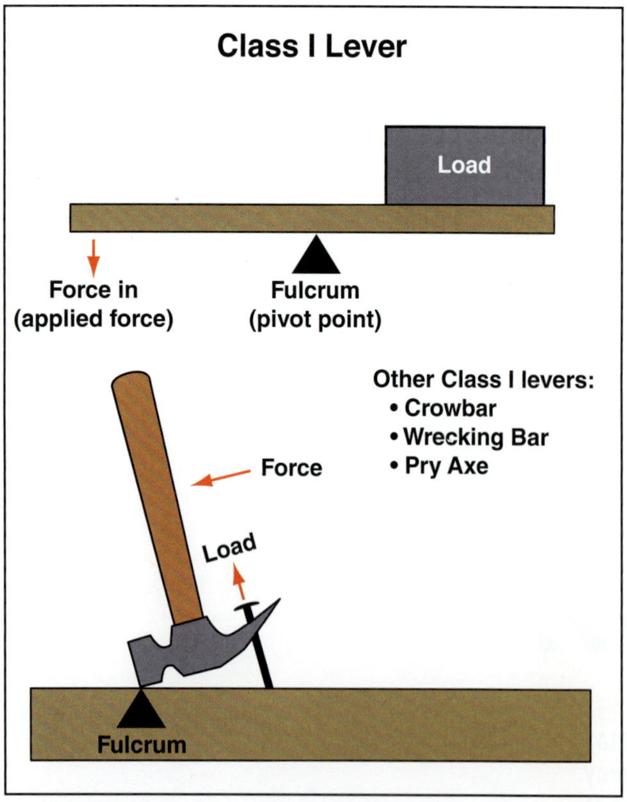

Class I Lever

The Class I lever is the most efficient to use for moving objects vertically. A Class I lever consists of an applied force at one end, a load at the opposite end, and a fulcrum between the two. Examples of Class I levers include crowbars, pry bars, and most fire service forcible entry tools (**Figure 7.14**).

When using a Class I lever, consider the stability and strength of the surface upon which the fulcrum rests. Both the fulcrum and the foundation on which it rests must be capable of holding twice the weight of the load to be lifted. If the load is 100 pounds (50 kg), it will take 100 pounds (50 kg) of force to lift it. That means that the fulcrum must be capable of holding 200 pounds (100 kg).

Skill Sheet 7-4 describes the steps for lifting a wheel-resting passenger vehicle using a Class I lever.

Figure 7.14 This illustration shows how a Class I lever works.

Section C • Chapter 7 – Passenger Vehicle Stabilization Operations

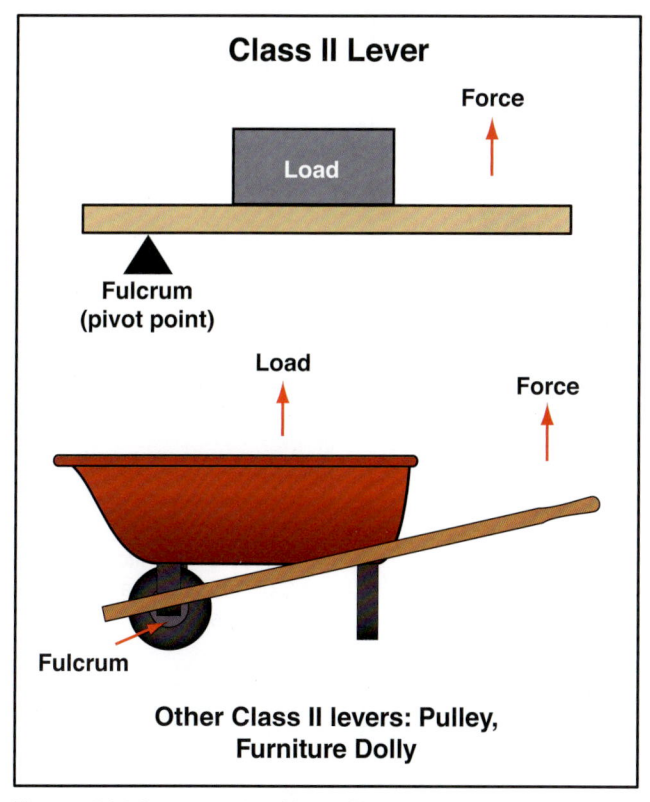

Figure 7.15 An example of how Class II levers work.

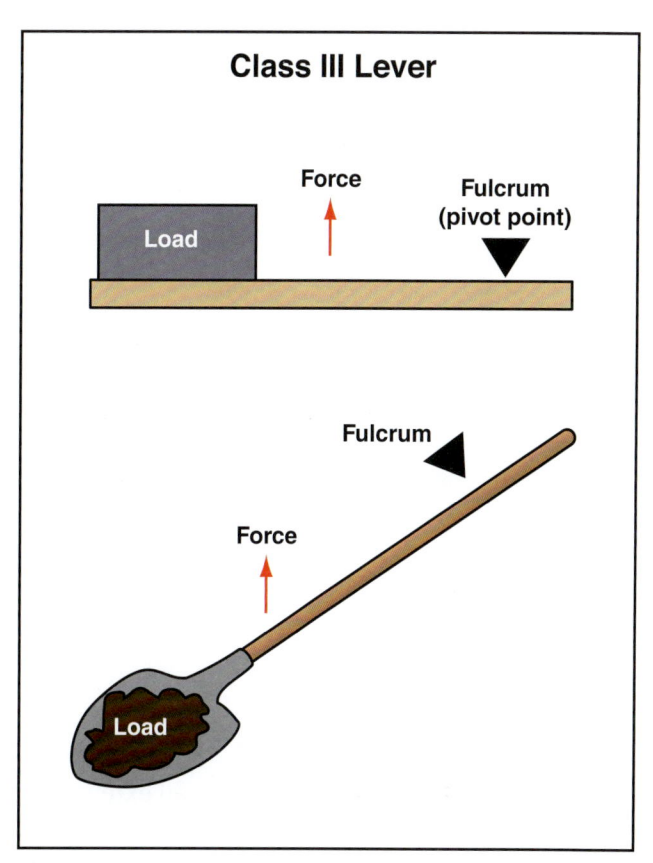

Figure 7.16 This is an example of a Class III lever.

Class II Lever

Class II levers move objects horizontally. A Class II lever consists of a fulcrum at one end, a load in the middle, and a force on the other end. Types of Class II levers include wheelbarrows, furniture dollies, and pulleys are types of Class II levers **(Figure 7.15)**.

Class III Lever

A Class III lever sacrifices force for distance. It places a load on one end, the fulcrum on the opposite end, and the force in the middle. Types of Class III levers include shovels and brooms. This class of lever is the least efficient method of lifting. It depends upon the rescuer's strength to move the load, not the multiplication of the force **(Figure 7.16)**.

Hitches

A hitch consists of a **sling**, regardless of type, attached to a load. In a hitch sling configuration the sling fastens either directly to or around an object or load. The following sections describe common hitches.

Vertical Hitch

A vertical hitch uses a single leg of rope, chain or webbing to support a load **(Figure 7.17, p. 248)**. A single leg (one straight piece of chain, rope or webbing) carries the full load. Rescuers should not use vertical hitches in the following cases:

- Load is hard to balance
- Center of gravity is hard to establish

Sling — Assembly that connects the load to the material handling equipment. There are four common types of slings: chain, wire rope, synthetic round, and synthetic web.

Section C • Chapter 7 – Passenger Vehicle Stabilization Operations

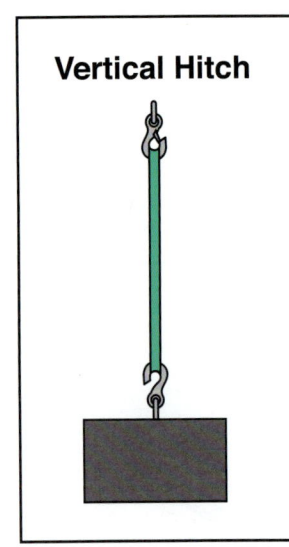

Figure 7.17 An example of a vertical hitch.

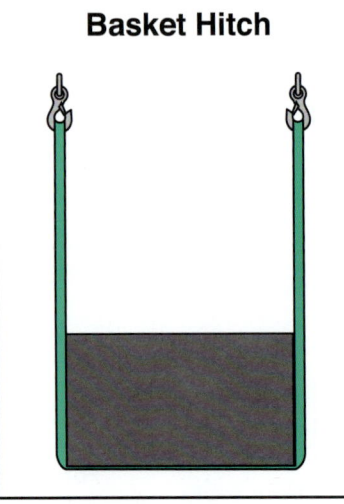

Figure 7.18 An example of a basket hitch.

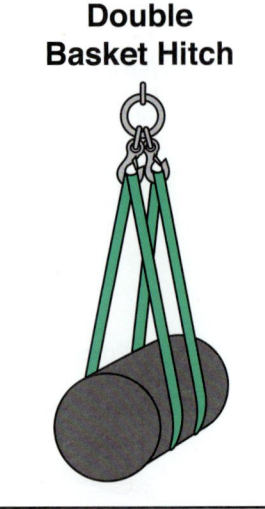

Figure 7.19 Double basket hitches are more stable than single basket hitches.

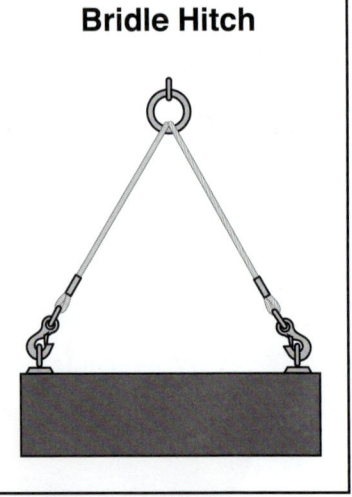

Figure 7.20 Bridle hitch slings have 2 or 3 legs that attach to the load to be lifted.

- Load is loose
- Load extends past the point of attachment

Basket Hitch

A basket hitch sling configuration passes the sling under the load and attaches both ends to the hook or a master link **(Figure 7.18)**. The design of a basket hitch does not keep a load balanced or stabilized.

Double Basket Hitch

A double basket hitch provides more stability than a single basket hitch. The double basket hitch uses two single slings, each attached to one central hook but each wrapped at separate locations around the load **(Figure 7.19)**. This hitch allows rescuers to locate the center attachment hook over the estimated center of gravity, and permits the wrapping of the slings to either side of the center of gravity. The slings of a double-wrap basket hitch make contact all the way around the load surface; this increases the security of the load, and works well for cylindrical loads.

Bridle Hitch

A bridle hitch sling configuration attaches two or three legs to the load. The slings are secured to a single point on the load, usually in line between the center of gravity and the anchor (lifting point). The bridle hitch provides stable lifting, stabilizing, moving, and pulling due to distribution of the load onto the multiple slings **(Figure 7.20).**

Choker Hitch

A choker hitch sling configuration passes one end of the sling under the load and through the other end of the sling. This sling is secured back onto itself and creates a vise-like grip on the load **(Figure 7.21)**. The choker hitch prevents a problem of load stability.

Figure 7.21 Choker hitches create a vise-like grip on the load being lifted.

248 Section C • Chapter 7 – Passenger Vehicle Stabilization Operations

Double Choker Hitch

A double choker hitch spreads two single slings spread apart around the load. This hitch does not make full contact with the load surface, but it can be double wrapped to help control or hold the load. When using straps in pairs, rescuers should arrange hooks on the straps so that the hooks will pull from opposite sides to create a better gripping action **(Figure 7.22)**.

Chains

Rescue chain is a minimum of three eighth-inch, Grade 8 or 10, also called Grade 80 or Grade 100, alloy steel chain for all rescue applications. Rescuers use rescue chain to help move wreckage away from a victim and to tie down unstable objects. Chain slings can be used for rugged applications in harsh environments that require flexibility, abrasion resistance, and long life. When using rescue chains, use hooks that have an equal rating. This grade can absorb shock loads better than other grades of chain rated at the same strength.

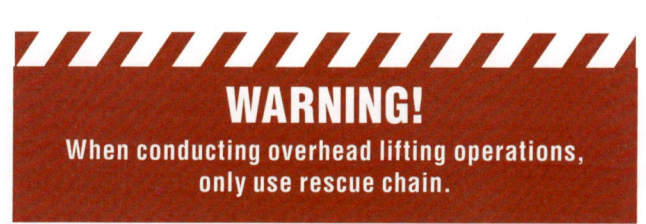

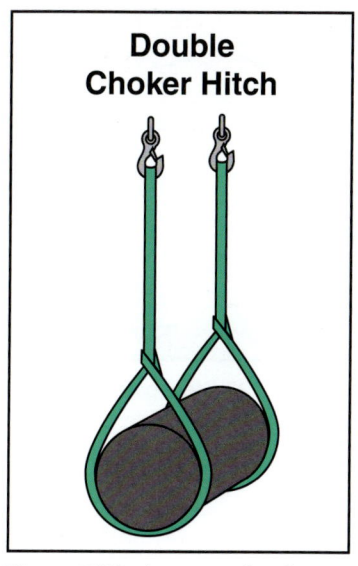

Figure 7.22 An example of a double choker hitch.

> **WARNING!**
> When conducting overhead lifting operations, only use rescue chain.

Precautions to take when using chains include the following:

- Do not exceed the listed safe working load of the chain. All chain should have an attached tag that lists the safe load weight.
- Remember that links break without warning.
- Place padding between the chain and the load to create a better gripping surface and to protect the chain from damage.
- Use padding, such as planks or heavy fabric, around sharp corners on the load to protect links from damage.
- Do not expose chain to cold temperatures for long periods of time.
- Do not permit chain to kink or twist while under stress.
- Seat the load in the hook.
- Do not attach chain hooks to the loads. Attach hooks only to the chain.
- Avoid sudden jerks in lifting and lowering the load. Do not shock load the chain.
- Remember that chains may create a sparking hazard.
- Do not tie a knot in a chain.
- Chain can be slippery when lifting steel. Watch for shifting loads.
- Use a chain gauge to check chain regularly for fatigue and stretching.
- Destroy damaged or worn-out chains.
- Do not re-weld broken links on alloy chain.

Inspect chain regularly; neglecting or abusing chains during use or storage can lead to chain failures. Metal fatigue and chain failure may result from improper treatment of chain components. When inspecting chains, look link by link for signs of cracks, nicks, gouges, bent links, corrosion, elongation, or any other defects. Remove defective chain from service.

Wire Rope

Wire rope, such as plow steel cable, is the strongest type of material used for slings **(Figure 7.23)**. Wire rope construction forms include:

- **Braided wire rope** — A wire rope formed by plaiting component wire ropes.
- **Cable laid rope** — A wire rope composed of six wire ropes wrapped around a fiber or wire rope core.
- **Strand laid rope** — A wire rope made with strands (usually six or eight) wrapped around a fiber core, wire strand core, or independent wire rope core.

A number of wire rope fitting and termination designs exist. The flemish eye is the most reliable and efficient termination and must be done in a shop **(Figure 7.24)**. The flemish eye does not reduce capacity. The wedge socket is the next most reliable type of termination. If properly manufactured and installed, the wedge socket will only reduce capacity 10 to 20 percent. The fold-back eye termination is the least reliable and should not be used for rescue work.

An incident may require rescuers to construct wire rope terminations using cable clips, so rescuers must familiarize themselves with positioning and tightening these useful devices. These clips reduce capacity by about 20 percent. The clips are installed in succession and torqued (tightened) according to manufacturer's specifications. Use a thimble when attaching the wire rope to a hang point that would cause the cable to bend sharply **(Figure 7.25)**. The thimble guides the cable into a natural curve and helps to protect the wire rope.

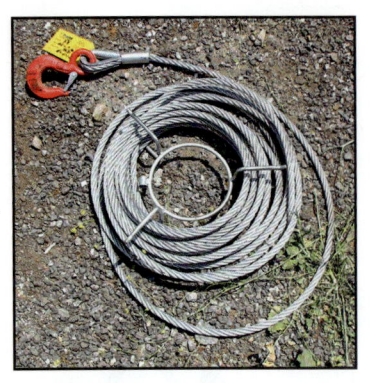

Figure 7.23 Steel cable is used for winches.

Wire Rope Terminations

Flemish Eye (100%)
Wedge Socket (90 to 75%)

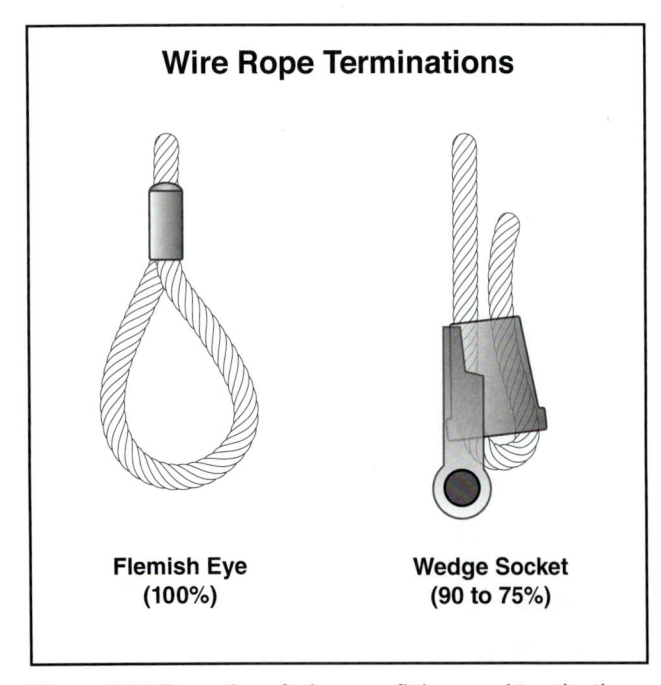

Figure 7.24 Examples of wire rope fittings and terminations.

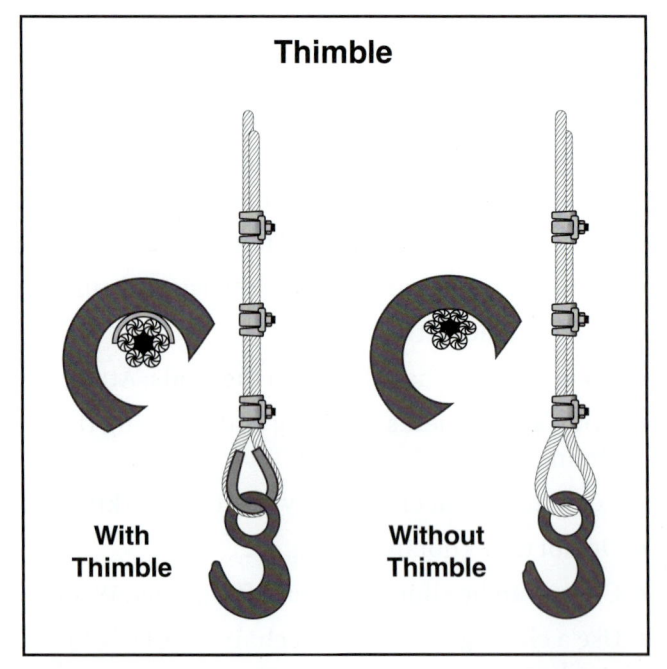

Thimble

With Thimble
Without Thimble

Figure 7.25 This illustration shows how a wire thimble can be used to protect wire rope.

Section C • Chapter 7 – Passenger Vehicle Stabilization Operations

Some important points about wire rope include:

- Keep it from kinking to avoid damage and loss of integrity.
- Sharp ends or edges will damage it. Use edge protection or softeners to protect it from this damage.
- Do not tie it into a knot. Knots place severe stress on the strands, breaking them
- Remember that wire rope stores kinetic energy during hauling. In the event of cable failure, it can whip around violently, and create a severe injury hazard.
- Destroy wire ropes when removing them from service due to wear or damage.

Inspect wire ropes on a regular basis and after each use. The following unsafe conditions provide signals to discard the wire rope:

- Broken wires – depends on location
- Crushed strands
- Kinks, birdcages (outer strands displace from the core forming a cage), and protruding core
- Stretch, diameter reduction
- Abrasion and corrosion
- Fatigue and electric arc

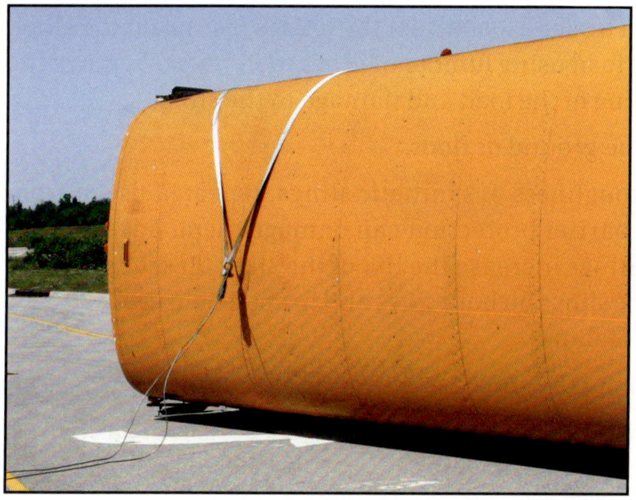

Figure 7.26 A synthetic sling material molds itself to the shape of this bus.

Synthetic Slings

Responders frequently use synthetic round slings and web slings in rescue work to quickly set up anchors and attachments for lifting, stabilizing, pulling, and moving operations **(Figure 7.26)**. Synthetic slings have the following characteristics:

- Tend to mold around the load, adding additional holding power
- Do not rust or spark
- Easier and safer to rig due to their light weight
- Have no sharp edges, thereby reducing injury potential
- Absorb shock loading better than wire rope or chain due to their elasticity

- Resist many chemicals and do not respond to moisture
- Are damaged more easily than cable slings
- Require protection from sharp edges in a rescue situation
- Unable to resist temperatures greater than 200°F (90°C) if made of Nylon or polyester

Whenever using any sling responders must observe the following practices

- Destroy any damaged or defective slings.
- Do not shorten slings with knots, bolts, or other makeshift devices.
- Prevent sling legs from kinking or twisting.
- Do not load slings in excess of their rated capacity.
- Balance the loads of slings used in a basket hitch to prevent slippage.
- Securely attach slings to their loads.
- Protect or pad slings from the sharp edges of their loads.
- Keep suspended loads clear of all obstructions.
- Keep all personnel clear of loads.
- Never place hands or fingers between the sling and its load while the sling is being tightened around the load.
- Avoid shock loading. Jerking the load could overload the sling, causing failure.
- Do not pull a sling from under a load when the load is resting on the sling. Create space under the load using lumber or other materials to remove the sling and prevent shifting of the load and damage to the sling.
- Do not drag slings on the ground or floor.

Despite the inherent toughness of synthetic slings, repeated use or from failure to provide proper barrier protection can damage them. Edge guards, movable sleeves, and coatings increase the life of the sling. Rescuers should inspect synthetic synthetic slings on both sides and in good light every 30 days and after each incident as follows:

- Pay particular attention to the stitching and ends for wear.
- Check the body of the sling for cuts, tensile damage, abrasion, punctures, snags, chemical damage, and heat damage.
- Remove any sling that shows excessive wear or damage from service.

Round Slings

A round sling, also known as an endless sling, is a synthetic sling — usually polyester fibers twisted into yarn bundles — made from a continuous loop of yarn and covered with a jacket. The yarn bundles are twisted into multiple, but separate continuous strands. These strands form the load-bearing members of the sling; the number of strands in the sling determines its strength. A polyester jacket acts as a protective covering over the continuous load-bearing strands. This covering reduces the potential of mechanical and physical damage to interior strands. Rescuers may use round slings for vertical, choker, basket, or bridle slings.

Web Slings
Commonly available web slings include endless, standard eye, and twisted eye. The endless sling has both ends of one piece of webbing lapped and sewn together to form a continuous piece. Rescuers can use them for vertical, bridle, choker, and basket hitches. The standard eye sling consists of a single piece of webbing sewn with an eye at either end in the same plane as the sling body. The twisted eye sling consists of a single piece of webbing with the eye at either end, sewn at 90 degrees to the plane (tapered or full width) of the sling. The twisting allows for better rigging of choker slings.

Rigging
Rigging is defined as a length of rope/chain/webbing attached to a load for the purpose of stabilizing, lifting, pulling, or moving objects. Basic rigging components include hooks and shackles/eyes for termination points to enable easily-made connections to the load. A heavy equipment company may supply the rigging; if so, the company will provide employees who will have responsibility for the care, maintenance, selection, and attachment of the rigging to the load and to the crane. Rescue personnel may be asked to assist with attaching the rigging to the load or manning guidelines. The following sections describe equipment associated with rigging: tighteners and rigging fittings.

> **Rigging** — Ropes or cables used with lifting or pulling devices such as block and tackle.

Tighteners
Rescuers have a choice of a number of different types of tighteners to adjust rigging including the following:

- **Wire rope tighteners** — Rescuers can use wire rope tighteners for lifting light loads or as tightening cable tiebacks and other rigging. Take care not to overload them.

- **Manual cable winch** — Because cable winches are 2 to 3 feet (600 to 900 mm) long, they may have limited use in confined spaces. When using a cable winch, the length of the handle and the strength of one person provide the overload limit **(Figure 7.27)**. Users should take care to avoid fouling the cable during rewinding. An example of a manual cable winch is a come-along or Griphoist®.

- **Powered cable winch** — Powered cable winches are generally either electric or hydraulic and utilize either wire cable or a synthetic winch rope **(Figure 7.28, p. 254)**. Nearly all winches obtain their rated capacity in straight line pull with a minimum of one layer of wire rope wrapped around the drum which creates a tensionless attachment that does not reduce the rated capacity of the wire rope. Rated capacities vary but common ratings for portable/pinned winches range up to 9,000 pounds (4 500 kg) and 12,000 pounds (6 000 kg) for stationary/mounted versions. Length of throw varies based on type of winch and manufacturer but may range up to 100 feet (30 m) or greater. The rated capacity of the winch decreases when the angle of pull does not align directly with the winch, and with each successive wrap placed on the drum. Rescuers may use rated pulleys and shackles to create mechanical advantage systems that increase the load capacity. The rescuer should follow all manufacturer recommendations regarding this practice.

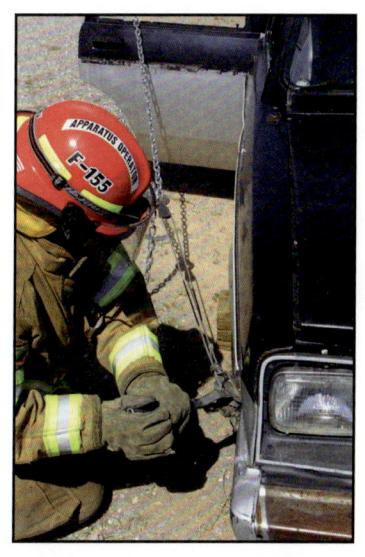

Figure 7.27 A rescuer prying a car door using a cable winch come-along.

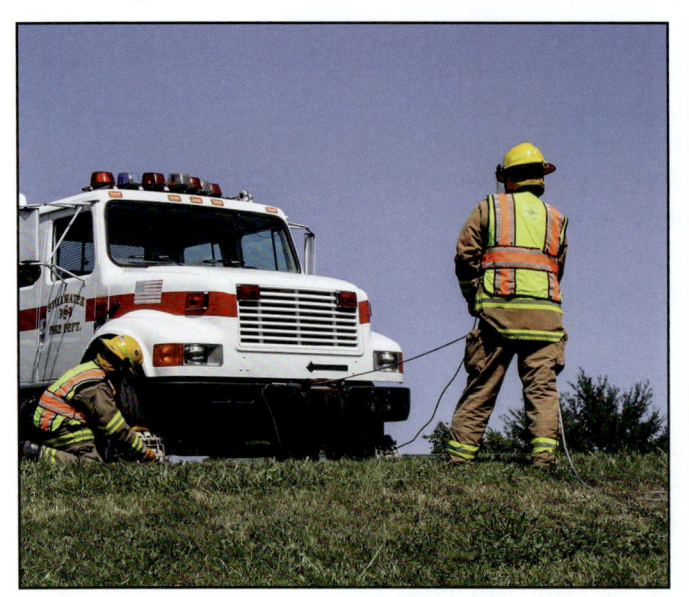

Figure 7.28 An example of a power cable winch on an apparatus.

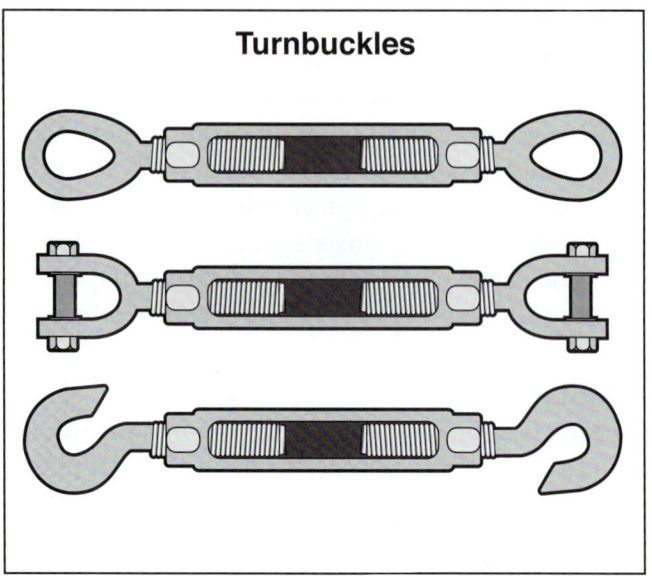

Figure 7.29 Examples of turnbuckles.

- **Load binder** — Load binders are most commonly used with chain assemblies. The ratchet type of load binder is more reliable, and responders should wire tie the handle for safety. Ratchet-type load binders have a 50:1 ratchet action, but only an 8-inch (200 mm) take-up.

- **Chain hoist** — A chain hoist can lift up to 6 tons with 100 pounds of force (50 N). Rescuers must not over pull by using more than one person. These tighteners have a large take-up (up to 10 feet [3 m]), and some only require a 12-inch (300 mm) clearance.

- **Turnbuckles** — Responders commonly use turnbuckles to do the final tightening of tiebacks, freeing a cable winch to do other jobs. The maximum take-up varies from 8 to 24 inches (200 to 600 mm), depending on the type **(Figure 7.29)**. The hook ends of turnbuckles are only 2/3 as strong as the eye or jaw ends.

> **WARNING!**
> Do not extend the handles of any tightening device or use additional people to operate any tightening device.

Rigging Fittings

Hooks, shackles and eyes make up the basic components of rigging. Hooks and shackles provide a way to lift loads without directly tying to the load. They attach to blocks, chains, or wire or fiber rope. The Clevis and eye-types enable rescuers to make rapid chain-to-hook connections. Hooks should have a latch or mouse closing device to keep slings or traps from slipping off the hook. Rescuers can use rope yarn, seizing wire, or shackles to mouse hooks.

Rescuers should use shackles when loads are too heavy for hooks to handle safely. Forged alloy steel should make up ring, hook, and shackle components of slings. The pins used in each shackle are not interchangeable with other shackles. Rescuers should screw the pin in all the way and back it off one-quarter turn before loading.

Struts

Rescuers may use struts to stabilize vehicles found on their side (side resting), upside down (roof resting), or on a slope. Each style of strut consists of three major components; a base, a strut, and a tip. All struts include a form of capture that locks the extension of the strut into place. Examples include inserting pins into manufactured holes or spinning locking collars.

Struts are used in combination with tension straps during stabilization operations. When using these stabilization systems, rescuers should practice the following:

- Use the number of struts in accordance with manufacturer's recommendations.
- Place struts at appropriate locations on the vehicle.
- Extend the struts from the ground to a high point on the vehicle in accordance with manufacturer's recommendations.
- Connect and tighten the tension straps.
- Use additional struts as required.

   NOTE: More information on strut systems can be found later in this chapter.

Recovery Vehicles

A recovery vehicle, such as a tow truck or rescue crane, may help stabilize vehicles. Rescuers may request these light, medium, and heavy-duty recovery vehicles to assist with rescue and recovery operations. They often require early identification and request due to the time delay in their response. In some cases, depending upon the situation and the other resources available, rescuers should prudently wait for a recovery vehicle to arrive before attempting to stabilize a vehicle. For example, if the vehicle is teetering on the edge of a high cliff or a bridge and the rescue units on scene do not have the necessary equipment to secure the vehicle, it may be safer for both the trapped occupants and rescue personnel to wait for a tow truck or rescue crane that is already responding. Attaching the cable from a tow truck or rescue crane winch to an un-stabilized vehicle can provide the initial stability needed for rescue personnel to safely access the trapped victims.

The Incident Commander (IC) or rescue personnel should maintain control of the scene while using tow trucks, rescue cranes, or other resources to assure a safe operation. They should not allow freelancing, even by other agencies. Rescuers control the scene until the completion of all extrication and rescue operations.

Passenger Vehicle Stabilization Operations

Rescuers must stabilize a crashed vehicle before entering it to conduct a more thorough assessment of the victims inside and properly package them for extrication. Rescuers should leave possible victim access areas open when stabilizing vehicles. The techniques employed to stabilize a passenger vehicle vary depending on the vehicle's position. Rescuers must follow the local AHJ

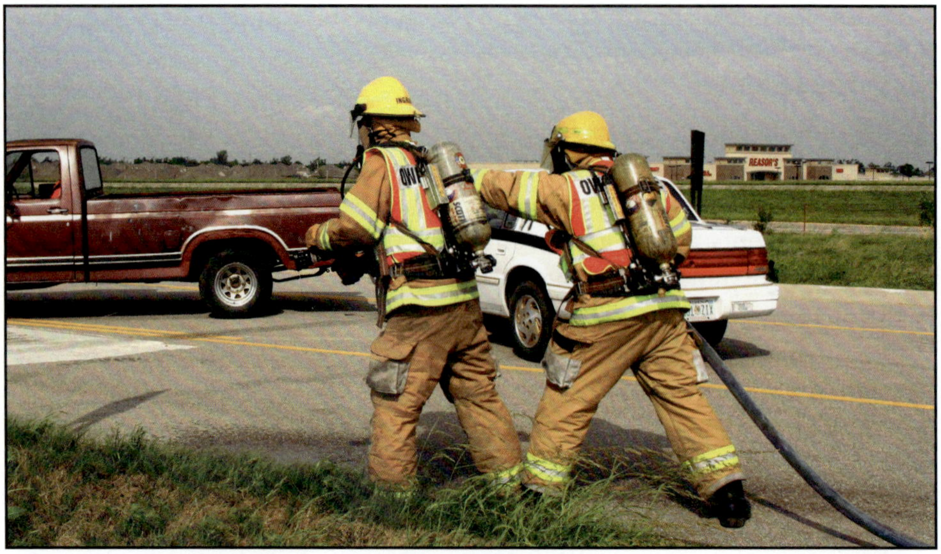

Figure 7.30 Firefighers extending a hoseline to provide fire protection during a vehicle incident.

policies and procedures for passenger vehicle stabilization. The following sections discuss the stabilization techniques used for wheel-resting, side-resting, roof-resting, and alternatively positioned vehicles.

Establishing fire protection is a high priority at vehicle incidents **(Figure 7.30)**. Those incidents involving side- or roof-resting vehicles are prone to leaking fluids. These fluids may come into contact with hot exhaust system components or electrical components that can serve as sources of ignition. Rescuers should have at least one 1 ½ inch (38 mm) or larger hoseline charged and ready. Responders should apply Class B foam to spilled fuel to suppress the production of flammable vapors.

Passenger Vehicle Structural and Damage Characteristics

Depending upon the size and type of vehicle involved, the speed of impact, and other variables, passenger vehicles may look significantly different than they did before the collision. For example, a passenger vehicle may have the following characteristics depending upon the type of impact:

- **Front-impact collision** — Front impacts may "accordion" the engine compartment and the rest of the front end straight back or to the side, making it difficult to locate and disconnect the battery. The collision may also displace the dashboard and steering column rearward into the passenger compartment, along with one or both kick panels. It may jam the doors shut. The windshield and other windows may or may not be intact following a front-impact collision. Fluids may leak from the engine compartment.

- **Rear-end collision** — A rear-ended passenger vehicle may have crumpled rear fenders and trunk. These vehicles may experience heavy fuel leaks if the fuel tank gets punctured. A rear-end collision may damage the tank of an LPG-powered vehicle which could result in a flammable gas leak. In addition, some modern passenger vehicles store their low and high-voltage batteries in the rear of the vehicle. If so, just like with frontal collision damage, this may make it difficult to locate and disconnect the battery.

- **Side-impact collision** —The chassis of a passenger vehicle may or may not be in one piece after a side-impact collision. The chassis may wrap around whatever it came into contact with. The doors and pillars on the impact side may be seriously damaged and virtually inaccessible, while the doors on the opposite side may be fully functional. For body-on-frame or solid-frame vehicles, the passenger compartment may become dislodged and separated from the frame and/or chassis.
- **Underrides and overrides** — Underrides and overrides commonly occur at vehicle incidents. Because they may involve two or more vehicles or commercial/heavy vehicles in addition to passenger vehicles, they will be described in Chapter 12, Special Extrication Situations.

Maintaining Vehicle Stability

Ongoing size-up of the incident site and operation is critical. Once rescuers perform the initial stabilization all on-scene personnel must reassess the stability of the vehicle(s) involved.

Each task rescuers perform may change the dynamic of the incident. Removing items such as doors or a roof may lighten the vehicle, causing vertical movement. The enormous pressures exerted by the extrication tools might force components into different locations, upsetting the center of gravity and rendering the vehicle unstable. Weather conditions such as rain or ice may cause changes in ground surfaces or topography, affecting contact points for stabilization equipment.

To avoid harming victims, rescuers should continuously evaluate a vehicle's stabilization, and make necessary corrections throughout the operation. The slightest push, pull, bounce, or sway, even from accidental contact in the wrong place, may cause a vehicle to move significantly. Any movement can compound or aggravate victims' injuries or even cause new injuries. By maintaining vehicle stability, rescue personnel will be less likely to aggravate or worsen victims' injuries.

Wheel-Resting Passenger Vehicle Stabilization

Most vehicles involved in collisions remain wheel-resting. Rescuers must stabilize wheel-resting vehicles to ensure maximum stability for extrication operations and to prevent any further movement in any direction.

The most common form of horizontal movement involves the vehicle rolling forward or backward on its wheels. To initially stabilize against and prevent this movement, rescuers can chock the wheels with conventional wheel chocks, pieces of cribbing, or other suitable objects.

Rescuers can also use the vehicle's mechanical systems, such as parking brake and transmission, to help prevent horizontal movement. Rescuers should place automatic transmissions in park, if possible, and leave manual transmissions in gear. Rescuers should also set the vehicle's parking brake.

CAUTION
Do not rely on mechanical systems – as the sole means of stabilization.

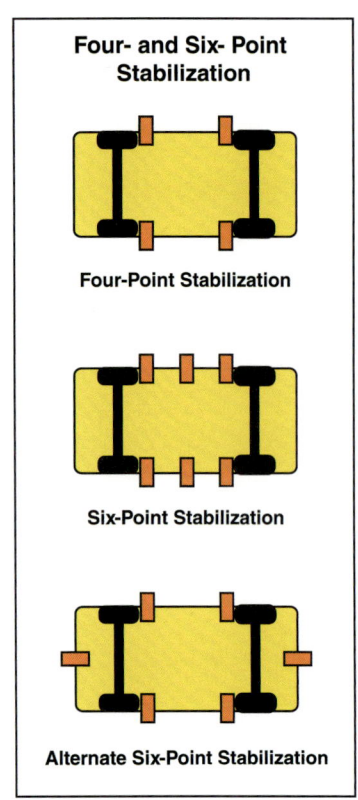

Figure 7.31 Examples of four- and six-point stabilization.

Rescuers can use both wooden and plastic step chocks on wheel-resting vehicles. They are effective and quick and easy to install. At least four step chocks are needed to provide adequate stabilization. **Skill Sheet 7-5** lists the procedures for stabilizing a wheel-resting passenger vehicle using step chocks.

Experience has shown that stabilization for most wheel-resting vehicles may require four to six points of contact (support) **(Figure 7.31)**. The situation will dictate the quantity of support and where to install it. Rescuers most commonly use the following two support methods:

1. **Four-point support** — Also called *four-points of contact*, the means employed may involve the use of cribbing or any of the other equipment described in this chapter. Regardless of what equipment rescuers use during this operation, support is placed behind the front wheel well and at the equivalent point forward of the rear wheel well on both sides of the vehicle.

2. **Six-point support** — Also called *six points of contact*, six-point support is most often needed to support a vehicle that is in danger of collapsing in the middle such as when the doors are opened or removed or when the roof is removed from a unibody vehicle. Support should be installed under the middle of both sides of the vehicle. However, it is possible the front and rear of the vehicle may need additional support.

Cribbing, especially when used with wooden or plastic wedges, is relatively easy to install. However, installing cribbing usually takes longer than using step chocks. Cribbing is most often installed in a box formation until enough cribbing is installed to support the vehicle. **Skill Sheet 7-6** describes the steps for stabilizing a wheel-resting passenger vehicle using cribbing.

When stabilizing a vehicle, rescue personnel must avoid placing body parts under the vehicle while installing the stabilization devices. To prevent any crush injuries rescuers should grasp each piece of cribbing from the sides, set it outside of the vertical plane of the vehicle, and push it into position under the vehicle with a tool or another piece of cribbing.

> **WARNING!**
> Never place body parts under a vehicle. Vehicles, even when stabilized, can suddenly shift and/or fall, potentially injuring or killing anyone beneath it.

Some department's standard operating procedures (SOPs) require rescuers to deflate all four tires to stabilize a wheel-resting vehicle. Removing the valve core, snipping off the valve stems with wire cutters, or pulling the stems out with pliers will quickly and safely accomplish deflation. However, this action also allows the vehicle to move as it settles onto its rims and thus could impart negative energy (potentially harmful movement) into the passenger compartment, so not all departments advocate this practice. Follow local agency protocols.

Deflating the tires prevents the vehicle from rising as it gets lighter when rescuers remove the roof and other components. Only deflate tires after installing cribbing to support the weight of the vehicle. For steps on deflating a wheel-resting passenger vehicle's tires, see **Skill Sheet 7-7**.

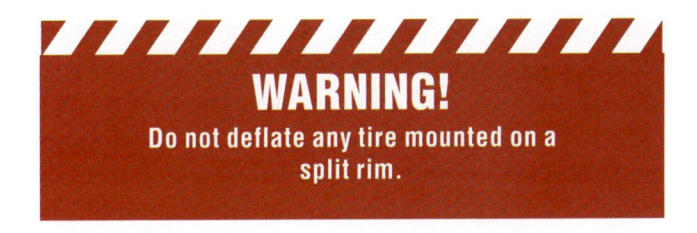

> **WARNING!**
> Do not deflate any tire mounted on a split rim.

> **WARNING!**
> Do not deflate any tire before adequately cribbing to support the vehicle's weight.

Side-Resting Passenger Vehicle Stabilization

When a vehicle comes to rest on its side, the exposed doors on the top side and rear may or may not be operable. If they are, occupants can escape through the door/window openings. If the vehicle is not on fire and rescue personnel will assist occupants through these openings, personnel should first stabilize the vehicle. Depending upon the situation, rescue personnel should use the best means available to quickly and safely prevent the vehicle from moving in any direction. This may involve the use of cribbing and/or step chocks as initial stabilization, and will also involve secondary stabilization.

When stabilizing a side-resting vehicle with struts, rescuers must assess the vehicle's construction, condition, and integrity. They must identify the support locations and purchase points on the vehicle. They should use wedges and/or cribbing to initially control the vehicle while setting up the stabilization system **(Figure 7.32)**. Rescuers use three common methods to stabilize a side-resting vehicle with struts:

- Same-side, opposing force system
- Opposite-side, opposing force system (tensioned buttress)
- Opposite-side, independent system

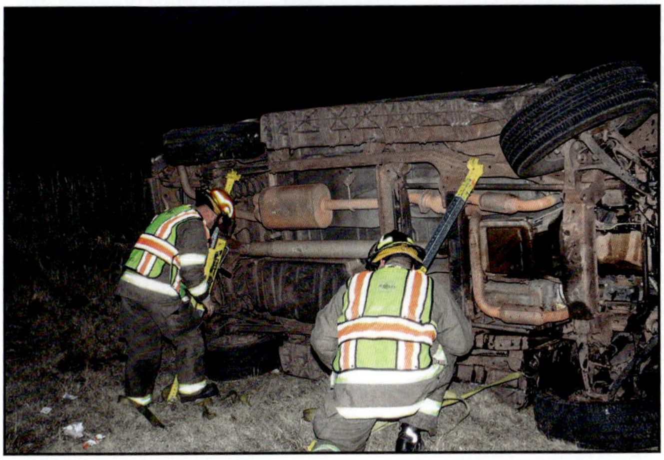

Figure 7.32
Responders stabilizing a side-resting vehicle using struts. *Courtesy of Mike Wieder.*

Section C • Chapter 7 – Passenger Vehicle Stabilization Operations

The same-side, opposing force system is considered to be the safest form of stabilization in a side-resting situation because the rescuers are performing a majority of the work on the undercarriage side of the vehicle. This system also provides a clear work space on the passenger compartment for extrication of the victim(s). Rescuers place initial stabilization around the vehicle to create multiple points of contact, preventing the vehicle from moving before completing secondary stabilization. To accomplish initial stabilization, rescuers use wedges, cribbing, and step chocks to fill voids in areas along the ground on both the undercarriage and passenger-compartment side of the vehicle. Secondary stabilization begins with capturing the vehicle on the undercarriage side using a system capable of tensioning. These systems most commonly consist of a mix of chains, chain attachments, and a tool capable of tensioning like a come-along, chain binder, or Griphoist®. The chain's attachment to the undercarriage needs to be at the highest possible point between the front and rear axles when possible, creating a bridle.

After making attachments to the undercarriage with the chain, rescuers secure a substantial anchor for the system with a chain wrap. Common anchors include guardrails, trees, and fire apparatus. Rescuers should then connect the chain attachment on the undercarriage to the anchor chain wrap using chain and a tensioning device. Rescuers should leave the system slacked and place two struts appropriately to the undercarriage of the vehicle. Once they place the struts, rescuers should tension the chain system until the vehicle loads the struts, and then rescuers should reassess initial stabilization. Rescuers should mark the area around the chain system to caution other rescuers working in and around the undercarriage side. **Skill Sheet 7-8** lists the steps for stabilizing a side-resting passenger vehicle using struts in a same-side, opposing force system.

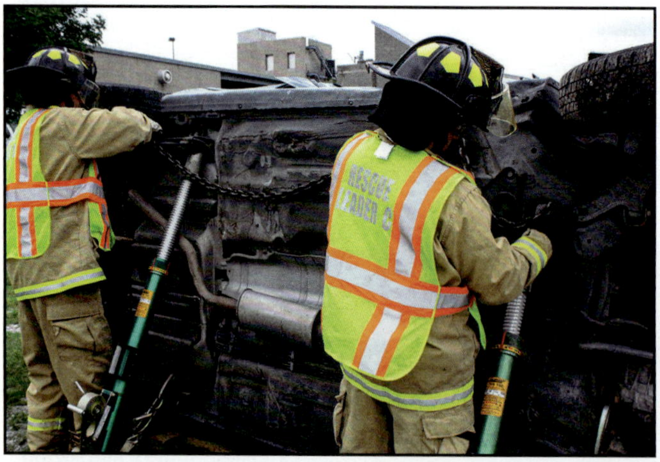

Figure 7.33 A vehicle on its side must be buttressed for stability.

The second stabilizing method – the tensioned buttress system — uses two struts placed on opposite sides of the vehicle, mirrored in position **(Figure 7.33)**. One strut will be placed to the undercarriage side of the vehicle, while the remaining strut is placed to the passenger-compartment side, most commonly at the firewall or trunk. Rescuers need to connect the bases of the mirrored struts (base-to-base) using a tensioning strap in order to tension the system. After rescuers place all the struts at the appropriate angles and make proper attachments to the bases, they should tension the system simultaneously until they have loaded the struts. Once the struts are loaded, rescuers should reassess initial stabilization and adjust where needed. Based on vehicle or accident dynamics, proper stabilization of a side-resting vehicle may require multiple tensioned buttress systems. **Skill Sheet 7-9** lists the procedures for stabilizing a side-resting passenger vehicle using struts in a tensioned buttress system.

The third common method for stabilizing a side-resting vehicle is an opposite-side, independent system. Similar to the tensioned buttress system, the opposite-side independent system connects the bases of the mirrored struts to a low point on the vehicle instead of to each other. Rescuers should pay close attention when attaching the straps on the passenger compartment side to ensure that the straps will not interfere with extrication efforts. Rescuers should tension the strut on the passenger compartment side first. Tensioning the passenger compartment side first will cause the strut to apply force to the vehicle at the point of contact (tip) loading the undercarriage side strut. This practice of loading the passenger side first will help counter the tendency of the vehicle to roll to the path of least resistance. Vehicle or accident dynamics may require multiple independent systems to adequately stabilize a side-resting vehicle.

When a vehicle has come to rest on a sloping, sandy, or other unstable surface, rescuers may need webbing/rope to stabilize the vehicle. Rescuers may use the webbing/rope alone or in combination with a stabilization system. Webbing, ropes, and/or chains can be attached to the vehicle and to a secure anchor point. Rescuers should protect ropes and webbing from chafing and/or contact with chemicals (such as battery acid) that may reduce their strength and cause them to fail. When deciding whether to backup rope or webbing with a second system, rescuers should weigh the need for redundancy against other factors in the situation.

Roof-Resting Passenger Vehicle Stabilization

With a roof-resting vehicle, the vehicle's roof posts may support the chassis more or less intact, or they may have collapsed. If the posts have collapsed, the normal window openings may have been reduced to narrow slits, too small to serve as access openings. If the A- and B-posts have collapsed but the vehicle has a rear door, rescuers may use an operable rear door to access the occupants, or they may remove a rear window. The occupants of roof-resting vehicles are likely to be hanging upside down, held in place by their seat belts.

The roofs of most vehicles are rounded above the door openings, and their surfaces have a smooth, painted finish, which provides less purchase for cribbing or step chocks in contact with the roof surface than with other parts of the vehicle. These rounded counters may necessitate further supporting the vehicle front and rear with cribbing, struts, chain slings, and/or Hi-Lift® jacks. **Skill Sheet 7-10** lists the steps for stabilizing a roof-resting passenger vehicle using struts in a tensioned buttress system.

Passenger Vehicles in Other Positions Stabilization

Because of the dynamic forces involved in collisions, vehicles can come to rest in a variety of positions other than those already described. For example, rescuers may find a vehicle at a steep angle resting against a tree, an embankment, other solid object or they may encounter a vehicle partially atop another

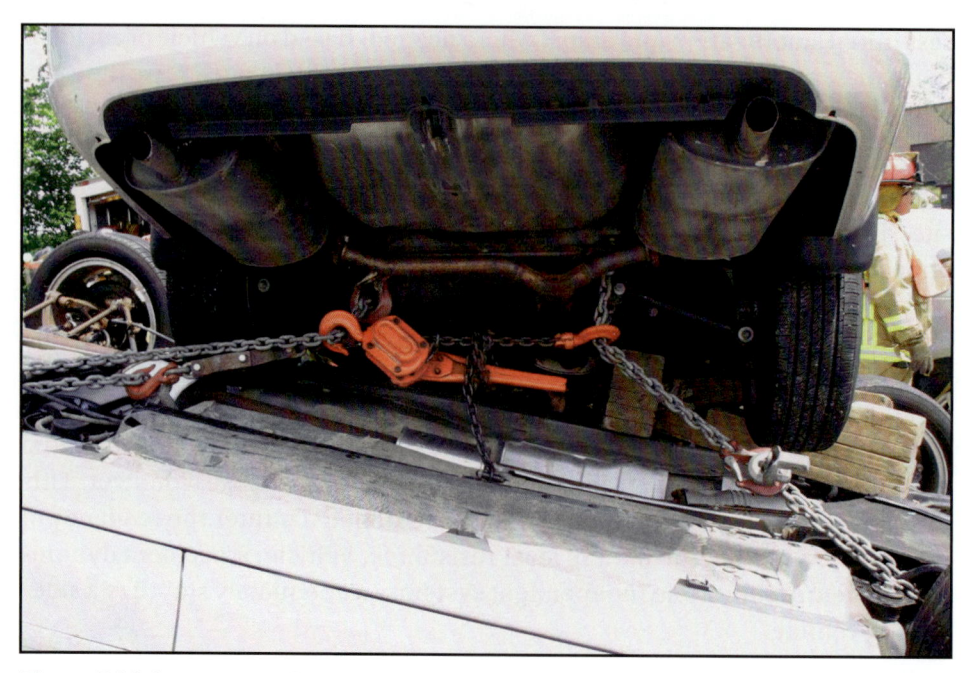

Figure 7.34 An example of two vehicles married together with chains and cribbing.

vehicle. Just as with spinal immobilization of an injured patient, rescuers face the challenge of stabilizing a vehicle in an unusual position as it is found without moving it.

In this situation, rescuers may practice the technique of marrying the vehicles or vehicles and objects together **(Figure 7.34)**. This technique is used when two or more vehicles and/or objects are in contact with each other. Under these conditions rescuers may secure the vehicles and/or objects in order to prevent them from moving and to make them safe throughout the rescue process. Sometimes, rescuers have no other option.

Marrying is the process of connecting multiple dynamic objects together into one fixed object, such as two vehicles. To successfully marry multiple objects, rescuers must provide additional support at key points between them. After completing the marrying operation, rescuers should proceed with stabilization operations between the married object and the ground or other solid surface.

Generally, rescuers use a combination of cribbing, struts, ropes, ratchet straps, come-alongs, and chains to accomplish this type of stabilization task. Sometimes they may need wreckers, cranes, and other large equipment to assist with stabilizing and marrying vehicles together, especially at incidents involving large buses, trucks, or other heavy duty vehicles. Rescuers should only use equipment with the manufacturer approved working load limits. **Skill Sheet 7-11** lists the steps to marry a vehicle to another vehicle or object.

Chapter Review

1. What happens during each of the three phases of vehicle stabilization?
2. How does a vehicle's center of gravity affect stabilization efforts?
3. What are the most likely directions of movement for an unstabilized vehicle?
4. Which parts of a passenger vehicle offer the most structurally sound points to utilize for stabilization?
5. How can rescuers modify the terrain to account for weather conditions or unsteady surfaces such as sand or mud?
6. When lifting an object off of a vehicle as part of stabilization, how can rescuers ensure that the object does not fall back onto the vehicle?
7. What safety precautions should rescuers take when using pneumatic lifting bags or cushions?
8. How do the three classes of lever differ with regards to stabilization operations?
9. Describe two common hitches.
10. What safety precautions should be taken when using chains to stabilize a vehicle?
11. List characteristics of synthetic slings.
12. What rigging components are used for stabilization?
13. How are struts used to stabilize a vehicle?
14. What role can recovery vehicles play at a vehicle incident?
15. What kind of damage are cars in a front-impact collision likely to sustain?
16. Where are stabilization tools and equipment placed when using the four-point or six-point support methods?
17. What methods are commonly used to stabilize side-resting vehicles?
18. What additional support do roof-resting vehicles often require?

Discussion Questions

1. What areas in your jurisdiction may make vehicle stabilization more challenging?
2. When a victim is in an unstabilized vehicle, how do rescuers balance the need for stabilization and the need for victim care?

SKILL SHEETS

7-1

Prevent horizontal movement of a wheel-resting passenger vehicle using chocks.

REMINDER: Not all agencies advocate the following practices. The following skill sheets present a snapshot of various procedures utilized during vehicle incident operations. Always follow manufacturer's recommendations and local SOPs. Rescuers must wear full PPE, including hand, eye, and respiratory protection. It is recommended that rescuers maintain communication with victims and make them aware of pertinent rescue information.

WARNING: Rescuers must ensure that the vehicle is properly stabilized and the scene is safe.

CAUTION: Rescuers must take necessary precautions to protect themselves and victims from hazards including, but not limited to, glass fragments and dust, jagged metal, SRS gas cylinders, undeployed airbags, and fire hazards.

NOTE: Monitor equipment throughout the operation, and make adjustments as needed.

Step 1: Identify vehicle's construction, condition, and integrity.

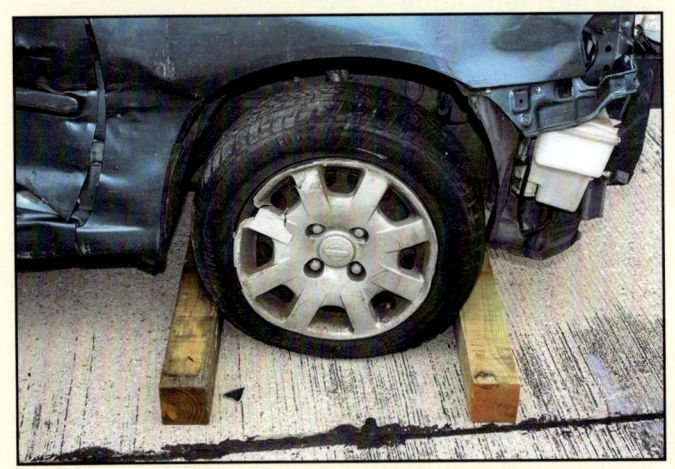

Step 2: Place chocks in front of and behind tires. Center chocks snugly and squarely against the tread of each tire.

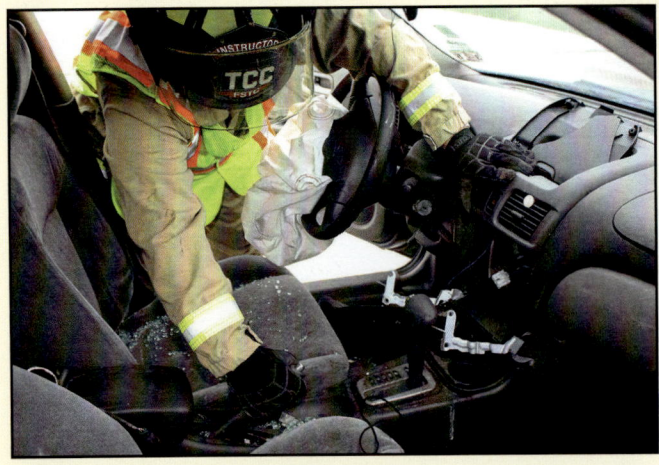

Step 3: Apply the parking brake.

Step 4: Inspect the vehicle and confirm that it is stabilized.

264 Section C • Chapter 7 – Passenger Vehicle Stabilization Operations

7-2
Lift a wheel-resting passenger vehicle using pneumatic lifting bags.

> **WARNING:** Rescuers must ensure that the vehicle is properly stabilized and the scene is safe.

> **CAUTION:** Rescuers must take necessary precautions to protect themselves and victims from hazards including, but not limited to, glass fragments and dust, jagged metal, SRS gas cylinders, undeployed airbags, and fire hazards.

NOTE: Inspect and maintain all equipment according to local SOPs and manufacturer's guidelines. Monitor equipment throughout the operation, and make adjustments as needed.

Step 1: Identify vehicle's construction, condition, and integrity.
Step 2: Provide initial stabilization.
Step 3: Identify a suitable lift point and support locations.
Step 4: Verify that the surface under the support locations will support weight of vehicle and equipment. Construct a solid base or use alternative actions to provide base support, if necessary.

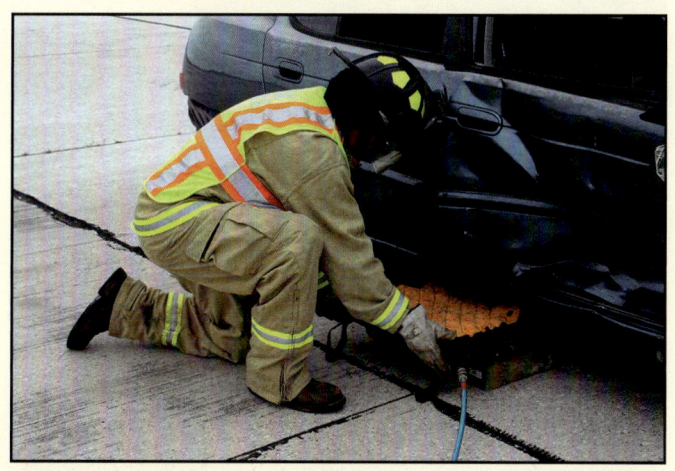

Step 5: Position the pneumatic lifting bags and cribbing.
Step 6: Inflate the bags slowly and in a coordinated manner.

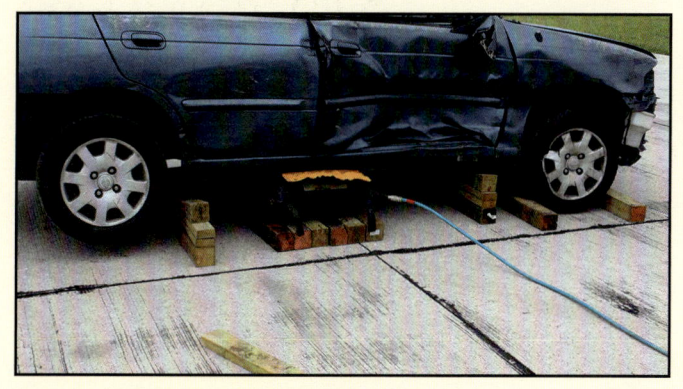

Step 7: Capture progress throughout the lift.

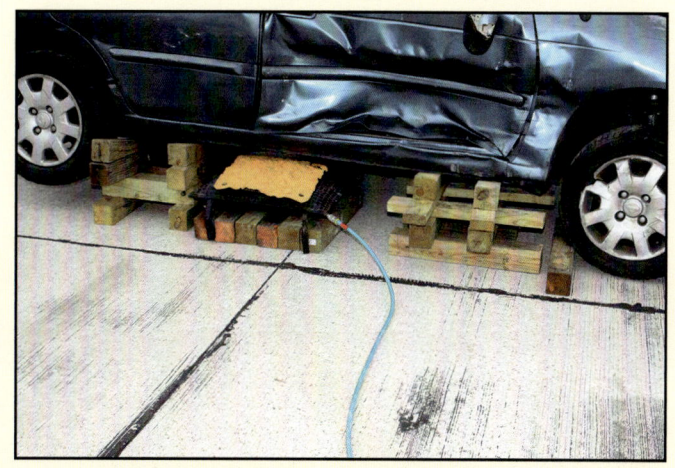

Step 8: Once lift is achieved, verify that progress has been captured, and deflate the lifting bags until the vehicle is resting firmly on the cribbing.

> **WARNING:** Improper use of a lifting bag can cause the bag to violently eject from under the load to be lifted. Always follow manufacturer's recommendations.

Step 9: Monitor and maintain the integrity of the cribbing.

Section C • Chapter 7 – Passenger Vehicle Stabilization Operations

SKILL SHEETS

7-3
Lift a wheel-resting passenger vehicle using a jack

WARNING: Rescuers must ensure that the vehicle is properly stabilized and the scene is safe.

CAUTION: Rescuers must take necessary precautions to protect themselves and victims from hazards including, but not limited to, glass fragments and dust, jagged metal, SRS gas cylinders, undeployed airbags, and fire hazards.

NOTE: Inspect and maintain all equipment according to local SOPs and manufacturer's guidelines. Monitor equipment throughout the operation, and make adjustments as needed.

Step 1: Identify vehicle's construction, condition, and integrity.
Step 2: Provide initial stabilization.
Step 3: Identify a suitable lift point and support locations.
Step 4: Verify that the surface under the support locations will support weight of vehicle and equipment. Construct a solid base or use alternative actions to provide base support, if necessary.
Step 5: Select the type of jack to be used and position the jack so it is directly beneath a suitable lift point.

WARNING: Do not lie beneath the vehicle while positioning the jack, as it may result in serious injury or death if the vehicle is improperly stabilized.

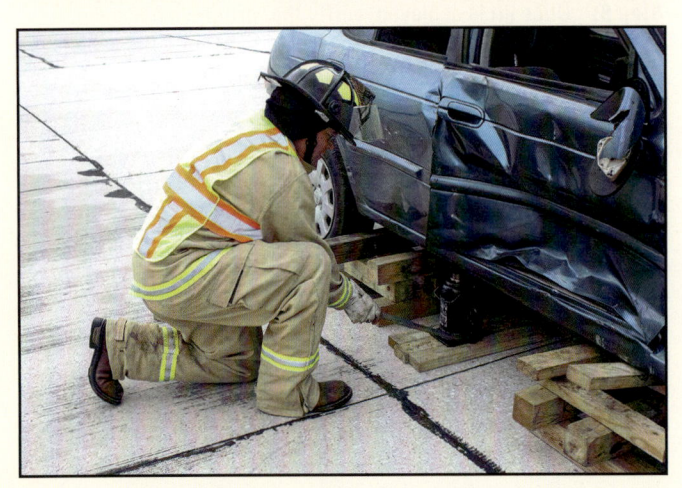

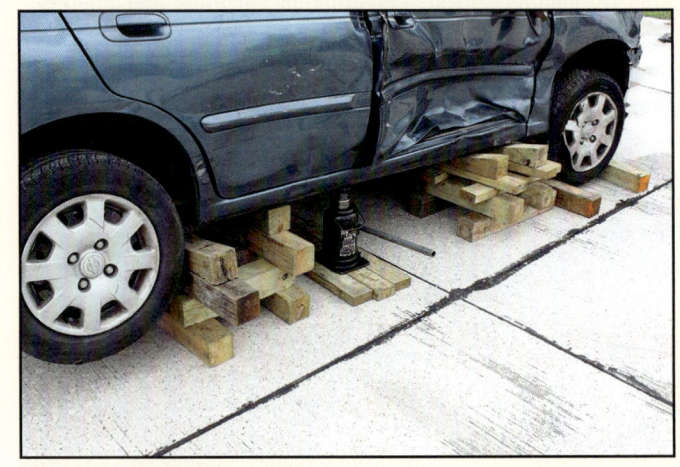

Step 7: Once lift is achieved, verify that progress has been captured, and lower the jack until the vehicle is resting firmly on the cribbing.
Step 8: Monitor and maintain integrity of the cribbing.

Step 6: Operate the jack until desired lift is achieved and capture progress throughout the lift.

266 Section C • Chapter 7 – Passenger Vehicle Stabilization Operations

7-4
Lift a wheel-resting passenger vehicle using a Class I lever.

SKILL SHEETS

> **WARNING:** Rescuers must ensure that the vehicle is properly stabilized and the scene is safe.

> **CAUTION:** Rescuers must take necessary precautions to protect themselves and victims from hazards including, but not limited to, glass fragments and dust, jagged metal, SRS gas cylinders, undeployed airbags, and fire hazards.

NOTE: Inspect and maintain all equipment according to local SOPs and manufacturer's guidelines. Monitor equipment throughout the operation, and make adjustments as needed.

Step 1: Identify vehicle's construction, condition, and integrity.
Step 2: Provide initial stabilization.
Step 3: Identify a suitable lift point and support locations.
Step 4: Verify that the surface under the support locations will support weight of vehicle and equipment. Construct a solid base or use alternative actions to provide base support, if necessary.

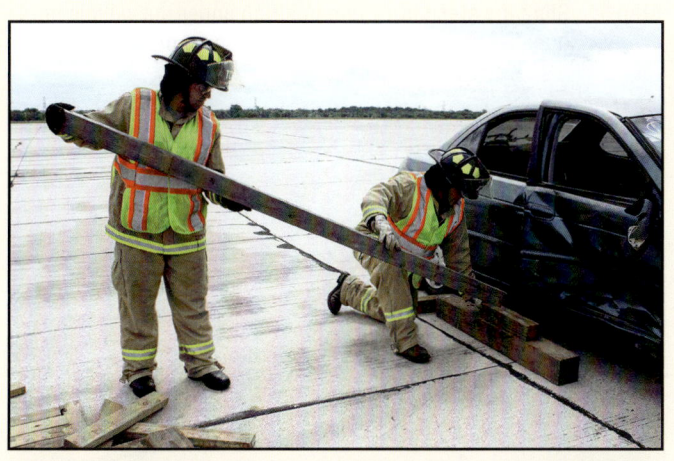

Step 5: Position prepared fulcrum or build a crib bed to act as a fulcrum.
Step 6: Place lever.

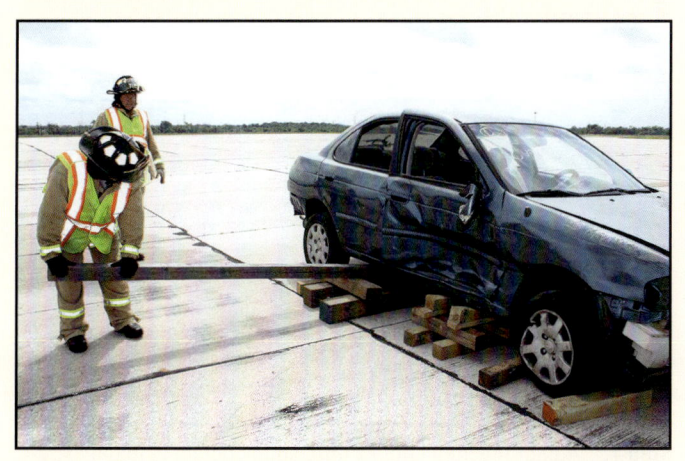

Step 7: Slowly add downward pressure to the end of the lever until the vehicle begins to lift.
Step 8: Capture progress throughout the lift.

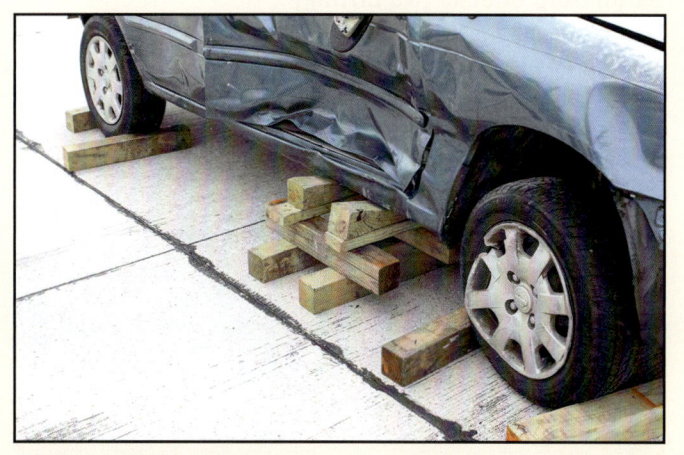

Step 9: Once lift is achieved, verify that the vehicle is resting firmly on the cribbing.
Step 10: Monitor and maintain integrity of the cribbing.

Section C • Chapter 7 – Passenger Vehicle Stabilization Operations **267**

SKILL SHEETS

7-5
Stabilize a wheel-resting passenger vehicle using step chocks.

WARNING: Rescuers must ensure that the vehicle is properly stabilized and the scene is safe.

CAUTION: Rescuers must take necessary precautions to protect themselves and victims from hazards including, but not limited to, glass fragments and dust, jagged metal, SRS gas cylinders, undeployed airbags, and fire hazards.

NOTE: Monitor equipment throughout the operation, and make adjustments as needed.

Using Step Chocks (No Lifting)

Step 1: Identify vehicle's construction, condition, and integrity.
Step 2: Provide initial stabilization.
Step 3: Identify support locations on the vehicle.

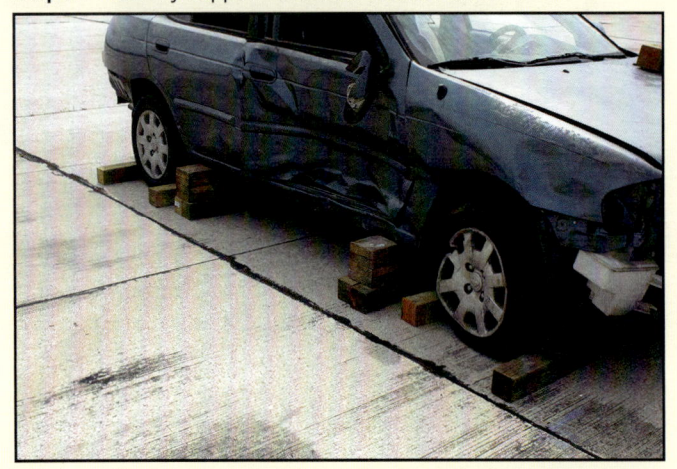

Step 4: Verify that the surface under the support locations will support weight of vehicle and equipment. Construct a solid base or use alternative actions to provide base support, if necessary.
Step 5: Slide the step chock into position under the vehicle until it makes solid contact with the vehicle's support point. Repeat until stabilization is complete.
Step 6: Deflate the tires.
Step 7: Inspect the vehicle and confirm that it is stabilized. Monitor and maintain the integrity of the step chocks.

Using Step Chocks (Lifting)

Step 1: Identify vehicle's construction, condition, and integrity.
Step 2: Provide initial stabilization.
Step 3: Identify support locations on the vehicle.
Step 4: Verify that the surface under the support locations will support weight of vehicle and equipment. Construct a solid base or use alternative actions to provide base support, if necessary.
Step 5: Slide the step chock into position under the vehicle until it makes contact with the vehicle's support point.

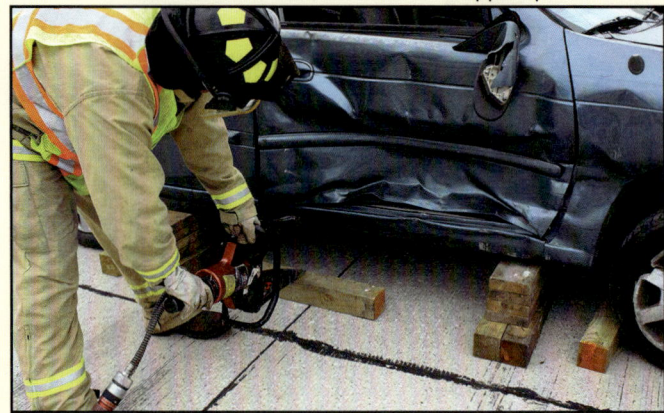

Step 6: Lift the vehicle at each point so that step chock will be loaded when vehicle is lowered.

CAUTION: Rescuers should use appropriate lifting devices rather than lifting with their body.

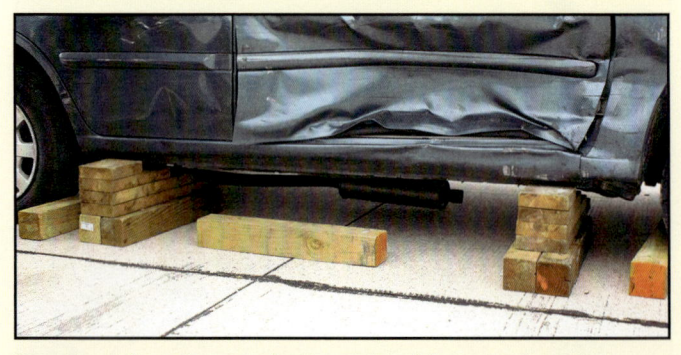

Step 7: Adjust the step chocks until solid contact is made.
Step 8: Lower the vehicle onto the step chocks.
Step 9: Inspect the vehicle and confirm that it is stabilized. Monitor and maintain the integrity of the step chocks.

7-6
Stabilize a wheel-resting passenger vehicle using cribbing.

SKILL SHEETS

> **WARNING:** Rescuers must ensure that the vehicle is properly stabilized and the scene is safe.

> **CAUTION:** Rescuers must take necessary precautions to protect themselves and victims from hazards including, but not limited to, glass fragments and dust, jagged metal, SRS gas cylinders, undeployed airbags, and fire hazards.

NOTE: Monitor equipment throughout the operation, and make adjustments as needed.

Step 1: Identify vehicle's construction, condition, and integrity.
Step 2: Provide initial stabilization.
Step 3: Identify support locations on the vehicle.
Step 4: Verify that the surface under the support locations will support weight of vehicle and equipment. Construct a solid base or use alternative actions to provide base support, if necessary.
Step 5: Position sufficient cribbing material at each support location.
Step 6: Crib the vehicle, allowing the ends of the cribbing pieces to extend at least four inches (100 mm) beyond the individual pieces of the base until the required height has been achieved.
Step 7: Use wedges to provide the maximum amount of contact between the crib and the vehicle.
Step 8: Deflate tires.
Step 9: Inspect the vehicle and confirm that it is stabilized. Monitor and maintain the integrity of the cribbing.

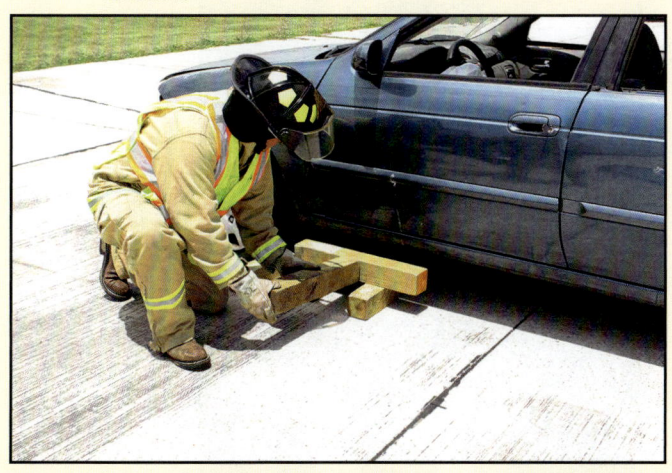

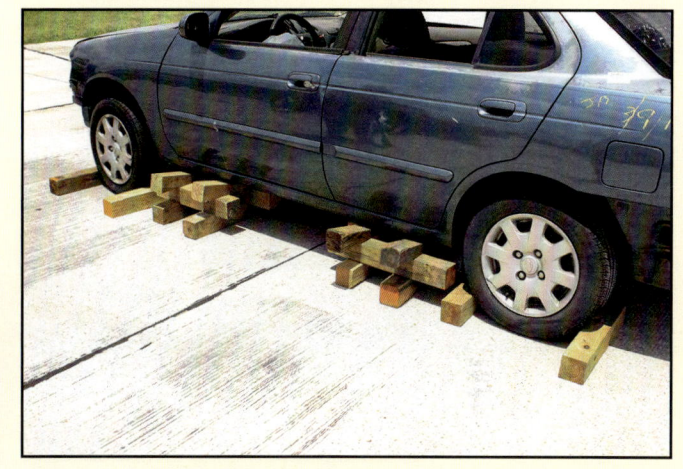

Section C • Chapter 7 – Passenger Vehicle Stabilization Operations 269

SKILL SHEETS

7-7
Deflate the tires of a wheel-resting passenger vehicle.

WARNING: Rescuers must ensure that the vehicle is properly stabilized and the scene is safe.

CAUTION: Rescuers must take necessary precautions to protect themselves and victims from hazards including, but not limited to, glass fragments and dust, jagged metal, SRS gas cylinders, undeployed airbags, and fire hazards.

NOTE: Monitor equipment throughout the operation, and make adjustments as needed.

Step 1: Provide initial stabilization.
Step 2: Identify support locations on the vehicle.
Step 3: Verify that the surface under the support locations will support weight of vehicle and equipment.
Step 4: Stabilize vehicle using cribbing.

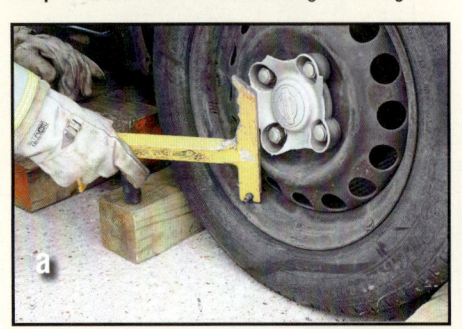

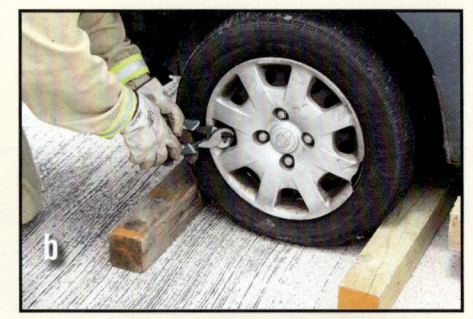

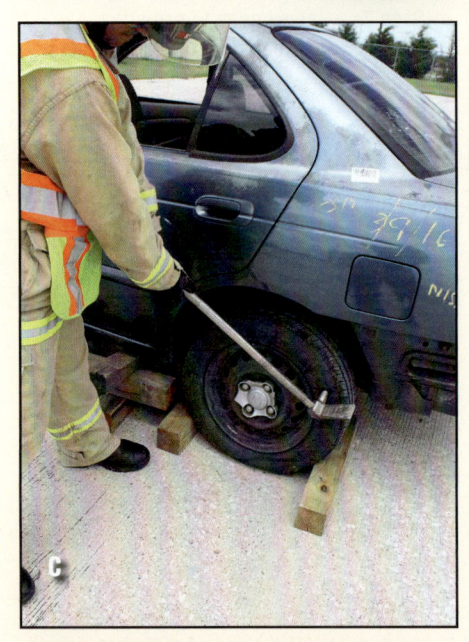

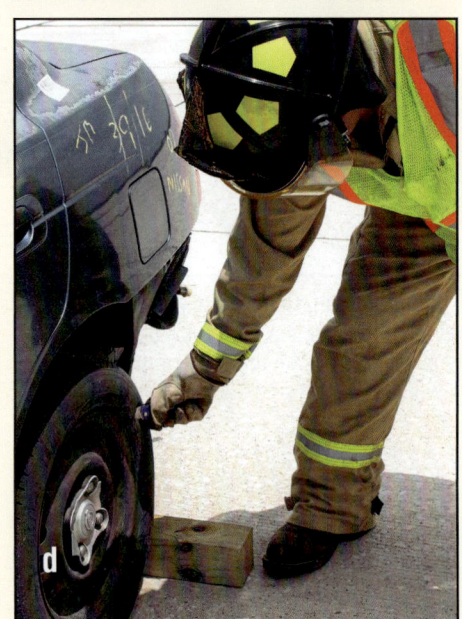

Step 5: Deflate the tires per local SOPs.

WARNING: Do not deflate any tire mounted on a split rim.

Step 6: Verify that the vehicle is resting on the cribbing and the weight is not resting on the suspension.

Section C • Chapter 7 – Passenger Vehicle Stabilization Operations

7-8
Stabilize a side-resting passenger vehicle using struts (same-side opposing force system).

> **WARNING:** Rescuers must ensure that the vehicle is properly stabilized and the scene is safe.

> **CAUTION:** Rescuers must take necessary precautions to protect themselves and victims from hazards including, but not limited to, glass fragments and dust, jagged metal, SRS gas cylinders, undeployed airbags, and fire hazards.

NOTE: Inspect and maintain all equipment according to local SOPs and manufacturer's guidelines. Monitor equipment throughout the operation, and make adjustments as needed.

Step 1: Identify vehicle's construction, condition, and integrity.
Step 2: Provide initial stabilization.
Step 3: Identify support locations and purchase points on the vehicle.
Step 4: Verify that the surface under the support locations will support weight of vehicle and equipment. Construct a solid base, or use alternative actions to provide base support, if necessary.

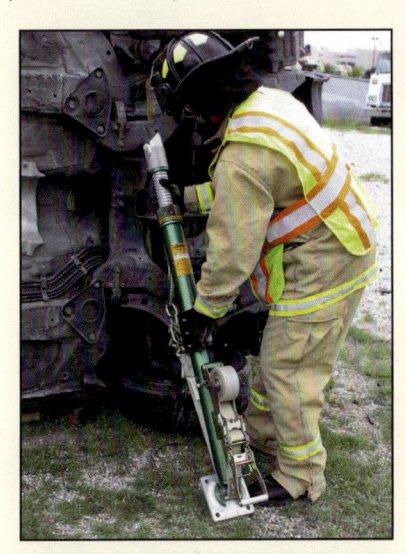

Step 5: Position struts on undercarriage.

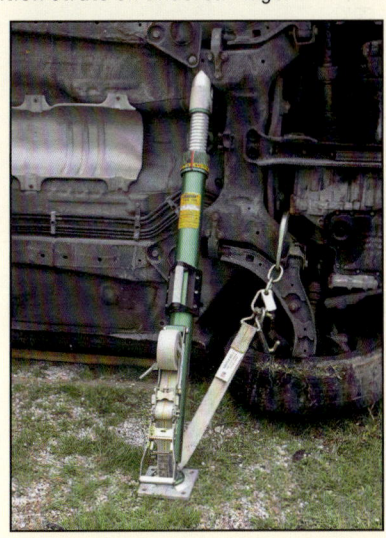

Step 6: Engage the stabilization system tip as high as possible, above the midline of the vehicle. Attach base strapping as low as possible, below the midline of the vehicle.
NOTE: Struts should lean at appropriate angles.

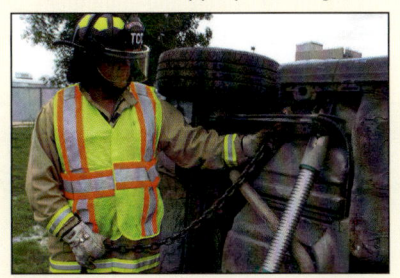

Step 7: Create a bridle hitch using static connection points.

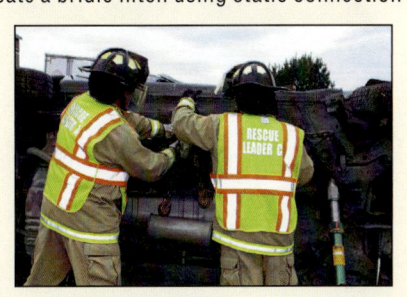

Step 8: Attach a tensioning device from the bridle hitch to a suitable anchor point.
Step 9: Check that straps and tip engagements are tight, and adjust if necessary.

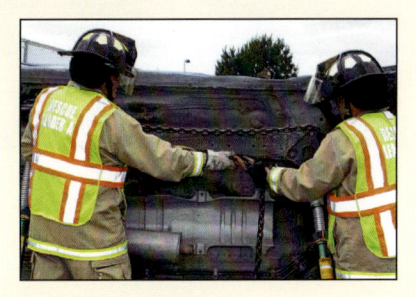

Step 10: Apply tension to the system.
Step 11: Reassess the vehicle and confirm that the vehicle is stabilized.

Section C • Chapter 7 – Passenger Vehicle Stabilization Operations

SKILL SHEETS

7-9

Stabilize a side-resting passenger vehicle using struts (tensioned buttress system).

> **WARNING:** Rescuers must ensure that the vehicle is properly stabilized and the scene is safe.

> **CAUTION:** Rescuers must take necessary precautions to protect themselves and victims from hazards including, but not limited to, glass fragments and dust, jagged metal, SRS gas cylinders, undeployed airbags, and fire hazards.

NOTE: Inspect and maintain all equipment according to local SOPs and manufacturer's guidelines. Monitor equipment throughout the operation, and make adjustments as needed.

Step 1: Identify vehicle's construction, condition, and integrity.
Step 2: Provide initial stabilization.
Step 3: Identify support locations on the vehicle.
Step 4: Verify that the surface under the support locations will support weight of vehicle and equipment. Construct a solid base or use alternative actions to provide base support, if necessary.

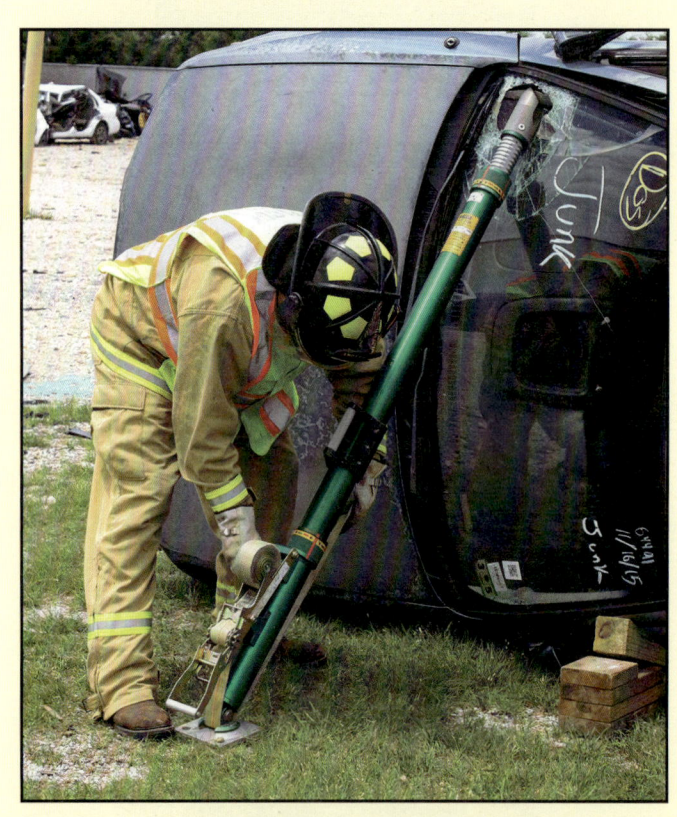

Step 5: Set and engage struts on least stable side of vehicle.

Step 6: Set and engage struts on opposite side of the vehicle

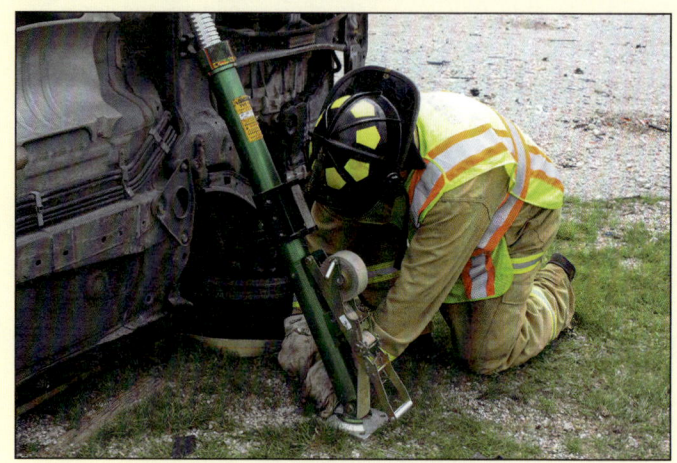

Step 7: Attach base strapping to opposing base plate.
Step 8: Apply tension to the system.
Step 9: Check that straps and tip engagements are tight. Adjust if necessary.

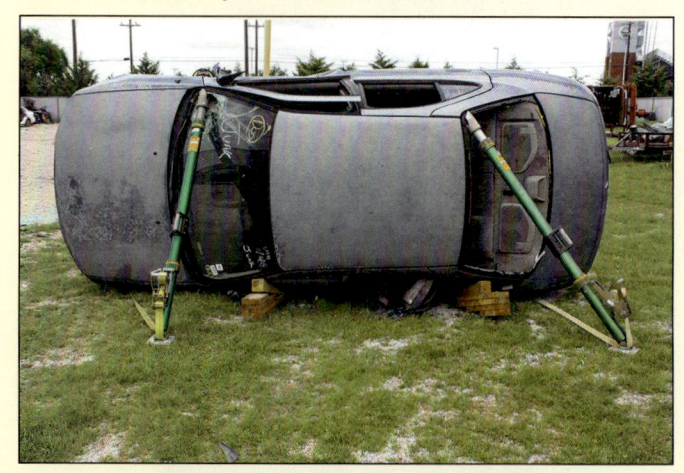

Step 10: Inspect the vehicle and confirm that it is stabilized.

Section C • Chapter 7 – Passenger Vehicle Stabilization Operations

7-10
Stabilize a roof-resting passenger vehicle using struts (tensioned buttress system).

🔥 **SKILL SHEETS**

> **WARNING:** Rescuers must ensure that the vehicle is properly stabilized and the scene is safe.

> **CAUTION:** Rescuers must take necessary precautions to protect themselves and victims from hazards including, but not limited to, glass fragments and dust, jagged metal, SRS gas cylinders, undeployed airbags, and fire hazards.

NOTE: Monitor equipment throughout the operation, and make adjustments as needed.

Step 1: Identify vehicle's construction, condition, and integrity.
Step 2: Provide initial stabilization.
Step 3: Identify support locations on the vehicle.
Step 4: Verify that the surface under the support locations will support weight of vehicle and equipment. Construct a solid base or use alternative actions to provide base support, if necessary.

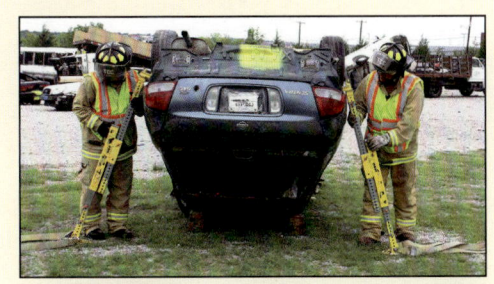

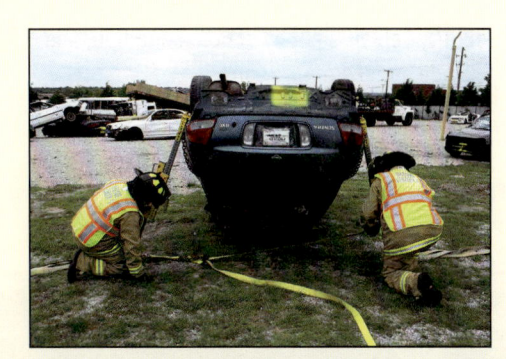

Step 6: Attach base strapping to the opposing base plate.
Step 7: Apply tension to the system.

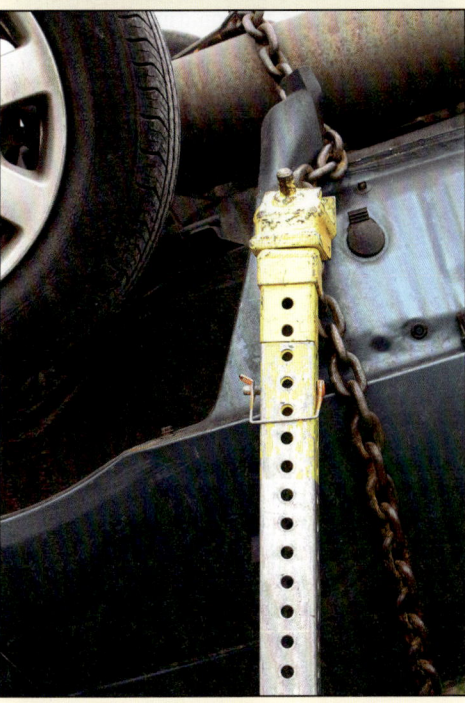

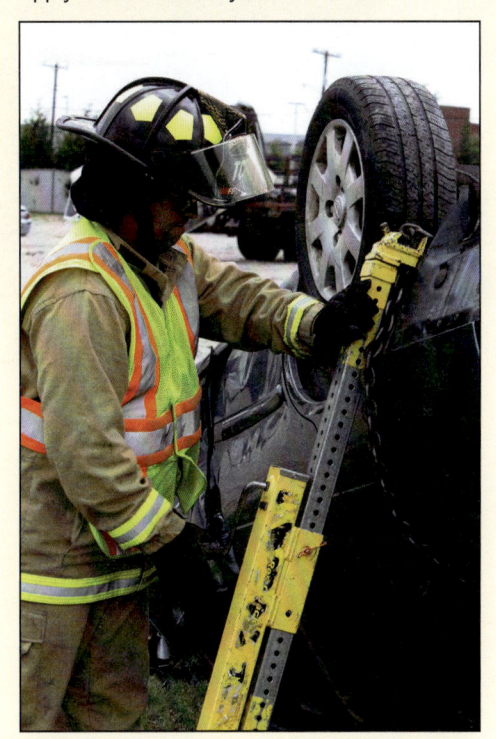

Step 5: Position struts.
   a. If using a chain cradle, set chain in the support location and attach to the strut.
   b. If not using chain, create or utilize existing purchase points in the vehicle.

Step 8: Check that straps and tip engagements are tight. Adjust if necessary.
Step 9: Inspect the vehicle and confirm that it is stabilized.

Section C • Chapter 7 – Passenger Vehicle Stabilization Operations 273

SKILL SHEETS

7-11

Stabilize a side-resting passenger vehicle using struts (tensioned buttress system).

WARNING: Rescuers must ensure that the vehicle is properly stabilized and the scene is safe.

CAUTION: Rescuers must take necessary precautions to protect themselves and victims from hazards including, but not limited to, glass fragments and dust, jagged metal, SRS gas cylinders, undeployed airbags, and fire hazards.

NOTE: Inspect and maintain all equipment according to local SOPs and manufacturer's guidelines. Monitor equipment throughout the operation, and make adjustments as needed.

Step 1: Identify the vehicle/object(s) to be stabilized and their construction, condition, and integrity.

Step 2: Provide initial stabilization on vehicles/objects as necessary.

CAUTION: Do not attach stabilization equipment or devices on movable or dynamic parts of the vehicle.

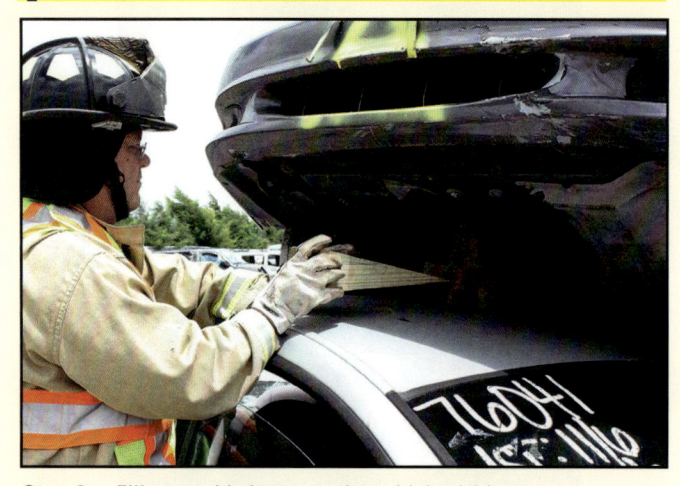

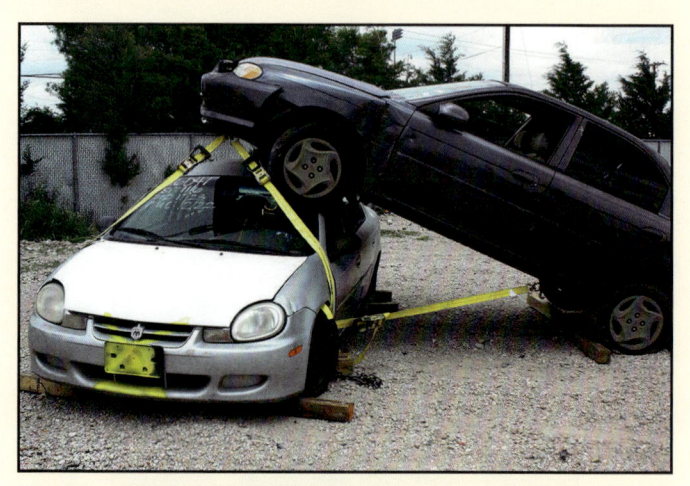

Step 4: Attach or "marry" the vehicles/objects together to minimize movement.

Step 5: Inspect the vehicle and confirm that it is stabilized. Monitor and maintain the integrity of the cribbing.

Step 3: Fill any voids between the vehicles/objects.

NOTE: Depending on the incident, voids may be filled prior to or after marrying the object or vehicles.

274 Section C • Chapter 7 – Passenger Vehicle Stabilization Operations

Victim Disentanglement and Extrication

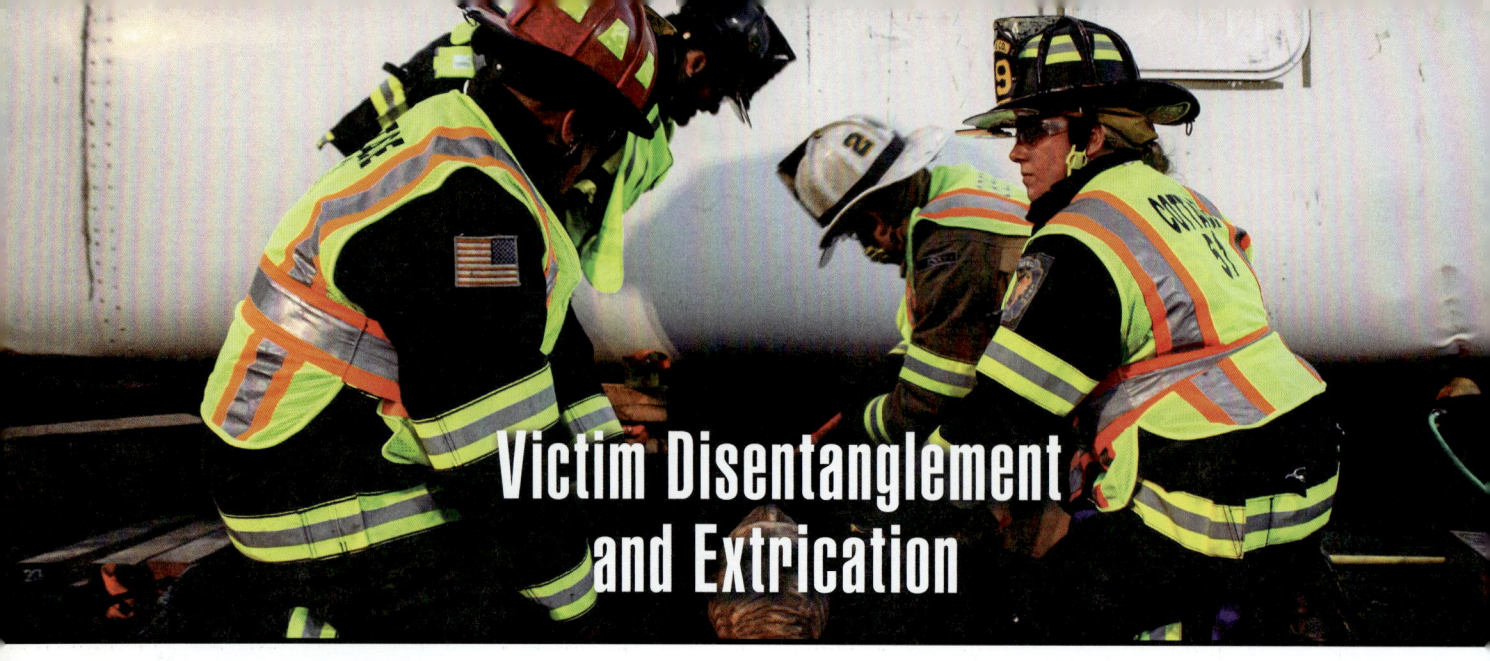

Chapter Contents

Victim Entrapment............................279
    Victim Locations.. 279
    Points of Entrapment 280
    Dynamics of Disentanglement 281
    Multiple Vehicle Incidents 285
    Minimizing Hazards to Victims................ 287

Passenger Vehicle Access and Egress Points 287
    Passenger Vehicle Access and Egress Routes......... 288
    Passenger Vehicle Entry Points 288

Passenger Vehicle Disentanglement and Extrication Operations................. 290
    Techniques for Creating Access and Egress Openings on Passenger Vehicles.. 290
    Alternative Techniques for Creating Access and Egress Openings on Passenger Vehicles with Advanced Steel 301
    Techniques for Disentangling Victims from Passenger Vehicles 303

Chapter Review 308
Discussion Questions 308
Skill Sheets..................................... 309

chapter 8

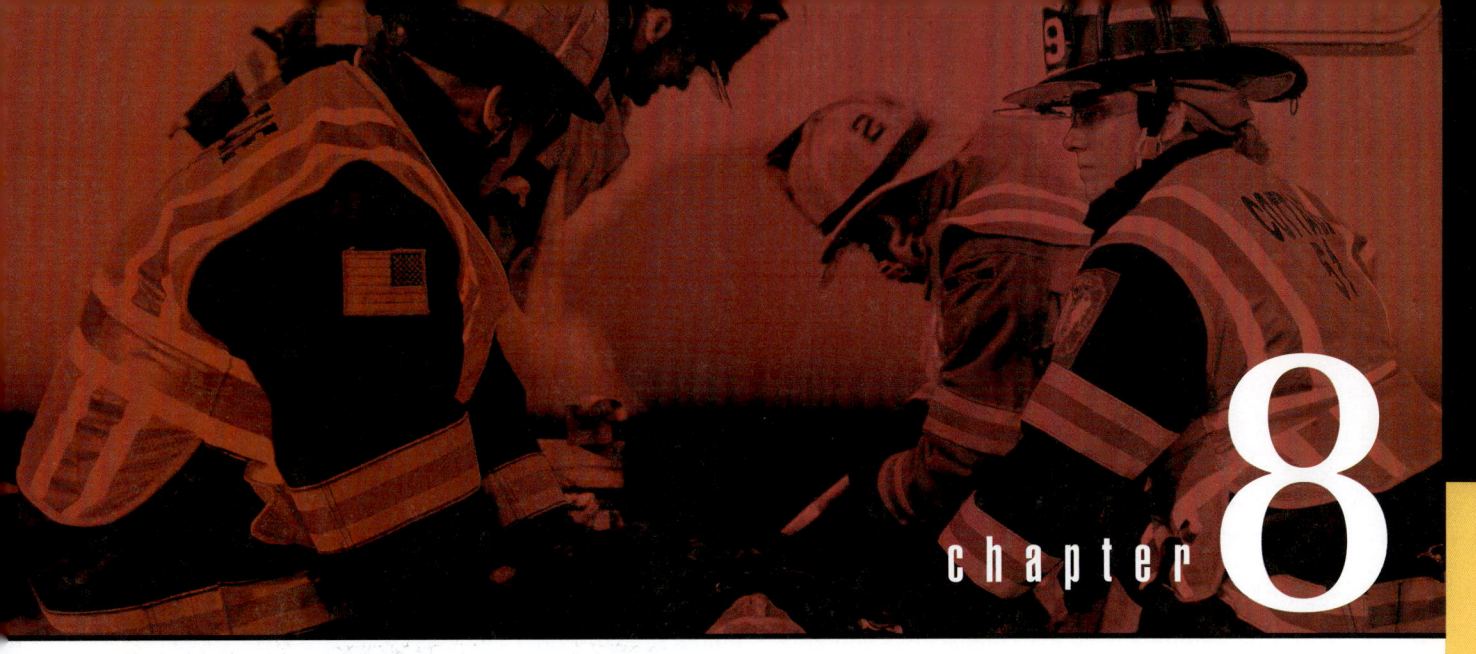

Key Terms

Access	288
Disentanglement	279
Egress	288
Entrapment	280
Mass Casualty Incidentals (MCI)	285

JPRs addressed in this chapter

This chapter provides information that addresses the following job performance requirements of NFPA 1006, *Standard for Technical Rescuer Professional Qualifications (2017)*.

8.2.1	8.2.5
8.2.2	8.2.6
8.2.3	8.2.7

Victim Disentanglement and Extrication

Learning Objectives

1. Identify common victim locations and points of entrapment. [8.2.5]
2. Explain how different types of vehicle collisions affect victim location and injury. [8.2.5]
3. Describe operational considerations at a multiple vehicle incident. [8.2.1, 8.2.2, 8.2.3, 8.2.6, 8.2.7]
4. Explain how to minimize hazards to victims. [8.2.6, 8.2.7]
5. Identify common passenger vehicle access and egress points. [8.2.5, 8.2.6]
6. Describe methods used to create access and egress points on passenger vehicles. [8.2.6]
7. Describe techniques for disentangling victims. [8.2.7]
8. Skill Sheet 8-1: Determine passenger vehicle access and egress points. [8.2.5]
9. Skill Sheet 8-2: Remove glass by removing the seal. [8.2.6]
10. Skill Sheet 8-3: Remove laminated vehicle glass. [8.2.6]
11. Skill Sheet 8-4: Remove tempered vehicle glass. [8.2.6]
12. Skill Sheet 8-5: Remove alternate types of vehicle glass. [8.2.6]
13. Skill Sheet 8-6: Open a door with a manually operated Hi-Lift® jack. [8.2.6]
14. Skill Sheet 8-7: Open or remove a door with a power ratchet, power impact wrench, or manual socket sets. [8.2.6]
15. Skill Sheet 8-8: Open or remove a door with hydraulic tools. [8.2.6]
16. Skill Sheet 8-9: Remove a sliding side door. [8.2.6]
17. Skill Sheet 8-10: Remove the side of a vehicle (total sidewall removal). [8.2.6]
18. Skill Sheet 8-11: Create an alternate (third-door) opening in a two-door vehicle. [8.2.6]
19. Skill Sheet 8-12: Create an alternate (fourth-door) opening in a vehicle (such as a panel van). [8.2.6]
20. Skill Sheet 8-13: Remove the roof of a wheel-resting passenger vehicle. [8.2.6]
21. Skill Sheet 8-14: Flap or remove the roof of a side-resting passenger vehicle. [8.2.6]
22. Skill Sheet 8-15: Create an access opening in the roof of a side-resting passenger vehicle. [8.2.6]
23. Skill Sheet 8-16: Remove the kick panel of a passenger vehicle. [8.2.6]
24. Skill Sheet 8-17: Create an access opening through the floor of a passenger vehicle. [8.2.6]
25. Skill Sheet 8-18: Tunnel through a trunk. [8.2.6]
26. Skill Sheet 8-19: Remove a windshield from around a victim. [8.2.7]
27. Skill Sheet 8-20: Displace a steering column. [8.2.7]
28. Skill Sheet 8-21: Displace a dashboard. [8.2.7]
29. Skill Sheet 8-22: Drop the floor pan of a vehicle. [8.2.7]
30. Skill Sheet 8-23: Displace or remove a front seat in a vehicle. [8.2.7]

Chapter 8
Victim Disentanglement and Extrication

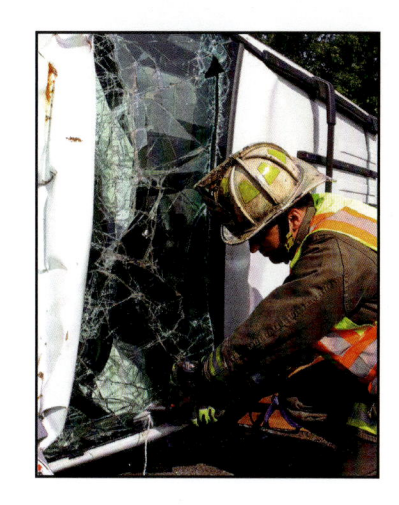

Vehicle collisions and other emergencies involving entrapped victims can present challenges to responders. Entrapment occurs when some part of a vehicle restrains the victim or part of the victim inside a vehicle. Rescuers attending to entrapped victims need proficient training in modern extrication techniques and need to provide highly skilled and competent medical care. These extrication techniques will disentangle the victim from whatever entraps them. Disentanglement, also known as *removing the vehicle from the victim*, relates to the removal and/or manipulation of vehicle components to allow the removal of a properly packaged victim from the vehicle.

Victim Entrapment

Once rescuers obtain access to trapped victims they can begin **disentanglement** procedures. Regardless of the trapped victims' location within the vehicle, rescuers must focus their efforts on disentangling the victims — removing the vehicle from the victims — and they must do so in a way that will not aggravate the victim's injuries. The extrication team must closely coordinate their efforts with the team that is stabilizing and packaging the victims.

Disentanglement — Aspect of vehicle extrication relating to the removal and/or manipulation of vehicle components to allow a properly packaged patient to be removed from the vehicle.

Victim Locations

Upon arrival, rescuers may encounter vehicles resting in many different positions and in various states of destruction. Several factors influence the final location of the victim within the wreckage:

- Collision damage
- Speed
- Vehicle construction
- Vehicle orientation (wheel-resting, side-resting, roof-resting)

In addition, rescuers may find victims who failed to wear proper restraints at any location within the passenger compartment. Unrestrained victims may get partially or fully ejected from the vehicle. Rescuers should conduct a thorough search in and around the area of the incident for these victims.

Rescuers may face challenges when disentangling and extricating victims from a side-resting vehicle. However, rescuers may face even greater difficulties in attempting to stabilize and package trapped victims in these vehicles. Rescuers may find these victims still belted into their seats or piled on top of each other at the bottom of the wreckage.

The occupants of roof-resting vehicles may have dire need of extrication. Unconscious victims hanging upside-down from their seat belts may not survive long, even if they have no other life-threatening injuries.

> **CAUTION**
> Side- and roof-resting vehicles have a greater possibility of catching fire than wheel-resting vehicles.

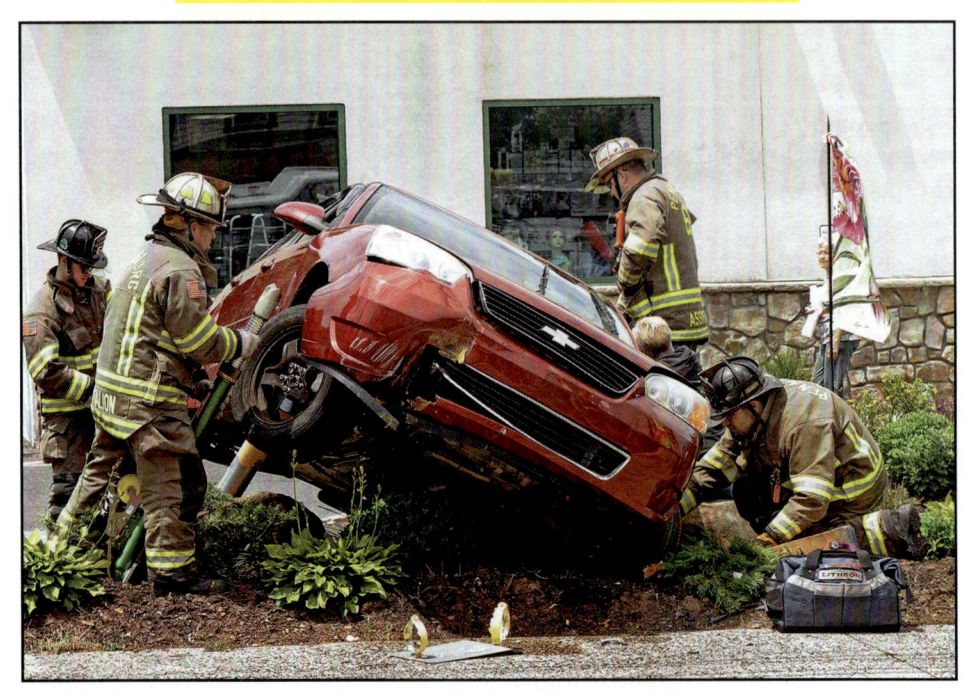

Figure 8.1 The position in which a vehicle is found is one factor in how rescuers determine their strategy for disentanglement and extrication. *Courtesy of Bob Esposito.*

Points of Entrapment

The type of **entrapment** encountered by the rescuers will vary with the type of collision. The point, direction, and speed of impact will dictate the level and severity of entrapment a collision will most likely produce. Rescuers will have to identify points of entrapment and determine ways to eliminate such points **(Figure 8.1)**.

Rescuers may encounter circumstances where one or more points of entrapment restrain a victim. The point of entrapment, also called the *disentanglement point*, is the exact location in which the metal or other object prevents or limits the victims from movement. Entrapped victims cannot free themselves. The type of intervention needed may depend on several factors:

- Number of victims
- Location of victims
- Collision damage to the vehicle (as determined by the traveling speed, force of impact, and construction method of the vehicle)
- Position in which the vehicle stops **(Figure 8.2)**

> **Entrapment** — When the victim or part of the victim is being mechanically restrained, or has restricted means of egress, by a damaged vehicle or machinery component.

280 Section C • Chapter 8 – Victim Disentanglement and Extrication

Points of entrapment after collision damage can be found in numerous locations within the passenger compartment of over-the-road transport vehicles, both commercial/heavy and passenger. Common points of entrapment may include:

- **Pedals** —Brake, gas, or clutch pedals may entrap feet.
- **Seats** — Seats may entrap passengers.
- **Steering wheel and dashboard** —These features may push rearward into the victim, resulting in entrapment.
- **Doors** — Damaged latches, hinges, or metal may prevent victims from opening the door.
- **Roof** — The roofs of vehicles involved in rollover incidents may collapse in on the victim.

Dynamics of Disentanglement

The type of entrapment rescuers encounter may differ depending upon the type of collision. A number of factors, including the ability to identify and determine the forces involved in the incident, can assist the rescuers with recognizing potential injuries, understanding the damage incurred, and knowing the most appropriate disentanglement technique. Knowing what type of injuries and damage front-impact, rear-impact, and side-impact, and rotational collisions produce, as well as the likely damage rollovers, underrides, and overrides, cause can help rescuers function more effectively at these incidents.

Figure 8.2 Rescuers must anticipate how their actions will affect the passengers. *Courtesy of Bob Esposito.*

Front-Impact Collisions

Front-impact collisions produce some of the worst injuries to vehicle occupants. During a front-impact collision, inertia forces the driver and any passengers forward as the vehicle recoils rearward in the split second following impact. Depending upon the speed of impact, as the front of the vehicle collapses, and the dashboard and steering column may displace rearward into the passenger compartment.

Front-impact collisions have different impacts on unrestrained and restrained occupants. Unrestrained occupants move with the forces applied to the vehicle. The face and chest of an unrestrained driver collide violently with the steering wheel/column and a deploying airbag, causing severe facial, head, spinal, and chest trauma. The driver's hands fly forward and strike the dashboard, and if the driver's legs stiffen in the moment before impact, they will likely break. An unrestrained front seat passenger will violently collide with the dashboard, perhaps breaking both arms and suffering massive facial, head, spinal, and chest trauma. The passenger will either propel over the dashboard and into the windshield (and perhaps through it), or wedge under the dashboard. The passenger may break one or both legs in the process. As the front of the vehicle collapses further, the kick panels, firewall, and tilt steering columns may collapse and entrap the feet, legs, and any other body parts wedged under the dashboard. The doors may crumple and jam or both front doors may fly open and occupants may eject from the vehicle through the doors.

Unrestrained rear seat passengers may be propelled forward into the backs of the front seats, perhaps slipping between the front seats and colliding with the dashboard. The forces generated by their weight impacting the backs of the front seats will contribute to the already tremendous forces acting on those in the front seats.

However, if the vehicle was equipped with airbags, and the occupants wear seat belts, the results could vary dramatically. Depending upon the speed of impact, a properly belted driver may survive the crash virtually unscathed or with only minor injuries. If one of the driver's hands rested at the top of the steering wheel when the airbag deployed, the force of the inflation could push that hand back into the driver's face. This may result in a broken nose and perhaps facial lacerations if the driver wore glasses. If a knee bolster airbag protects the driver's lower legs as the front of the vehicle collapses, the driver may suffer little if any injury.

Properly restrained front seat passengers could expect similar protection in a vehicle equipped with passenger airbags. Their extremities may flail about until the vehicle comes to rest, but they will likely sustain relatively minor injuries. Properly restrained rear seat passengers may also flail about some, but will similarly sustain relatively minor injuries.

Rear-Impact Collisions

Rear-impact collisions can create unique problems for vehicle occupants and rescuers, depending upon the speed of impact. In relatively low speed impacts, the rear-end structure of large sedans and station wagons act as a crumple zone and soften the impact on those inside. In higher speed impacts, those inside may suffer whiplash trauma resulting in spinal injuries. Rear-impact collisions can throw unrestrained and improperly restrained occupants upward, causing them to make violent contact with the roof of the vehicle. Additionally, the impact can cause the seatbacks to collapse, complicating the injuries sustained by the occupants. Also, since the rear of most passenger vehicles is lighter than the front, a rear-end collision can raise the rear of the vehicle off the ground while pushing the vehicle forward. This can result in the rear-ended vehicle rolling over. When this happens, it adds the physical effects of being thrown about inside the passenger compartment to any other rear-impact injuries.

Side-Impact (Lateral) Collisions

Side-impact collisions can also produce serious injuries. Side-impact collisions have the same result whether the impact results from a T-bone collision, or the vehicle slides sideways into a tree or other solid object. T-bone collisions can also result in the struck vehicle rolling over. A vehicle that is struck in the side tends to fold itself around the point of impact. This type of impact may produce intrusion into the passenger compartment and may cause more injuries to the occupants. High-speed impacts may cause side-impacted vehicles to tear completely apart, causing significant injury to anyone inside the vehicle.

While side-impact airbags and head protections systems may prevent or reduce side-impact injuries, many passenger vehicles still do not have these safety features. Vehicle occupants on the impacted side may suffer head, spinal, chest, abdominal/pelvic, and extremity injuries from the intrusion into the passenger compartment.

Rotational Collisions

Rotational collisions occur when off-center front or side impacts forcefully turn the impacted vehicle horizontally inducing a spin to one or more of the accident vehicles. Collisions of this nature occur when a vehicle strikes a stationary object (such as a tree, guardrail, or post) or is struck by another vehicle. Generally, occupants in rotational collisions experience the kinds of injuries associated with front, rear, and side impacts.

Rollovers

When vehicles roll over one or more times, vehicle occupants typically sustain a variety of serious injuries. The most common type of rollover involves a vehicle rolling sideways — onto its side and perhaps continuing to roll onto its roof, its other side, and back onto its wheels. Depending upon the terrain, the speed at which the vehicle was traveling, and other variables, a vehicle may roll several times before coming to rest. If the vehicle occupants are properly restrained by their seat belts, they may survive a rollover with relatively minor injuries — provided that the roof does not collapse **(Figure 8.3)**. If the occupants are unrestrained and/or the roof of the vehicle collapses on them, the occupants will likely suffer much more serious, perhaps fatal injuries. In addition to being tumbled over and over inside the vehicle, unrestrained occupants can be thrown out of the vehicle openings.

Less common, although not rare, are incidents involving a vehicle rolling end-over-end. Vehicles must travel at a high rate of speed to generate the force necessary to flip end-over-end repeatedly. However, the environment in which

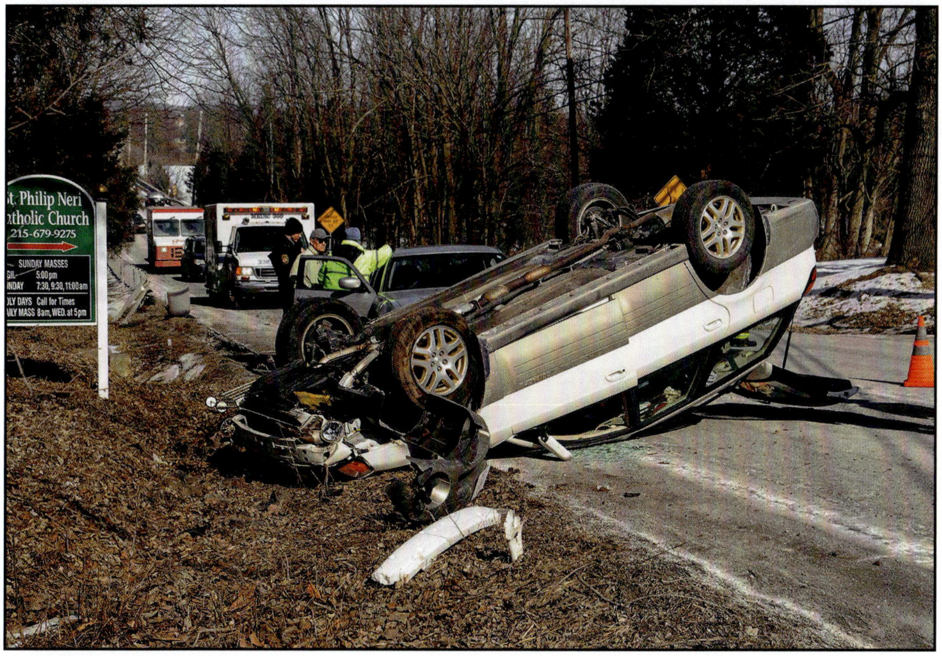

Figure 8.3 Rollover accidents can become more serious if the roof collapses. *Courtesy of Bob Esposito.*

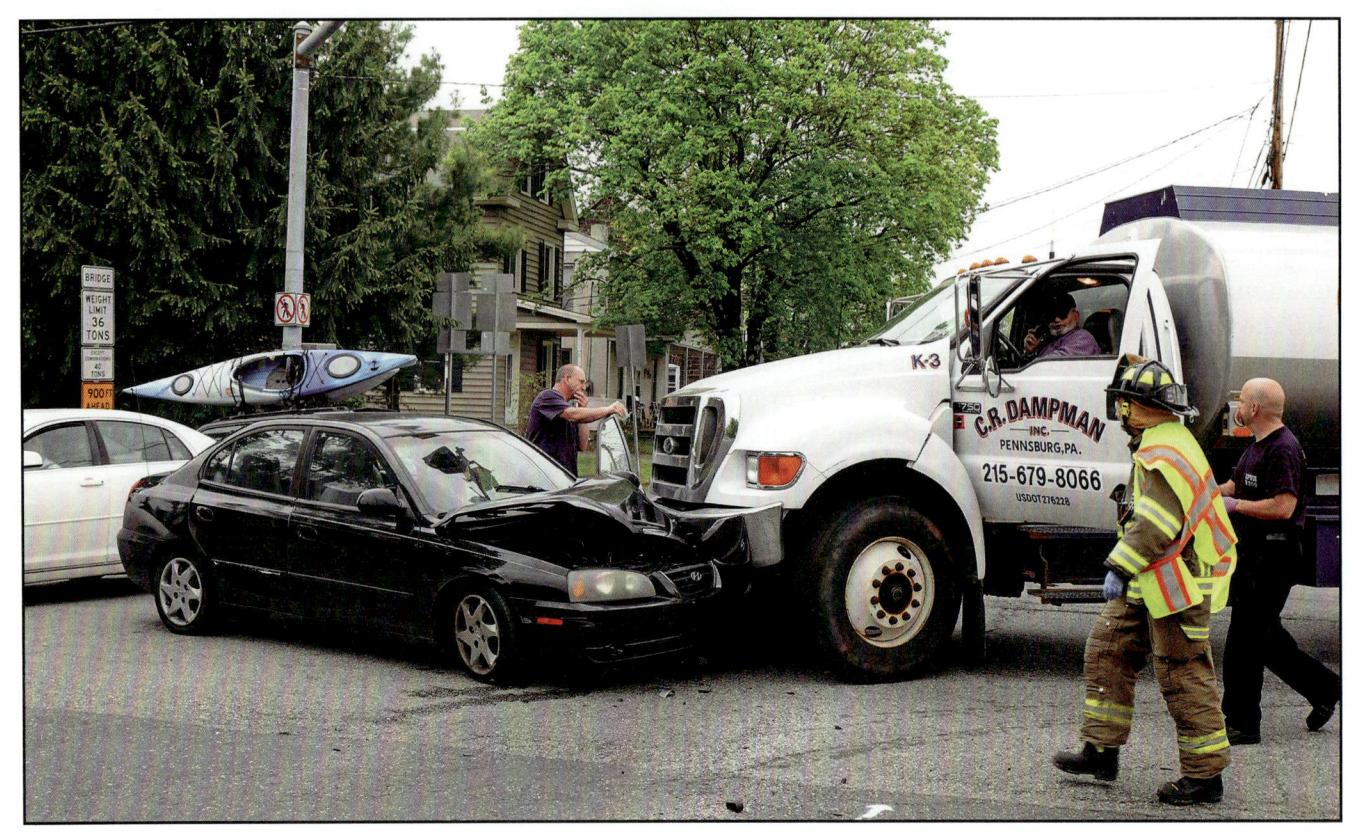

Figure 8.4 An example of an override/underride collision. *Courtesy of Bob Esposito.*

the rollover occurs can contribute to this type of incident. For example, if a vehicle traveling at normal highway speed plunges down a steep slope and strikes a boulder or other solid object, inertia may cause it to flip once and the effects of gravity and the angle of the slope may cause it to continue to flip until it reaches the bottom of the slope. Because the roof of a vehicle involved in this type of incident will likely collapse, even properly restrained occupants may suffer head and spinal injuries.

Underride and Override

Underride and override incidents occur when a passenger vehicle is forced underneath another vehicle that sits higher off the ground than the passenger vehicle. For example, the front end of most passenger vehicles is typically lower than the bottom of commercial/heavy vehicles **(Figure 8.4)**. Consequently, when a passenger vehicle crashes into a truck's trailer, the bed of the trailer typically enters the vehicle's passenger compartment. Without the front end of the car to absorb any impact from the collision, these accidents often cause severe injuries to the occupants of the passenger vehicle.

Underride incidents can occur in a number of ways, including both rear-end collisions and collisions with the side of a truck's trailer. Rear underride incidents occur when a passenger vehicle rear-ends a commercial/heavy vehicle. The passenger vehicle may become wedged underneath the commercial/heavy vehicle and present occupant access difficulties. Side underride incidents occur when a passenger vehicle strikes the side of a commercial/heavy vehicle, and becomes wedged underneath the side of the commercial/heavy vehicle.

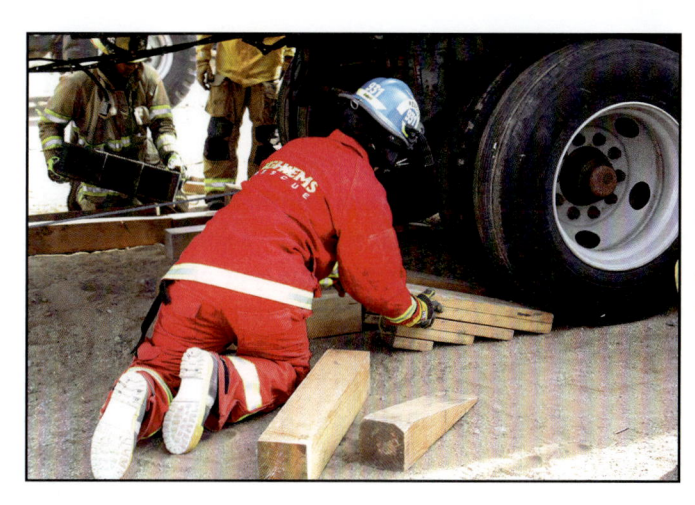

Figure 8.5 A rescuer stabilizing a heavy vehicle involved in an override incident.

Override occurs when a striking vehicle collides with another vehicle and comes to rest on top of the vehicle being struck, such as when a commercial/heavy vehicle runs over a smaller vehicle. The force of impact and weight of the upper vehicle can remove or collapse the roof of the lower vehicle as well as prevent the vehicle's door from opening. Passengers in the override vehicle can receive injuries to the head, neck, arms, torso, and legs.

Most modern commercial/heavy vehicles have safety features to alleviate these problems, however they are often insufficient. Any trailer built after 1993 is required to have reflective tape on its sides. When this tape is dirty, it yields almost no advantage. Any trailer built after 1996 is required to have a rear underride guard that is 22 inches (550 mm) above the ground or lower. However, in many accidents, this height can still be extremely dangerous.

Special considerations for underrides and overrides include:

- Capturing the suspension of the underride vehicle(s)
- Stabilizing the override vehicle **(Figure 8.5)**
- Identifying lifting points
- Mitigating fuel and other fluid leaks
- Monitoring fuel tanks for leaks
- Accounting for victims who may have been ejected between the vehicles
- Maintaining control of air and hydraulic systems so that there is no movement in the systems

Multiple Vehicle Incidents

Multiple vehicle incidents (MVIs) resulting in multiple victims and or casualties are also referred to as **mass casualty incidents (MCIs)**. MCIs are those incidents where the first-responding resources are insufficient to handle the incident. Rescuers should recognize this type of incident early so they can call additional resources to assist with mitigation. Rescuers should establish sources of additional resources should during preincident planning.

MVI Considerations

When sizing up MVIs, rescuers should first ask: Is there anything in the situation that would put rescue personnel or others at greater risk than any other vehicle incident? If so, rescuers should call the needed resources immediately.

Mass Casualty Incident — Incident that results in a large number of casualties within a short time frame, as a result of an attack, natural disaster, aircraft crash, or other cause that is beyond the capabilities of local logistical support. See Multi-Casualty Incident.

While waiting for the additional resources to arrive, on-scene personnel should be used to establish and maintain control of the scene, and perform any other duties for which they have the resources and training.

The problems associated with assessing the condition of multiple vehicles involved in an incident have less to do with the environment and more to do with the number of vehicles involved. Vehicular triage — a sorting of the vehicles into categories of damage — is the first step of this type of rescue. Some vehicles may have superficial damage to the front and rear; others may have suffered significant structural damage and deformation that will require major manipulation to provide access to their occupants. These types of collisions present a greater than normal threat of fires due to the uncontrolled release of flammable liquids close to a variety of ignition sources. Fire crews with portable fire extinguishers and charged hoselines (1½-inch [38 mm] minimum) with foam capability should stand ready.

A multiple-vehicle incident will likely involve multiple casualties. This may indicate a need for several medical teams working at once. Depending upon the number of vehicles involved, weather conditions, visibility, and other factors, rescuers may have a challenge identifying the exact number of trapped victims may be a challenge, especially at night. It is critical that the IC organize and conduct MCI operations using the ICS to reduce the chances of overlooking any victims.

MVI Operations

The prospect of stabilizing a large number of damaged vehicles at the same time can be daunting. Making decisions based on the results of the vehicular triage can make the process organized and efficient. Each team should stabilize one vehicle at a time.

Because these incidents often involve a series of rear-end collisions, rescuers may have extremely limited access to the front and rear of the vehicles. Otherwise, the tools and techniques rescuers will use to access into many vehicles are the same as those used to gain access into a single passenger vehicle.

Rescuers may have challenges disentangling and extricating victims because the vehicles may be in a variety of positions and environments **(Figure 8.6)**. Some vehicles may be accordioned between other vehicles at their front and rear. Other vehicles may be wedged under or resting on top of other vehicles, while other vehicles may be on their sides or upside down. Some vehicles may be pushed into a ditch, off a bridge or cliff, or into a body of water.

Figure 8.6 An example of a multiple vehicle accident. *Courtesy of Chris Mickal.*

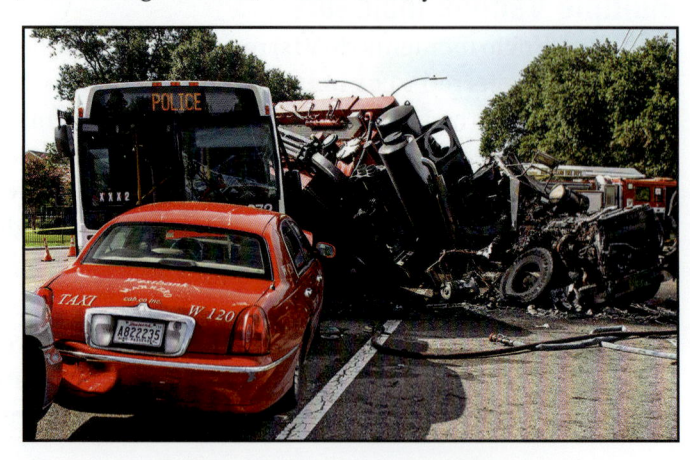

Each extrication team must focus on one vehicle at a time. Based on the condition of the victims and the vehicle, the team must determine the best way to remove the vehicle from around the victims and to remove the victims from the wreckage.

Minimizing Hazards to Victims

Contact victims prior to any extrication activity. If any victims are conscious, tell them what is happening and what is about to happen. Informing victims of the activities, sounds, and smells that will occur during extrication may decrease their anxiety level.

Stabilizing the vehicle increases the safety of the emergency responders and the victims. Shifting loads or movement can transfer negative energy into the passenger compartment, creating a potential for further injury.

Provide victims with respiratory protection and cover them with fire retardant protective coverings before performing any glass management activity. When possible, break the glass furthest away from victims to minimize exposure to glass particles.

Make every effort to protect accident victims from inclement weather conditions. This may involve using salvage covers or rapidly erected canopies to shelter victims from precipitation or the sun. Use blankets and heating or cooling packs to control the temperature directly around the victim(s). In many circumstances, leaving windows and roofs intact and in place will provide victims with protection from inclement weather conditions.

Passenger Vehicle Access and Egress Points

The number of rescue and support personnel working in a confined area can make vehicle incident scenes chaotic. Vehicle incidents typically occur on active roadways, which creates further complications for rescue personnel. Rescue personnel should coordinate their efforts to move tools and equipment from the rescue vehicle to the accident vehicle, and to move around the accident vehicle and incident scene. Bumping into people or tripping over tools and equipment can easily slow personnel. Organizing equipment and the flow of personnel will enable rescuers to give the most efficient and effective possible care to victims **(Figure 8.7)**.

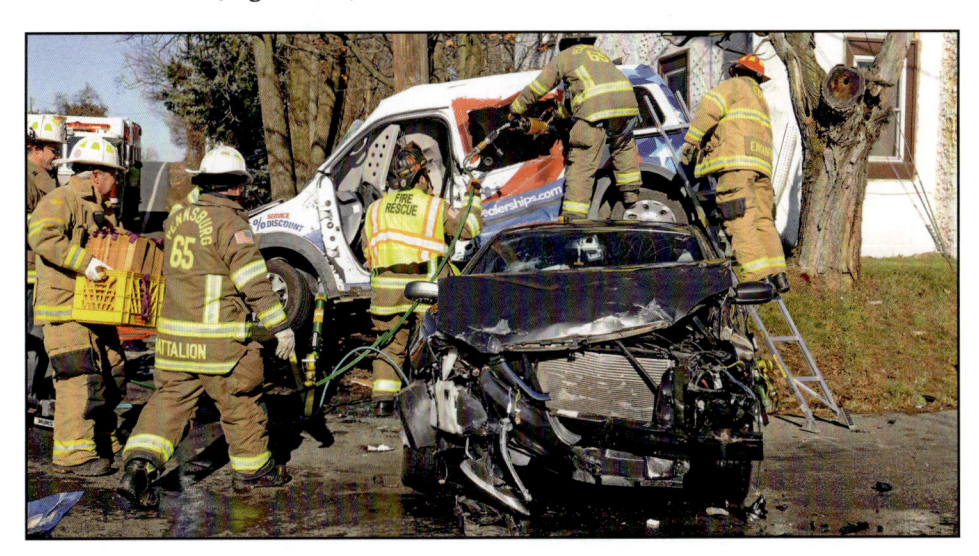

Figure 8.7 Rescuers must organize equipment and personnel to provide the most effective care possible to accident victims. *Courtesy of Bob Esposito.*

Access — (1) Place or means of entering a structure or vehicle. (2) Roadways allowing fire apparatus to travel to an emergency. *See* Egress.

Egress — Place or means of exiting a structure or vehicle.

When vehicle incidents leave passengers trapped in their vehicles, rescuers will have to identify the appropriate victim **access** and **egress** points on a vehicle. This operation is all part of passenger vehicle extrication and will require a level of coordination between rescue personnel, tools and equipment, and the victim(s). Rescuers must follow the local AHJ policies and procedures for identifying passenger vehicle access and egress points. This section will cover passenger vehicle access and egress routes as well as the various vehicle entry points.

Passenger Vehicle Access and Egress Routes

The rescuer must survey the vehicles in which victims are trapped to determine how best to gain access to and remove the victims. This may mean deciding between several possible actions, including:

- Removing one or more doors
- Removing or penetrating the roof
- Making entry/egress through a rear hatch

Rescuers' decision making will also need to take into account the vehicle's location and position, the number and location of victims, the known and unknown hazards, available tools and equipment, and the skill set of the rescue personnel. Rescuers should make all personnel aware of the influencing factors and the decided-upon access and egress route. For example, rescuers may decide that the most effective way to access a vehicle and extricate a victim is to perform a third-door conversion. After making this decision, rescuers should inform all personnel of the decision so that everyone present focuses all efforts on coordinating the flow of personnel, tools and equipment, and, eventually, the victim(s) to support the operation.

> **CAUTION**
> When accessing and egressing vehicles, rescuers should watch out for sharp objects such as broken glass or jagged metals. Identify, cover, and/or remove these objects from the vehicle whenever possible.

Passenger Vehicle Entry Points

The easiest way for rescuers to access passenger vehicles is to use the existing entry points. These points include:

- Windows
- Doors
- Roofs
- Floor panels

Windows

If the doors are locked or jammed, rescuers may need to remove the side windows to allow access to the door locks/handles. Rescuers may attempt to lower the window prior to attempting removal of the window to minimize potential for flying glass and injury. Once they have removed the windows, rescuers can reach the door lock or handle through the window opening. Depending upon the specific situation, they may or may not need to remove the vehicle's windshield **(Figure 8.8)**.

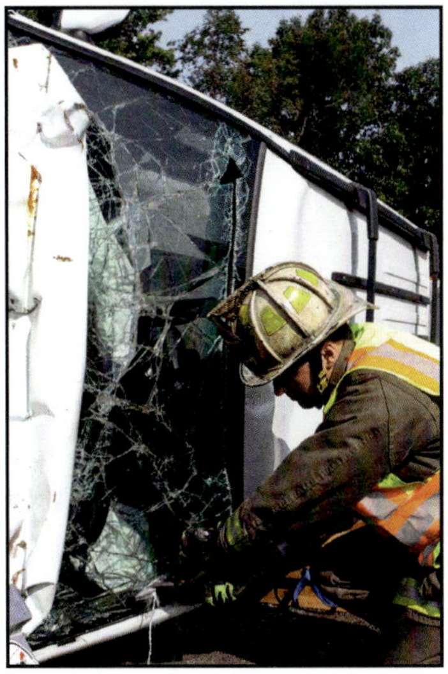

> **WARNING!**
> Rescuers should look out for undeployed airbags when reaching through open windows.

Figure 8.8 A rescuer removing a windshield on a side resting vehicle.

Doors

After unlocking the door, try to operate the door handle. If the door opens, hold it in the open position to prevent it from latching again if it closes when released. Rescuers may use various tools, such as a wedge or a racquet ball, to hold the door handle in the open position.

Rescuers must force jammed doors open. The specific situation will dictate whether rescuers need to remove or merely open doors. In two-door passenger vehicles, even opening or removing the doors may still not provide sufficient working room for safe and efficient extrication operations. These situations may require a third-door conversion.

Third-door conversions involve cutting and spreading tools to flap back the side panel between the B-post and the rear fender well. This creates an unobstructed opening from the A-post back to the rear fender well.

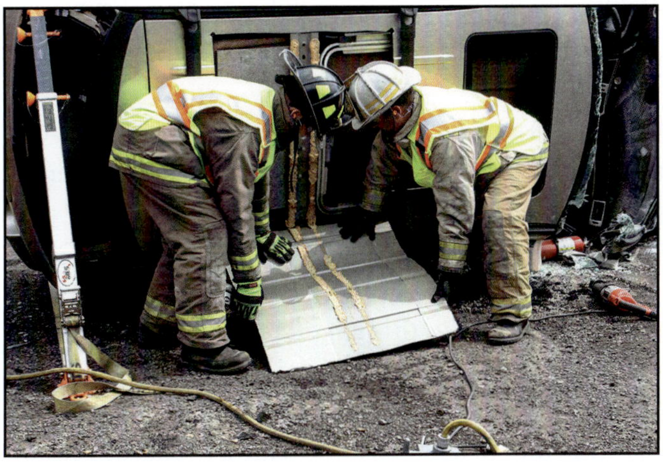

Figure 8.9 Rescuers removing a roof to access passengers.

Depending upon how the vehicle rests, responders can use cutters or other suitable cutting tools to cut through accessible roof posts. Rescuers can cut all the posts and remove the roofs of side-resting vehicles with accessible door and roof posts. If the vehicle is lying on the roof posts on one side of the vehicle, the opposite posts can be cut and the roof flapped down to the ground **(Figure 8.9)**. A cut around the edge of the roof and removing of the sheet metal and any cross members will create a relatively large opening through which rescuers can extricate trapped victims. However, compared with roof removal, cutting through the roof will probably be more time consuming.

> **CAUTION**
> Flapping or removing the roof of a side-resting passenger vehicle may compromise the vehicle's integrity.

Floor Panels

Unibody vehicles use the floor panels and the undercarriage as structural elements and thus do not require a full chassis to provide body support. The strength and configuration of these panels may make them more difficult to penetrate and remove in order to gain access to the interior of the vehicle. **Skill Sheet 8-1** provides practice determining passenger vehicle access and egress points.

Passenger Vehicle Disentanglement and Extrication Operations

After stabilizing the vehicle, rescuers must gain access to its interior to extricate any victims. The extrication techniques rescuers use will vary depending upon a number of factors, such as, but not limited to, the position of the vehicle and the location of any victims. Rescuers will typically extricate victims using four basic methods: manipulative extrication, disassembly, cutting, and forcing. They will usually apply these methods to the most common points of entrapment, which include pedals, seats, dashboard and steering wheel/column, doors, and the roof.

The remainder of this chapter discusses the following features of extricating victims from passenger vehicles:

- Techniques for creating access and egress openings on passenger vehicles
- Alternative techniques for creating access and egress openings on passenger vehicles with advanced steel
- Techniques for disentangling victims from passenger vehicles

NOTE: Responders can best follow instructions for gaining access to the interior of passenger vehicles described in this chapter if they use the tools as described in Chapter 4, Tools and Equipment.

NOTE: Refer to Chapter 8 for information on patient care. The following extrication techniques assume that rescuers will provide patient care simultaneously with extrication operations, if possible.

NOTE: Rescuers may use several of the passenger vehicle extrication skills in this chapter for commercial/heavy vehicles. Always follow local SOPs. Refer to Chapter 11 for more information on commercial/heavy vehicle extrication techniques.

Techniques for Creating Access and Egress Openings on Passenger Vehicles

This section will cover the following techniques for creating access and egress openings on passenger vehicles:

- Glass removal
- Door removal
- Factory third and fourth doors
- Total sidewall removal
- Third-door conversion
- Fourth-door conversion
- Roof displacement and removal
- Kick panel removal
- Entry through the floor
- Trunk tunneling

Glass Removal

Rescuers can remove glass from a passenger vehicle to quickly and easily gain access to a vehicle's interior. Removing the glass may be necessary if rescuers cannot operate or unlock the doors, cannot retract, lower or otherwise open the glass or need to remove or flap the roof. Rescuers should protect vehicle occupants from any glass dust and chips that the removal process produces. To protect themselves, rescue personnel should wear full PPE to include eye and respiratory protection. If rescuers need to break a window to access a victim, they should choose a window as far away from the victims as possible.

Vehicles use multiple types of window materials. Rescuers should know how to remove the following types of window materials:

- Laminated safety glass
- Tempered glass
- Polycarbonate
- Transparent armor
- Enhanced protective glass (EPG)

NOTE: Rescuers should continuously monitor new developments in automotive glass.

Removing laminated safety glass. Removing windshields and other laminated windows is more complicated and time-consuming than removing tempered side or rear windows. During many extrication operations, rescuers may decide to leave the windshield in place. **Skill Sheet 8-2** lists the steps for removing the window seal to remove vehicle glass.

Windshields and other windows constructed of laminated safety glass do not shatter and fall out. Rescuers can use the following hand tools to remove or cut laminated glass:

- Reciprocating saw
- Commercial glass removal tools
- Air chisel
- Axe
- Long-handled hook

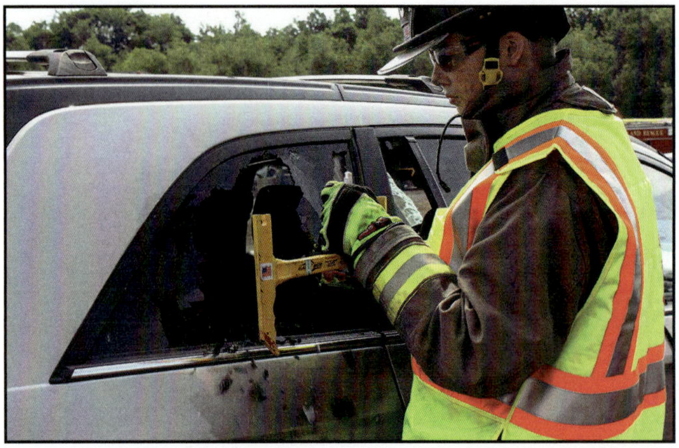

Figure 8.10 A glass hammer is sometimes used to remove vehicle glass.

In most modern vehicles, the windshield, the two A-posts, and the forward edge of the roof compose part of the structural integrity of the vehicle body and should remain in place unless they hinder rescue and extrication efforts. If rescuers must remove the windshield, they should remove the glass while leaving the A-posts and roof edge intact to maintain structural integrity. If rescuers need to remove the windshield or other laminate glass, they may need to cut the glass on all four sides. **Skill Sheet 8-3** lists the steps for removing laminated vehicle glass.

Under some circumstances, rescuers may remove the windshield with the roof. To perform this operation, rescuers should make a single cut along the bottom of the windshield from A-post to A-post, and then make the roof removal cuts. Rescuers can then remove the roof and the windshield together.

Removing tempered glass. To break and remove side and rear tempered glass windows, rescuers should strike them with a sharp, pointed object such as a glass hammer **(Figure 8.10)**. They may also press a spring-loaded center punch against the glass. Rescuers should usually apply these tools at a lower corner of the glass but they may work at any point on the glass surface. When using a spring-loaded center punch, rescuers should brace the hand holding the tool with the other hand to increase control of the tool. Having control prevents the rescuer's hand from going into the glass when it breaks. It also prevents the center punch from pushing through the window opening and possibly striking any vehicle occupant located near the window. Rescuers may also use a standard center punch or Phillips head screwdriver. They must drive both of these tools into the glass with a hammer or other striking tool. A controlled strike with the pick end of a pick-head axe or Halligan tool in the corner of the window will also work if rescuers have no other available tools.

To control the glass fragments, rescuers may apply a sheet of self-adhering contact paper to the surface of the glass. Once broken, the glass adheres to the contact paper. Alternatively, rescuers may place duct tape on the windows and then spray the glass surface with an aerosol adhesive that forms a coating on the glass. This coating sets up in seconds and allows rescuers to break the glass and retain it in a sheet. Then rescuers can remove the glass in sheets instead of tiny pieces. **Skill Sheet 8-4** lists the steps for removing tempered glass.

CAUTION
Do not use hands to clear glass from the window.

Some rear windows are tempered glass and some are laminated. If a window does not respond to removal techniques for tempered glass, rescuers must treat it as laminated glass and remove it in the same way as a windshield.

Removing alternative types of glass. Rescuers should know how to remove other types of glass such as enhanced protective glass, polycarbonates and transparent armor. **Skill Sheet 8-5** lists the steps for removing alternative types of vehicle glass.

Door Removal

When removing the glass from a crashed vehicle does not allow sufficient access to those inside the vehicle, rescuers must use other means. In some situations, rescuers can open the vehicle's doors to provide this access. If the doors will not open because they are locked, rescuers can reach the interior door lock release through the window opening. If unlocking the doors does not allow them to open when using both the inside and outside latches simultaneously, rescuers must either force the doors open or remove them from the vehicle entirely. Rescuers can unintentionally deploy frontal airbags, side-impact airbags, head protection systems, and seat belt pretensioners can be unintentionally deployed when forcibly opening or removing doors.

> **WARNING!**
> Keep rescuers, victims, and loose objects (including seat belt buckles) out of the deployment path of any airbags, head protection systems, or seat belt pretensioners.

If rescuers cannot open the doors, they will have to force or remove them. Opening the door makes its eventual removal easier. Rescuers can implement a number of methods to force open or remove a door.

- Use spreaders and/or cutters (fastest and most common)
- Total sidewall removal or side out (the removal of both doors and the B-post along one side of the vehicle)
- Remove the bolts on the door's hinges using power ratchets, power impact wrenches, or manual socket sets
- Third door conversion (create a wider door opening on two-door vehicles) **(Figure 8.11)**
- Fourth door conversion (create another door in a panel or work van)

Prior to conducting any door removal operation, rescuers should peel away any trim or plastic components on the vehicle's interior around the area to be removed. This operation, commonly known as *peel and peek*, helps rescuers identify the location of any seat belt pretensioners, airbag gas cylinders, or other safety devices. It also helps prevent the trim and plastic pieces from breaking loose and striking victims or rescuers during extrication operations.

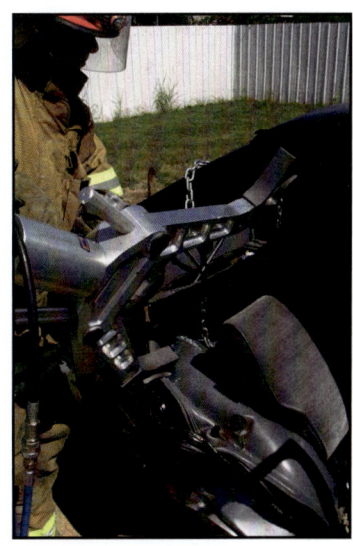

Figure 8.11 A rescuer performing a third door conversion.

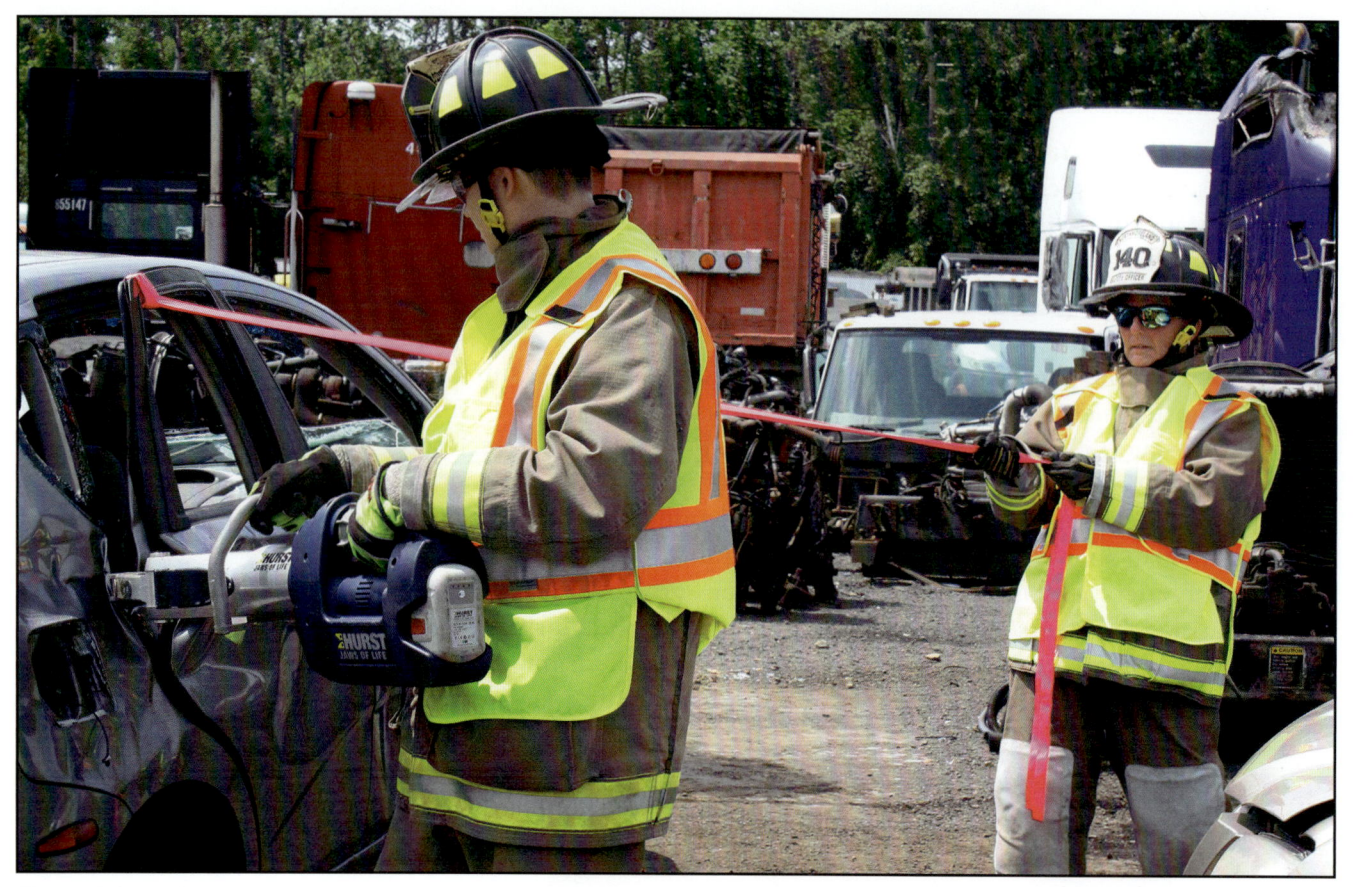

Figure 8.12 Webbing can be attached to a door to maintain control of the door while it is being opened or removed.

> **WARNING!**
> Always peel back the interior trim along the roof rails and all pillars to expose supplemental restraint system compressed gas cylinders, pretensioners, and other devices that could cause injury. If accidentally cut, these devices can cause severe injury and death.

Rescue personnel should always maintain control over a door they are attempting to open or remove to prevent injury to victims and rescuers. To accomplish this, rescuers should attach webbing, straps, rope, chains, or other materials to the door and maintain tension on the material and door to prevent it from striking personnel **(Figure 8.12)**.

> **WARNING!**
> Do not lose control of a door while trying to open or remove it.

If the vehicle door contains an airbag, rescuers will expose a cable (possibly yellow) between the door and the A-post when they remove the door is removed. If rescuers must cut the wires between the door and the A-post, after the battery has been disconnected and the reserve power dissipatedif at all possible the rescuers should cut and separate the wires one at a time with handheld cutters. Cutting the yellow wire in these situations may deploy supplemental restraint systems.

> **WARNING!**
> All undeployed airbags must be considered live, and rescuers should be aware of their potential for sudden deployment.

When removing a door from a vehicle, rescuers must first determine whether to start on the hinge side or the latch side. Conditions of the incident, such as vehicle damage and victim location, will dictate which side rescuers start on first.

Whichever side rescue personnel plan to start with, they must first gain a purchase point to use the tools selected to open the door. Rescuers can use several tools to gain purchase points, including:

- Hydraulic spreaders
- Halligan tools or pry bars
- Hydra rams or rabbit tools

Using hydraulic spreaders to create purchase points. The majority of the time, rescuers can use hydraulic spreaders to gain a purchase point **(Figure 8.13)**. Rescuers should use a fender crush technique to gain an opening between the fender and the door. This allows the rescuers to spread the fender out of the way and cut or spread the hinges to remove the door. This method also enables rescue personnel to bring only a spreader and cutter to the vehicle.

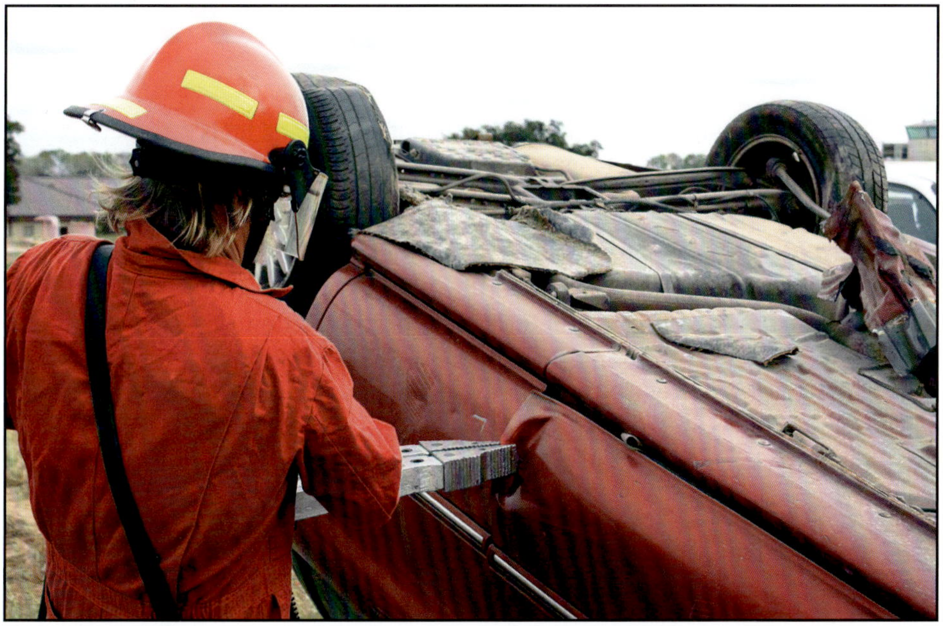

Figure 8.13 Hydraulic spreaders being used to create a purchase point on a rear door of a passenger vehicle.

Section C • Chapter 8 – Victim Disentanglement and Extrication

To use this technique, a rescuer should open the spreaders and place one arm in the wheel well on the front fender behind the shock/strut tower. The rescuer should place the other arm on top of the fender and then close the spreaders. Closing the spreaders will crush the fender and create an opening between the door and the fender. This action will compromise the front fender/support to allow for future dashboard displacement, if needed.

Rescuers must practice this method before using it during an actual extrication. When trying this for the first time, the spreader often slides off the top of the fender before it crushes the fender. When this happens it makes it difficult for rescuers to make a second attempt at the same location, so rescuers will need to move to another spot on the fender and attempt to crush it again.

To avoid this error, rescuers can fit the spreader tip edge into the space between the fender and the hood. If rescuers can fit this tip edge into this space, the spreader arms will not slide off the hood and instead will bite down onto the fender and crush. Raising the back end of the spreader slightly above a 90-degree angle will help prevent the tool from slipping.

Rescuers can also use a spreader in the window opening to spread the upper and lower parts of the door away from the roof rail and pillars. Many leading rescue technicians recommend using this vertical spread technique to create purchase points and even pop open doors. This method forces the door away from the victim and often pops open a door without needing to reposition the spreader or use any other tools, thus making it quicker to extricate the victims.

Rescuers should make safety a concern when performing extrication, especially with the latest technology. Always exercise caution when operating around airbags.

Using a Halligan tool or pry bar to create purchase points. Place the adz end of the Halligan either between the door and the fender for the hinge side or the door and the post for the latch side and rotate the tool up and down vertically to create an opening to use the tool to open the door. When using the pry bar, place the bar in the same place as the Halligan, and move the bar left to right to create an opening to use the tool to open the door.

> **CAUTION**
> Avoid rocking the victims when using hand tools to make purchase points.

Using a hydra ram or rabbit tool to create purchase points. Rescuers can use these manually operated hydraulic spreaders to create purchase points. Agencies use these tools often for forcible entry on residential and commercial doors, but they are also good for gaining purchase points on doors, hoods, and trunks. To use this tool, rescuers place the spreader tips into the space between the door and the fender and/or post and manually pump the handle until they increase the size of the opening.

Using tools to remove doors. Rescuers can use a Hi-Lift® jack to crush or weaken the door's collision bar and then open a door. Once rescuers crush the collision bar, they should reposition the jack over the latching mechanism to roll the door down and off the latching mechanism. **Skill Sheet 8-6** describes the steps for using a Hi-Lift® jack to open a door. Use caution with Hi-Lift® jacks. If not deployed properly, they can slip easily and be dangerous.

Another door removal method uses power ratchets, power impact wrenches, or manual socket sets to remove the bolts on the door's hinges **(Figure 8.14)**. Rescuers may also cut door hinges with a variety of tools. With the hinges disconnected, rescuers can operate the door latch mechanism to unhook the door from the latching mechanism and remove the door. This method works well for removing doors on vehicles equipped with airbags in the doors. **Skill Sheet 8-7** lists the steps for opening or removing a door with a power ratchet, power impact wrench, or manual socket set.

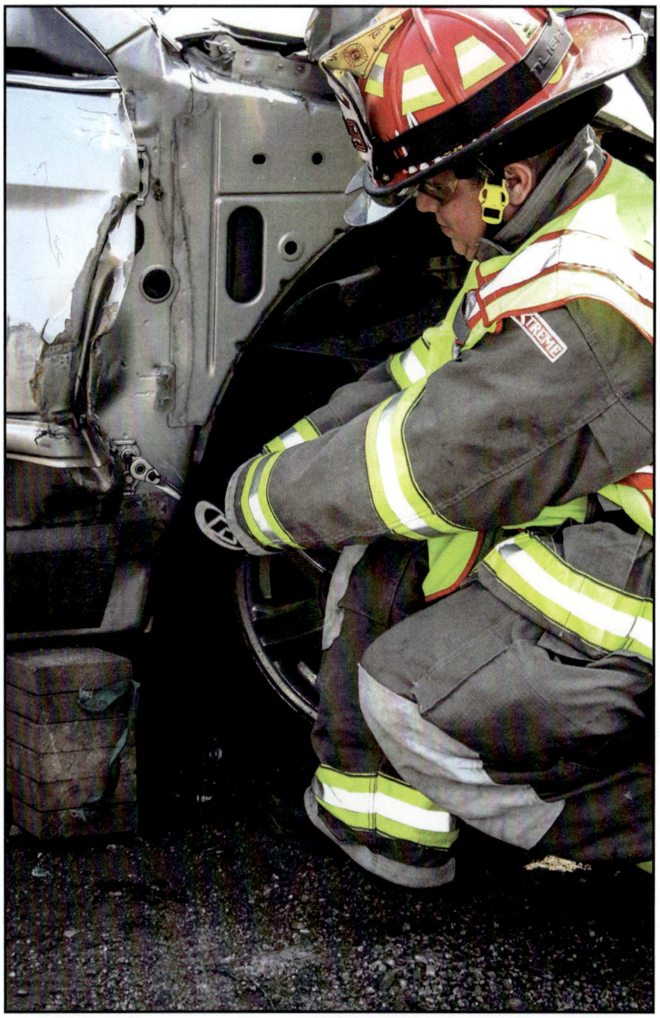

Hydraulic tools, such as spreaders and cutters provide the fastest and most commonly used method of forcing or removing a jammed door. Rescuers insert the spreader tips into the seam between the door and the B-post above the door lock. They then open the spreader in a downward and outward direction. This motion allows the door latch to roll off the latching mechanism and open the door. Rescuers should maintain the control of the door using webbing, ropes, or chains. **Skill Sheet 8-8** describes the procedures for using hydraulic tools to open or remove a door.

NOTE: On vehicles with pressed metal hinges, it may be quicker to cut the hinges, as opposed to spreading them.

Figure 8.14 A rescuer using a socket wrench to remove door hinge bolts.

Factory Third and Fourth Doors

Some manufacturers build automobiles and light trucks with a third (and sometimes fourth) door that is smaller than the regular door. On automobiles and light trucks, manufacturers locate the third door directly behind the driver's door. Some light trucks now have this type of door on both sides of the vehicle. Regardless of how many of these doors a vehicle has, there is no B-post between the front door(s) and the third and fourth door. Since these frames have no B-post, the front door latches to the leading edge of the third/fourth door. Therefore, rescuers cannot open the third and fourth doors unless they first open the adjacent front doors.

Factory third and fourth doors latch at the top and bottom, and even though some of them have inside door handles, they can normally be opened only when the front door is open. On some light trucks (but not all), the third and fourth door hinges are slightly exposed behind the trailing edge of the door. This exposure allows access to these hinges, and rescuers can cut them from outside the vehicle with powered cutters. All factory third and fourth doors have tempered glass windows. However, since the inside door handle (if so equipped) will not work with the front door closed, rescuers will have no advantage in breaking this window in an attempt to gain access into the vehicle.

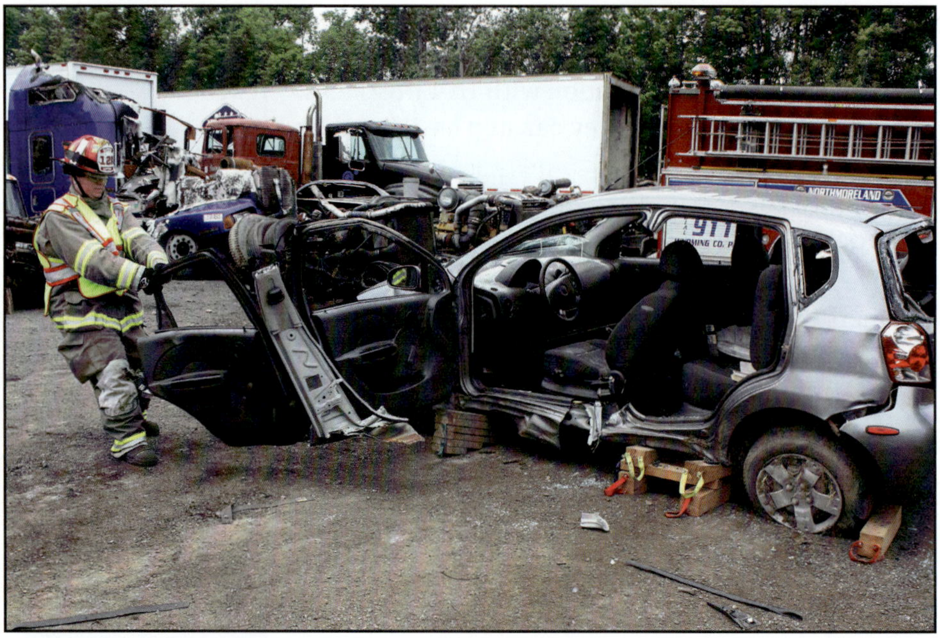

Figure 8.15 A total sidewall removal is an advanced extrication technique.

Minivans also come with factory third and fourth doors. Minivans also have a sliding door, or dual sliding doors, that extend outward/away from the vehicle and then slide along a track, usually toward the rear of the vehicle. Rescuers may encounter manual or powered versions of these doors. If rescuers cannot open these doors manually, or the door is blocked, rescuers may have to create an alternate opening to access the vehicle's passengers. **Skill Sheet 8-9** lists the steps for removing a vehicle's sliding side door.

Total Sidewall Removal

Rescuers may remove the vehicle's total sidewall or both doors and the B-post along one side of the vehicle in order to access victims. This technique is also known as the B-post blowout and side out. This method has the advantage of providing a wide access way to the victim to perform extrication and disentanglement as well as providing wide access for victim removal. **Skill Sheet 8-10** describes the steps for performing a total sidewall removal.

The total sidewall removal is an advanced extrication technique that has numerous methods of completion. Rescuers should seek additional training to learn other techniques to perform a total sidewall removal **(Figure 8.15)**.

Third-Door Conversion

The term third-door conversion refers to the technique that rescuers use to create a wider door opening on two-door vehicles. Because rear seat passengers in two-door vehicles are trapped as long as the front seats are intact and in place, rescuers may need to remove the wall of the vehicle to allow the passengers to escape or to allow rescuers to gain access to them for medical evaluation and stabilization.

Rescuers often use reciprocating saws, spreaders, and air chisels to perform third-door conversions. **Skill Sheet 8-11** lists the steps for creating an alternate (third-door) opening on a two-door vehicle.

Fourth-Door Conversion

The term fourth-door conversion refers to the technique that creates an alternate opening on a panel van or work van that only has one operating door for cargo loading and off-loading. Rescuers make cuts between the B- and C-posts in the side panel, creating a large opening for rescue access and victim removal. **Skill Sheet 8-12** lists the steps for creating an alternate (fourth-door) opening in a vehicle.

Roof Displacement and Removal

Rescuers frequently remove part, or all, of a vehicle's roof to gain access to trapped victims. Flapping or removing the roof also eliminates the possibility of Side Impact Protection Systems (SIPS) or inflatable window curtains deploying. The roof of a vehicle may collapse or compress as a result of the collision or a rollover event. These vehicles may come to rest on their wheels, sides, or roofs. When roofs are the point of entrapment, rescuers may have to displace or remove the roof to access the victim(s).

Rescuers may perform most roof-removal techniques with cutters, reciprocating saws, or air chisels. The needs of the victim and access for the rescuers will ultimately determine the technique used. Rescuers can use rams or spreaders to expand an opening and create more space in the passenger compartment. Wheel resting vehicles may require total roof removal or the roof to be flapped. If the vehicle is side resting, a roof flap or removal probably will provide the best option for creating a clear opening through which rescuers can extricate the victims.

Rescuers should peel and peek prior to cutting to avoid cutting into the seat belt pretensioners or side airbag gas cylinders. They should make cuts at the most advantageous place to access the victim(s) and avoid SRS components.

Roof removal. Engineers design unibody vehicles to function as a unit; therefore, removing the doors and roof can seriously compromise the vehicle's structural integrity. Therefore, rescuers should place a step chock or other support under the B-post of unibody vehicles before removing the roof. The windshields, A-posts, and forward edge of the roof on modern cars compose the structural integrity of the vehicle body, so they should remain intact and rescuers should cut the roof just behind the A-posts. Rescuers can then cut the remaining door posts and lift the entire roof off as a unit **(Figure 8.16)**.

Rescuers may have difficulty cutting through larger rear posts with hydraulic cutters because the posts are often wider than the opening of the cutters. When rescuers encounter wide posts, they can cut and remove a triangular section from one side of the post. This allows rescuers to insert the cutters deeper to make additional cuts. Rescuers can also compress and compact the posts into a smaller size with spreaders. **Skill Sheet 8-13** lists the steps to remove the roof from a wheel-resting vehicle.

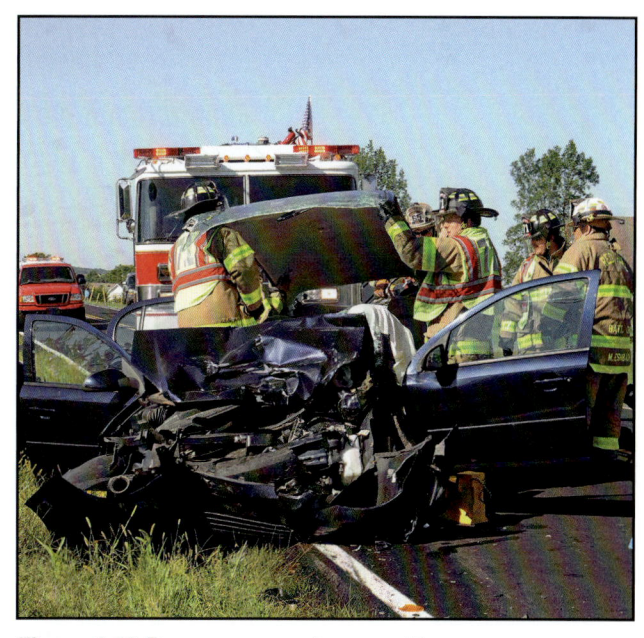

Figure 8.16 Rescuers removing a roof from a passenger vehicle to access the victim. *Courtesy of Bob Esposito.*

Flapping a roof. Historically, some agencies folded the roof back onto the trunk or forward onto the hood rather than remove it. These procedures were sometimes called *making a roof flap* or simply *flapping the roof.*

Rescuers sometimes need to flap a roof because of the complications involved in removing the roof on some vehicles. Rescuers also flap a roof when they cannot access all areas of the roof to perform total roof removal. In addition, the materials used in the construction of some newer vehicles may prevent rescuers from folding the roof. Rescuers will have to determine whether to flap the roof forward or backward, make applicable cuts, then flap the cut section of the roof.

Entry through the roof of side-resting vehicles. Rescuers can gain access to the passenger compartment through the roof of a side-resting vehicle. **Skill Sheet 8-14** lists the steps for flapping or removing the roof of a side-resting vehicle. Rescuers may need to add cribbing under the roof flap, between the flap and ground, to create a stable and secure platform and to reduce movement caused by a void space.

To gain entry through the roof, rescuers can use an air chisel or reciprocating saw. **Skill Sheet 8-15** lists the steps to create an access opening in the roof of a side-resting vehicle.

Kick Panel Removal

When the pedals pin a vehicle driver's feet and legs, rescuers often need to move the kick panel out of the way to allow access to the victim's feet. **Skill Sheet 8-16** lists the steps for removing the kick panel from a passenger vehicle.

CAUTION
Rescuers should avoid cutting the fuse box panel when performing kick panel removal.

Entry through the Floor

Rescuers may need to gain access through the floor of roof-resting vehicles that allow limited access to the windows. In these situations, entry through the sides of the vehicle is difficult if not impossible.

Prior to cutting, rescuers should identify the locations of any fuel and hydraulic lines. On hybrid cars, rescuers should look for high-voltage cables that run from the high-voltage batteries (usually in the rear of the vehicle) forward to the engine compartment. Battery packs on electric vehicles may consume the entire floor area underneath the vehicle, making entry through the floor impossible.

Rescuers should check the interior of the vehicle before cutting to ensure that victims are not in contact with the portion of the floor that is about to be cut. If rescuers cannot determine the location of victims through conventional openings, they should remove the drain plugs in the bottom of the floor pan. They may see the victims through the resulting holes. Do not use cutting torches to gain entry because of the fire hazard presented by floor covering materials and any fuel that may have spilled.

> **WARNING!**
> Do not use cutting torches to make entry through the floor of a vehicle.

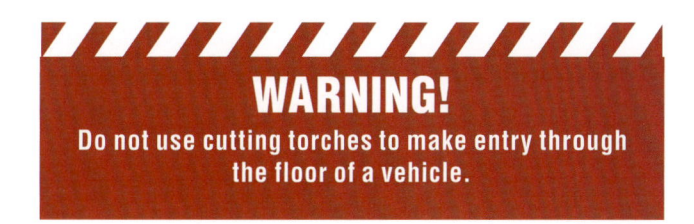

Rescuers can use two methods to enter a vehicle through its floor. The choice of entry is best determined by the type of vehicle, the number of trapped occupants, their locations within the vehicle, and their conditions. **Skill Sheet 8-17** lists two methods of creating an access opening through the floor of a passenger vehicle.

Trunk Tunneling

Due to the position and condition of the vehicle, rescuers may need to tunnel through the trunk area of a passenger vehicle to gain access to the passenger compartment. Rescuers may need this technique after a rear or side underride or when they encounter obstructions to both sides and the top of the vehicle, making door and roof removal impossible. **Skill Sheet 8-18** lists the steps for tunneling through a trunk.

> **CAUTION**
> Trunks or other vehicle compartments may contain hazards.

Alternative Techniques for Creating Access and Egress Openings on Passenger Vehicles with Advanced Steel

Improved crashworthiness in newer passenger vehicles has resulted from changes in the Federal Motor Vehicle Safety Standards designed to improve side impact and roof crush resistance. Vehicle manufacturers have responded to this engineering challenge in two basic ways. Some manufacturers reinforce the side and roof structure areas of a vehicle with more layers or thicker layers of steel. Other manufacturers make areas such as B-posts, roof rails, and rocker panels of ultra-high-strength steels otherwise known as advanced steels.

With increasing frequency, some fire departments, especially those with outdated or older tools, cannot cut through structural areas such as the B-posts of late model vehicles. The tools that have worked well for so many years may not cut the steel found in new model vehicles produced within recent years. This section will describe several alternative techniques that rescuers have successfully used to gain access to passenger vehicles with advanced steels, such as:

- Pie cut
- B-pillar lift
- Cross ramming
- Ramming the roof off
- Partial or total sunroof

Pie Cut
Often times, only the B-posts contain advanced steel and not the roof rail. In these situations, rescuers may cut the roof rail at the top of the B-post, on both sides, in a pie cut fashion and lay the pillar down.

B-post Lift
In contrast to the above maneuver, sometimes the B-posts and the entire roof rail consist of advanced steel that the rescue team cannot cut through. Rescuers should attempt to cut all along the roof rail first, just in case the structure contains soft steel somewhere. However, if those attempts fail, rescuers may succeed with efforts to cut through the post at the bottom, near the rocker panel. One popular manufacturer's structural design has mild steel at the bottom of the B-post, spot-welded to the main portion of the pillar. Once rescuers detach the B-post at the bottom, they can lift it up and away from the vehicle, creating access to the victim(s).

Cross Ramming
If rescuers cannot cut through the advanced steel B-posts or rescuers encounter increased intrusion into the passenger compartment from a lateral/side impact, they can ram the B-post away from the trapped occupants. With this technique, rescuers will push the post out and away from the passenger compartment of the vehicle using a hydraulic ram placed on the transmission tunnel/hump and extending to the vehicle's B-post. Additionally, if rescuers have a long enough hydraulic ram, they can use a spread from B-post to B-post to move a crash-damaged pillar off the victims trapped inside. Rescuers should monitor roof movement because the roof may begin to lower into the vehicle as the B-posts move outward.

Ramming the Roof Off
When a rescue team cannot cut through a B-post or roof rail that contains advanced steel, they may attempt to ram the roof off the top of the B-post. Even though advanced steel may be present, a powerful ram may be able to push the roof rail up until it begins to tear at the spot welds. After an initial push behind the B-post, a second push along the front side may completely tear the B-post from the roof rail. Rescuers will need to place cribbing beneath the rocker panel to support the push of the ram.

Partial or Total Sunroof
When rescuers encounter a passenger vehicle with advanced steel located in key locations of the roof pillars, roof rail, and rocker panel, they can attempt a partial sunroof or total sunroof evolution. The partial sunroof technique is similar to a roof flap; however, the roof hinges on the side as opposed to the front or back. First, rescuers cut the roof from the front windshield header to the rear window, inside the roof rail. They make a relief cut at the front and rear on the hinge side of the roof and lift the entire roof panel up and away from the victim(s). Rescuers may accomplish a rapid extrication once they open the partial sunroof. If needed, rescuers can make a second cut on the opposite side from the windshield header to the rear window and can remove the entire roof panel, creating a total sunroof.

Techniques for Disentangling Victims from Passenger Vehicles

Rescuers may need to disentangle victims from passenger vehicles. Depending on the circumstances, they may find the following techniques useful when performing these operations:

- Removing a windshield from around a victim
- Displacing a steering column
- Displacing a dashboard
- Dropping a floor pan
- Displacing a B-post
- Displacing and removing seats
- Removing pedals

Removing a Windshield from Around a Victim

Sometimes a vehicle occupant impacts the windshield and rescuers must remove the windshield from around the victim. **Skill Sheet 8-19** describes two methods for removing a windshield from around a victim. Rescuers must exercise extreme care when performing this operation.

Displacing a Steering Column

Front-end collisions can cause victims to become entrapped under the dashboard and/or steering wheel/column. To free such victims, rescuers must displace the dashboard and/or steering wheel/column. Rescuers can perform a dashboard push/roll using a ram in the door jamb along with the appropriate relief cuts. They can use the spreaders in the kick board to perform a dashboard lift; this technique also requires appropriate relief cuts.

Rescuers will displace a steering column in order to lift the steering column off a victim. Rescuers pierce the windshield and wrap a rescue hook or chain around the steering column. They place the hook or chain as close to the dashboard as possible, in order to prevent the steering wheel from flying into the victim. Rescuers can then lift steering column, allowing them to disentangle the victim. This process can relieve respiratory compromise safely and in much less time than other methods. **Skill Sheet 8-20** lists the steps for displacing a steering column.

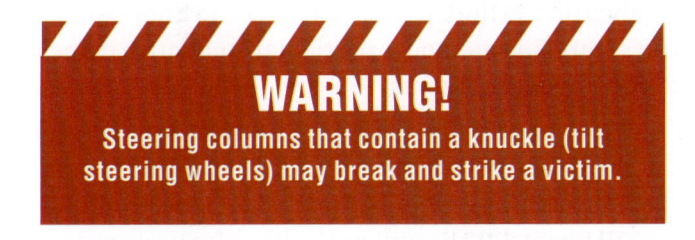

WARNING!
Steering columns that contain a knuckle (tilt steering wheels) may break and strike a victim.

Displacing a Dashboard

Displacing a dashboard lifts the dashboard up and away from victims in the front seat. Rescuers may use several methods to displace a dashboard. Each method depends upon the vehicle's condition, the available tools, and the local policies and procedures.

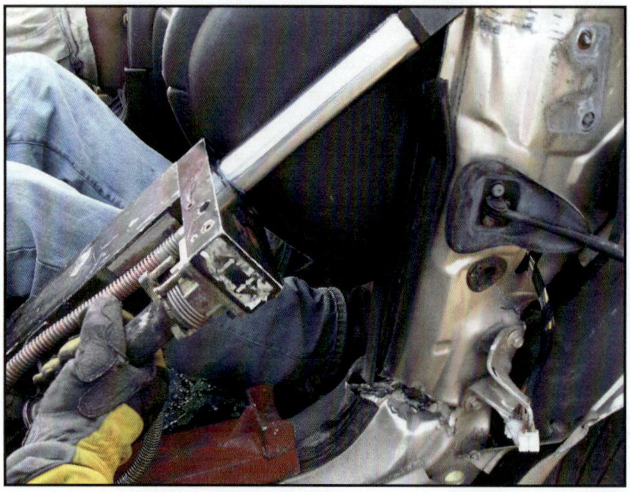

Figure 8.17 A hydraulic ram being used to roll a dashboard. *Courtesy of Alan Braun, University of Missouri Fire and Rescue Training Institute.*

Rescuers can perform a dashboard push/roll using a ram in the door jamb along with the appropriate relief cuts **(Figure 8.17)**. They can use the spreaders in the kick board to perform a dashboard lift; this technique also requires appropriate relief cuts. They may also lift (jack) the entire assembly vertically or use a procedure called a dashboard push (roll) which raises the assembly up and away from the victim.

After displacing the dashboard, rescuers must prevent it from returning to its original position. To accomplish this, rescuers should insert cribbing or other suitable stabilization equipment under the base of the A-post on unibody vehicles, or between the frame and the body on full-frame vehicles. **Skill Sheet 8-21** describes three methods of displacing a dashboard.

> **CAUTION**
> When displacing a dashboard, rescuers must protect themselves and the entrapped victims from any undeployed front-impact or knee-bolster airbags.

Dropping a Floor Pan

Rescuers may drop the floor pan to disentangle the victim's feet. Instead of raising the dashboard, the floor pan drop moves the floor pan down and away from the victim's feet. This method is particularly effective in incidents involving front and side impact collisions.

Dropping the floor pan involves making cuts that greatly resemble a dashboard lift but with no cuts made to the upper A-post or fender rail **(Figure 8.18)**. Rescuers make cuts in the lower A-post and rocker panel to allow them to lower the floor pan. **Skill Sheet 8-22** describes the steps for performing the floor pan drop. Rescuers should identify vehicle power cables (hybrid vehicles), brake lines, fuel lines, and other cables that extend along the inner side of the rocker panel under the vehicle before beginning this technique to avoid increasing the risks to the rescuers and victims.

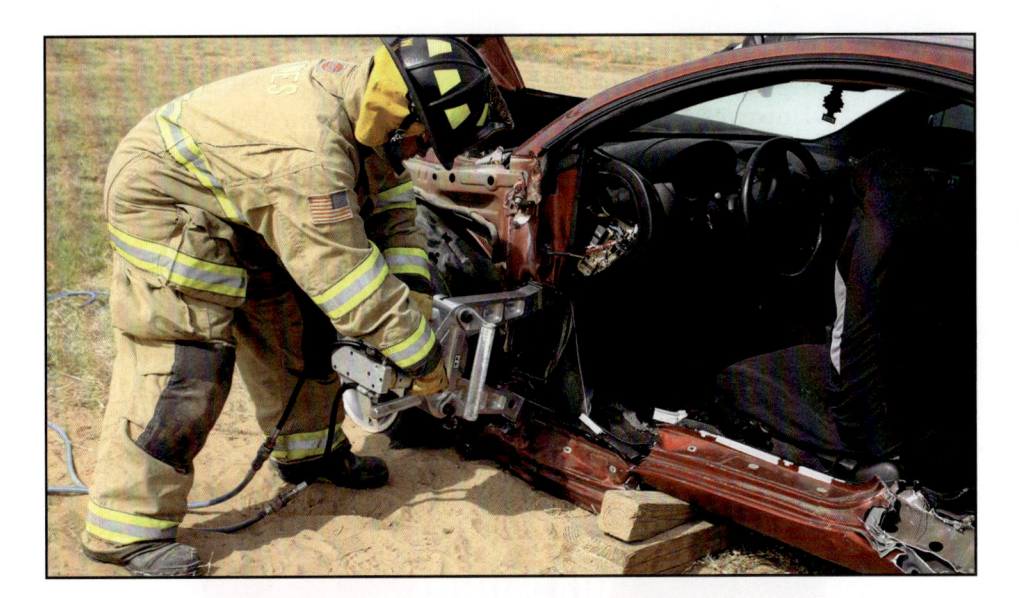

Figure 8.18 This rescuer is dropping the floor plan.

> **WARNING!**
> Do not damage the electronic controls for the front-impact airbags.

> **WARNING!**
> Keep rescuers, victims, and any loose objects out of the airbag deployment path.

Displacing the B-Post

Some techniques enable rescuers to alleviate intrusion and displace the impacted side outward. This allows rescuers to remove doors and the B-post without causing further injury to victims. Two of these techniques are cross ramming and interior spreading. Cross ramming was described earlier in this chapter. Interior spreading positions the spreaders behind the victim, usually from the rear floorboard to the lower B-post. Rescuers should use cribbing on the floorboard to provide an adequate base for the spreader arm. Operating the spreaders in this fashion will apply force to the compromised B-post, forcing the intrusion outward and relieving pressure to the trapped/pinned victim.

Displacing and Removing Seats

The driver's seat and front passenger's seat are usually adjustable. The method of adjustments vary from a simple mechanical system for moving the seat forward or backward or adjusting the angle of the seatback, to electrically operated systems with 8-way movement and adjustable lumbar support. The seats in some newer automobiles also contain side-impact airbags. These features, designed to increase passenger comfort and safety, can sometimes cause injuries to passengers and rescuers during extrication operations if rescuers do not take precautions.

Adjustable vehicle seats slide forward and back in tracks mounted on the floor of the vehicle. Small metal teeth hold the seats in the desired position in the tracks. However, the inertial forces generated by a high-speed impact often break the teeth of these mechanisms, allowing the seats to move rapidly forward and carrying the seat occupants with them. If the vehicle lacks front-impact and knee-bolster airbags, the driver may submarine under the dashboard — become wedged under the dashboard and/ or entangled in the steering wheel and brake pedal. In these cases, rescuers may need to move the seats to access the victims.

In many vehicles, the seatbacks on bucket seats can recline several degrees. On bucket seats that do not recline, rescuers will need to cut the seat frame on both sides in order to lower the seatback. Rescuers should use caution when cutting or pushing off seats because of the hazards presented by the SRS systems.

> **WARNING!**
> All undeployed airbags must be considered live, and rescuers should be aware of their potential for sudden deployment.

Rescuers can eliminate seat entrapment by using spreaders to displace the front seat. To lay the seat back to a horizontal position, rescuers must cut the seat frame at its base on both sides of the seat. It is sometimes necessary to remove a front seat entirely — such as to provide room to work on a rear seat passenger. In this case, rescuers can cut the seat mounts at the point of attachment to the tracks with hydraulic cutters. If rescuers can properly package and monitor the victim they can move the seat to facilitate removing the victim from the vehicle.

Before moving a seat, rescuers must properly package any victims as dictated by their injuries and closely monitor them during the seat movement. If a rescuer cannot package a victim without moving the seat, rescuers must leave the seat must in position and remove the vehicle from around the victim. In general, rescuers should try to displace or roll dashboard to disentangle a victim instead of moving the seat. If rescuers can properly package and monitor the victim, they can move the seat to facilitate removing the victim from the vehicle. **Skill Sheet 8-23** lists the methods for displacing or removing a front seat in a passenger vehicle.

Displacing or Removing Pedals

Pedals commonly pin the driver's feet in a vehicle crash. To free a trapped victim, rescuers must either move the pedal away from the victim's foot or remove the pedal entirely. Once rescuers gain access to the pedal area — either through the door opening or after a kick panel roll-up — they can either cut the pedals or move them out of the way. Rescuers may use hydraulic spreaders, cutters, straps, or ropes to move the pedals away from the victim's foot or completely remove the pedals. When the brake and/or clutch pedal pins a vehicle driver's legs rescuers may need to move the kick panel out of the way to allow access to the victim's feet and legs. Rescuers may instead perform a floor pan drop. Instead of raising the dash, the floor pan drop moves the floor pan down and away from the victim's feet and legs.

CAUTION
When cutting pedals, the pedals may break or shatter and turn into projectiles because they are often made of cast materials.

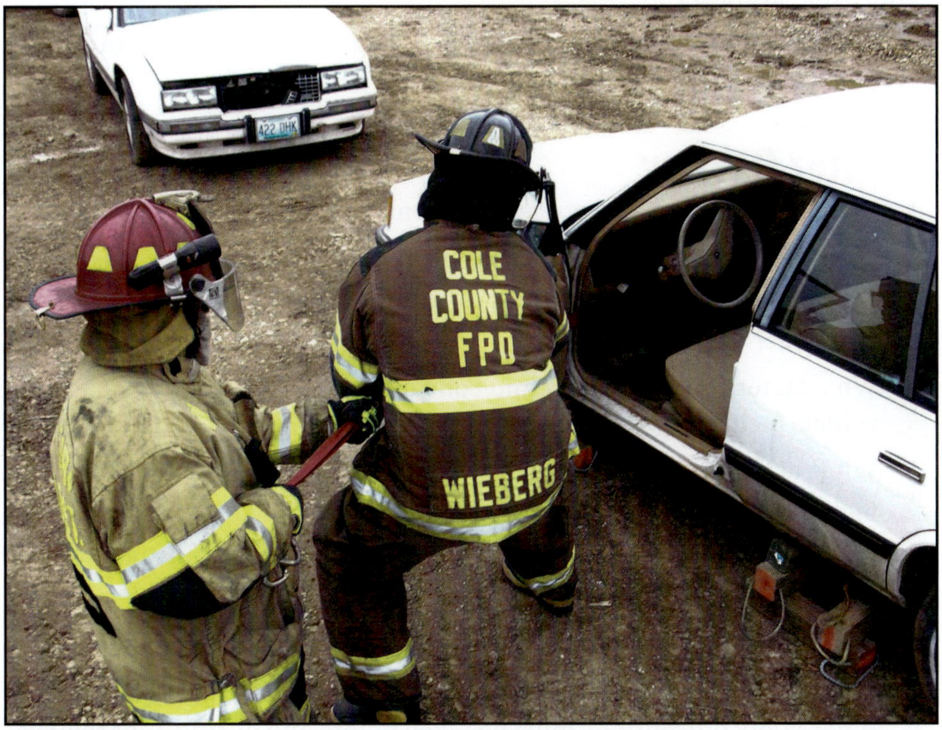

Figure 8.19 Rescuers can use webbing to pull vehicle pedals away from a victim's feet. *Courtesy of Alan Braun, University of Missouri Fire and Rescue Training Institute.*

Cutting pedals. If available, rescuers can use a hydraulic pedal cutter to quickly cut the pedal arms and free the victim's feet **(Figure 8.19)**. Extrication personnel should exercise caution when operating hydraulic pedal cutters around a victim's legs and feet to avoid causing injury to the victim. The tool may roll during the cutting operation, causing further injury. To prevent a pedal from twisting and pinching the victim's leg or foot, rescuers should wrap a web strap around the pedal and place tension on the strap to pull the pedal away from the victim's extremities. To cut the pedals, rescuers should cut the pedal arm as needed with the cutting tool and then remove the pedal from the area around the victim's leg or foot.

Displacing pedals. Rescuers can use one of the following methods to displace pedals:

- Bending the pedals with a hydraulic spreader
- Attaching a chain, web strap, or rope around the pedal arm near the foot pad and pulling laterally:

Section C • Chapter 8 – Victim Disentanglement and Extrication **307**

- Rescuers can pull manually
- Rescuers can form the attachment into a short loop, slip one end of the loop over a spreader tip, place the other tip against the rocker panel near the A-post, and spread the tips to move the pedal
• Strapping the pedal to a functional, partially opened door and fully opening the door
• Strapping the pedal to the steering wheel and then turning the wheel to bend the pedal upwards
• Using the same tools used in jacking or lifting the steering column and dashboard to move the pedals.

Chapter Review

1. What are common points of entrapment in passenger vehicles?
2. What kinds of injuries are victims involved in rollovers likely to sustain?
3. What special considerations must rescuers make for underride/override incidents?
4. What factors must be taken into consideration when working at a multiple vehicle incident?
5. What actions can rescuers take to protect victims during extrication operations?
6. What must rescuers take into account when determining access and egress points on a vehicle?
7. What are four common existing entry points on passenger vehicles?
8. What methods exist for removing different types of vehicle glass?
9. What safety precautions must be taken before and during door removal?
10. How can rescuers create purchase points in vehicles in order to better facilitate extrication?
11. Describe three methods for gaining access to victims through the roof of a passenger vehicle.
12. What alternate methods may be used to gain access to victims if rescuers are unable to cut through thick steel components of a passenger vehicle?
13. What methods may be used to disentangle victims who are trapped by the steering column?
14. How can rescuers disentangle victims who are trapped by the pedals of the vehicle?

Discussion Questions

1. You arrive at the scene of a side-impact collision. The driver of the vehicle that was impacted is trapped by the steering column, and the door is jammed. What methods can you use to access and disentangle the victim?
2. What protocols does your jurisdiction have in place for multiple vehicle incidents (MVIs) or mass casualty incidents (MCIs)?

8-1
Determine passenger vehicle access and egress points.

🔥 **SKILL SHEETS**

Directions: Read each scenario and study the accompanying diagram. Complete the steps below for each scenario.
NOTE: There may be multiple access locations and methods for each scenario. Refer to local SOPs to determine the method used in your jurisdiction.

Scenario 1
You respond to the scene of a two-vehicle incident involving a pickup truck and a van. The pickup truck was driving west on a one-way street. The van was travelling north on an intersecting two-way street, and it failed to stop at the intersection. As it was turning left, the van struck the front of the pickup on the driver's side and pushed it into a row of cars parallel parked at the curb. There are two victims pinned inside each vehicle. The driver's side door of the van is inoperable, and the passenger door and sliding door allow minimal space for access. The cars parked at the curb are unoccupied but sustained considerable damage.

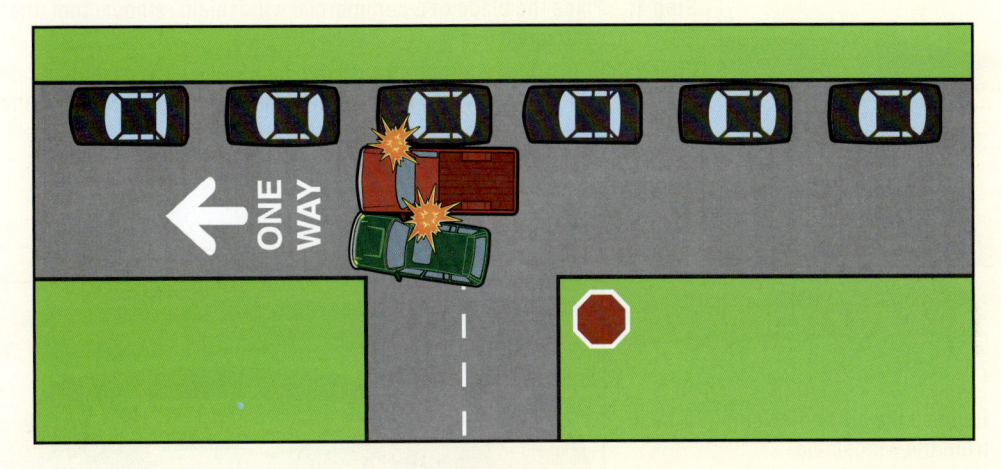

Scenario 2
You respond to an incident involving a single-car rollover. A midsize car was traveling on a two-lane highway when it hit a patch of ice as it came around a bend. The car rolled several times and came to rest on its side. A driver and a small child are trapped inside the car. No other cars were involved.

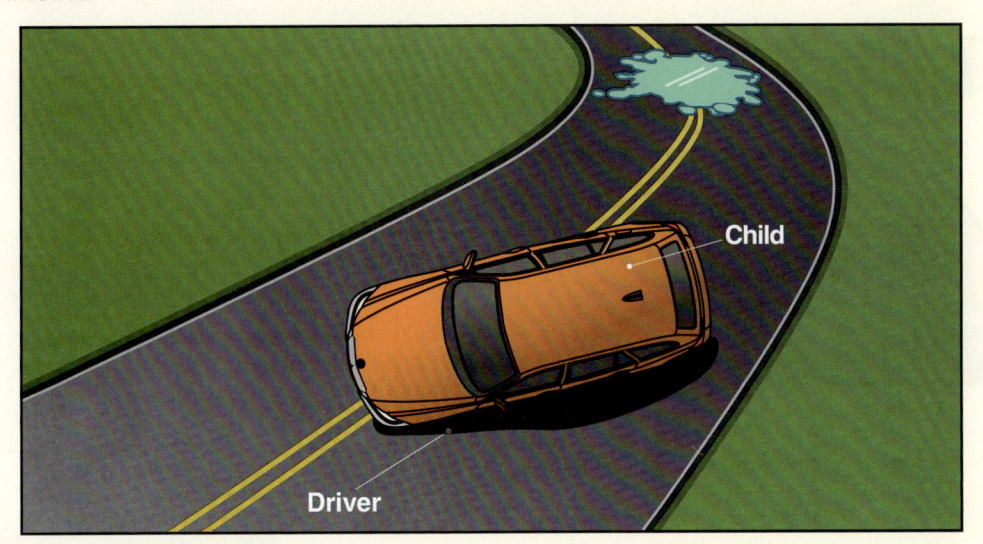

Step 1: Identify probable victim locations and points of entrapment.
Step 2: Determine the appropriate locations for rescuer and equipment access and for victim removal.
   a. Factor in time constraints and available resources.
   b. Ensure that vehicle stability will not be compromised.
Step 3: Assess the impact that the vehicle's stability and position will have on the victim(s) and on rescue operations.
Step 4: Describe the safety precautions that must be taken before extrication can begin.
Step 5: Describe the method of stabilization that will be used.

Section C • Chapter 8 – Victim Disentanglement and Extrication   309

SKILL SHEETS

8-2 Remove glass by removing the seal.

WARNING: Rescuers must ensure that the vehicle is properly stabilized and the scene is safe.

CAUTION: Rescuers must take necessary precautions to protect themselves and victims from hazards including, but not limited to, glass fragments and dust, jagged metal, SRS gas cylinders, undeployed airbags, and fire hazards.

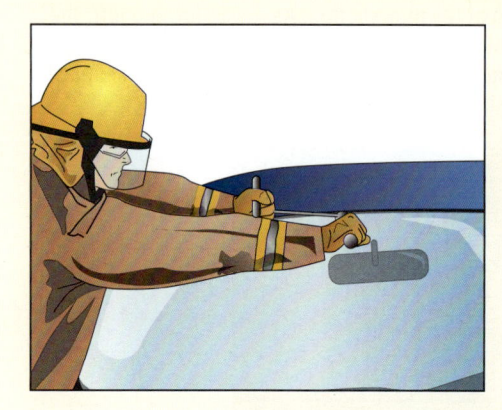

Step 1: Place the blade of a commercial windshield removal tool under the windshield seal.

Step 2: Hold and stabilize tool with one hand. Place the other hand on the attached cable and handle and begin to pull, ensuring that the blade of the tool remains against the windshield and under the seal at all times. Continue until the entire seal has been cut.

Step 3: Remove the outer portion of the seal from the windshield.

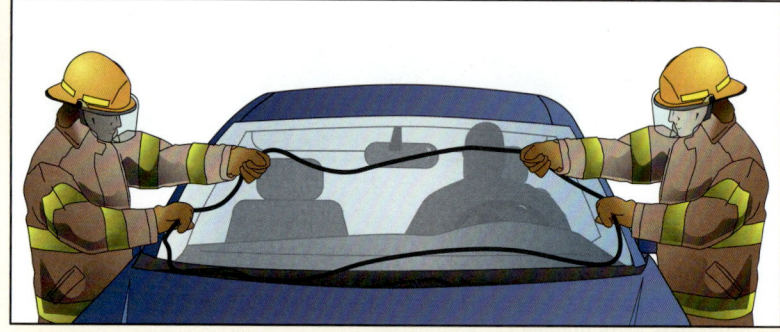

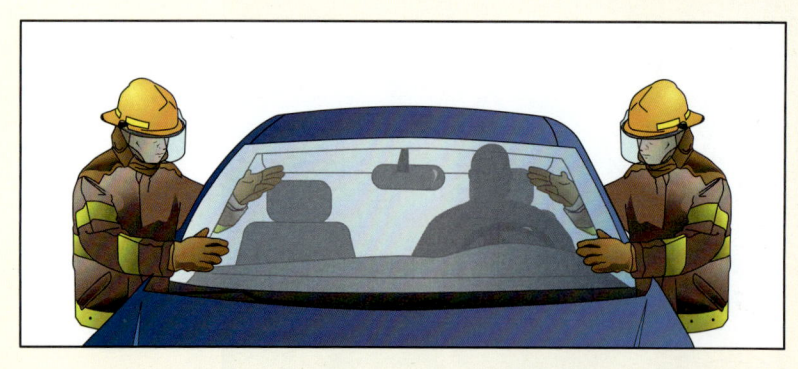

Step 4: Push the windshield outward from the interior of the vehicle.

NOTE: An alternative removal option is to place duct tape handles or suction cups onto the outer portion of the windshield and pull to remove.

Step 5: Position the windshield away from the rescue scene.

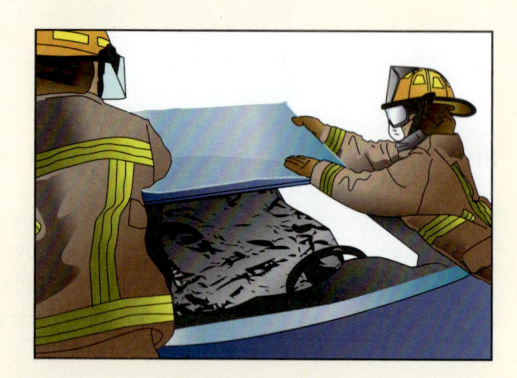

Section C • Chapter 8 – Victim Disentanglement and Extrication

8-3
Remove laminated vehicle glass.

WARNING: Rescuers must ensure that the vehicle is properly stabilized and the scene is safe.

CAUTION: Rescuers must take necessary precautions to protect themselves and victims from hazards including, but not limited to, glass fragments and dust, jagged metal, SRS gas cylinders, undeployed airbags, and fire hazards.

Step 1: Two rescuers position on opposite sides of the vehicle.

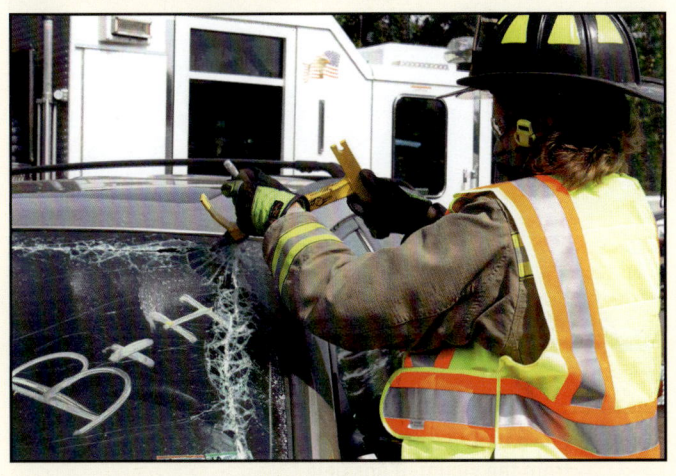

Step 2: Make a vertical cut on each side of the glass.

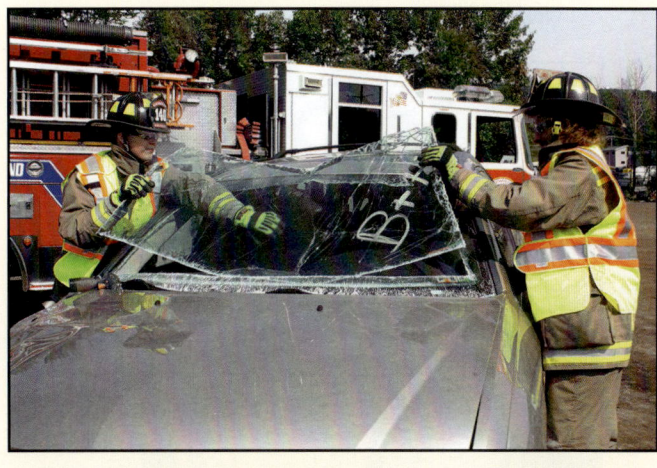

Step 6: Remove the glass and position it away from the rescue scene.

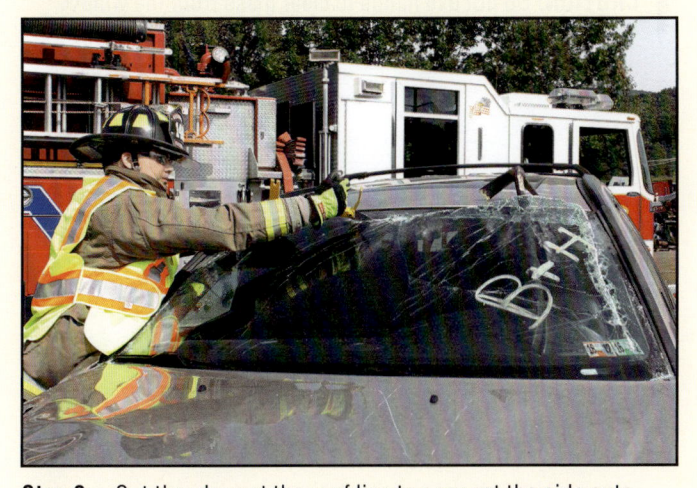

Step 3: Cut the glass at the roof line to connect the side cuts.
Step 4: Rescuers grasp the glass on each side near the roof line cut.
Step 5: Cut bottom side of glass to connect each vertical side cut.

Section C • Chapter 8 – Victim Disentanglement and Extrication

SKILL SHEETS

8-4
Remove tempered vehicle glass.

WARNING: Rescuers must ensure that the vehicle is properly stabilized and the scene is safe.

CAUTION: Rescuers must take necessary precautions to protect themselves and victims from hazards including, but not limited to, glass fragments and dust, jagged metal, SRS gas cylinders, undeployed airbags, and fire hazards.

Step 1: Place a center punch or other tool in the lower corner of the window.

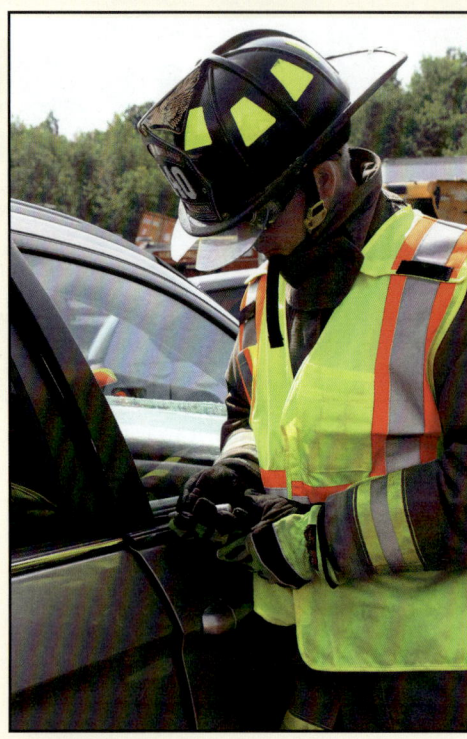

Step 2: Brace the hand holding the center punch with the opposite hand to prevent it from pushing through the glass.

Step 3: Break the window.

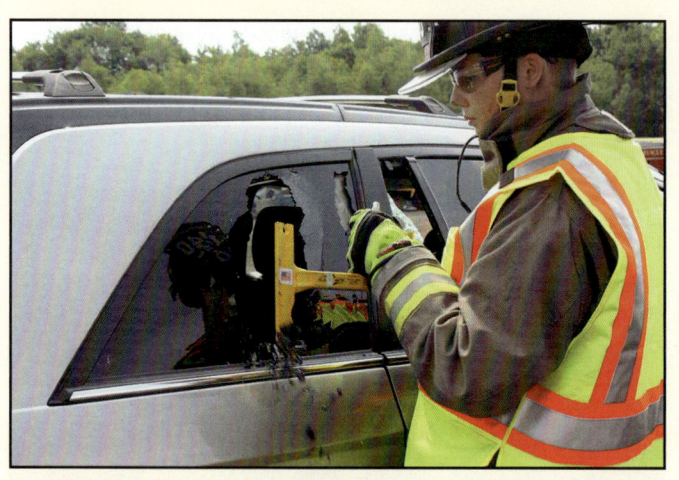

Step 4: Use a tool to clear the remaining glass outward and away from the victim, if possible.

CAUTION: Do not use hands to clear glass from the window

8-5
Remove alternate types of vehicle glass.

> **WARNING:** Rescuers must ensure that the vehicle is properly stabilized and the scene is safe.

> **CAUTION:** Rescuers must take necessary precautions to protect themselves and victims from hazards including, but not limited to, glass fragments and dust, jagged metal, SRS gas cylinders, undeployed airbags, and fire hazards.

NOTE: Inspect and maintain all equipment according to local SOPs and manufacturer's guidelines.

Step 1: Two rescuers position on opposite edges of the glass.

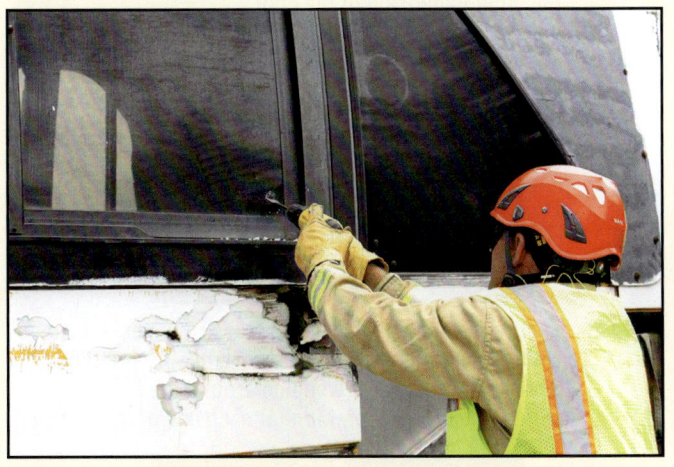

Step 2: Drill a starting hole in one corner of the glass on each side.

NOTE: This may require drilling several holes in close proximity to each other.

Step 3: Insert the saw blade in the starting hole and make a vertical cut on each side of the glass.

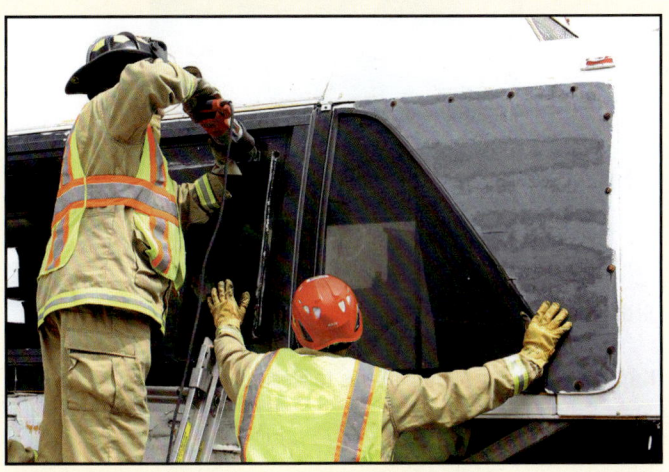

Step 4: Cut the glass horizontally at the roof line to connect each vertical cut.

Step 5: Rescuers grasp the glass on each side near the roof line cut.

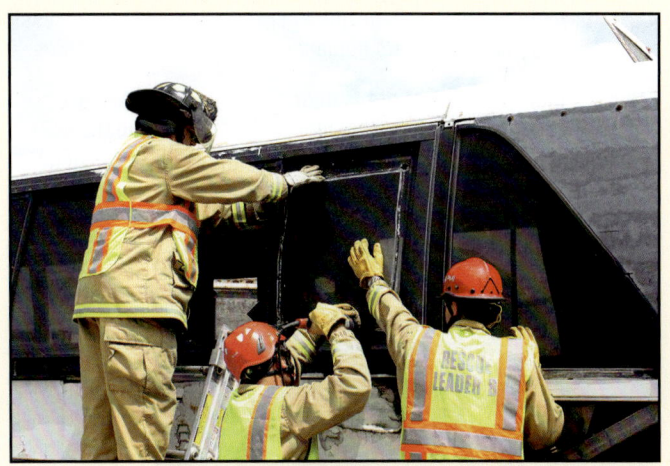

Step 6: Cut bottom side of glass to connect each vertical side cut.

Step 7: Remove the glass and position it away from the rescue scene.

Section C • Chapter 8 – Victim Disentanglement and Extrication

SKILL SHEETS

8-6
Open a door with a manually operated Hi-Lift® jack.

> **WARNING:** Rescuers must ensure that the vehicle is properly stabilized and the scene is safe.

> **CAUTION:** Rescuers must take necessary precautions to protect themselves and victims from hazards including, but not limited to, glass fragments and dust, jagged metal, SRS gas cylinders, undeployed airbags, and fire hazards.

NOTE: Only use Hi-Lift® jacks that are designed for and dedicated to extrication tasks. In this method, the jack is inverted in order to maintain the carriage and operating handle at an accessible level. Inspect and maintain all equipment according to local SOPs and manufacturer's guidelines.

Step 1: Maintain control of the door opening by deploying cribbing or lashing the door to the adjacent post.

Step 2: If the window is framed with a solid frame attached to the door, separate the frame from the roof line, and cut or remove it.

Step 3: Place the jack's operating lever in the raised position.

NOTE: Place the jack's operating lever in the raised position prior to positioning the jack.

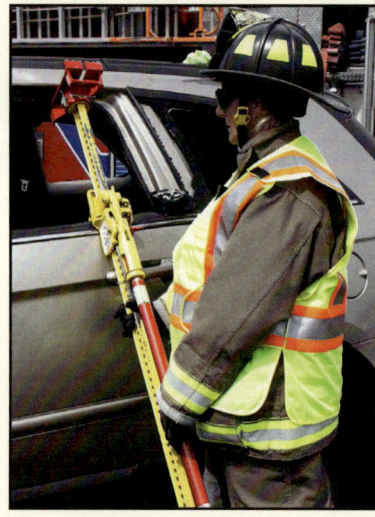

Step 4: Place the base of the jack on the upper section of the door at the roof line.

Step 5: Move the jack to a position over the latching mechanism.

Step 6: Place the carriage of the jack in position for it to "grab" the inner panel/skin of the door.

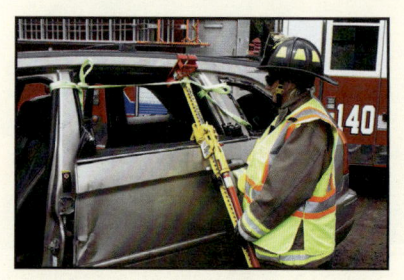

Step 7: Secure the main bar of the jack toward the base plate with 1 inch (25 mm) tubular rescue quality webbing. Secure one end of the webbing around the posts on either side of the door. Monitor each end of the webbing.

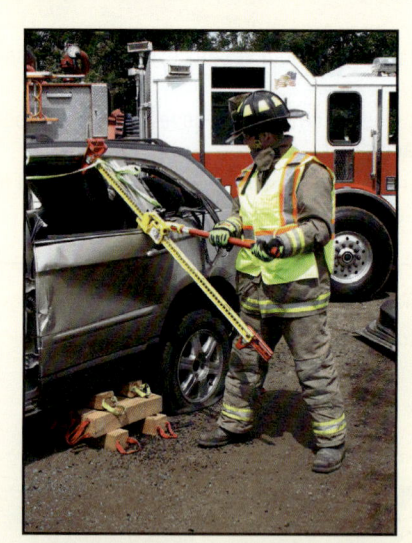

Step 8: Operate the jack to push the door down and off the latching mechanism.

NOTE: Look for opportunities to free the pin or latching mechanism during this operation.

8-7
Open or remove a door with a power ratchet, power impact wrench, or manual socket set.

> **WARNING:** Rescuers must ensure that the vehicle is properly stabilized and the scene is safe.

> **CAUTION:** Rescuers must take necessary precautions to protect themselves and victims from hazards including, but not limited to, glass fragments and dust, jagged metal, SRS gas cylinders, undeployed airbags, and fire hazards.

NOTE: Inspect and maintain all equipment according to local SOPs and manufacturer's guidelines.

Step 1: Gain access to hinge side of the door.

Step 2: Identify how the door hinges are bolted onto or attached to the post. If the hinge is bolted to the post, determine the bolt head size.

Step 3: Select the appropriate socket size and the appropriate type of socket.

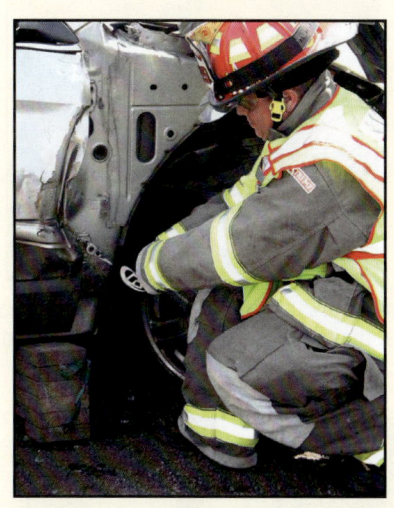

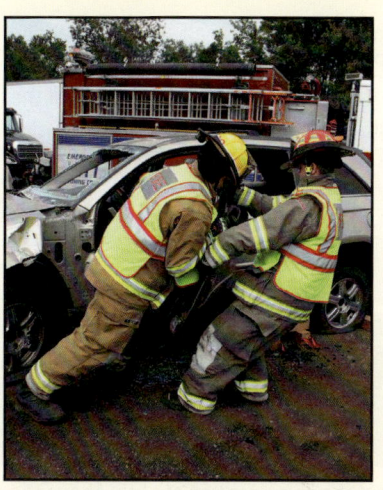

b. If the door does not release from the latching mechanism, it may be necessary to bend the door back away from the victim using the latching mechanism as a hinge.

Step 4: Attempt to unscrew the bolt to release the hinge from the post.
    a. If bolts will loosen, remove them.
    b. If the bolts will not loosen, attempt to snap them off by over-tightening them.

Step 5: Attempt to open the door latch mechanism to release the door from the latching mechanism.
    a. If the door latch mechanism works, remove door.

Section C • Chapter 8 – Victim Disentanglement and Extrication   **315**

SKILL SHEETS

8-8
Open or remove a door with hydraulic tools.

WARNING: Rescuers must ensure that the vehicle is properly stabilized and the scene is safe.

CAUTION: Rescuers must take necessary precautions to protect themselves and victims from hazards including, but not limited to, glass fragments and dust, jagged metal, SRS gas cylinders, undeployed airbags, and fire hazards.

NOTE: Inspect and maintain all equipment according to local SOPs and manufacturer's guidelines.

Step 1: Create a purchase point at the edge of the door near the latch.

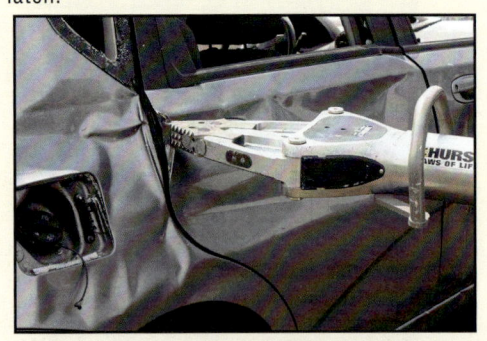

Step 2: Insert the spreader tips slightly above the door lock in such a position that they will push the door outward.

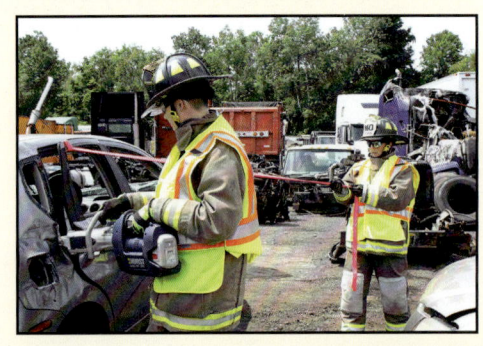

Step 3: Maintain control of the door using equipment such as a strap, rope, chain, or webbing in order to prevent the door from striking anyone.

Step 4: Open the spreader arms until the door opens.

NOTE: It may be necessary to reposition the spreader tips in order to free the latching mechanism. If door materials begin to tear, cutters may be necessary to complete the operation.

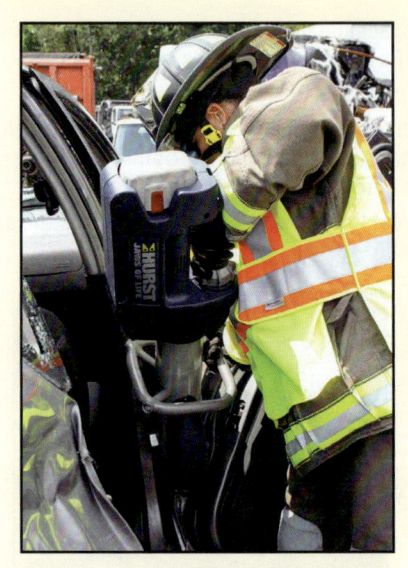

Step 5: Insert spreader tips at the hinges in such a position that they will force the door down and away from victims and rescue personnel.

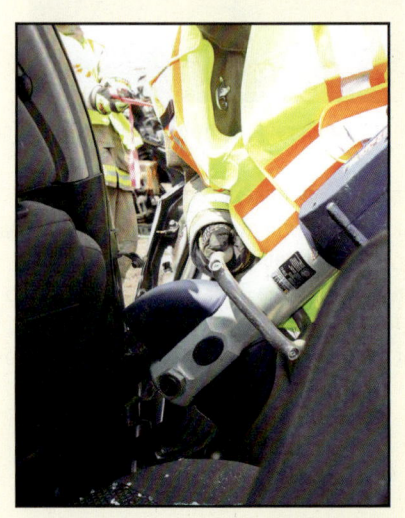

Step 6: Open the spreaders until the first hinge fails or can be cut.

Step 7: If the top hinge was addressed first and the tool is properly positioned, attempt to break the second hinge without repositioning. If not possible, reposition the tool and spread to break the bottom hinge.

Step 8: If the bottom hinge was addressed first, reposition the spreaders above the top hinge and open the spreaders until the top hinge fails or can be cut.

NOTE: On vehicles with pressed metal hinges, it may be quicker to cut the hinges as opposed to spreading them.

Step 9: Remove the door.

316   Section C • Chapter 8 – Victim Disentanglement and Extrication

8-9 Remove a sliding side door.

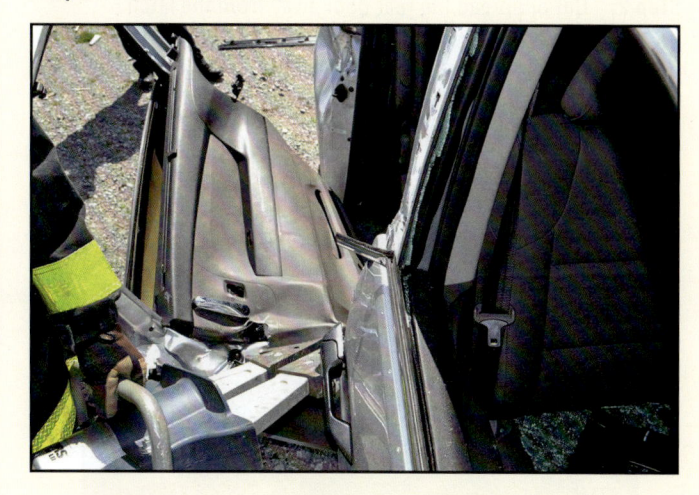

SKILL SHEETS

WARNING: Rescuers must ensure that the vehicle is properly stabilized and the scene is safe.

CAUTION: Rescuers must take necessary precautions to protect themselves and victims from hazards including, but not limited to, glass fragments and dust, jagged metal, SRS gas cylinders, undeployed airbags, and fire hazards.

NOTE: Inspect and maintain all equipment according to local SOPs and manufacturer's guidelines.

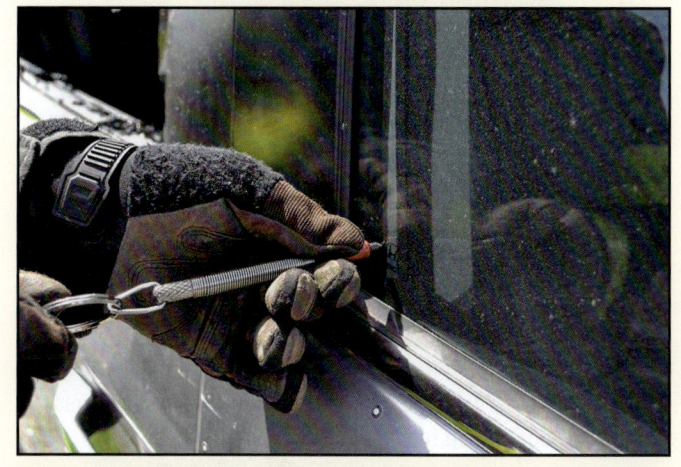

Step 1: Remove glass.

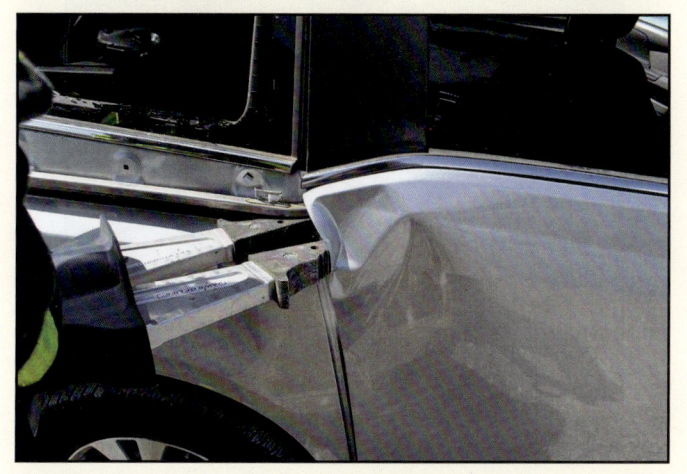

Step 2: Create a purchase point at the rear edge of the sliding side door.

Step 3: Spread the rear edge of the sliding side door outward.

Step 4: Create a purchase point at the front edge of the sliding side door.

Step 5: Spread the door outward and rearward so that the sliding brackets and hinges release the door from the side body of the van.

Step 6: Remove the door.

Section C • Chapter 8 – Victim Disentanglement and Extrication 317

SKILL SHEETS

8-10
Remove the side of a vehicle (total sidewall removal).

> **WARNING:** Rescuers must ensure that the vehicle is properly stabilized and the scene is safe.

> **CAUTION:** Rescuers must take necessary precautions to protect themselves and victims from hazards including, but not limited to, glass fragments and dust, jagged metal, SRS gas cylinders, undeployed airbags, and fire hazards.

NOTE: Inspect and maintain all equipment according to local SOPs and manufacturer's guidelines.

Step 1: Create a purchase point to access the latch on rear door.
Step 2: Cut or spread the rear door away from the latch.
Step 3: Identify location of seat belt pretensioner.
Step 4: Cut seatbelts and disentangle any seatbelt webbing from attachment points on the vehicle.
Step 5: Cut the B-post above or below the pretensioner, preferably below the bottom door hinge.
Step 6: Position the spreaders between the rocker panel and the base of the rear door on the hinge side of the door.
Step 7: Operate spreaders until the base of the B-post separates from the rocker panel.
Step 8: Cut the top of the B-post at the roofline, enabling the entire side to pivot on the front door or A-post hinges.
Step 9: Cut or spread the front two hinges.
Step 10: Remove the sidewall.

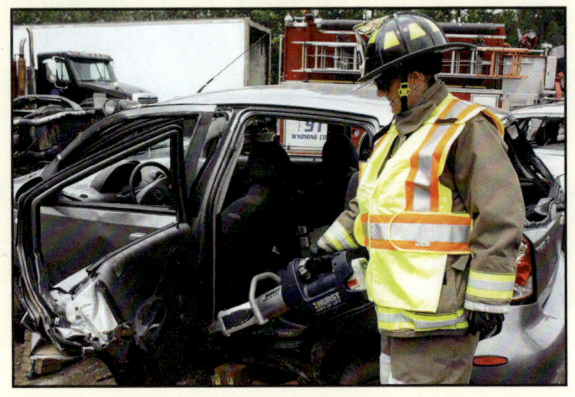

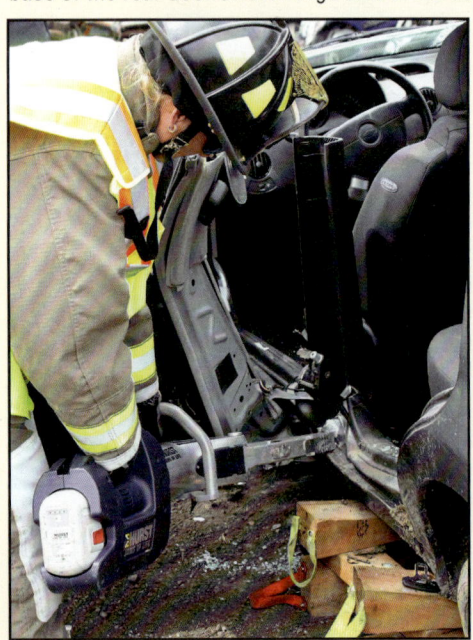

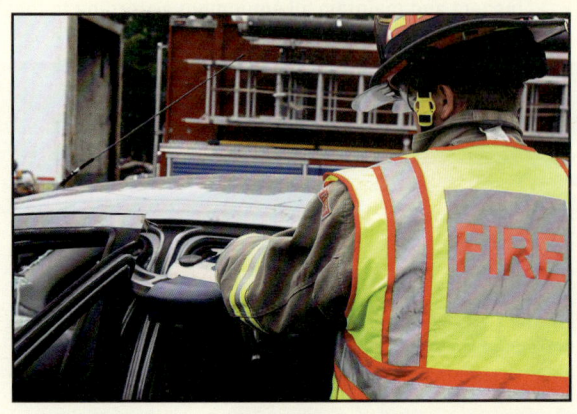

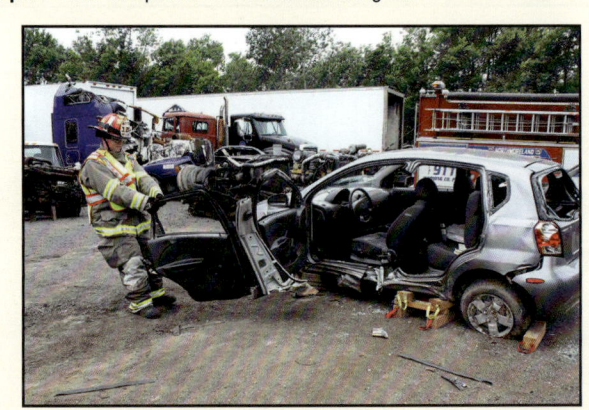

318   Section C • Chapter 8 – Victim Disentanglement and Extrication

8-11
Create an alternate (third-door) opening in a two-door vehicle.

> **WARNING:** Rescuers must ensure that the vehicle is properly stabilized and the scene is safe.

> **CAUTION:** Rescuers must take necessary precautions to protect themselves and victims from hazards including, but not limited to, glass fragments and dust, jagged metal, SRS gas cylinders, undeployed airbags, and fire hazards.

NOTE: Inspect and maintain all equipment according to local SOPs and manufacturer's guidelines.

Step 1: Remove glass.

Step 2: Make a vertical cut from the lower rear corner of the rear side window down as far as the cutter will go.

NOTE: If using a reciprocating saw or air chisel, the cut may be continued to the rocker panel.

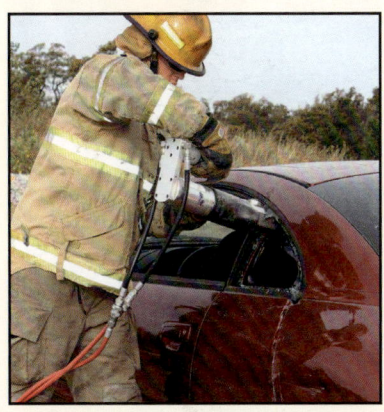

Step 3: Cut the B-post at the roofline.

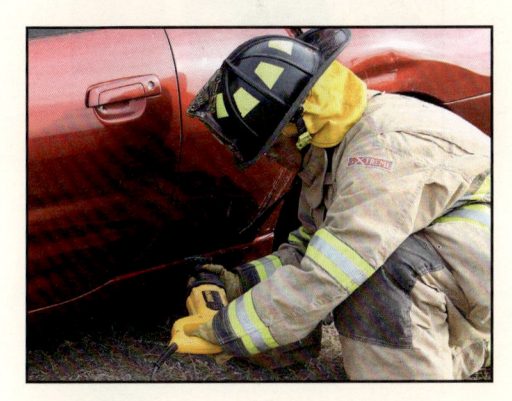

Step 4: Make a flat cut along the rocker panel into the lower B-post.

NOTE: Additional cuts may be necessary.

Step 5: Position the spreaders at either the lower rear corner of the window or between roof rail and the bottom window rail.

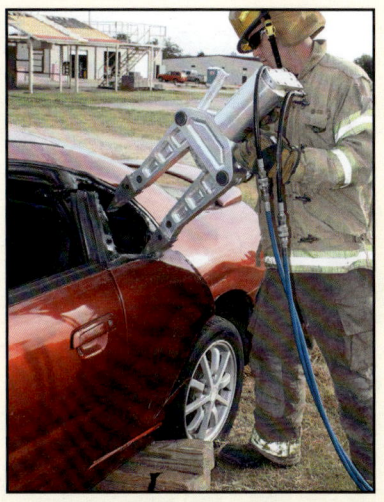

Step 6: Operate the spreaders to displace the sidewall downward and away from the vehicle. If the roof is already removed, slowly pry the section down without moving the vehicle.

NOTE: As an alternative, a reciprocating saw or air chisel may be used to cut the entire section out. If using the reciprocating saw or air chisel, second cuts may be needed behind the exterior cuts due to the separate walls of the vehicle.

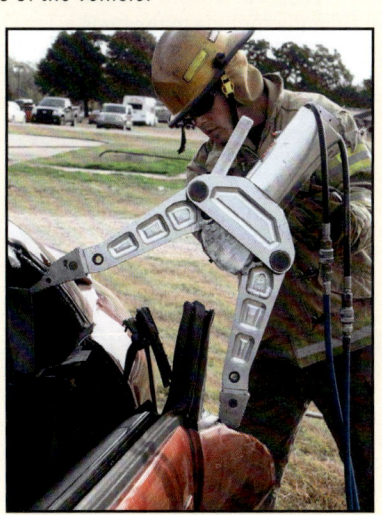

Section C • Chapter 8 – Victim Disentanglement and Extrication

SKILL SHEETS

8-12

Create an alternate (fourth-door) opening in a vehicle (such as a panel van).

> **WARNING:** Rescuers must ensure that the vehicle is properly stabilized and the scene is safe.

> **CAUTION:** Rescuers must take necessary precautions to protect themselves and victims from hazards including, but not limited to, glass fragments and dust, jagged metal, SRS gas cylinders, undeployed airbags, and fire hazards.

NOTE: Inspect and maintain all equipment according to local SOPs and manufacturer's guidelines.

Step 1: Remove glass.

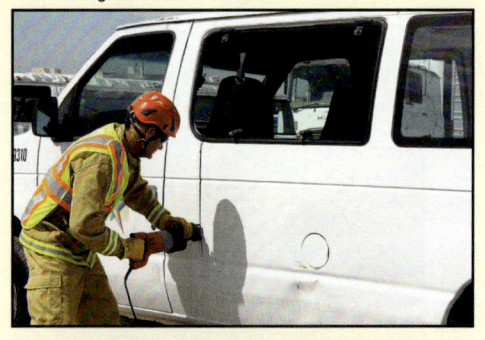

Step 2: Make a vertical cut behind the B-post in the side body panel from the roofline to the floor.

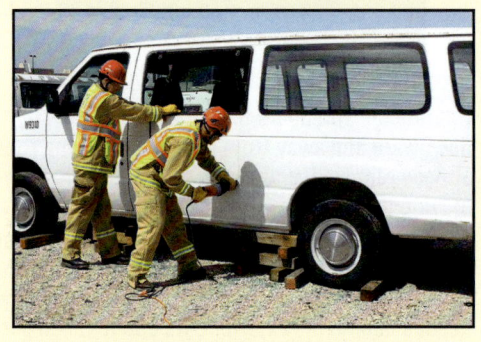

Step 3: Make a vertical cut in front of the C-post in the side body panel from the roofline to the floor.

Step 4: Make a horizontal cut that joins the vertical cuts.

Step 5: Spread the panel down and out or proceed with total removal.

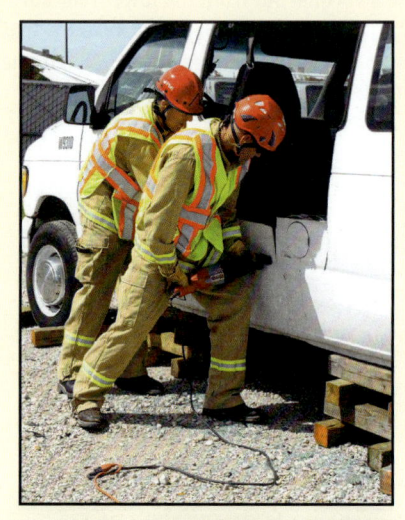

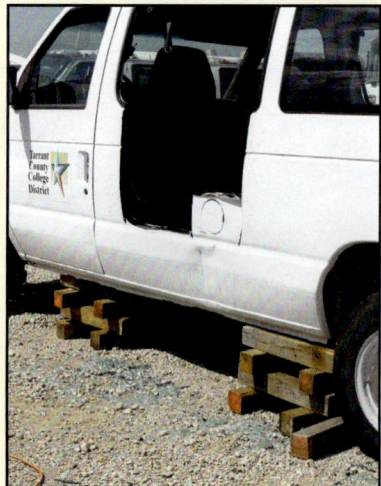

Step 6: For total removal, make a horizontal cut along the rocker panel that joins the vertical cuts, and then remove the panel.

320   Section C • Chapter 8 – Victim Disentanglement and Extrication

8-13
Remove the roof of a wheel-resting passenger vehicle.

SKILL SHEETS

> **WARNING:** Always peel back the interior trim along the roof rails and all posts to expose supplemental restraint system compressed gas cylinders. If accidentally cut, these devices can cause severe injury and death. All undeployed airbags must be considered live. Ensure that the vehicle is properly stabilized and the scene is safe.

> **CAUTION:** Rescuers must take necessary precautions to protect themselves and victims from hazards including, but not limited to, glass fragments and dust, jagged metal, SRS gas cylinders, undeployed airbags, and fire hazards.

NOTE: Damage to the vehicle and victim location will dictate the order in which the posts are cut. Inspect and maintain all equipment according to local SOPs and manufacturer's guidelines.

Step 1: Remove glass.

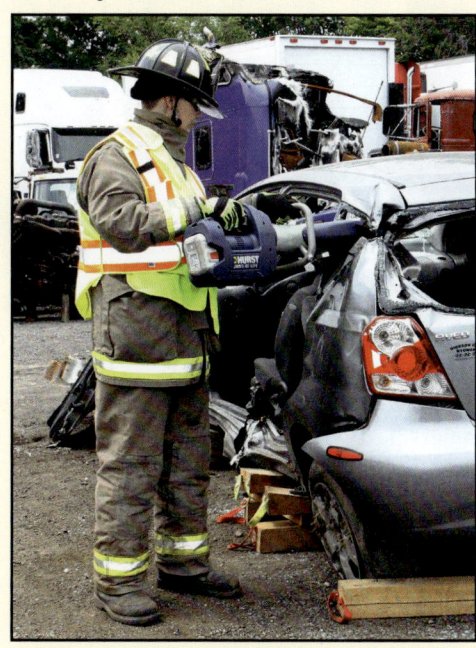

Step 2: Cut the first post at the furthest point from the victim.

Step 3: Cut remaining posts, with the final cut on the post closest to the victim. Support the roof throughout the removal.

Step 4: If the posts are too large to place the cutters, use one of the following removal methods.

   a. Cut a triangular section from one side of the post. Remove the triangular section and reinsert the cutters, allowing the blades to be inserted deeper to make additional cuts.

   b. Cut one side of the post, then position the cutters on the other side of the post and make a second cut that joins the initial cut.

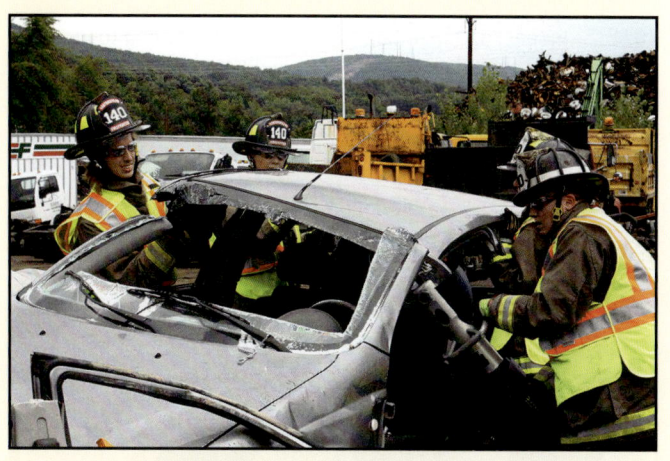

   c. Compress the post with spreaders, compacting it into a smaller size. This may allow the cutters to cut the post in one try.

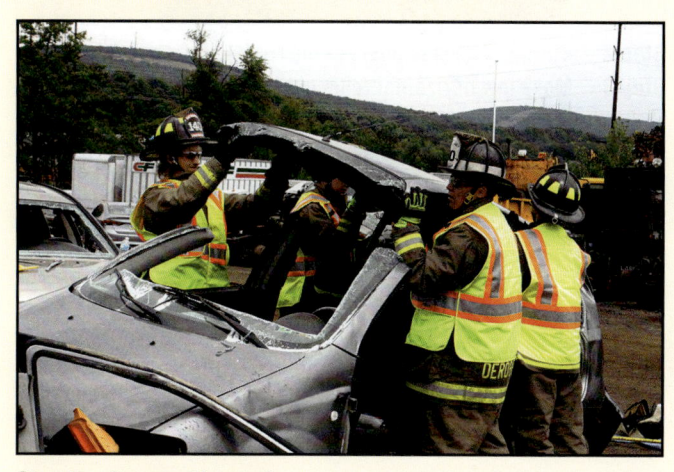

Step 5: Remove the roof.

Section C • Chapter 8 – Victim Disentanglement and Extrication

SKILL SHEETS

8-14
Flap or remove the roof of a side-resting passenger vehicle.

WARNING: Always peel back the interior trim along the roof rails and all posts to expose supplemental restraint system compressed gas cylinders. If accidentally cut, these devices can cause severe injury and death. All undeployed airbags must be considered live. Ensure that the vehicle is properly stabilized and the scene is safe.

CAUTION: Rescuers must wear full PPE including hand, eye, and respiratory protection. Protect vehicle occupants from glass and dust fragments.

NOTE: Inspect and maintain all equipment according to local SOPs and manufacturer's guidelines.

Step 1: Remove glass.

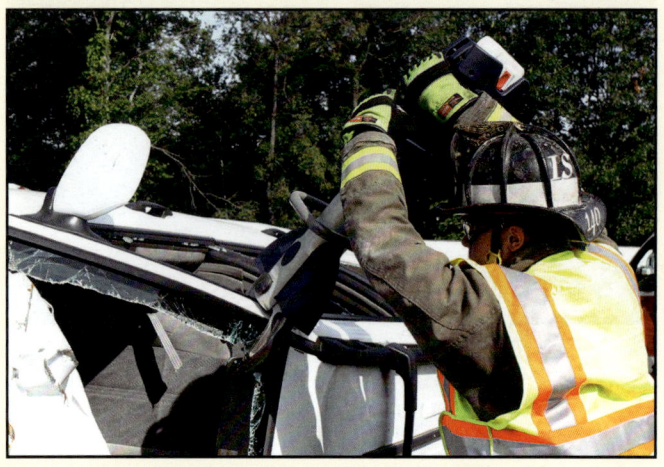

Step 2: Cut the high side posts at the roof line.

Step 3: Make low horizontal relief cuts at the front and rear of the lower roof posts.

Step 4: Place cribbing between the roof and surface below as needed to support the roof.

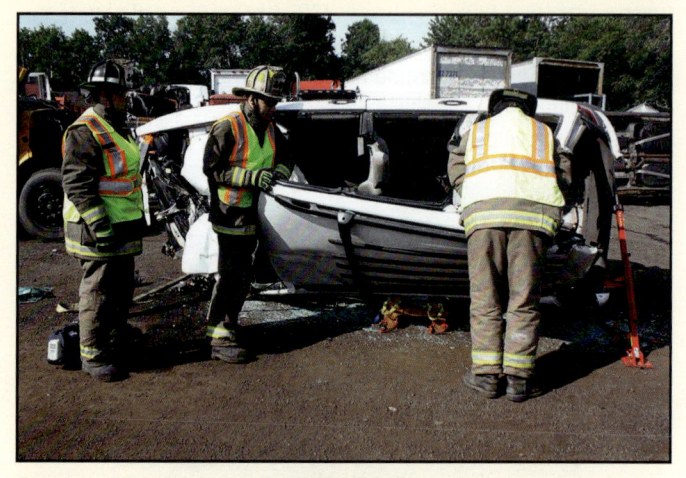

Step 5: Flap the roof outward and down, making deeper or additional relief cuts if needed.

Step 6: For total roof removal, cut through lower posts and remove the roof.

322 Section C • Chapter 8 – Victim Disentanglement and Extrication

8-15
Create an access opening in the roof of a side-resting passenger vehicle.

WARNING: Rescuers must ensure that the vehicle is properly stabilized and the scene is safe.

CAUTION: Rescuers must take necessary precautions to protect themselves and victims from hazards including, but not limited to, glass fragments and dust, jagged metal, SRS gas cylinders, undeployed airbags, and fire hazards.

NOTE: Inspect and maintain all equipment according to local SOPs and manufacturer's guidelines.

Step 1: Create a purchase point near the top of the roof on one side of the vehicle.

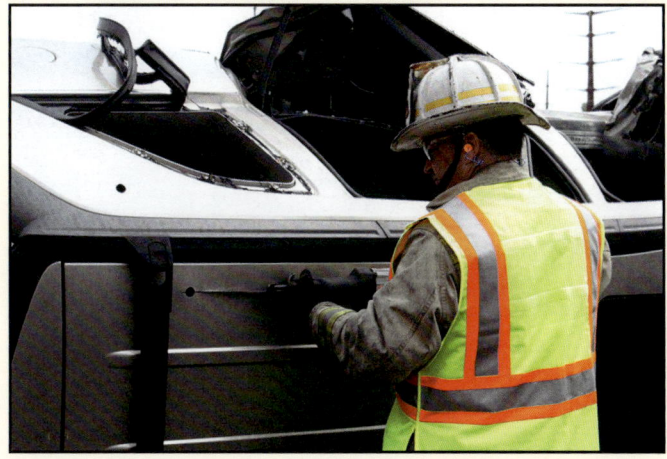

Step 2: Insert the cutting tool into the purchase point and cut horizontally across the top of the roof.

Step 3: Make a vertical cut from the end of the horizontal cut to the bottom of the roof.

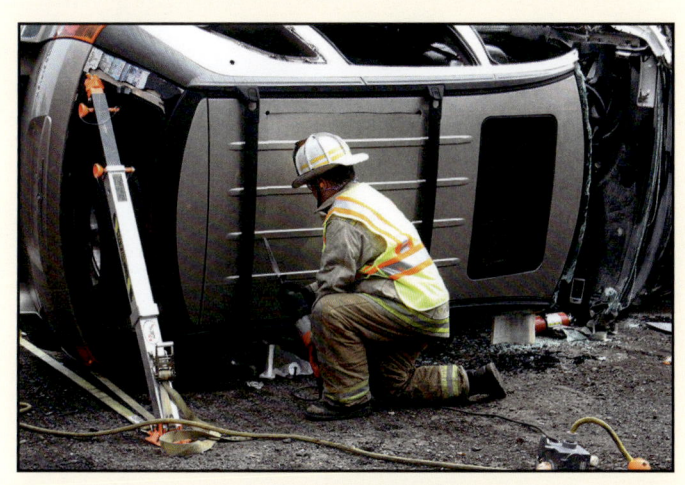

Step 4: Make a second vertical cut from the point of the original purchase point to the bottom of the roof.

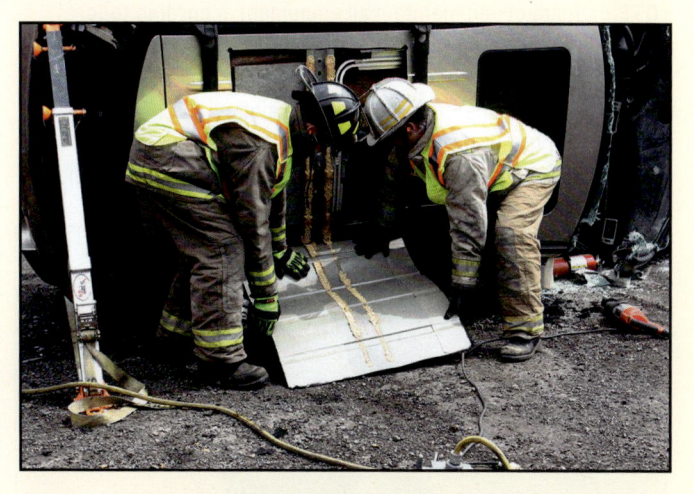

Step 5: Fold the roof panel down to the ground. Remove the headliner and any remaining roof members.

Step 6: To completely remove the flap, make a horizontal cut across the bottom of the roof that joins the two vertical cuts.

SKILL SHEETS

8-16
Remove the kick panel of a passenger vehicle.

WARNING: Rescuers must ensure that the vehicle is properly stabilized and the scene is safe.

CAUTION: Rescuers must take necessary precautions to protect themselves and victims from hazards including, but not limited to, glass fragments and dust, jagged metal, SRS gas cylinders, undeployed airbags, and fire hazards. Do not cut the Engine Control Module (ECM).

NOTE: Inspect and maintain all equipment according to local SOPs and manufacturer's guidelines.

Step 1: Remove the door.
Step 2: Remove the front fender, if possible.
Step 3: Cut through the base of the A-post.
Step 4: Make a relief cut in the A-post at the dashboard level.

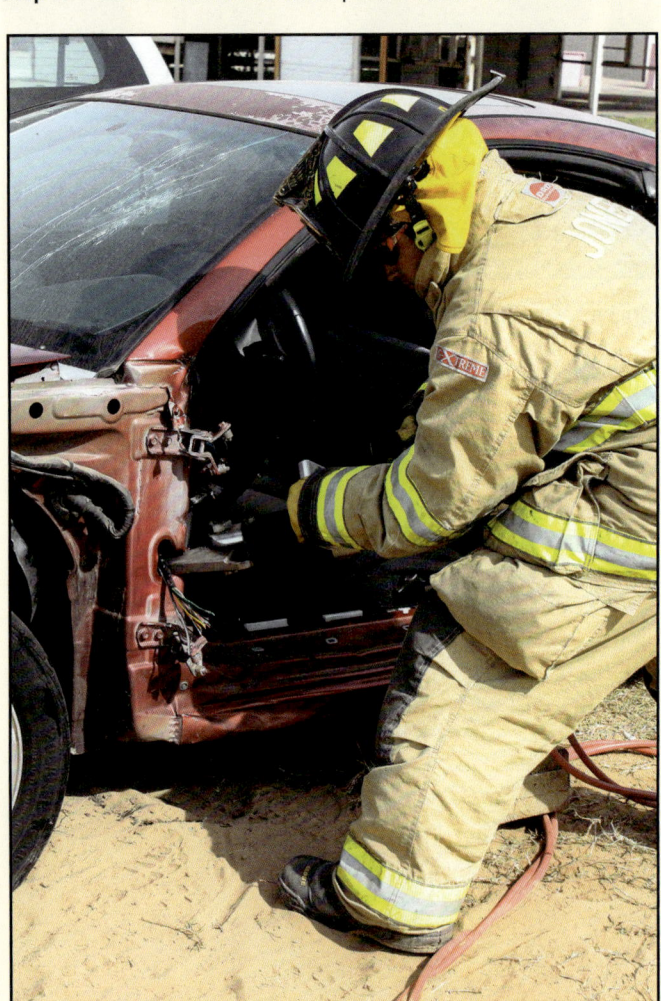

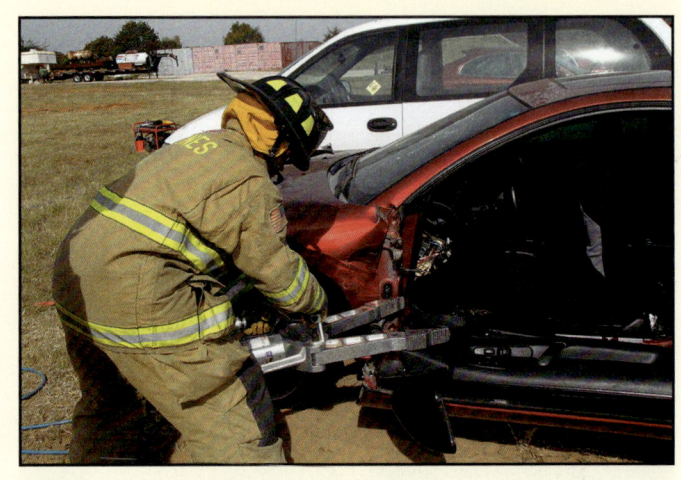

Step 6: Use the spreaders to fold the kick panel upward or to the side to expose the foot well area.

Step 5: If the fender was not removed, cut the kick panel from the base of the A-post forward to the wheel well and vertically to the level of the top door hinge.

324 Section C • Chapter 8 – Victim Disentanglement and Extrication

8-17
Create an access opening through the floor of a roof-resting passenger vehicle.

WARNING: Rescuers must ensure that the vehicle is properly stabilized and the scene is safe.

CAUTION: Rescuers must take necessary precautions to protect themselves and victims from hazards including, but not limited to, glass fragments and dust, jagged metal, SRS gas cylinders, undeployed airbags, and fire hazards.

NOTE: Inspect and maintain all equipment according to local SOPs and manufacturer's guidelines.

Method 1

Step 1: Mark an area approximately 2 x 2 feet (600 x 600 mm) over the rear foot well between the rocker panel on unibody vehicles or the inside of the frame vehicles and the centerline of the vehicle.

Step 2: Create purchase points at the corners of the square, if necessary.

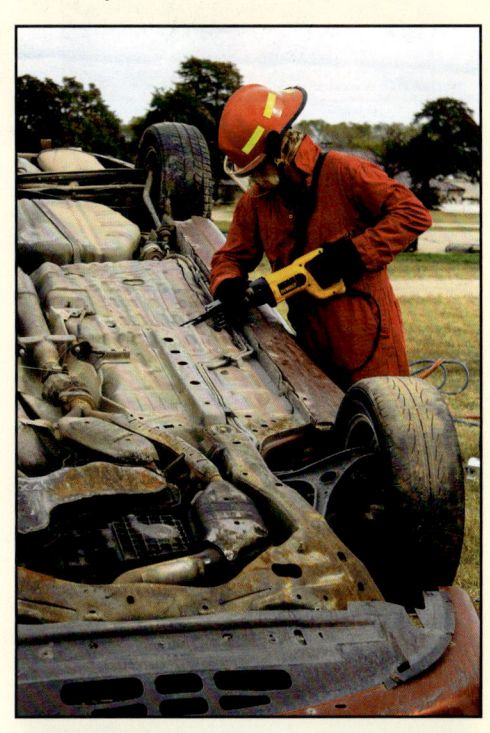

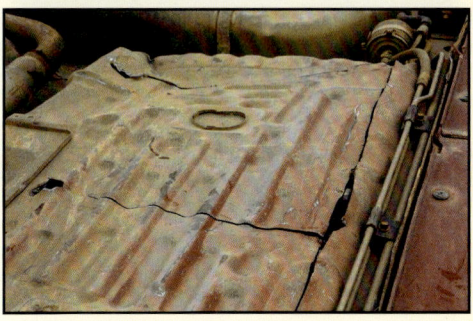

Step 3: Cut three sides of the marked square.

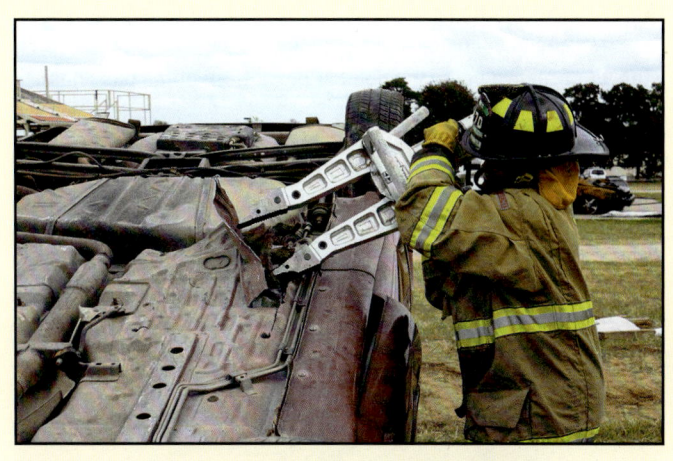

Step 4: Bend the flap to allow access to the interior.

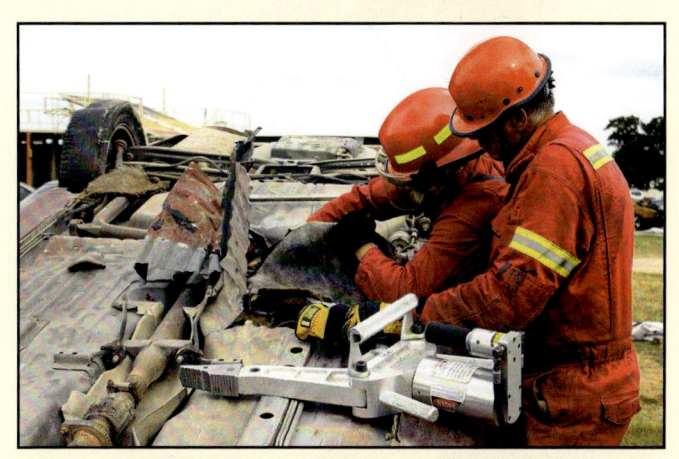

Step 5: Pull or cut away any interior floor coverings in the area of the access opening.

Section C • Chapter 8 – Victim Disentanglement and Extrication

SKILL SHEETS

8-17

Create an access opening through the floor of a roof-resting passenger vehicle.

WARNING: Rescuers must ensure that the vehicle is properly stabilized and the scene is safe.

CAUTION: Rescuers must take necessary precautions to protect themselves and victims from hazards including, but not limited to, glass fragments and dust, jagged metal, SRS gas cylinders, undeployed airbags, and fire hazards.

Method 2

NOTE: This method can only be used on unibody vehicles with an unoccupied front passenger seat.

Step 1: Create a purchase point at the bottom of the passenger door.

Step 2: Insert the spreader tips and pry the bottom of the door as far away from the rocker panel as possible.

NOTE: The opening must be large enough to allow the blade of an open cutter to be inserted.

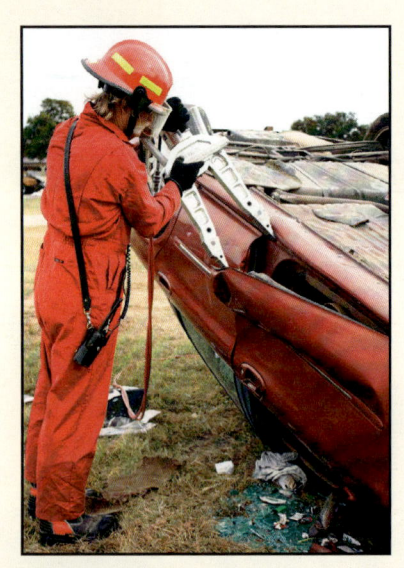

Step 3: Insert the cutter blades into the void between the door and rocker panel.

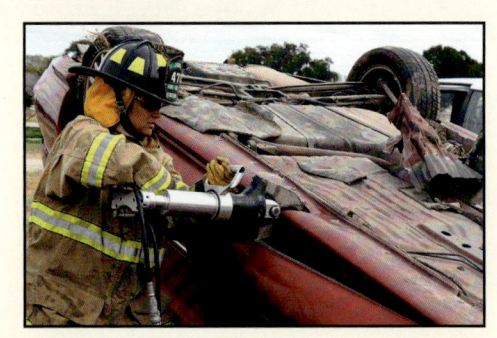

Step 4: Cut through the rocker panel at a point near the A-post and at a point near the B-post.

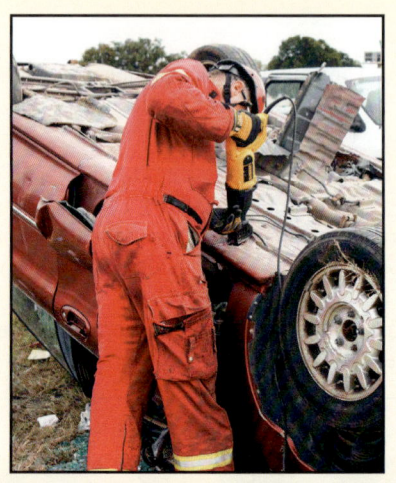

Step 5: Using a reciprocating saw, extend the cuts toward the centerline of the vehicle.

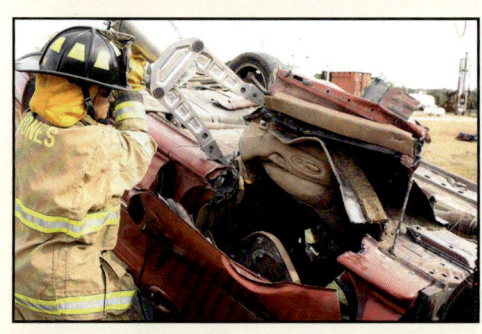

Step 6: Lift the flap of the floorboard with the passenger seat attached and fold it toward the centerline of the vehicle.

NOTE: It may be necessary to cut the seatback from the passenger seat as it is being rotated out of the vehicle.

326   Section C • Chapter 8 – Victim Disentanglement and Extrication

8-18
Tunnel through a trunk.

WARNING: Rescuers must ensure that the vehicle is properly stabilized and the scene is safe.

CAUTION: Rescuers must take necessary precautions to protect themselves and victims from hazards including, but not limited to, glass fragments and dust, jagged metal, SRS gas cylinders, undeployed airbags, and fire hazards.

NOTE: Inspect and maintain all equipment according to local SOPs and manufacturer's guidelines.

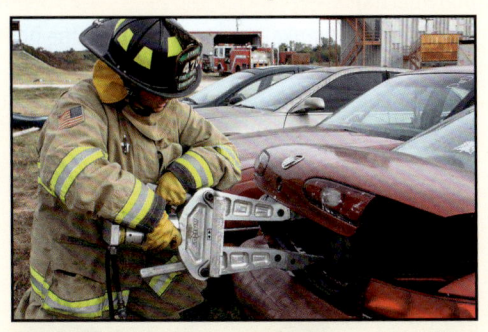

Step 1: Open and remove the trunk lid.

CAUTION: The trunk may contain a variety of hazards.

Step 2: Remove the contents of the trunk.

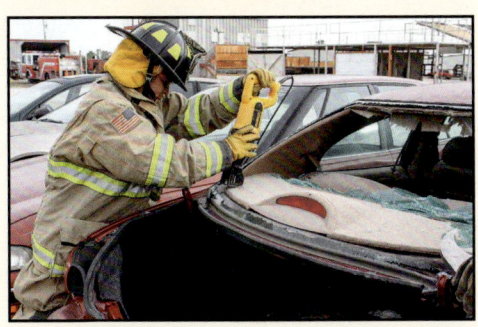

Step 3: Cut and remove the deck lid and support structures to allow sufficient access to the passenger compartment.

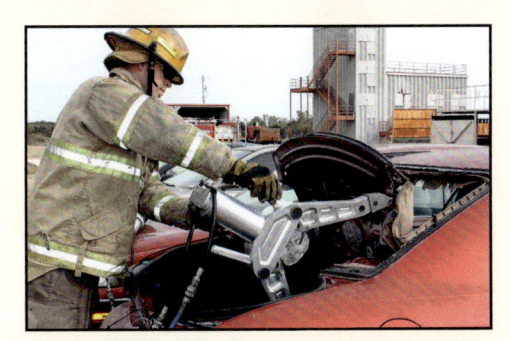

Step 4: Remove the seat back by pushing it into the passenger compartment or pulling it out through the trunk opening, if possible.

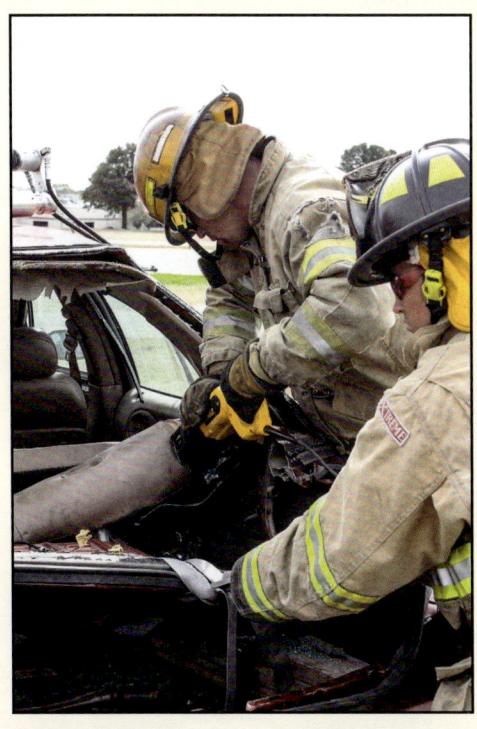

Step 5: Make entry into the passenger compartment.
Step 6: Remove or cover any objects that may interfere with victim care and removal.

Section C • Chapter 8 – Victim Disentanglement and Extrication

SKILL SHEETS

8-19
Remove a windshield from around a victim.

WARNING: Rescuers must ensure that the vehicle is properly stabilized and the scene is safe.

CAUTION: Rescuers must take necessary precautions to protect themselves and victims from hazards including, but not limited to, glass fragments and dust, jagged metal, SRS gas cylinders, undeployed airbags, and fire hazards.

Pulling Glass

Step 1: Stabilize the weight of the victim's body and protruding body part(s).

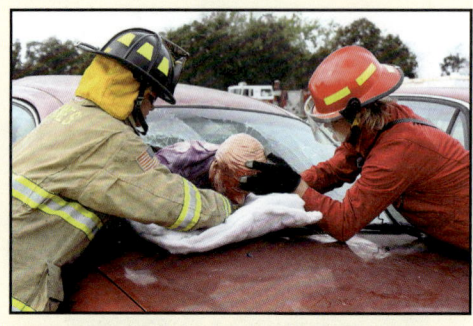

Step 2: Work a towel, blanket, or sheet between the body part(s) and the windshield.

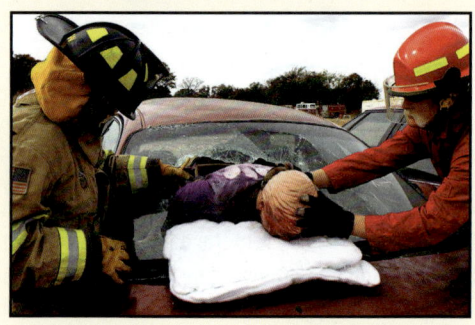

Step 3: Pull glass from around the body part(s) using pliers or another suitable tool, creating a space between the body part(s) and glass that is large enough for the impaled part(s) to travel through.

NOTE: It may also be necessary to cut the plastic laminated sheet away using tin snips or shears.

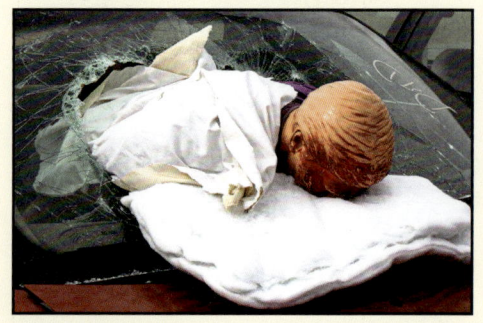

Step 4: Pad any adjacent sharp edges.

Step 5: Carefully move the body part(s) back through the windshield under the supervision of EMS personnel.

Pulverizing Glass

Step 1: Stabilize the weight of the victim's body and protruding body part(s).

Step 2: Work a towel, blanket, or sheet between the body part(s) and the windshield.

Step 3: Place the face of one ball peen hammer on the inside of the windshield adjacent to the impaled body part.

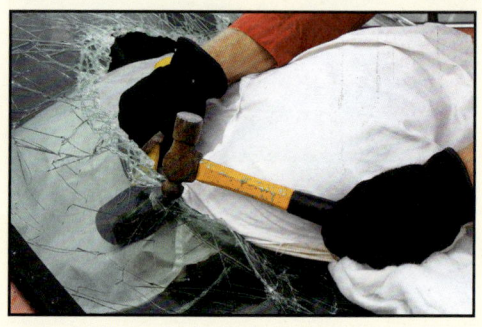

Step 4: Gently tap the outside of the glass (opposite of the hammer face on the inside) with the peen of a second hammer.

Step 5: Remove the plastic laminate, creating a space between the body part(s) and the glass that is large enough for the impaled part(s) to travel through.

Step 6: Pad any adjacent sharp edges.

Step 7: Carefully move the parts part(s) back through the windshield under the supervision of EMS personnel.

Section C • Chapter 8 – Victim Disentanglement and Extrication

8-20
Displace a steering column.

SKILL SHEETS

WARNING: Rescuers must ensure that the vehicle is properly stabilized and the scene is safe.

CAUTION: Rescuers must take necessary precautions to protect themselves and victims from hazards including, but not limited to, glass fragments and dust, jagged metal, SRS gas cylinders, undeployed airbags, and fire hazards.

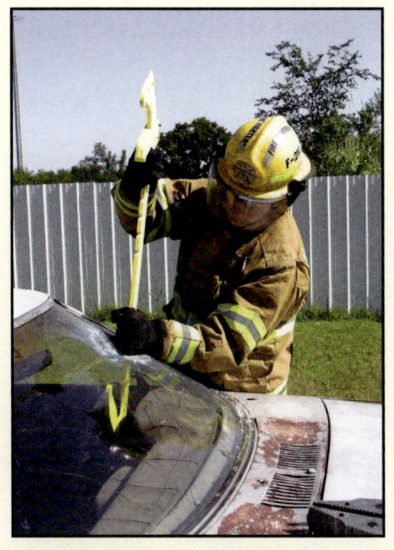

Step 1: Pierce the windshield above the steering column.

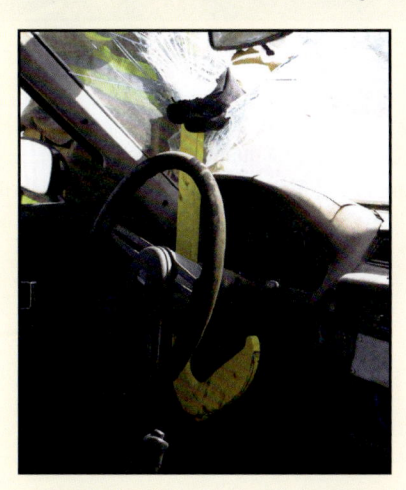

Step 2: Hook a rescue hook or wrap a chain around the steering column as close to the dash as possible.

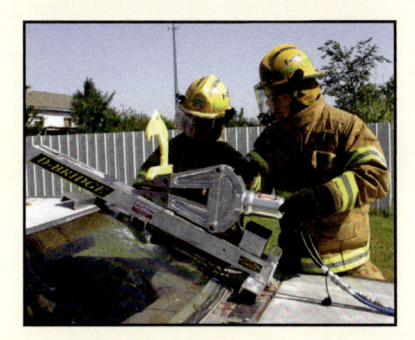

Step 3: Place a bridge device across the windshield, extending from the firewall to the top of the roof.

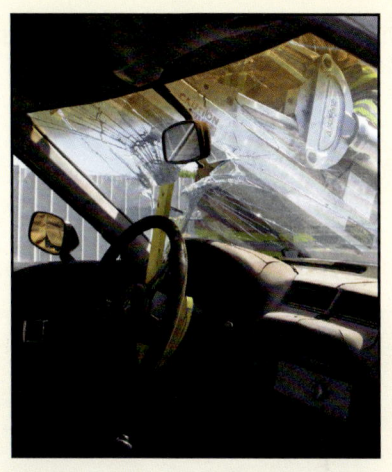

Step 4: Place a lifting device on the bridge in line with the steering column and dash.

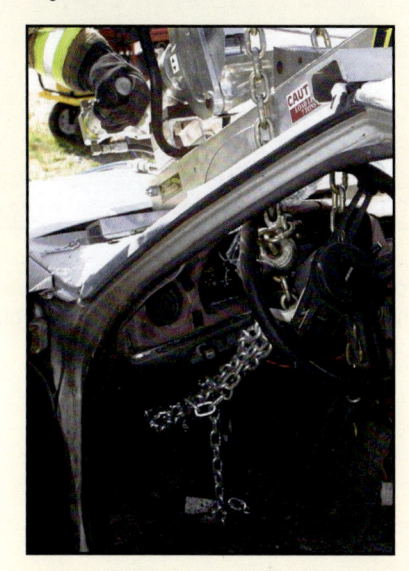

Step 5: Connect the hook or chain to the lifting device.
Step 6: Lift the steering column and wheel enough to create sufficient space for disentanglement.
NOTE: A piece of webbing can also be wrapped around the pedals to lift them at the same time.

Section C • Chapter 8 – Victim Disentanglement and Extrication

SKILL SHEETS

8-21
Displace a dashboard.

WARNING: Rescuers must ensure that the vehicle is properly stabilized and the scene is safe.

CAUTION: Rescuers must take necessary precautions to protect themselves and victims from hazards including, but not limited to, glass fragments and dust, jagged metal, SRS gas cylinders, undeployed airbags, and fire hazards.

NOTE: Additional cuts may be necessary, depending on the vehicle and incident situation.

Jacking or Lifting with Spreaders

Step 1: Remove the front door.
Step 2: Make relief cuts behind the strut mounts to eliminate movement of the front end of the vehicle.
Step 3: Cut the upper portion of the A-post if the roof is intact.

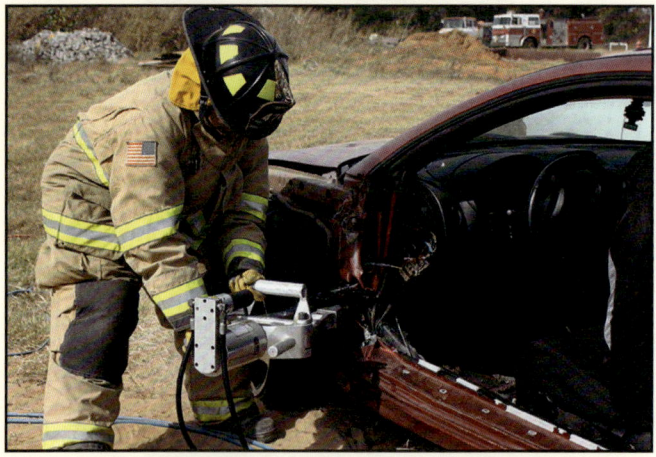

Step 4: Create a purchase point in the lower portion of the A-post large enough to accommodate the spreader tips to the desired depth. Create the purchase point between the door hinges, if possible.

Step 5: Place cribbing between the base of the A-post and the surface beneath.
Step 6: Insert spreader tips into the purchase point on the A-post.

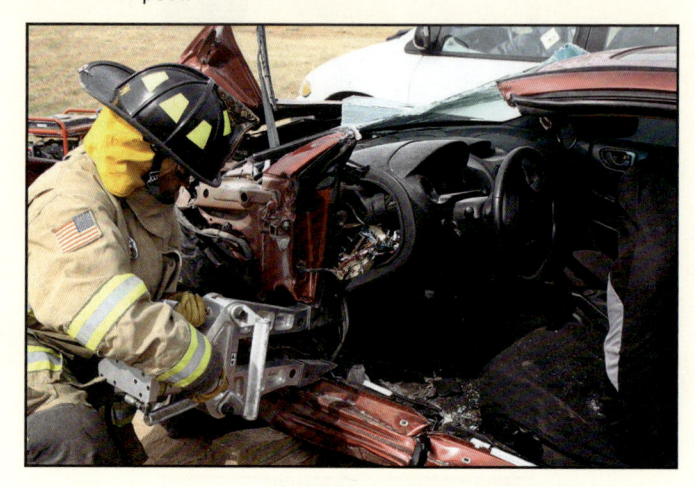

Step 7: Open spreaders to lift the dash until sufficient clearance is achieved while maintaining capture.
Step 8: Monitor and maintain the integrity of the cribbing.

8-21
Displace a dashboard.

SKILL SHEETS

Jacking or Lifting with Alternative Tools

Step 1: Remove the front door.
Step 2: Make relief cuts behind the strut mounts to eliminate movement of the front end of the vehicle.
Step 3: Cut the upper portion of the A-post if the roof is intact.

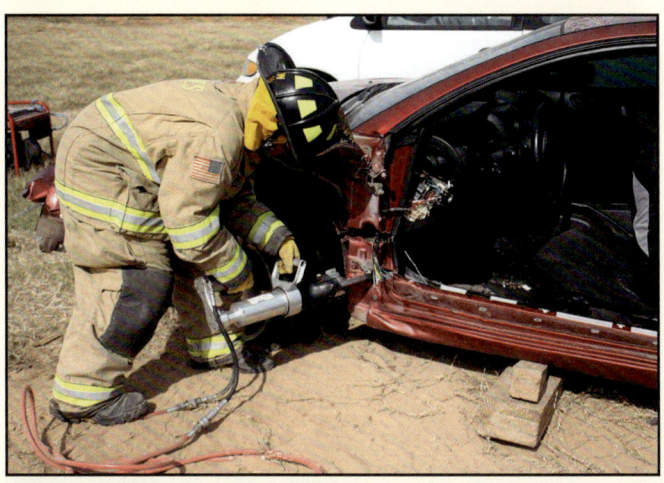

Step 4: Make one cut to the bottom of the A-post, as deep as possible.
Step 5: Place cribbing between the base of the A-post and the surface beneath.
Step 6: Position jacking or lifting device base on the rocker panel, supported by the cribbing.

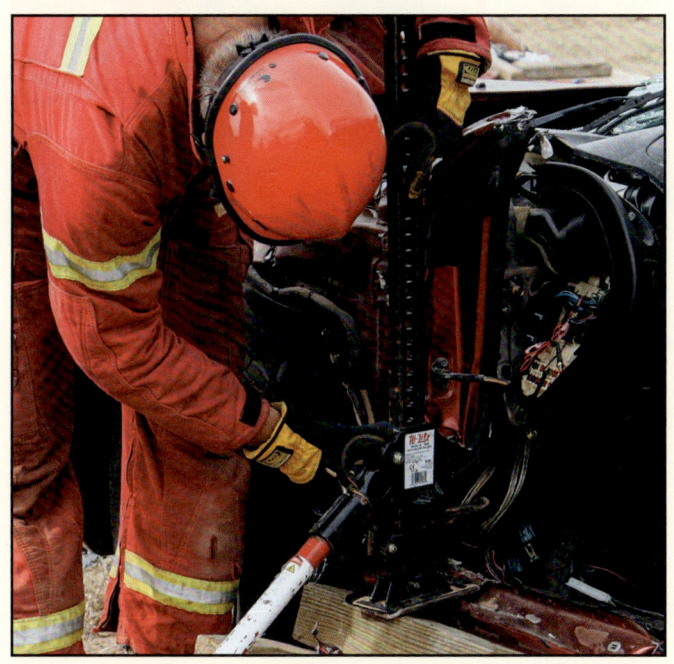

Step 7: Place the working end of the jacking or lifting device on the remaining section of the A-post.
Step 8: Operate the tool until sufficient clearance is achieved.
Step 9: Monitor and maintain the integrity of the cribbing.

Pushing or Rolling a Dashboard

Step 1: Remove the front door.
Step 2: Make relief cuts behind the strut mounts to eliminate movement of the front end of the vehicle.

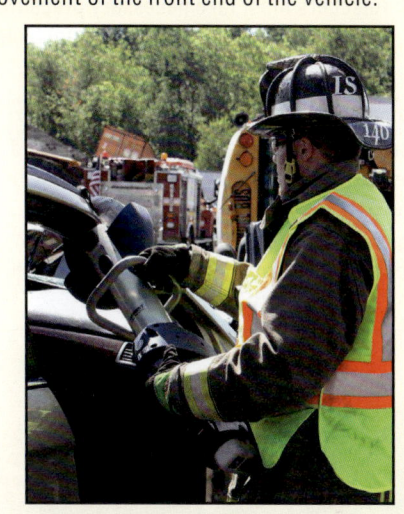

Step 3: Cut the upper portion of the A-post if the roof is still intact.
Step 4: Cut the bottom portion of the A-post, below the bottom door hinge if possible.
Step 5: Place cribbing between the rocker panel and the surface beneath.
Step 6: Position ram between base of the B-post and on an area just above the top hinge on the A-post.

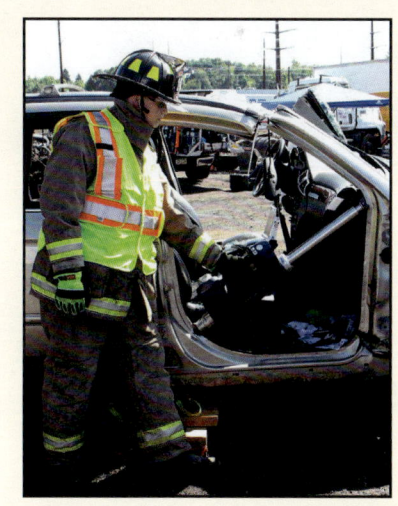

Step 7: Extend the ram to move the dash until sufficient clearance is achieved.
NOTE: Additional relief cuts may be needed during the operation. If tools need to be removed, a wedge can be placed within the void to prevent the return or lowering of the dash.

Section C • Chapter 8 – Victim Disentanglement and Extrication   331

SKILL SHEETS

8-22
Drop the floor pan of a vehicle.

WARNING: Rescuers must ensure that the vehicle is properly stabilized and the scene is safe.

CAUTION: Rescuers must take necessary precautions to protect themselves and victims from hazards including, but not limited to, glass fragments and dust, jagged metal, SRS gas cylinders, undeployed airbags, and fire hazards.

Step 1: Remove the door.

Step 2: Place cribbing between the rocker panel and the surface beneath in an area that will not restrict the downward travel of the floor pan.

Step 3: Create a purchase point in the lower portion of the A-post large enough to accommodate the spreader tips to the desired depth.

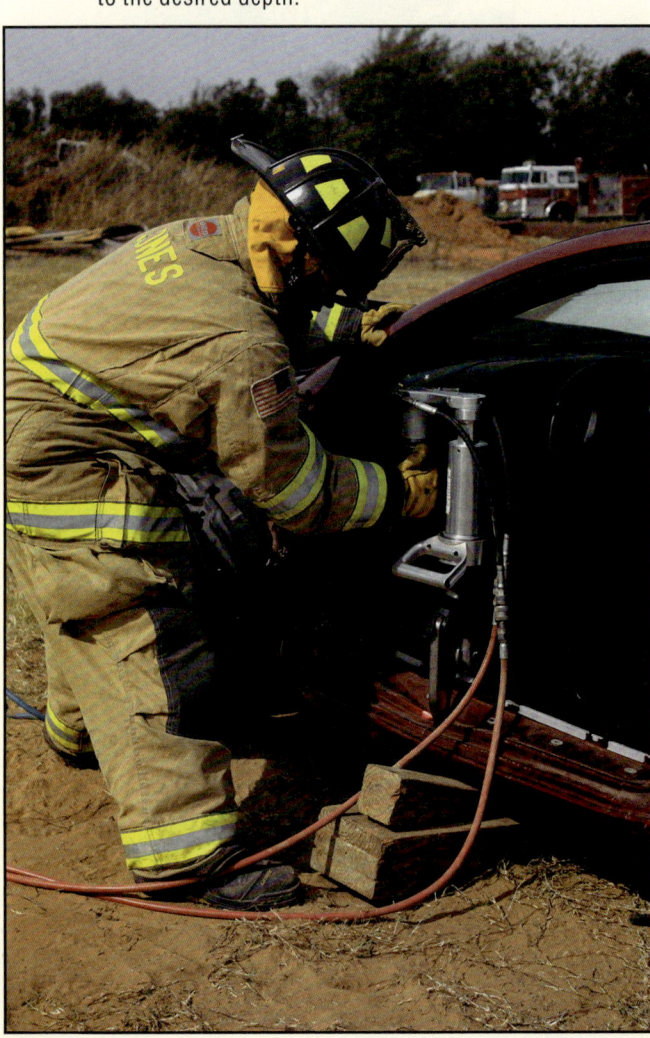

Step 4: Make a cut to the rocker panel parallel to the front of the seat.

Step 5: Insert spreader tips into the purchase point on the A-post.

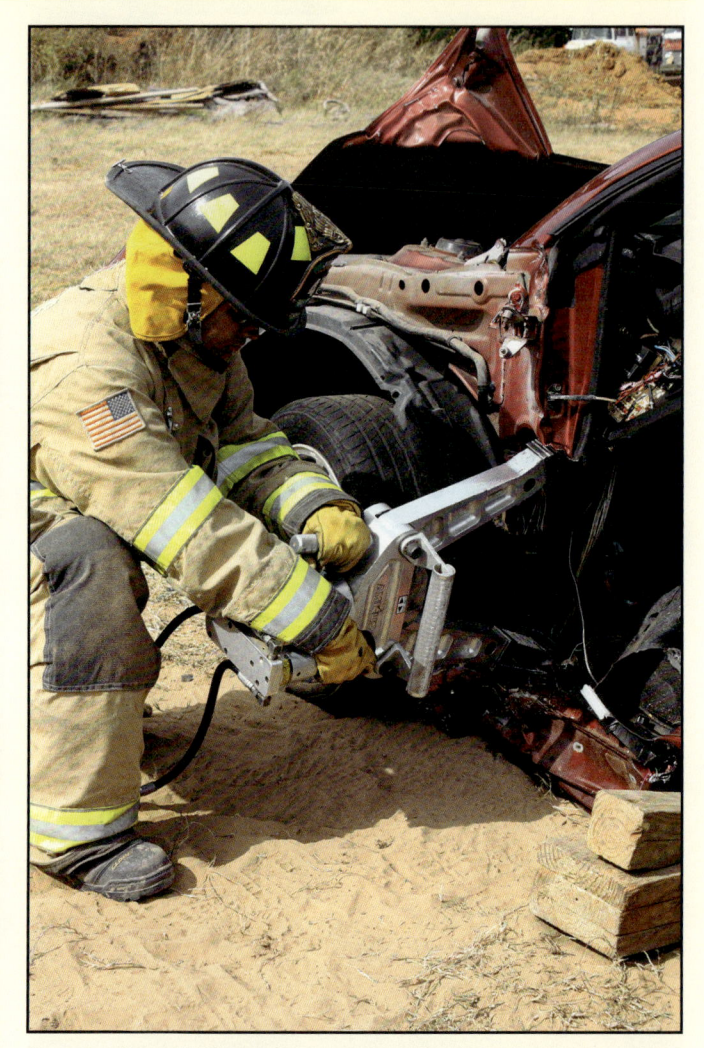

Step 6: Open the spreaders and push the floor down until sufficient clearance is achieved.

Step 7: Monitor and maintain integrity of the cribbing.

NOTE: If using other pushing devices such as rams or Hi-Lift® jacks, use the upper portion of the A-post or roof rail as the anchor point to push against, allowing the floor pan to be pushed downward. Additional cuts to the A-post, firewall area, and the floor pan may be required.

Section C • Chapter 8 – Victim Disentanglement and Extrication

8-23
Displace or remove a front seat in a vehicle.

> **WARNING:** Rescuers must ensure that the vehicle is properly stabilized and the scene is safe.

> **CAUTION:** Rescuers must take necessary precautions to protect themselves and victims from hazards including, but not limited to, glass fragments and dust, jagged metal, SRS gas cylinders, undeployed airbags, and fire hazards.

NOTE: Victims must be properly packaged before displacing the seat.

Front Seat Displacement with Spreaders

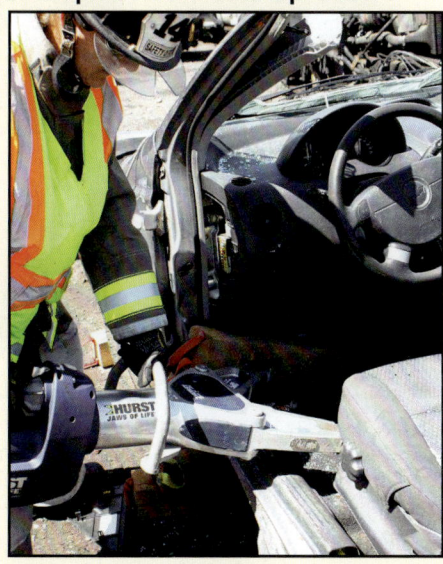

Step 1: Place a piece of cribbing between the spreader tip and the post to prevent the post from buckling.

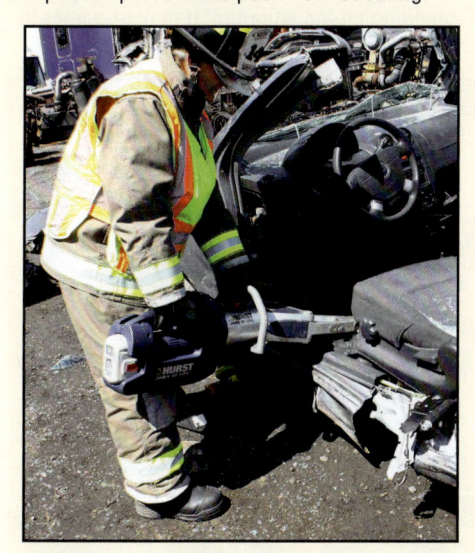

Step 2: Position one spreader tip on the seat's lower frame, directly above the seat runner. Place the other tip against the A-post at a point higher than the seat frame.

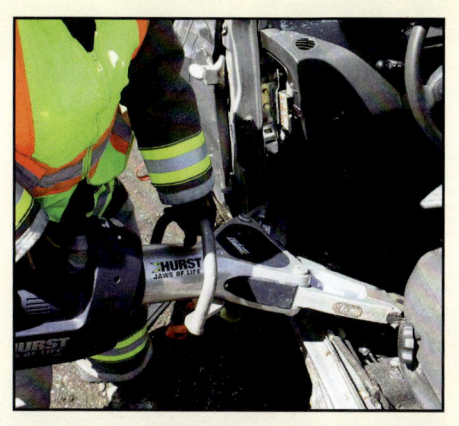

Step 3: Open the spreader arms to move the seat toward the rear of the vehicle.

Front Seat Displacement with a Hydraulic Ram

Step 1: Position the ram between the corner of the seat's lower frame and directly above the seat runner and firewall or A-post.

Step 2: Place a piece of cribbing between the firewall and the heel of the ram to prevent it from pushing through the firewall.

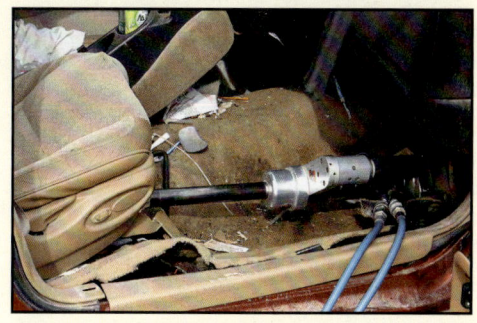

Step 3: Extend the ram to move the seat toward the rear of the vehicle.

NOTE: This method is more effective if two rams are used at the same time, one on each side of the seat.

8-23
Displace or remove a front seat in a vehicle.

Seatback Displacement or Removal

Step 1: Expose the seat frame by cutting or removing the upholstery.

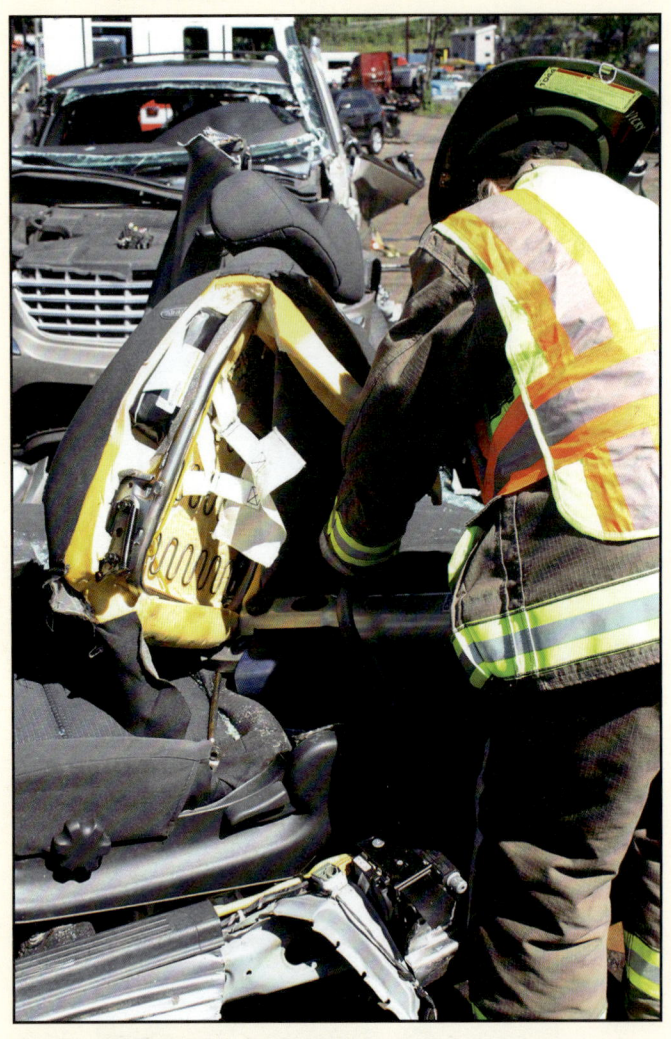

Step 2: Cut both sides of the seat frame at its base.

Step 3: Lay the seatback horizontal or remove it, if necessary.

Front Seat Removal

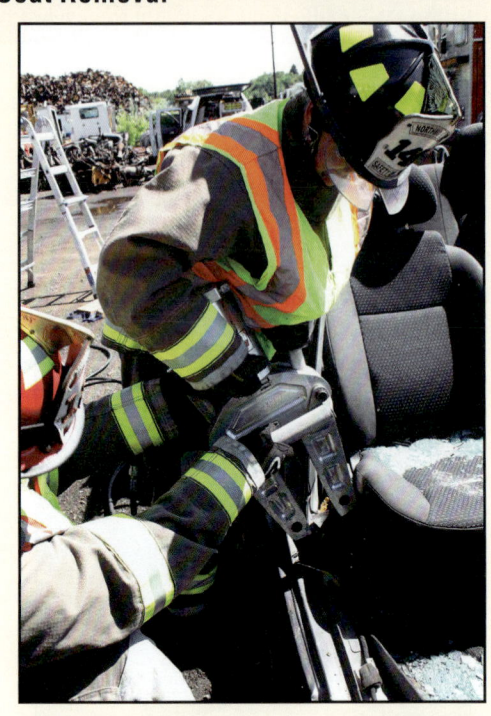

Step 1: Cut or break away the seat mounts at the point of attachment to the outer track. To break away the seat mounts, insert the spreader tips between the rocker panel and bottom of the seat frame.

Step 2: Insert the tool between the seat and transmission hump on the inside and separate the seat mounts from the inside track.

NOTE: Depending on the situation, it may be easier to unbolt the seat mounts from the brackets.

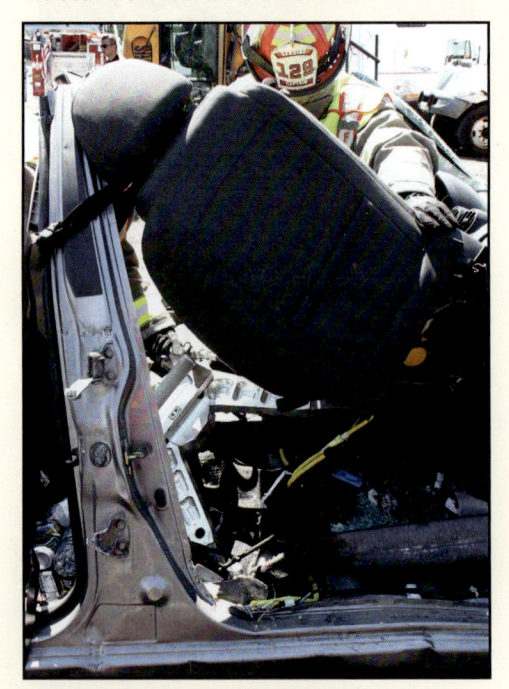

Step 3: Remove the seat.

SECTION D: TECHNICIAN LEVEL RESCUERS — HEAVY VEHICLE EXTRICATION

Commercial/ Heavy Vehicles

Courtesy of Chris Mickal.

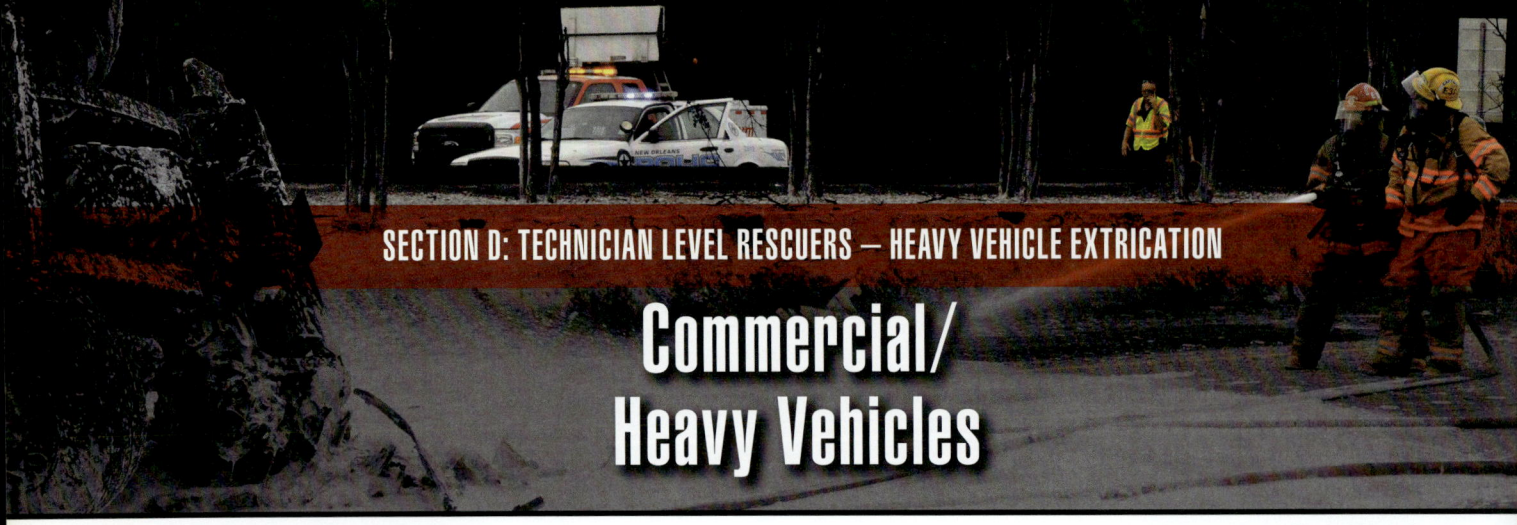

Chapter Contents

Medium and Heavy Vehicles 339
Medium and Heavy Trucks 339
    Straight Trucks 340
    Truck and Semitrailer Combinations 341
    Specialty Trucks 341
Medium and Heavy Truck Anatomy 343
    Cabs 343
    Trailers 346
Medium and Heavy Truck Construction 350
    Medium and Heavy Truck Construction Components 350
    Medium and Heavy Truck Battery Systems 350
    Medium and Heavy Truck Fuel Systems................... 350
    Medium and Heavy Truck Conventional Electrical Systems 351
    Medium and Heavy Truck Auxiliary Power and Hydraulics Systems 351
    Medium and Heavy Truck Brake Systems 353
    Medium and Heavy Truck Suspension Systems 354
    Medium and Heavy Auxiliary Lift Axles 354
Medium and Heavy Truck Safety Features 355
    Medium and Heavy Truck On-Board Safety Systems (OBSS) 355
    Fifth Wheels... 355

Buses 356
    School Buses 356
    Transit Buses 357
    Commercial Buses 358
    Specialty Buses 359
Bus Anatomy 360
    Bus Doors 361
    Bus Windows 363
    Bus Seats 365
    Bus Aisles 366
Bus Construction and Safety Features ... 367
    School Bus Construction Components 367
    Transit Bus Construction Components 370
    Commercial Bus Construction Components 370
    Hydraulic Lifts 371
    Bus Battery Systems 371
    Bus Electrical Systems 372
    Bus Fuel Systems 374
    Bus Suspension Systems 376
Chapter Review 378
Discussion Questions 378

336   Section D • Chapter 9 – Commercial/Heavy Vehicles

chapter 9

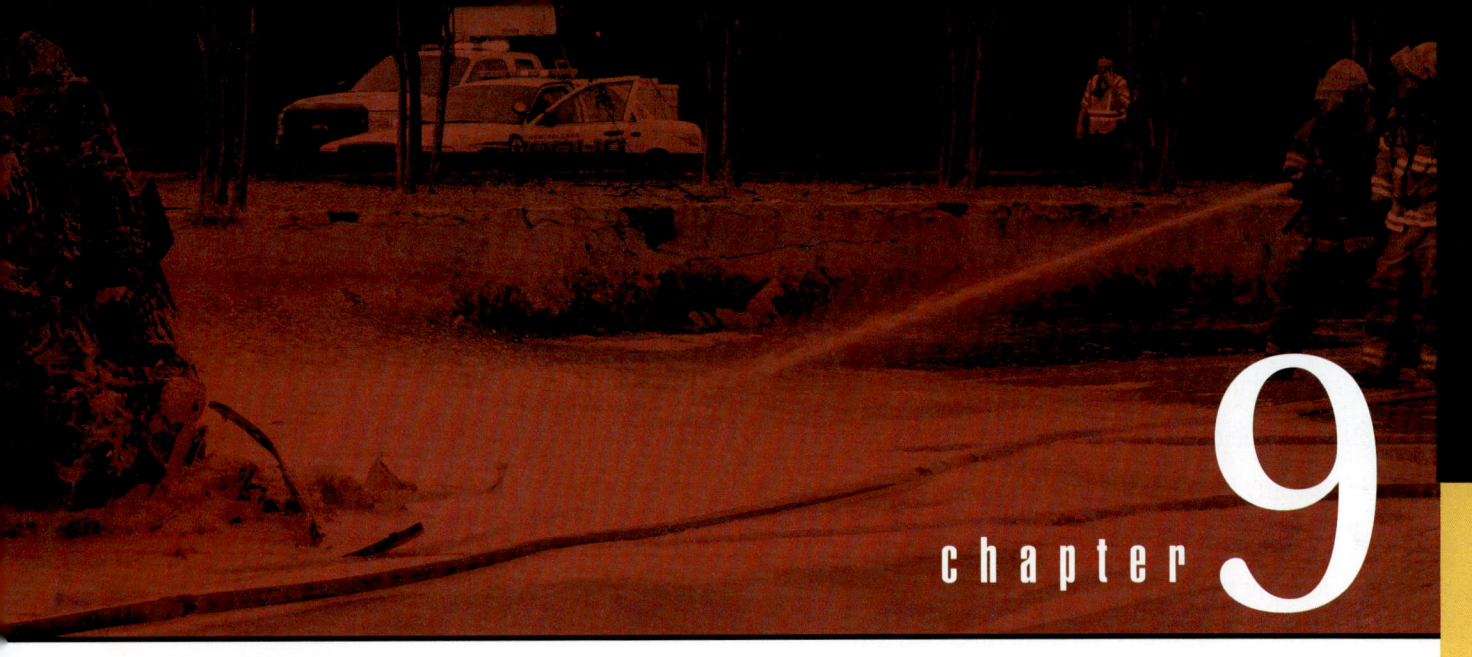

Key Terms

Coil Spring Suspension	354
Fairing	346
Kneeling	377
Placard	341
Pantograph	376
Pneumatic	354
Sleeper	345
Trailer	346

JPRs addressed in this chapter

This chapter provides information that addresses the following job performance requirements of NFPA 1006, *Standard for Technical Rescuer Professional Qualifications (2017)*.

- 8.3.1
- 8.3.3
- 8.3.4

Commercial/Heavy Vehicles

Learning Objectives

1. Differentiate among types of medium and heavy trucks. [8.3.1]
2. Describe common elements of medium and heavy truck anatomy. [8.3.1, 8.3.3, 8.3.4]
3. Identify components used to construct medium and heavy trucks. [8.3.3, 8.3.4]
4. Identify characteristics of systems found in medium and heavy trucks. [8.3.3, 8.3.4]
5. Identify safety features found in medium and heavy trucks. [8.3.3, 8.3.4]
6. Differentiate among types of buses. [8.3.1]
7. Describe common elements of bus anatomy. [8.3.1, 8.3.3, 8.3.4]
8. Describe bus construction and safety features. [8.3.3, 8.3.4]

Chapter 9
Commercial/Heavy Vehicles

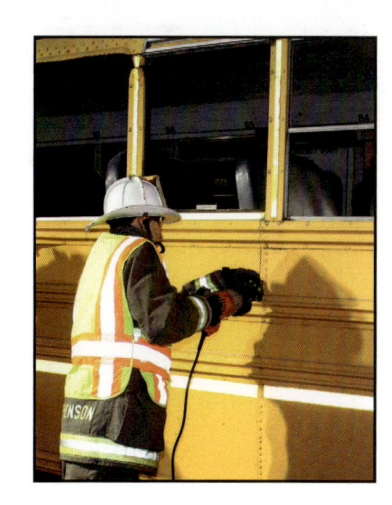

Vehicle incidents may become more complex when commercial/heavy vehicles are involved. There are many different types of commercial/heavy vehicles, but this chapter will focus on medium and heavy trucks and buses. Medium and heavy trucks and buses are constructed differently due to their intended purpose and use. Rescuers may encounter different vehicle anatomy, construction, and features, depending on the type of commercial/heavy vehicle. If possible, rescue personnel should identify a subject matter expert for training and emergency response assistance with the commercial/heavy vehicles common to their jurisdiction.

Medium and Heavy Trucks

Medium and heavy trucks are used for a variety of jobs and are generally configured based on need or task. Rescuers may encounter many types of trucks including tractors, semis, combination trucks, doubles, triples and more. These vehicles carry a variety of commodities and materials using a variety of methods such as tanks, hoppers, boxes, containers, van trailers, and flatbed/heavy hauling trailers.

Not every type of truck, trailer, or body style can be described in this manual. However, the most common types will be covered in this chapter. Rescuers and instructors should look in their geographic area for specialty transportation vehicles not described in this text. The following sections will cover medium and heavy trucks, including:

- Types of medium and heavy trucks
- Medium and heavy truck anatomy
- Medium and heavy truck construction and safety features

Medium and heavy trucks are designed to haul cargo or to serve as the chassis for special vehicles such as fire apparatus and tow trucks. The following are characteristics of medium trucks:

- The U.S. defines medium trucks as weighing between 13,000 and 33,000 pounds (6 500 and 16 500 kg).
- Common local delivery and garbage trucks are generally medium trucks.

Heavy trucks are defined in the U.S. as weighing more than 33,000 pounds (16 500 kg). The axle assemblies of heavy trucks may include two or more axles, some of which are powered. Medium and heavy trucks include:

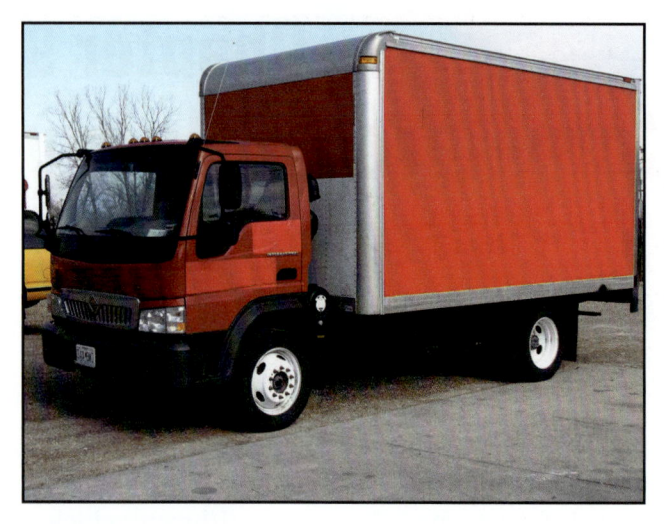

Figure 9.1 This delivery vehicle is an example of a straight truck. *Courtesy of Alan Braun, University of Missouri Fire and Rescue Training Institute.*

- Straight trucks
- Truck and semitrailer combinations
- Specialty trucks

Straight Trucks

The straight truck is perhaps the most common of all the truck types. The straight truck is built on a rigid frame and is not intended to pull a trailer **(Figure 9.1)**.

The straight truck may have the following features:

- They may have either two or three axles, all attached to one frame.
- They may have a gross vehicle weight rating (GVWR) between 10,000 and 40,000 pounds (5 000 - 20 000 kg).
- They may weigh significantly more than other straight trucks.
- They may have large, rather boxy bodies.
- They may be used as local delivery vans.
- They may have flatbeds or large box bodies mounted on their frames.

One common type of straight truck is the dump truck, which is often used for transporting loose materials such as sand, gravel, or dirt. Most dump trucks have an open-box body that is equipped with hydraulic pistons to lift the front vertically, allowing the contents to dump via a hinged rear onto the ground behind the vehicle. However, there are variations of dump trucks that empty their contents from underneath or the side. Rescuers should know the types and operational abilities of all dump trucks in their jurisdiction. Rescuers should be aware of dump trucks that are in the elevated position at incidents.

WARNING!
Be aware of overhead hazards, such as power lines, when working around dump trucks in the elevated position. If the vehicle comes in contact with a power line, it may become electrically charged.

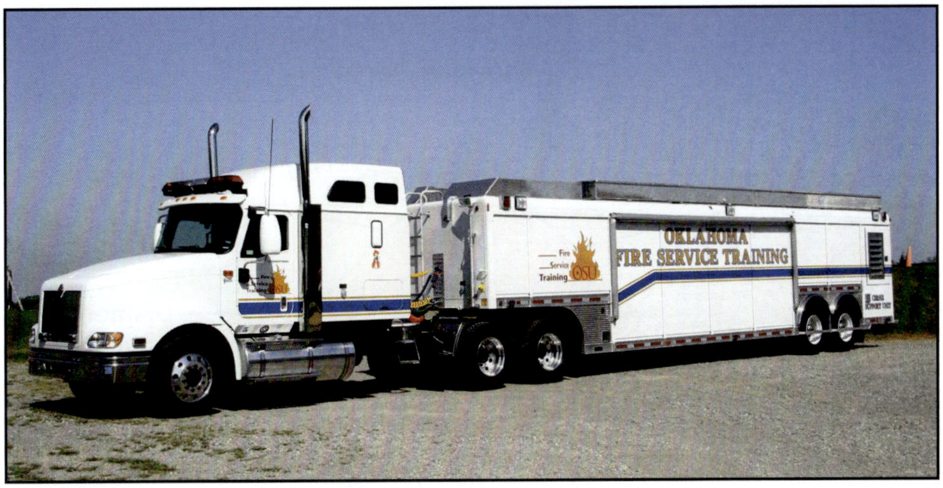

Figure 9.2 A tractor/trailer combination.

Truck and Semitrailer Combinations

Truck and semitrailer combinations are jointed vehicles composed of a motorized tractor designed to pull one or more trailers. A fifth-wheel device, mounted on the motorized tractor, serves as the attachment point for a semitrailer and allows the tractor and trailer to rotate independently from each other. In some countries, truck tractors may pull more than one trailer **(Figure 9.2)**.

The entire truck and semitrailer combination may weigh up to 140,000 pounds (70 000 kg). The tractors may have either two or three axles and may weigh up to 18,000 pounds (9 000 kg). The trailers may be flatbeds, enclosed box trailers, tankers, or specialized to functions such as grain or vehicle transport. While some of these vehicles will be labeled or **placarded** to indicate the nature of their cargo, others will not. Truck and semitrailer combinations may be carrying almost any commodity, including up to 440 pounds (220 kg) of hazardous materials. The load may be made up of combinations of commodities without being placarded for each commodity **(Figure 9.3, p. 342)**.

Truck and semitrailer combinations are referred to in a variety of ways depending on one's location. The following list provides various names for truck and semitrailer combinations:

- In the U.S, they are called *semitrailer trucks*, *tractor-trailers*, *18-wheelers*, *semis*, or *big-rigs*.
- In the U.K., Ireland, and New Zealand, they are called *articulated lorries*, *artics*, or *trucks and trailers*.
- In Australia and Canada, they are called *semi-tractor trains*, *semis*, and/or *land trains*.

These land trains can vary in length and may be as long as 175 feet (50 m).

Specialty Trucks

Specialty trucks are differentiated only by their unique purposes, as they are designed for specific functions **(Figure 9.4, p. 343)**. Otherwise, they may have the same configuration as any of the medium and heavy trucks already described. Specialty trucks are likely to weigh as much as any other truck of the same type and size. They may be straight trucks or truck and semitrailer combinations and include, but are not limited to:

> **Placard** — Diamond-shaped sign that is affixed to each side of a structure or a vehicle transporting hazardous materials to inform responders of fire hazards, life hazards, special hazards, and reactivity potential. The placard indicates the primary class of the material and, in some cases, the exact material being transported.

DOT Placard Parts

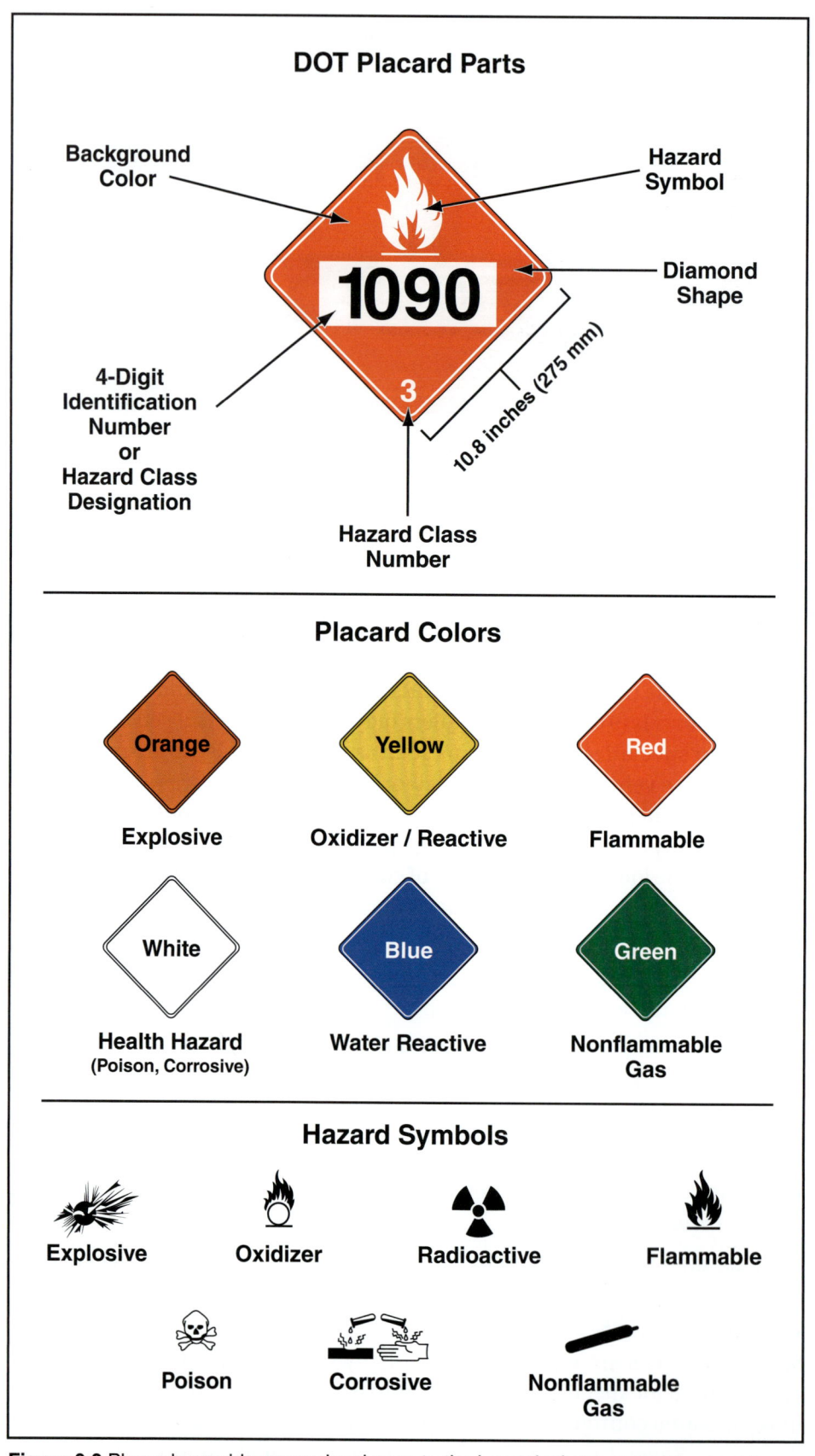

- Background Color
- Hazard Symbol
- Diamond Shape
- 10.8 inches (275 mm)
- 4-Digit Identification Number or Hazard Class Designation
- Hazard Class Number

Placard Colors

- **Orange** — Explosive
- **Yellow** — Oxidizer / Reactive
- **Red** — Flammable
- **White** — Health Hazard (Poison, Corrosive)
- **Blue** — Water Reactive
- **Green** — Nonflammable Gas

Hazard Symbols

- Explosive
- Oxidizer
- Radioactive
- Flammable
- Poison
- Corrosive
- Nonflammable Gas

Figure 9.3 Placards provide many visual cues to the hazards that a material presents.

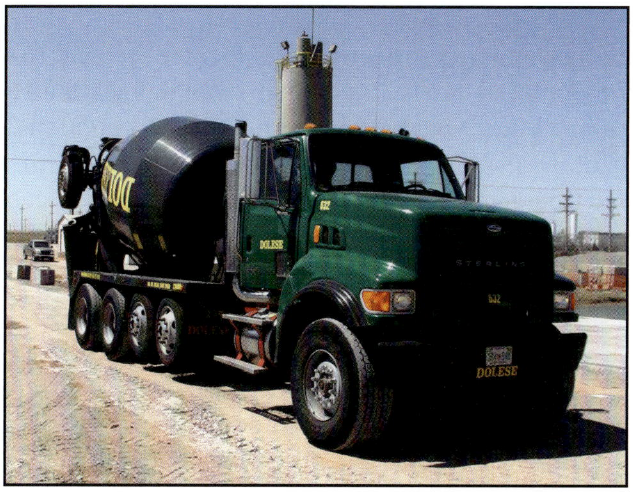

Figure 9.4 This cement mixer is an example of a specialty truck.

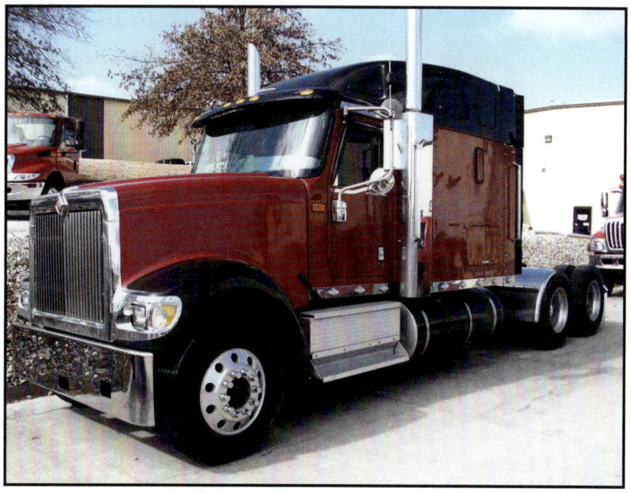

Figure 9.5 A conventional cab on a tractor. *Courtesy of Alan Braun, University of Missouri Fire and Rescue Training Institute..*

- Fire apparatus
- Military vehicles
- Logging trucks
- Large motor homes
- Book mobiles
- Medical treatment vehicles
- Highway repair vehicles

Medium and Heavy Truck Anatomy

All types of medium and heavy trucks are relatively large and often extremely heavy. Their sheer size and weight can complicate extrication and may necessitate the use of specialized resources such as booms, cranes, or other massive lifting devices. This section will describe medium and heavy truck anatomy:

- Cabs
- Trailers
- Medium and heavy truck systems

Cabs

Except for delivery vans, all medium and heavy trucks have a cab. In delivery vans, the cab is merely the front portion of the vehicle's body, separated from the cargo area only by a bulkhead on either side of the center aisle. The two most common types of cabs are conventional and cab-over units, although a cab-beside-engine may also be found in certain industrial areas **(Figure 9.5)**. The sections that follow describe these three types of cabs and the following aspects of cab anatomy:

- Sleepers
- Cab doors
- Cab windows
- Cab roofs

Conventional Cabs

In a conventional cab, the passenger compartment is located behind the engine compartment. A conventional cab is longer from front to back than a cab-over unit. The engine may be accessed by raising the sides of a hood that is hinged down its midline, or by tilting forward a single-unit hood and front fenders composed of molded fiberglass. The remainder of a conventional cab is usually made of steel, aluminum, or a combination of fiberglass panels over a steel framework.

Air-Ride Cabs

Some medium and heavy trucks are equipped with air-ride cabs. An air ride cab is a truck's cab that has air bags to allow the cab and sleeper of a truck to cushion the driver while driving the truck up and down the highways.

The concern with securing the cab is to put blocks of cribbing between the frame and cab so if the air bleeds off the truck's cab, it does not lower and hinder extrication or inadvertently air up during the extrication. Rescuers would capture the cab with chains or straps to secure the cab from any hazard and make the cab safe to work with in either situation.

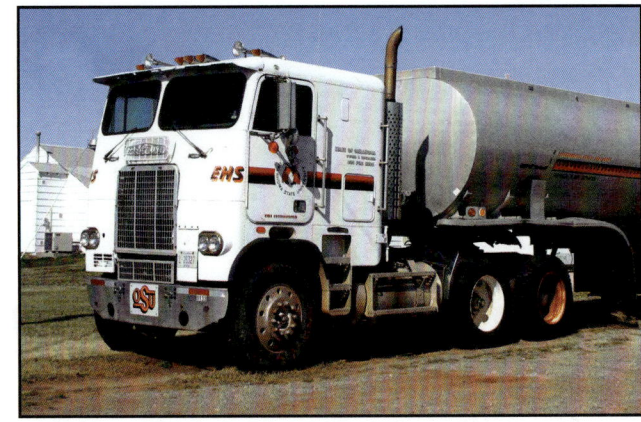

Figure 9.6 A cab-over unit on a tractor

Cab-Over Units

In cab-over units, the engine is located directly under the midline of the passenger compartment, roughly between the seats. The cab-over unit is designed to tilt forward to allow access to the engine. Generally, the cab is attached to the chassis at three points — in the center behind the cab (latch point) and by a hinge at the front of each frame rail. Cab-over units may be made of steel, aluminum, fiberglass, or a combination of these materials **(Figure 9.6)**.

Cab-Beside-Engine

In the mid-1950s, Kenworth produced its cab-beside-engine design. Also called the *bullnose* or *half-cab*, the cab-beside engine design is rarely seen on the roadways today. However, it can still be used on industrial sites and shipyards.

Sleepers

Because many long-haul trucks are driven great distances, the law limits the number of hours a driver can operate a commercial vehicle without a rest period. Many heavy trucks are equipped with a sleeping compartment in or behind the cab **(Figure 9.7)**.

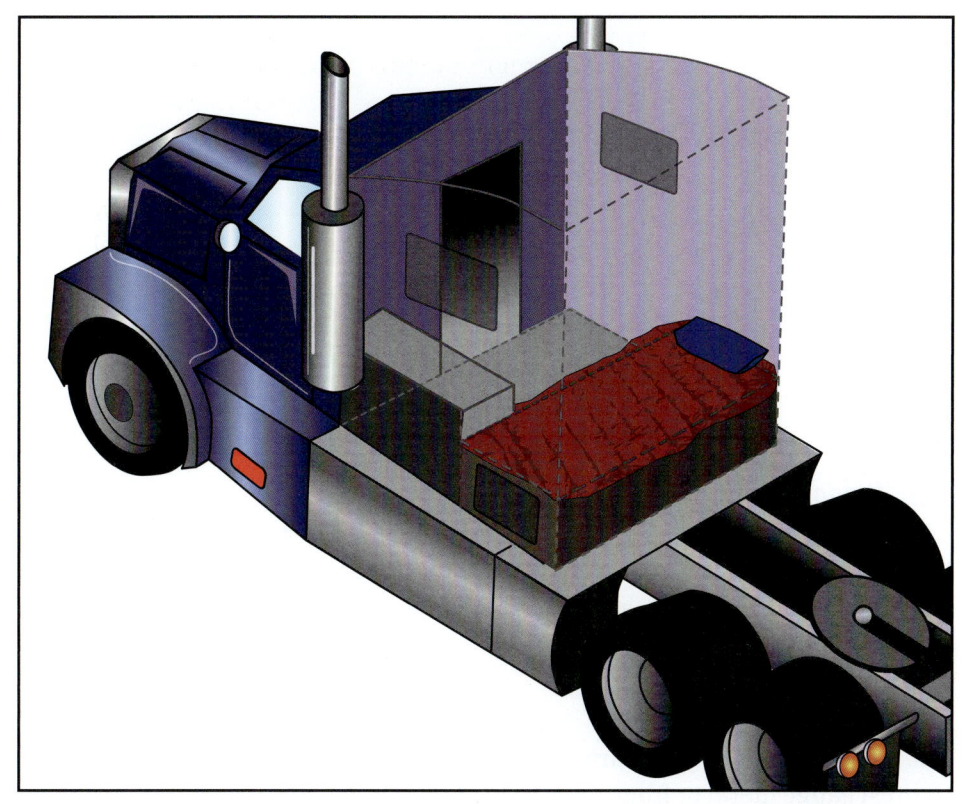

Figure 9.7 A sleeping compartment attached to the rear of a conventional cab.

The vast majority of **sleepers** are merely an extension of the cab and not a separate unit. Rescuers access these units through the cab or by forcing entry through the required exterior door. Sleepers that are separate units must have an intercom between the sleeper and the cab. The access door to the sleeper may be on either side of the unit. Because the occupant of a sleeper is not required to be restrained, rescuers should expect any passenger found in a sleeper to have sustained injuries following a collision.

If a truck has a sleeper attached to the cab, rescue personnel should check there for another occupant during the size-up of a heavy vehicle incident. Often, team drivers will have a sign indicating the driving team on the driver's door area.

Sleeper — Compartment built into or behind the cab of a large truck, to be used by the driver for rest and relaxation.

Cab Doors

The forward doors on most delivery vans are pocket doors that slide rearward into the vehicle's sidewall to open. These doors have a single latch point at the center of the front edge of the door. Newer delivery vans have conventional front-hinged doors.

The doors on both conventional and cab-over units are much heavier and stronger than those on automobiles and light trucks. These doors are equipped with either conventional or piano-type hinges. Most cabs have a single latch with a two-step locking action. Because of the height of the doors above the ground, the door latch handle is usually located in the lower rear corner of the door.

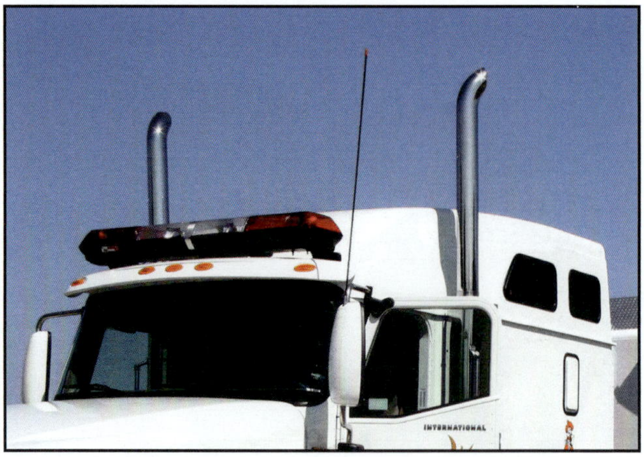

Figure 9.8 The roof configuration of a conventional cab.

Cab Windows

The windshields and rear windows of medium and heavy trucks are made of laminated safety glass, and they are set in center-bead rubber gaskets. The cab side windows are made of tempered glass that is heavier than that used in automobiles and light trucks.

Cab Roofs

The cab roofs of most medium and heavy trucks are usually covered with the lightest gauge metal or fiberglass on the vehicle, and the skin is supported by two or more ribs running from front to rear. Many heavy trucks have a large fiberglass **fairing** (wind deflector) mounted on the roof, often with an air horn and an air-conditioning unit behind it **(Figure 9.8)**.

Trailers

Trailers are available in a wide variety of shapes and sizes, depending upon their intended use. The most common trailers seen on the highways are:

- Huge box trailers hauling almost anything that will fit inside the box. These box trailers may be insulated.
- Flatbed trailers hauling cargo that can be secured to the bed.
- Trailers with bottom-dump capability hauling sand, gravel, grain, and other dry products.
- Long, cylindrical tankers whose styles vary depending upon their cargo.
- Trailers with spherical tanks for carrying cryogenic (extremely low temperature) materials.

No matter their shape, all trailers are one of two basic styles: trailers or semitrailers **(Figure 9.9)**. A trailer is a freestanding unit with wheels front and rear. These trailers are usually shorter than semitrailers. The front axle on a trailer is connected to a turntable that can be turned from side to side for better tracking, and the rear axle is fixed. A trailer couples to a tractor or another trailer with a long tow bar, often called a *dolly*.

Semitrailers only have wheels at or near the rear end, and the front end is supported by the tractor when locked into the fifth wheel described later in this chapter. When a semitrailer is not coupled to a tractor, its front end is supported by a pair of small wheels or plates, sometimes called *landing gear*, that are attached to the underside of the trailer by two struts. When not in use, the trailer's landing gear can be lowered with a hand crank.

Fairing — An auxiliary structure or the external surface either attached to, or a part of the roof of a large truck that serves to reduce drag.

Trailer — Highway or industrial-plant vehicle designed to be hauled/pulled by a tractor.

Trailer Configurations

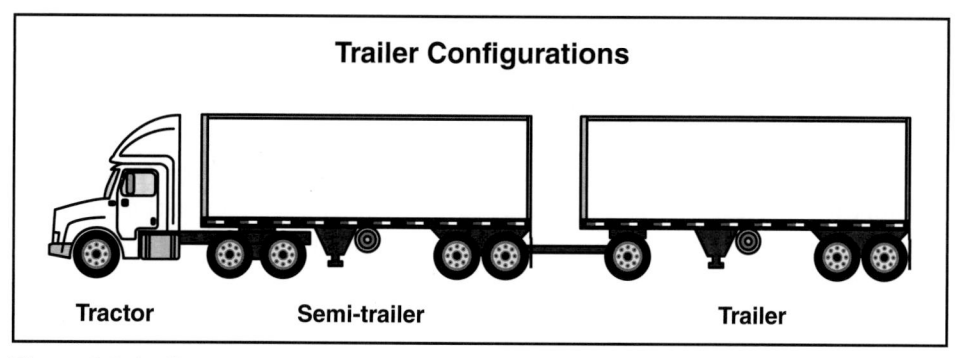

Figure 9.9 An illustration showing the difference between a semi-trailer and a trailer.

On many of these semitrailers, the hand crank has two speeds:

- Push in and crank for slow raising or lowering
- Pull out and crank for fast raising or lowering

If undamaged, the landing gear can be used for additional temporary stabilization, as well as for lifting/lowering in conjunction with proper stabilization.

Many different types of trailers are equipped with axles that may be designed to move (slide) along a track or the frame rail system. The axles may slide in tandem (pairs) or may move individually. These sliding axles are used to manage trailer loads, improve close quarters maneuverability of the trailer, or allow loading and unloading of the trailer.

One or more of the axles may be designed to move along the track/frame rail either manually or by means of a powered system. In either case, secure the mechanical locking pin on both track/frame rails to lock the axle(s) into position.

Low-load bed trailers and heavy-equipment trailers, often have a powered system to slide entire axle assemblies along the track or frame rails of the low-slung trailer. This action lowers one end of the trailer to the ground. Use this system to drive the equipment off the rear of the trailer to load and unload the equipment.

Responders should secure movable trailer axles against unplanned/unintentional movement. In some trailer designs, multiple lock pins may be secured or released by activating a single lever or actuator. While this feature is convenient for the operator under normal conditions, unintentional release of axle lock pins at an emergency incident could have deadly consequences. Even where a single action is designed to engage or disengage multiple trailer axle slide lock pins, the emergency responder charged with securing trailer axles should check each individual lock pin.

Many trailers and semitrailers are equipped with air suspension systems. The same precautions apply to working under these trailers as apply to working under trucks with similar suspension systems. The sections that follow provide rescuers with more detailed information about various types of trailers they will encounter at accident scenes.

Box Trailers

With the exception of refrigerated trailers that have heavily insulated walls and roofs, most box trailers have a relatively lightweight metal frame that is covered by thin metal or fiberglass or a combination of the two. There may be rub rails along the inside walls of the box to protect it and add strength. The roof of the box trailer is the area most easily penetrated because the covering material is thinnest and there are the fewest structural members. While there are many exceptions, most box trailers have 110 inches (2 750 mm) of vertical clearance inside, from front to rear. The following doors are common to box trailers:

- **Rear cargo doors** — Rear cargo doors on box trailers may be one of two types: swinging or roll-up. Trailers with swinging doors usually have two single-leaf doors that latch near the middle and swing outward on conventional or piano-type hinges. Most roll-up doors on trailers are constructed in sections similar to a garage door. Most types of roll-up doors latch in the center at the bottom of the door.

> **CAUTION**
> Opening rear cargo doors may compromise the structural integrity of the trailer.

- **Side cargo doors** — Some box trailers have one or two side cargo doors, usually located at the midpoint of the trailer's length on one or both sides. These doors are generally swinging doors on conventional or piano-type hinges. These doors may consist of a single-leaf door or two single-leaf doors that latch near the middle.

Livestock Trailers

While not as numerous as other types of trailers on the roadways, rescuers should be aware of livestock trailers. Unlike most other trailers, they often contain a significant life hazard. Horses or other livestock that are already frightened because of the collision can be further agitated by the sounds of power tools being used in the extrication operation. In their panic, they can seriously injure themselves, other animals, or rescue personnel.

It may be possible to calm an animal by blindfolding it and/or restricting its hearing. If this is not successful, it may be best to free the animal as quickly and as quietly as possible. A frightened animal that is freed from the confines of a wrecked trailer may attempt to flee. Fleeing animals can create a traffic hazard for motorists and may harm themselves. It is sometimes advisable to call a veterinarian to the scene to tranquilize any animal that cannot be extricated quickly.

Tanker Trailers

Tanker trailers are made of steel, aluminum, stainless steel, and other materials and have capacities that range from 200 to 14,000 gallons (8 000 to 56 000L). There are many different types and styles of tanker trailer on the roads. Responders should be concerned with the contents of the tank during the response and upon arrival. The contents of tankers can shift during extrication efforts.

Lowboys

Lowboy trailers, also known as heavy-duty trailers, feature a low center deck area designed to carry large, heavy loads up to several hundred tons. Trailers may also have a heavy steel beam framework that the load is mounted to for transportation. Lowboy trailers commonly have two or three rear axles with two wheels per side. Trailers may also have additional sections with multiple axles to support especially heavy loads. These loads may be over 175 feet (50 m) long and/or over width (greater than 8 feet [2.5 m] wide). Rescuers may experience difficulty in stabilizing the large size and heavy weight of lowboy loads. These types of loads may overwhelm available resources due to the large volume of material needed to stabilize them.

Lowboys are made with most of the same equipment as other standard over-the-road trailers. They have air brakes supplied by the tractor. Most are hydraulically operated. Some operate from the cab of the tractor while others are operated by generators and electric hydraulic pumps. These methods are used to split them apart to unload equipment.

Dump Trailers

Dump trailers are common on highways and the interstate system. In the U.S., the DOT limits their gross vehicle weight to 80,000 pounds (40 000 kg). Dump trailers may have a frame structure or the trailer body may be used as the frame. Trailers can be constructed of steel, aluminum, or stainless steel. Dump trailers can carry many different loads including rock, dirt, scrap metal, and hazardous materials. Responders should take care when assessing dump trailers due to the many different possible load types and weights and due to potential load shifting during extrication.

These trailers contain most of the same equipment as standard over-the-road trailers. They have air brakes supplied by the tractor. Most dump trailers are hydraulically operated from the cab of the tractor. Some of the smaller trailers are operated by generators or battery powered electric hydraulic pumps.

Car Carrier/Hauler Trailers

Car carrier/haulers have ramps for loading/offloading. Many have multiple decks for storing vehicles, which increases the number of vehicles that can be transported at one time. Hydraulic systems are used to tilt and lift the ramps and decks. Most of these trailers can carry as many as eight vehicles, which are normally secured to the trailer with chains or straps.

Some car carrier/hauler trailers are enclosed. These may be towed by any transport medium and typically transport luxury vehicles or race cars. The enclosed car carrier/hauler may be more than 50 feet (15 m) in length, may have multiple decks, and may house living and mechanic quarters.

Dry Bulk Trailers

Also referred to as hoppers, these enclosed trailers are used throughout North America to transport dry bulk materials. They are easily recognized due to their V-shaped bottom-unloading compartments. Rescuers should be aware of the potentially hazardous cargo inside these trailers.

Medium and Heavy Truck Construction

Medium and heavy trucks contain a variety of systems that rescue personnel should be familiar with. These systems include the following:

- Construction components
- Battery systems
- Fuel systems
- Auxiliary power and hydraulics systems
- Brake systems
- Suspension systems
- Auxiliary lift axles

Medium and Heavy Truck Construction Components

The construction of medium and heavy trucks utilizes steel, aluminum, and fiberglass. The foundation begins with two large steel frame rails, and onto that frame the cab, chassis, suspension, and brake systems are mounted. The hood and front fenders are typically molded in plastic or fiberglass to enable intricate aerodynamic shapes. The front bumper may be stamped and extruded from steel or aluminum, or it may be molded plastic and backed with a steel substructure. The roof is one of the weaker components of the cab.

In modern vehicles, a fairing, which is usually made of fiberglass, will be mounted above the cab for aerodynamics and fuel savings. Additionally, air-conditioning units, air horns, and possibly a GPS locater will be located on top of the cab.

NOTE: The frame and/or chassis provide points on the vehicle for rescuers to perform stabilization.

Medium and Heavy Truck Battery Systems

Medium and heavy trucks have either a 12-volt or 24-volt electrical system supplied by one or more banks of batteries. The battery banks may be in more than one location on the vehicle. Those with 24-volt systems normally have four 6-volt batteries in series, with a negative ground.

Medium and Heavy Truck Fuel Systems

Most medium and heavy trucks operate on diesel fuel rather than gasoline. Use of diesel fuel reduces, but does not eliminate, the danger of a flash fire following a collision. While the flashpoint of diesel fuel varies from 126° to 204° F (50° to 95° C) it can easily be heated to that point if it leaks onto exhaust system components, which may exceed 1,200° F (650° C), or even onto very hot pavement. Personnel should be aware that this presents an extreme fire hazard.

The diesel fuel is usually contained in large external saddle tanks attached to either side of the frame. The capacity of these saddle tanks may vary from 50 to 300 gallons (200 to 1 200 L) each. Many vehicle saddle tanks are interconnected by a small tube that equalizes the volume of fuel in both tanks. At one or both ends of this tube is a small valve that can be used to isolate the tanks from each other if one tank is leaking. This will limit the amount of fuel that can escape **(Figure 9.10)**.

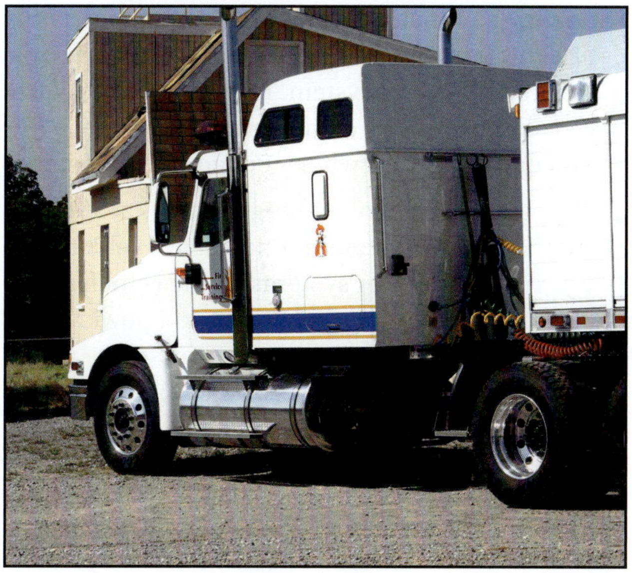

Figure 9.10 This truck is equipped with large saddle tanks to carry the truck's fuel supply.

Some medium and heavy trucks operate on alternative fuels — either liquefied petroleum gas (LPG) or compressed natural gas (CNG). A small number of trucks now operate on liquefied natural gas (LNG) or hydrogen. Decals or other signs should be visible to alert rescue personnel that a particular vehicle uses an alternative fuel. The locations of the fuel tanks vary considerably. Leaking fuel may present more than fire and explosion hazards.

> **WARNING!**
> Contact with LPG and LNG can cause frostbite to exposed skin.

Medium and Heavy Truck Conventional Electrical Systems

Medium and heavy trucks generally have more electrical requirements than passenger vehicles. They use either a 12-volt or 24-volt electrical system supplied by one or more banks of batteries. These batteries are usually parallel wired together to produce a higher amperage flow. The battery locations may be in more than one location on the vehicle, depending on the manufacturer or specifications of the truck. Master battery shutoff or disconnect switches are not generally found on heavy trucks, however, some owners may have installed after-market switches. Separate batteries may exist to power optional devices such as generators.

Just as with any other vehicle, search for and locate the battery compartment(s) and isolate the electrical system without delay if the task can be safely performed. The negative (ground) cable should either be disconnected or double cut first, followed by the positive cable. Due to the higher amperage required, these cables may be much bigger in diameter than those of passenger vehicles.

Medium and Heavy Truck Auxiliary Power and Hydraulics Systems

Some larger trucks are equipped with auxiliary power systems. These may include generators and inverters, as well as hydraulic systems. Some vehicles have a generator or battery-powered inverter to provide 110-220 volt power.

This power may be used to operate climate control and other electrically powered equipment while the vehicle is traveling or parked overnight. Some vehicles are equipped with a separate hydraulic system. This system may power vehicle components such as a concrete truck's drum or a dump trailer's lift. These systems may be running continuously or when needed by the operator.

Auxiliary power sources are potentially harmful energy sources at a vehicle incident. Medium and heavy trucks and other commercial/heavy vehicles are equipped with varying types of auxiliary power systems. Some vehicles have a generator or battery-powered inverter to provide 110-220 volt power. This section discusses the following types of auxiliary power sources:

- Mechanical
- Hydraulic
- Pneumatic

Mechanical Systems

Mechanical power, such as the Power Take-Off (PTO), transfers power from the tractor to any implement or attachment. PTO shafts can rotate at more than 1,000 revolutions per minute and can easily entangle rescuers and/or bystanders. Isolate mechanical power by locking/tagging out the piece of equipment.

> **Lock-out/Tag-out Procedures**
>
> Lock-out/tag-out procedures ensure that the position of certain valves and switches are not changed at a critical moment in the rescue operation. These procedures can be implemented on vehicles that use electrical, hydraulic, or pneumatic power. Opening a valve or flipping a switch could re-energize the machine in which a victim is trapped. This could cause sudden and unexpected movement of the machine and place the victim and rescue personnel in jeopardy.
>
> Personnel should follow their local lock-out/tag-out procedures when appropriate. If lockout/tag-out devices are not available, a rescuer with a portable radio should be assigned to stay at the valve or switch to prevent anyone from turning the power back on before it is safe to do so.

Hydraulic Systems

Commercial and heavy vehicles often use hydraulic systems to power various vehicle components. It is also common to find hydraulic fluids in the struts and suspension systems of most passenger vehicles. Hydraulic systems may be running continuously or when needed by the operator. Pressure in hydraulic lines can reach pressures capable of penetrating protective clothing. Mitigate the hydraulic pressure in any hydraulic lines prior to any rescue attempt. Hydraulic systems need to be shut down, locked out, and tagged out.

Pneumatic Systems

Many types of vehicles have pneumatic (air) systems. Some implements, attachments, and ancillary equipment may be operated by pneumatic pressure. A breached high-pressure pneumatic line can easily pierce PPE and even sever fingers. Pneumatic systems need to be shut down, locked out, and tagged out.

Medium and Heavy Truck Brake Systems

Medium and heavy trucks are equipped with either hydraulic brakes, air brakes, or a combination of the two **(Figure 9.11)**. These systems usually operate drum brakes, although disc brakes are becoming more common. The hydraulic brake systems are heavier-duty versions of those in automobiles and light trucks. Some trucks have hydraulic brakes that are assisted by air pressure. In the air brake systems, compressed air is used to apply the brakes under normal operation. Under abnormal conditions, such as a complete loss of air pressure in the braking system, heavy-duty springs automatically apply the rear brakes.

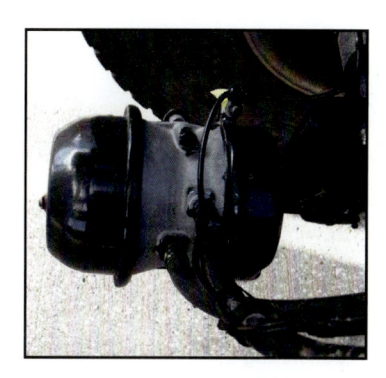

Figure 9.11 A double chamber air brake unit on a heavy truck. *Courtesy of Alan Braun, University of Missouri Fire and Rescue Training Institute.*

Because the trailers on tractor/trailer rigs also have air brakes, the trailer's air system is connected to that of the tractor by a breakaway valve at the rear of the cab, commonly called a glad-hand connection. The flexible air line connecting the tractor and trailer is often supported on a vertical stand, sometimes called a pogo stick, mounted on the rear of the tractor or by some other securing device.

Both trucks and tractor/trailer combinations with air brakes have air brake chambers mounted under each axle. The double chambers (called piggyback chambers) under the rear axles contain large compressed springs. These springs apply the brakes mechanically for parking or if there is a loss of air pressure. The parts of each double chamber are held together with a metal clamp. Loosening this clamp can release a spring that has sufficient force to cause serious injury.

Rescuers should never loosen the clamp on an air brake chamber. Loosening this clamp can release a spring that has sufficient force to cause serious injury or even death. Rescuers should also stay clear of the rear of air brake chambers when they are involved in fire. If the chamber melts, the compressed spring can break. Rescuers should avoid all brake components. Stay clear of the rear of air brake chambers when they are involved in fire. If the chamber melts, the compressed spring can break.

> **WARNING!**
> Never loosen the clamp on an air brake chamber.

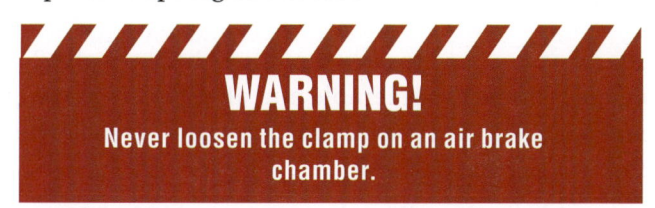

NOTE: The buses discussed in this chapter include brakes identical or very similar to those described in this section. Rescuers should take similar precautions when working with any vehicle with air brakes.

> **WARNING!**
> Never loosen the clamp on an air brake chamber. Severe injury or death can occur.

> **WARNING!**
> Stay clear of the rear of air brake chambers when they are involved in fire. Severe injury or death can occur.

Medium and Heavy Truck Suspension Systems

Most medium and heavy trucks have conventional heavy-duty suspension (leaf and/or **coil springs**). However, a growing number of heavy trucks are equipped with air suspension systems. In these systems, the conventional metal springs are replaced with compact rubber air bags that are somewhat similar to a bellows. At each wheel, there are air suspension bags — two on each axle. An on-board compressor maintains the air pressure within the bags as high as 120 psi (840 kPa). Depending upon the load of the vehicle and the condition of the road, the pressure within each bag is automatically increased or decreased to maintain the vehicle in a level state. If the pressure in an air suspension bag is lost because of damage to the bag or its associated piping, the truck chassis can suddenly drop several inches.

Medium and Heavy Auxiliary Lift Axles

Auxiliary lift axles can be found either in front of (pusher axle) or behind (tag axle) the drive axle on the truck, mounted directly to the frame. The auxiliary lift axles that are located in front of or behind the drive axle are straight drop down axles designed to operate in an air down/air up or air down/spring up manner.

Stingers, the auxiliary lift axles that are located only behind the drive axles, operate in a fold-down manner. Stingers are either **pneumatic** (operated by air) or hydraulic, and are assembled with much heavier construction than the tag or pusher axles. Stingers are commonly found on cement mixers and dump trucks.

Auxiliary lift axles are used to carry and distribute weight. They raise and lower when needed. Some are steerable and all have air brake chambers for braking. Depending upon the type of axles, they can weigh between 6,000 and 10,000 pounds (3 000 kg and 5 000 kg).

Straight trucks with auxiliary lift axles can exceed 120,000 pounds (54 431 kg) in off-road use such as construction sites and mining locations. Some trucks can have several lift axles.

Major concerns for rescuers include the rear lift axles, specifically the stinger type, in rear-collision incidents. When a vehicle impacts the hinge locations or damages the lifting mechanism, the 6,000- to 10,000-pound (3 000 kg and 5 000 kg) lift axle could potentially fall on the impacting vehicle or rescuers.

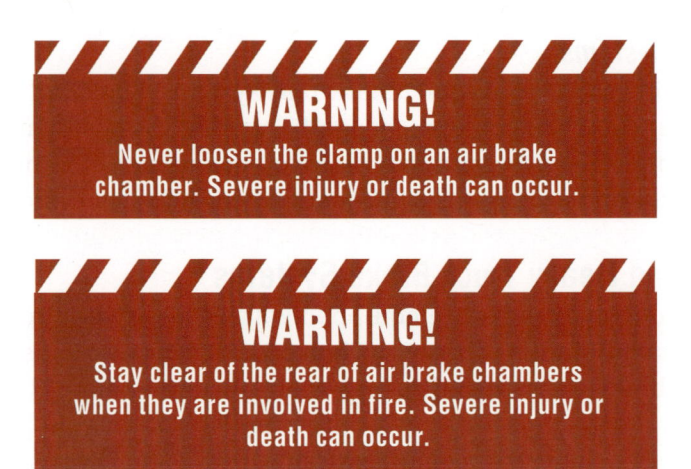

Coil Spring Suspension — Suspension system consisting of numerous spirally-bound, elastic steel bodies that recover their shape after being compressed, bent, or stretched.

Pneumatic — Operated by air or compressed air.

The lift axle should be secured forward of the affected area, with chains and chain binders. Rescuers should also look out for trucks, such as log trucks, which have a lift axle that is not equipped with emergency air brake chambers. If the truck's load is lost and the pneumatics are still operational, then the lift axle may raise the truck off of its brakes and the vehicle may roll. Rescuers must ensure the vehicle is stabilized before engaging in extrication procedures.

Medium and Heavy Truck Safety Features

Medium and heavy trucks have specific construction and safety features that rescue personnel should be familiar with, such as:

- Medium and heavy truck on-board safety systems
- Fifth wheels

Medium and Heavy Truck On-Board Safety Systems (OBSS)

A modern truck may have one or more on-board safety systems (OBSS) to mitigate or avoid a crash. The OBSS include lane departure warning (LDW) systems, roll stability control (RSC) systems, and forward collision warning (FCW) systems. In addition, the OBSS in medium and heavy trucks are equipped with seat belts, supplemental restraint systems, and rollover protection systems (ROPS) to protect the driver and any passengers riding in the vehicle.

In recent years, just as with passenger vehicles, great strides in technology have improved the crashworthiness of medium and heavy trucks, especially with ROPS. According to the Federal Motor Carrier Safety Administration (FMCSA), more than half of occupant fatalities in large trucks involve a rollover. Features such as the RollTek® system have been installed in many commercial trucks. This system includes sensors that detect imminent rollover and deploy a three phase protection system which activates the airbags and seatbelt pre-tensioners and also pulls down the suspension seat to its lowest position. Lowering the seat increases survivable space in the cab of the vehicle. These systems operate in much the same manner as those found in passenger vehicles and present the same types of concerns.

Fifth Wheels

Mounted on the rear of every highway tractor is a heavy-duty circular steel plate called a fifth wheel. The fifth wheel allows the trailer to rotate more than 90 degrees from center in both directions. The fifth wheel turntable can pivot approximately 15 degrees front to rear. On some vehicles, it can be adjusted fore and aft. The fifth wheel has a wedge-shaped slot in its rear aspect to receive the trailer's king pin. When the king pin reaches the center of the fifth wheel during coupling, the pin is locked into place by two spring-loaded jaws. A pull handle on the driver's side of the tractor opens the jaws to allow the trailer to be uncoupled from the tractor. On some vehicles, the jaws can be opened from the cab via a pneumatic system **(Figure 9.12)**.

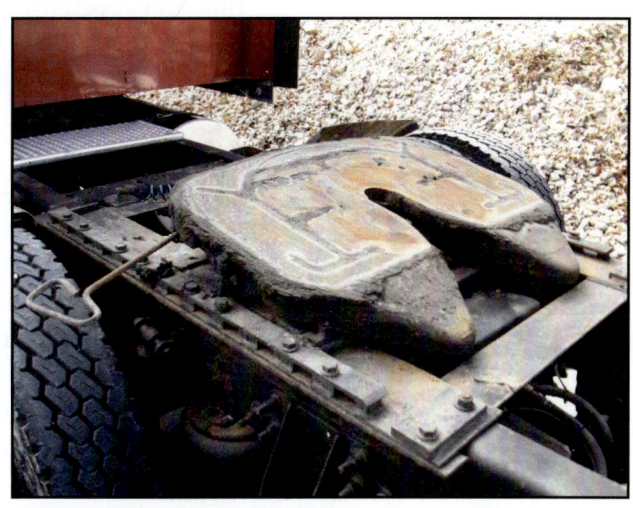

Figure 9.12 A fifth wheel mounted on a rear of a tractor. *Courtesy of Alan Braun, University of Missouri Fire and Rescue Training Institute.*

Buses

Buses are all designed for the same purpose – to transport a relatively large number of passengers from one point to another safely and comfortably. They are commonly used to transport children to and from school, citizens between their homes and workplaces, and travelers from city to city. Buses are used to provide transportation in many environments including:

- Rural
- City
- Intercity
- Tourism

Buses are one of the largest types of commercial/heavy vehicles that rescue personnel may encounter which contain a significant passenger capacity. Rescue personnel should be familiar with the following bus classifications:

- School buses
- Transit buses
- Commercial buses
- Specialty buses

School Buses

A school bus is defined as a passenger motor vehicle designed to carry more than ten passengers, and is used to transport students to or from schools or school-related events. School buses have the following characteristics:

- Variety of sizes and configurations
- At least one entry/exit door
- At least one additional emergency exit, usually at the rear of the vehicle, which may or may not be an exit door

By definition, buses are designed to carry more than ten passengers, but often carry significantly more based on the type of bus, the manufacturer, and the end-user's needs. Rescuers may encounter buses with passenger counts that far exceed their intended passenger capacity. Personnel should become familiar with the typical buses and passenger totals for their jurisdiction. In North America, school buses are divided into four types: A, B, C, and D.

Type A

These are the smallest type of school buses **(Figure 9.13)**. Type A bus passenger counts vary, but some are capable of carrying up to 36 passengers. They are a standard SUV or van conversion built on a heavy duty, van-type front section chassis. The bus entry/exit door is located behind the front wheels, and the bus also has a driver-side door. The engine is located under the windshield or between the front seats. Type A school buses come in two varieties: A-1 and A-2. A-1 buses have a GVWR of 10,000 pounds (5 000 kg) or less. A-2 buses have a GVWR of 10,000 pounds (5 000 kg) or more.

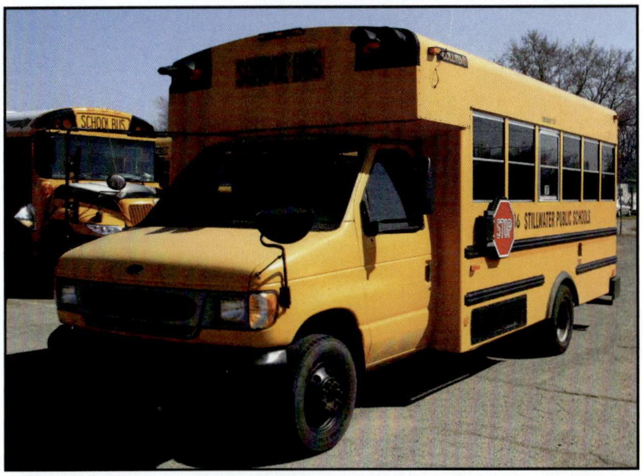

Figure 9.13 An example of a Type A-2 school bus.

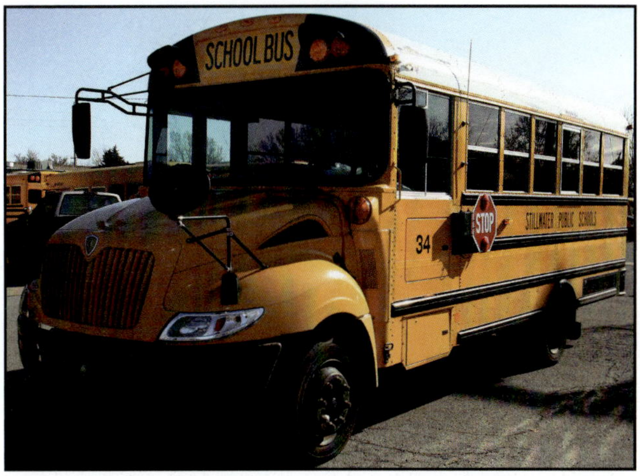

Figure 9.14 An example of a Type C school bus.

Type B

Passenger counts on type B buses vary, but some are capable of carrying up to 36 passengers. Type B school buses are either a conversion or their body is constructed on a front-section vehicle chassis. The entry/exit door is located aft (in front of) of the front wheels. The engine is located beneath the windshield and/or beside the driver's seat. Type B school buses have a GVWR of more than 10,000 pounds (5 000 kg).

Type C

This type of school bus is the model Americans usually think of when they think of a school bus **(Figure 9.14)**. Some type C buses are capable of carrying up to 78 passengers. The passenger body is installed on a flat-back cowl chassis.

The entry/exit door is located aft of the front fender, and there is no driver-side door **(Figure 9.15, p. 358)**. The engine compartment protrudes from the front of the vehicle. Type C school buses have a GVWR of more than 10,000 pounds (5 000 kg), and have an average weight of 20,000 to 30,000 pounds (10 000 to 15 000 kg).

Type D

These buses are full-size vehicles with a boxy appearance. Some type D school buses are capable of carrying up to 90 passengers **(Figure 9.16, p. 358)**. The entry/exit door is located forward of the front wheels, and there is no driver-side door. Roof hatches may also be provided, one toward the front of the bus and a second toward the rear. The engine location varies, but could be located in the front, midship, or rear of the vehicle. Type D school buses have a GVWR of more than 10,000 pounds (5 000 kg), and many of these weigh more than 30,000 pounds (15 000 kg).

Transit Buses

Transit buses are designed to move a large number of people over relatively short distances. They have capacities for both seated and standing passengers **(Figure 9.17, p. 358)**. These buses are most commonly found in urban or metropolitan areas that operate mass transit systems. In some cases, these bus routes extend far into the suburbs surrounding the core coverage area. Similar types of buses are often used for the following:

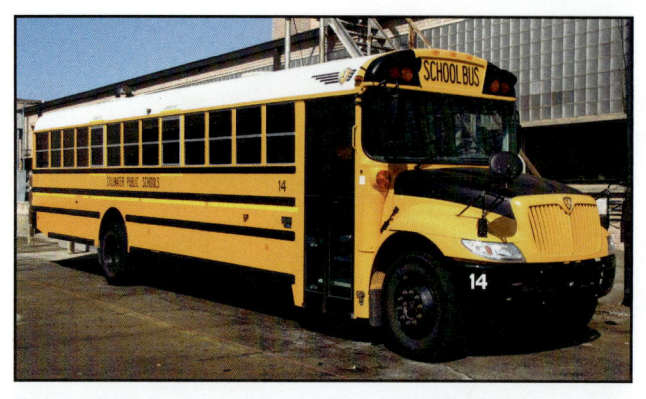

Figure 9.15 Another view of a Type C school bus.

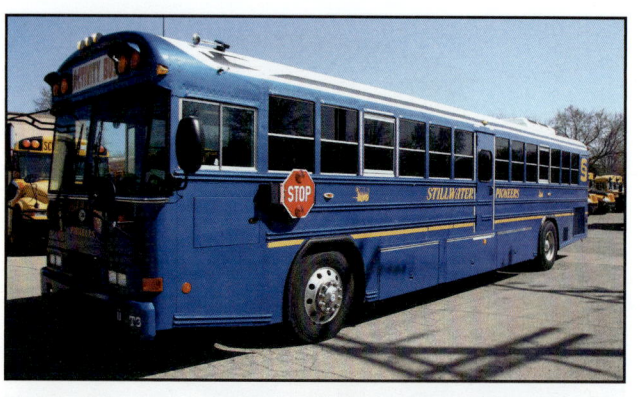

Figure 9.16 An example of a Type D school bus.

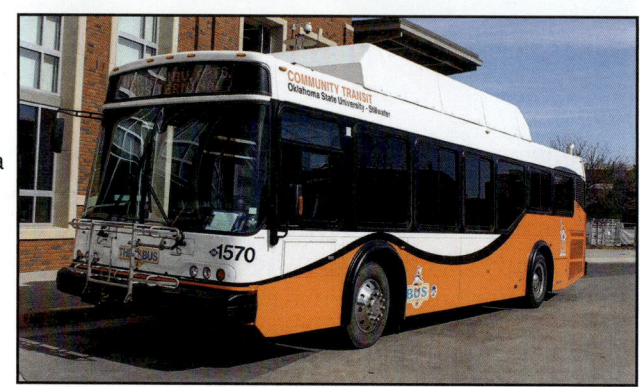

Figure 9.17 An example of a transit bus.

- Parking shuttles at airports
- Large amusement or entertainment facilities
- Employee shuttles within large business or industrial complexes

Transit buses generally operate in heavy traffic, which increases the potential for involvement in an accident. The potential for a large number of casualties is present because of high passenger loads and the fact that passengers may be sitting or standing in an irregular and unrestrained manner.

This classification includes articulated transit buses. In some areas, budget limitations have forced transit systems to reduce the frequency of bus service. To offset this reduction, some areas use larger buses that can transport more passengers per trip. Because it is impractical to design a single chassis vehicle longer than about 40 feet (12 m), some transit authorities have switched to articulated buses **(Figure 9.18)**. The advantages in maneuverability offered by these buses are similar to those that the tractor-tiller aerial apparatus offers to the fire service. The vehicle's ability to flex in the middle makes it able to maneuver extremely well in areas that single-chassis vehicles of comparable size could not.

Commercial Buses

Commercial buses, also called motor coaches, charter buses, and touring buses, are primarily designed to transport up to 50 passengers over relatively long distances. These buses may travel regularly scheduled routes or may be chartered to a specific location. Because charter buses travel through almost every region, every organization responsible for extrication must be prepared to deal with this type of vehicle **(Figure 9.19)**.

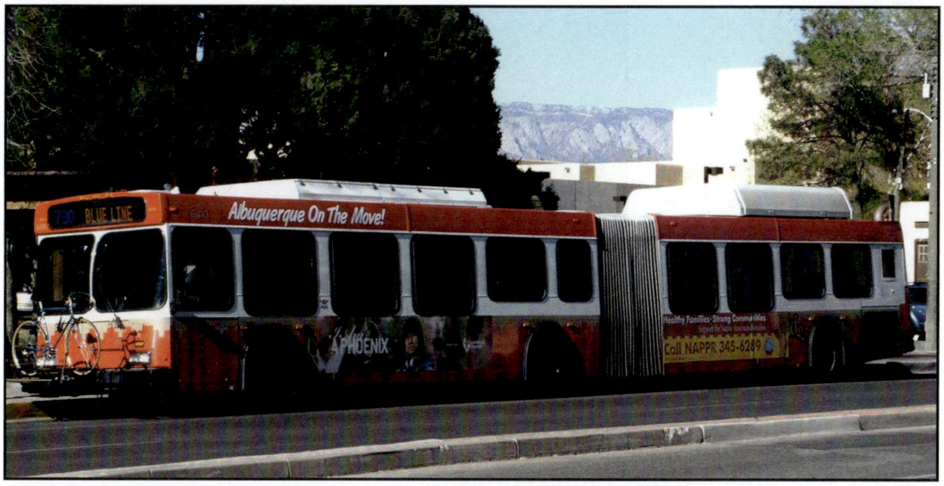

Figure 9.18 An example of an articulated transit bus. *Courtesy of John Perry, Albuquerque, N.M.*

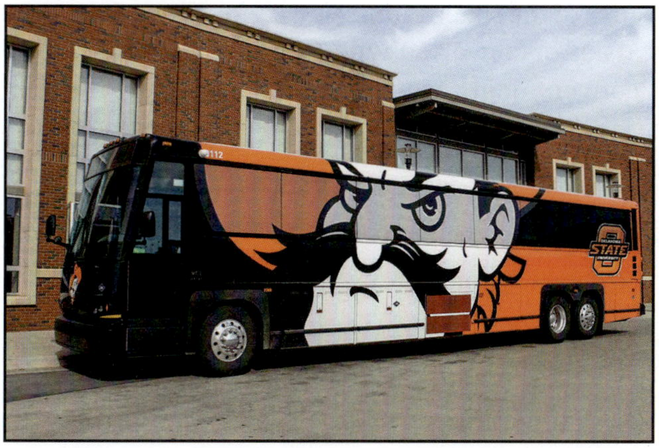

Figure 9.19 An example of a commercial bus, also called a motor coach, charter bus, or touring bus.

NOTE: Some buses may have bathrooms, kitchens, and sleeping areas. The kitchens may have propane-fueled equipment.

CAUTION

Although commercial buses should not transport hazardous materials, the bus operator does not check the contents of passengers' bags and cannot be certain that no hazardous materials are present. Many of these buses contain personal oxygen cylinders and/or oxygen generators for passengers with special needs.

Specialty Buses

Specialty buses are typically conversions of other bus classifications. Converted buses have the same general construction features as the conventional vehicles from which the conversions were made, with a few exceptions. The following sections discuss some of the exceptional features of bus conversions.

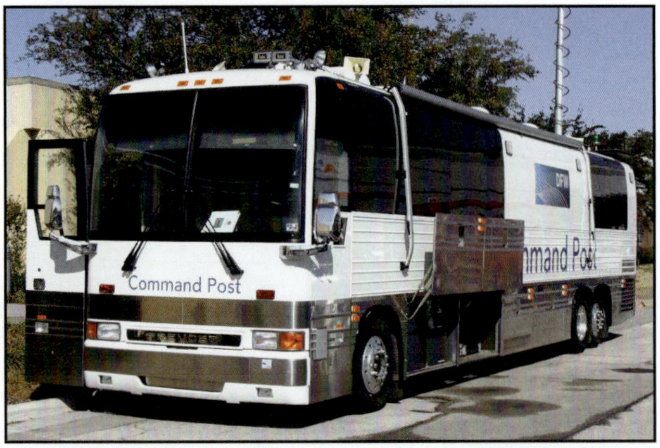

Figure 9.20 An example of a commercial bus converted into a department of public safety mobile command post.

Type A and B School Bus Conversions

Many type A and B school buses have been converted into transports for individuals with disabilities. These conversions are usually designed to carry fewer total passengers because of the space requirements for wheelchairs and other devices. The center aisles in converted type A and B buses are significantly wider than those in conventional buses in order to make more room for Emergency Medical Service (EMS) personnel to maneuver inside the vehicle **(Figure 9.20)**.

Commercial Bus Conversions

Commercial buses have been converted into a variety of specialty buses including the following:

- Prisoner transports
- Mobile field hospitals and ambulances
- Mobile command posts and communications vehicles
- Mobile living quarters
- Mobile business offices
- Limo buses or party buses

In most cases, these buses vary from standard commercial buses mainly in the configuration of their interiors. Those converted as prisoner transports may have conventional seating but the windows may be covered with bars, heavy-gauge wire screens, or even metal plates with louvers to allow for air circulation. Those converted for use as mobile offices may have most of the original seating removed and office furniture in its place. There may or may not be separate sleeping quarters. Those that have been converted into mobile living quarters may be more like motor homes than buses, but their basic structure is still that of a commercial bus, and rescue personnel should follow the protocols and procedures recommended for that type of bus. Bus conversions can often be identified by their blacked-out windows and customized paint schemes.

Bus Anatomy

Even though all buses are intended for similar purposes, there are significant differences in how the various types of buses are constructed. The level of familiarity that rescue personnel have with the anatomy of a bus will dictate how effectively they can handle extrication problems in that type of vehicle. Rescue personnel should be able to identify different types of:

- Bus doors
- Bus windows
- Bus seats
- Bus aisles
- Bus battery systems
- Bus battery systems
- Bus electrical systems
- Bus fuel systems
- Bus suspension systems

Bus Doors

Bus doors vary based on the classification of bus. The following types of bus doors will be described in this section:

- School bus front doors
- School bus rear doors
- Transit bus doors
- Commercial bus doors

School Bus Front Doors

There are various types of entry doors on school buses, each serving a specific function. The doors are strategically located to maximize exit paths during an emergency. Entry doors on some type A and type B school buses are stock versions provided by the original manufacturer. The latch and lock mechanism is the Nader safety lock found on most motor vehicles since 1973.

The passenger side front door may be drastically altered to suit the needs of the school bus owner/operator. It may have the same general design as a standard passenger vehicle door, but the window glass is typically permanently fixed in a closed position. The door handles, armrests, and window cranks may be removed.

The passenger side front doors on the full-size type C and D school buses open in a variety of ways. Some are two-part, split-type doors that open inwardly or outwardly, with outward being most common **(Figure 9.21)**. When operated, these doors split in the middle, with each half of the door swinging to its respective side.

Another common type of door is a center-hinged door that opens by folding forward or rearward **(Figure 9.22)**. Regardless of the type of door, the most common way to open it or secure it in the closed position is with the manual control arm mechanism. When open, school bus front doors typically have a horizontal opening between 22 and 24 inches (550 and 600 mm) and a minimum vertical opening approximately 68 to 72 inches (1 700 to 1 800 mm).

On older buses, the only way to open or close the front passenger exit door is a manual control arm operated by the driver. Newer buses have a powered door opening mechanism operated by the driver and an emergency release

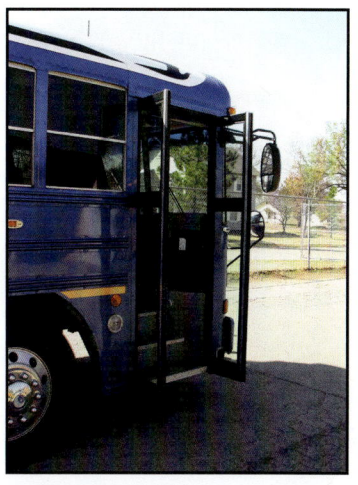

Figure 9.21 Outward opening, two-part, split-type doors on a Type D school bus.

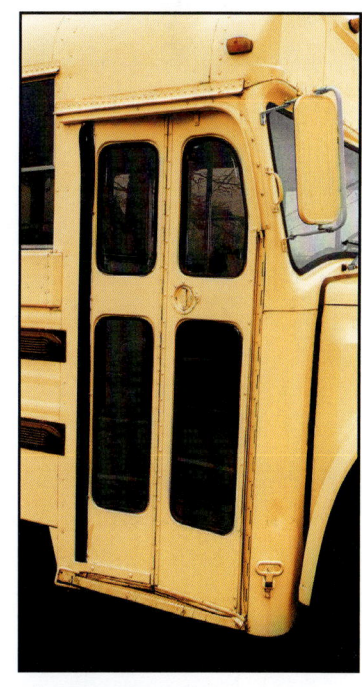

Figure 9.22 A center-hinged, forward folding door.

handle mounted on the inside of the door. School buses of all types used to transport special needs passengers may be equipped with electric lifts at the side doors.

Some school buses use air-operated mechanisms to control the front door. The main switch is usually located to the left of the driver on the instrument console. There will also be a backup emergency release mechanism in the exit stairwell inside the vehicle. The readily identifiable release button or switch causes the air lock device to release the door. Rescue personnel can then manually move the door through its normal path of travel. There may not be an air override release mechanism if there are two similar doors located along the same side of the bus.

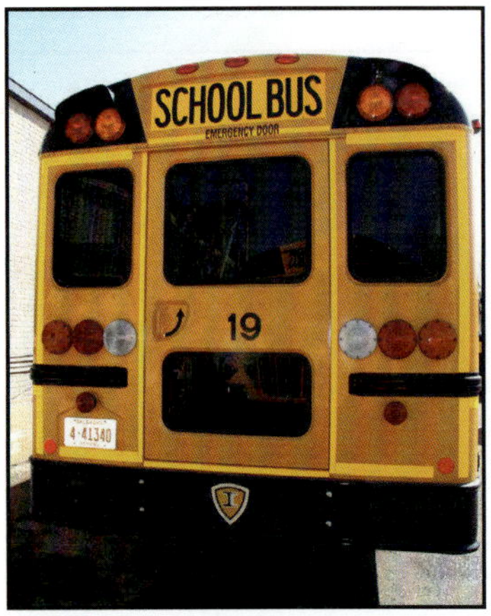

School Bus Rear Doors

The rear exit door is designed to give occupants inside the vehicle a way to exit if the front door does not function or is blocked. On type A school buses, there may be one or two rear exit doors. On type B, C, and some D school buses, there is usually one large rear exit door. There is no locking device on these rear doors, and they open outwardly by manipulation of a lever to release a latch mechanism **(Figure 9.23)**. These doors may be opened from the exterior as well as from the interior.

The rear exit door is secured by a one-point or three-point latch system. The main latch is at the edge of the door near the control handle. The other two latches, if present, are found at the top and bottom of the door, engaging the bus body and the floor assembly.

Figure 9.23 A rear exit door on a Type C school bus.

NOTE: Rear-engine type D buses do not have a rear exit door but are required by U.S. Motor Vehicle Safety Standards to have a rear emergency window exit.

In some states, buses with larger capacities are required to have an additional exit door along the driver's side of the vehicle. This third door, or left-hand door, provides an opening of 24 x 48 inches (600 x 1 200 mm) and is secured with the same one-point or three-point latch mechanism as the rear door. Access is easier from the exterior, since the interior access to the latch mechanism may be obstructed by the passenger seats.

Transit Bus Doors

Nearly all transit bus doors are two-pieces and center-opening. While most swing toward the outside, some slide laterally. The opening mechanism may be pneumatic, hydraulic, or electric, depending upon the manufacturer. The operating control is usually located at the driver's left side. Most transit buses are constructed with two passenger side doors. One is at the front of the vehicle, directly opposite the driver; the other is midship, or slightly aft of midship. Both doors are intended for normal entry and exit by passengers. These doors normally open and close simultaneously. Unlike school buses, transit buses generally do not have a specific emergency exit door. Instead, all transit buses are equipped with window exits in addition to the regular exits.

Commercial Bus Doors

All commercial buses have a single passenger-side door at the front. This door is usually a one-piece, single-hinged door with hinges located on the forward edge of the door. A few models have a two-piece center-opening door, or a folding door. The folding door is not a center opening door like those found on school or transit buses. It has a hinge along one edge and in the center allowing it to fold to one side. The door folds toward the front of the bus instead of swinging open like a one-piece door.

Many commercial bus doors use air-operated opening mechanisms. When the driver operates a dash-mounted control device, compressed air pressure opens the door. In the event of air compressor failure, or any other emergency, the driver can open these doors by operating an emergency release that allows the door to be manually operated. Interior emergency releases are located near the top of the door. Exterior releases are usually located in one of the following places:

- In the right front wheel well
- Under or to the left of the door on the outside of the vehicle
- Directly below the center of the windshield

Some motor coaches have mechanical pivot arm openers similar to those used on school buses. The emergency release for these doors is a knob or latch located directly under the center of the windshield on the front of the bus.

Most commercial buses do not have emergency exit doors, although a few import models do. Most rely on window exits for emergencies.

Bus Windows

Bus windows vary based on the classification of bus. The following types of bus windows will be described in this section:

- School bus windows
- Transit bus windows
- Commercial bus windows

School Bus Windows

The openings for the side and rear windows are defined by the vertical frame members, the roof edge, and the top of the sidewall. The vertical posts between the windows are either extensions of the roof bows or are hollow tubular structures consisting of several layers of sheet metal. These posts can be removed with powered cutters or reciprocating saws.

The windows may be laminated or tempered safety glass framed in extruded aluminum. The windows are of the split-sash design and are affixed to the rough openings with screws, rivets, or similar fasteners. Typical school bus windows open from the top down, providing an opening of approximately 9 x 22 inches (225 x 550 mm), or one-half the total size of the window area.

Some states have regulations requiring that certain side windows be designed as emergency exits and labeled as such inside the vehicle. From the exterior, rescuers can identify these exits by the hinges located along the top side of the window frames **(Figure 9.24, p. 364)**. Once opened, these windows provide a larger opening through the side of the vehicle than standard windows.

On smaller conversion-type school buses, the stock one-piece laminated safety glass windshields are set into the vehicle body with a multi-piece rubber mounting gasket. Windshields on full-size buses are mounted the same way but consist of two or more sheets of laminated safety glass.

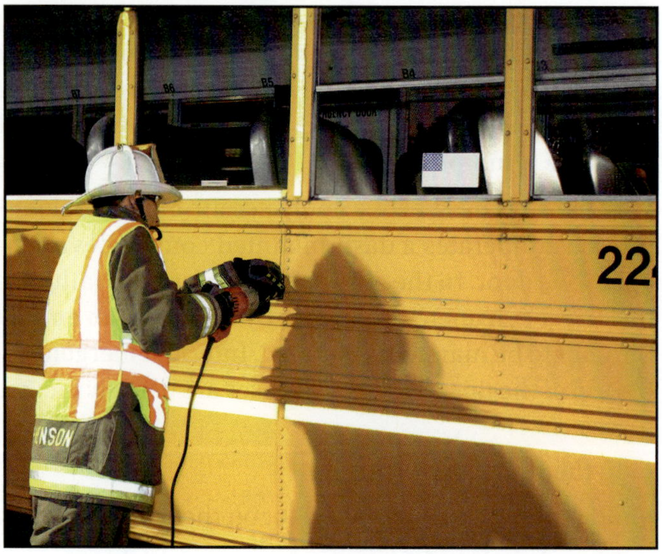

Figure 9.24 The center window of a school bus. The silver colored frame can be removed and the opening used as an emergency exit.

Rear windows are flat sheets of laminated safety glass and are mounted with removable rubber gaskets. The mounting components for both the windshield and the rear windows are similar to those described in Chapter 6, Passenger Vehicles. Types C and D buses may also be equipped with fixed windows and air conditioning systems.

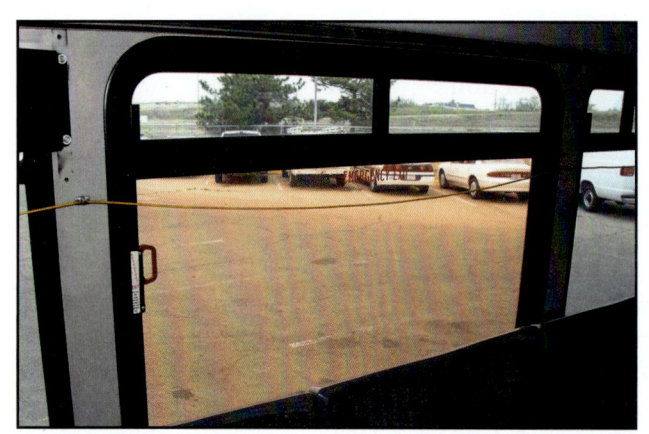

Figure 9.25 An example of a transit bus window looking outward from the interior.

Transit Bus Windows

Transit buses most commonly have windows made of laminated safety glass. Some transit buses have side windows of tempered glass, Plexiglas®, or other synthetic material. Transit bus windshields and rear windows are similar to those in school buses or other large vehicles. The large windshields are typically of two-piece design. Transit bus windshields are held in place by a simple locking rubber filler strip **(Figure 9.25)**.

Types of transit bus side windows vary greatly, depending on the age of the bus and the manufacturer. Older buses without air conditioning may have windows that can only be opened by sliding to one side or the other. The glass in sliding windows is set into aluminum or another lightweight metal frame designed to slide open a distance equal to one-half the width of the entire window unit. Transit buses are now commonly equipped with windows that are hinged at the top and are designed to tilt out when the latch on the lower side is released. Some transit buses have windows that are designed to slide open during normal operation, and tilt out to provide an emergency exit. These windows will not stay open by themselves and have to be propped open.

Commercial Bus Windows
Most commercial buses are air-conditioned, with little or no need for windows that open. Because of this, all modern motor coaches are designed with single-piece side windows, some of which can be opened in emergencies. These exit windows are set in metal frames that are hinged at the top. These windows can be opened by lifting a horizontal bar located across the bottom of the window frame. Releasing this mechanism allows passengers to push out the bottom of the window and provides an exit path. These emergency exit window openings are 20 x 48 inches (500 x 1 200 mm) or larger. Rescuers must prop these window exits to keep them open. Pike poles are well suited for this purpose.

Commercial bus windshields and rear windows are set in a rubber molding. Windshields and rear windows are usually constructed of laminated automotive safety glass. Side windows may be laminated glass, tempered safety glass, Lexan®, or other synthetic material.

Bus Seats
Bus seats vary based on the classification of bus. The following types of bus seats will be described in this section:

- School bus seats
- Transit bus seats
- Commercial bus seats

School Bus Seats
The two types of seats found in school buses are driver's seats and passenger seats. The driver's seat is an adjustable bucket-type seat with a floor-mounted seat belt and/or shoulder harness assembly. Passenger seats are framed with 1-inch (25 mm) tubular steel. The seats are bolted into the bus floor and into the sidewall. Detachable foam rubber seat cushions and seat backs are covered with vinyl upholstery. Since 1977, school bus seat backs have been required to be 24 inches (600 mm) high.

All types of school bus passenger seats may be equipped with lap-style seat belts if mandated by local ordinance or state law, but all type A buses under 10,000 pounds (5 000 kg) GVWR must have lap belts. Buses used to transport people with physical or mental disabilities may have positive body restraint harnesses in specially designated seats.

Transit Bus Seats
Nearly all passenger seats found on transit buses are molded from some type of plastic. They may be further covered by a vinyl or plastic covering or cushions. Transit bus seats are supported by a metal framework that is bolted to the floor and the sides of the bus. Some buses have handrail systems bolted to their ceilings **(Figure 9.26, p. 366)**.

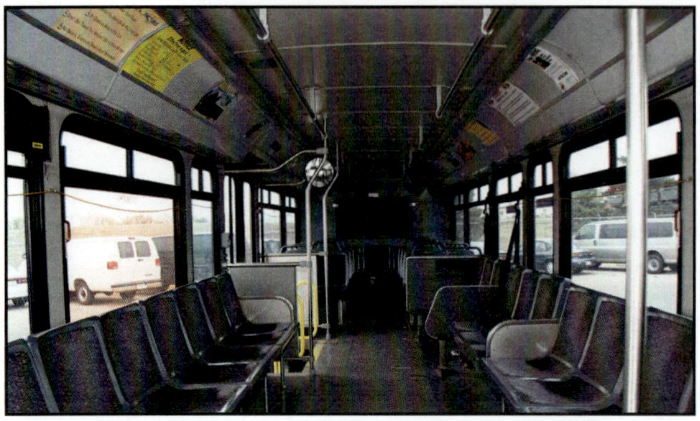

Figure 9.26 The front seats in this transit bus face the center while those in the back face forward.

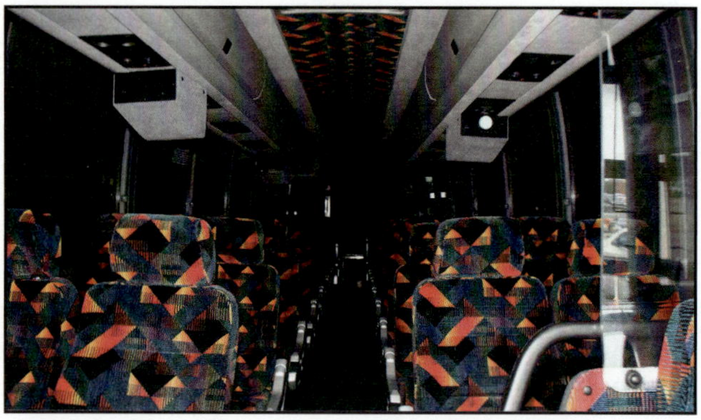

Figure 9.27 Commercial bus seats are designed for passenger comfort.

Transit bus seating has a different layout than other types of buses. Most transit buses do not have the standard, uniform front-facing seat arrangement. The seats in a transit bus may face forward, toward the center aisle, or toward the rear of the bus. The layouts vary depending on the owner/operator's specifications. They may vary within the same transit fleet, depending on the age of individual buses and prevailing trends at the time the vehicles were purchased. The driver's seat in a transit bus is similar to the driver's seat in a school bus.

Commercial Bus Seats

Commercial buses are generally equipped with individual bucket-type seats for each occupant, similar to those on commercial airliners **(Figure 9.27, p. 366)**. These seats have high backs, can be reclined, and may or may not have armrests between the seats. They are usually mounted four to a row, two on each side of the center aisle. Seat mounting varies from manufacturer to manufacturer. Some seats are connected and mounted like the bench seats in a school bus. The legs on the aisle side are bolted to the floor, and the window side of the seat is bolted to the floor and/or the sidewall. Other seats may be mounted on a pedestal that is bolted to the floor. Most drivers' seats are pedestal mounted. Some motor coaches have a bench at the rear of the bus; this bench is usually molded into the rear frame design and removing anything other than the cushions is extremely difficult.

Bus Aisles

Bus aisles vary based on the classification of bus. The following types of bus aisles will be described in this section:

- School bus aisles
- Transit bus aisles
- Commercial bus aisles

School Bus Aisles

The position of the seats inside the school bus dictates the width of the vehicle's center aisle. The aisle of Suburban-type buses can be as narrow as 10 inches (250 mm). Aisle space in van-conversion buses increases to approximately 12 inches (300 mm). Full-size school buses may have aisle widths between

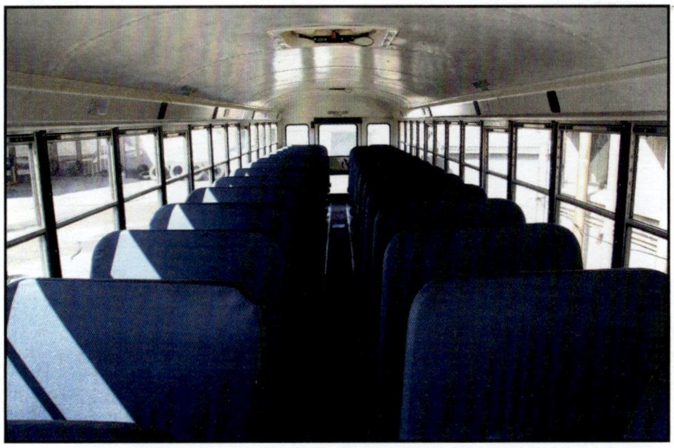

Figure 9.28 An example of the aisle space provided between passenger seats on either side of the school bus.

12 and 15 inches (300 and 375 mm). Since the width of a typical backboard is 18 inches (450 mm), a narrow center aisle can make the process of removing victims difficult **(Figure 9.28)**.

Wheelchair-equipped vehicles generally have a 30-inch (750 mm) wide aisle in the area where the chair will be maneuvered. The aisle may not be that wide throughout the entire vehicle.

Transit Bus Aisles
In most transit buses, the width of the center aisle is considerably wider than typical school bus aisles. This is because transit buses are designed for adults who may be carrying items such as packages and briefcases. The wider aisle also results from different seating arrangements. Depending on seat layout, transit bus aisles vary in width from about 20 inches (500 mm) to about 5 feet (1.5 m). This extra width makes transit buses somewhat easier than school buses for rescue personnel to work and maneuver in.

Commercial Bus Aisles
Most commercial buses have a uniform aisle width for most of the length of the seating area. Some buses may have some variation in aisle width toward the rear of the bus near the rest room. The center aisle is usually between 13 and 18 inches (325 and 450 mm) wide. This narrow width creates problems for rescuers trying to remove victims on backboards, scoop stretchers, or other litters. The ceiling height in commercial bus aisles is generally 75 to 78 inches (1 900 to 1 950 mm). Because of the high seat backs and low overhead luggage racks, it may be difficult to carry the litters over the seat tops. In some cases, rescuers may have to remove seats to make passage possible.

Bus Construction and Safety Features
Buses have specific construction and safety features that rescue personnel should be familiar with, such as:

- School bus construction components
- Transit bus construction components
- Commercial bus construction components
- Hydraulic lifts

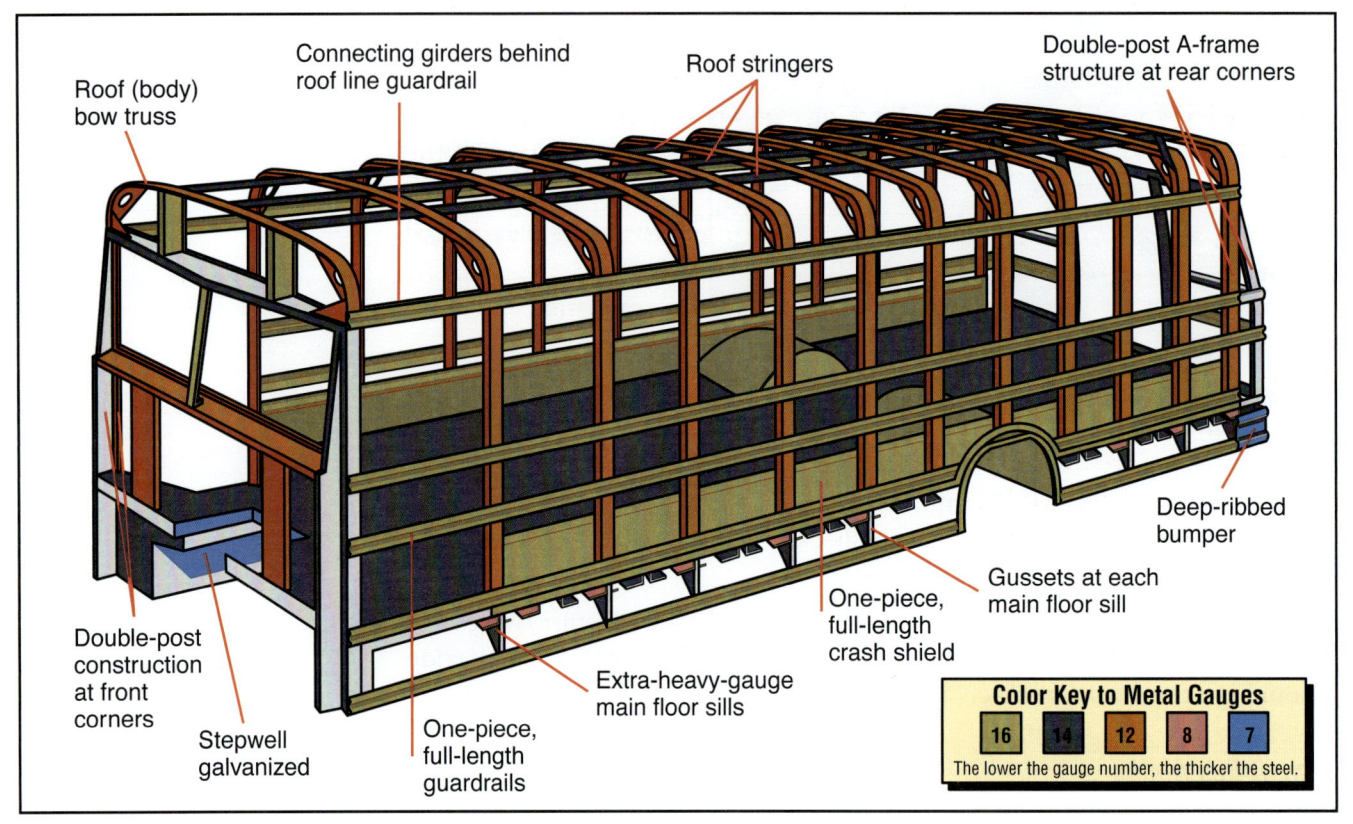

Figure 9.29 An in-depth look at the skeletal system of a school bus body. *Courtesy of the Wayne Corporation.*

- Battery systems
- Electrical systems
- Fuel Systems
- Suspension systems

NOTE: Construction components such as the frame and chassis provide stabilization points for rescuers. However, on buses that do not have a rigid frame, rescuers should look for specially designed jack plates to use for bus stabilization.

School Bus Construction Components

Major school bus manufacturers use two basic construction methods:

- **Integral construction** — The body and chassis are formed as a unit. The manufacturer assembles the vehicle starting with the frame and chassis assembly and proceeds item by item to the finished vehicle.

- **Body-on-chassis** — The body and chassis are manufactured as separate units and joined by the bus manufacturer.

School Bus Skeletal System

All school bus body units are comprised of a roof, floor, two sidewalls, and front and rear assemblies. The finish and trim components of each area of the body are supported by a skeletal system beneath. This skeletal system forms the basic structure of the entire bus. It dictates how the vehicle will respond during a collision and forms the basis of the protective envelope designed to provide occupant safety and survival **(Figure 9.29).**

Sidewalls are comprised of vertical load-bearing frame members. In some models, the roof bows extend down to form the support members. These vertical members serve as partitions between window openings. Running horizontally along the base of each sidewall is a framing element referred to as a collision beam. This heavy-gauge steel beam limits penetration of an object into the passenger compartment.

Finish panels of 20-gauge steel are typically mounted on the exterior and 22-gauge on the interior of the sidewall frame members. To meet requirements for interior noise attenuation and temperature control, insulation materials may be sandwiched between the interior and exterior panels.

Additional impact resistance is added to the exterior sidewall. Formed rub rails (4.75-inch [120 mm] wide) of 16-gauge steel run the full length of the sidewalls. They are intended to minimize penetration during collision and can also be used for identifying occupant location from the exterior. One rub rail will indicate the seat cushion level; if a second rail is present, it will identify the floor level. Some school buses have as many as four rub rails from the bottom of the windows down to the bottom of the skirts.

The rear skeletal system is similar to the sidewall, with additional reinforcement installed to provide protection from rear-end collisions. Some buses use a double-post A-frame structural member built into their rear corners.

The skeletal framework of the school bus roof commonly consists of 11-14 gauge steel frame members called roof bows. Roof bows span the roof structure from side to side. Within this frame are 14-16 gauge girders (known as stringers) running from front to rear, strengthening and spacing the bows. There may be as many as three stringers in the roof skeleton.

Insulation material and electrical wiring are located within the framework of the roof. The outside and inside of the framing members are generally covered with sheet metal panels. If breaching the roof structure becomes necessary, rescuers can determine the location of the roof bows and stringers by the rows of rivets used to secure the roof panels.

Emergency escape hatches may also be located in the roof structure. These hatches are made of fiberglass or other lightweight materials, and they open by the activation of a release mechanism from inside or outside of the bus. If necessary, they may be forced open using conventional prying techniques. These hatches open fully to provide a clear opening of at least 11 x 14 inches (275 x 350 mm). Some buses may have larger hatches, especially if they are used to transport passengers with physical disabilities **(Figure 9.30 a and b, p. 370)**.

School Bus Floor and Undercarriage

The floor of a school bus consists of several components. In most full-size buses, a heavy-duty vinyl or rubber floor covers plywood decking and 14 gauge metal flooring panels. The smaller conversion-type vehicles may have one half or five eighth-inch (12.5 or 15.5 mm) plywood sheets placed on top of the existing vehicle floor. Structural members, acting as floor joists, are spaced as close as every 9 inches (225 mm) along the underside of the floor **(Figure 9.31, p. 370)**.

The undercarriage of a typical school bus is substantially reinforced with 8 gauge angle bar, 12 gauge channel stock, and 14 gauge sheet metal. Guard loops around the entire length of the driveshaft prevent the driveshaft from falling to the ground if it breaks or becomes disconnected.

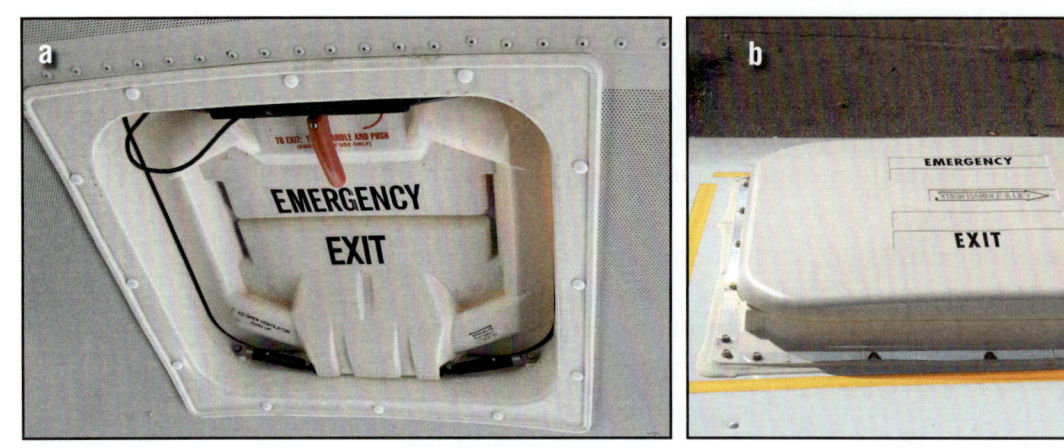

Figure 9.30 a. An emergency escape hatch in the roof of a school bus as seen from the interior. **b.** An exterior view of a roof mounted emergency escape hatch on a school bus.

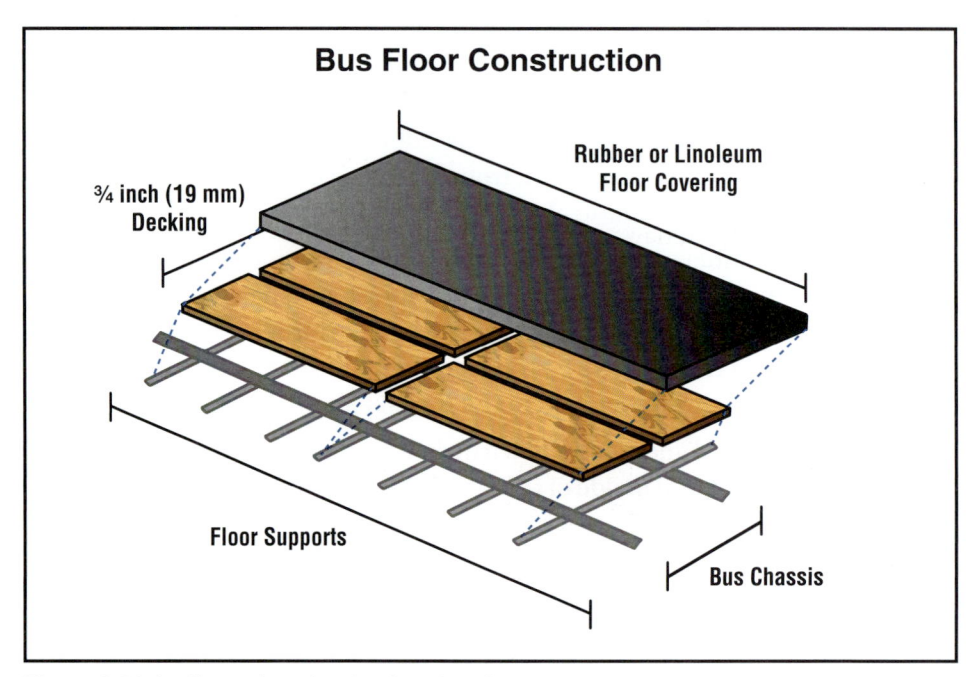

Figure 9.31 An illustration showing how bus floors are constructed.

NOTE: Forcible entry through the floor is difficult and time consuming. Floors should not be considered as a primary entry point.

Transit Bus Construction Components

In general, transit buses are of integral body construction. This construction combines the chassis framing and the body understructure into one integral module. The main undercarriage structure consists of longitudinal beams that support horizontal and vertical beams made of carbon steel, mild steel, and other materials.

All other structural components are made of either galvanized or stainless steel or aluminum. These components include tubular support members, cross bracing, inner or outer panels, plates, and any other formed members.

Formed tubular members support the upper body portion of the bus. This upper body structure is welded to the vertical carline supports located near the floor of the bus. Carline supports are gussets that strengthen the sidewall of a bus at the level most likely to be struck by a vehicle. The roof is constructed of inner and outer panels that sandwich insulation and electrical wiring and fixtures between them. The most common material used for transit bus floor decking is three fourth-inch (19 mm) plywood. The decking may be covered with floor coverings such as rubber or linoleum.

Commercial Bus Construction Components

Most manufacturers of commercial buses construct the entire frame of the vehicle as one integral unit. The majority of the frame is constructed of low carbon, square steel tubing 1 to 2 inches (25 to 50 mm) in diameter. The frame is covered with either aluminum or stainless steel sheeting. On some buses, the panels covering the front and rear modules are made of fiberglass.

Framing members that support the roof are generally separated by about 24 to 26 inches (600 to 650 mm) on center. The outer (roof) and inner (ceiling) panels sandwich wiring and insulation. Unlike other types of buses, panels in a commercial bus may not be riveted to every structural member. Some manufacturers rivet the panels to every other roof rafter; therefore, there is a structural member about halfway between each row of rivets. If the rows of rivets are more than about 2 feet (0.7 m) apart, a rafter is likely to be located between the two riveted members.

Commercial bus floors are constructed in a manner similar to those on transit buses. Most are one half- or three fourth-inch (12.5 or 19 mm) plywood covered with a composite rubber or other synthetic covering.

Hydraulic Lifts

Many type A and B school bus conversions are equipped with double entry/exit doors located midship on the passenger side that also convert to an electrically operated wheelchair lift. Some transit buses are designed to accommodate passengers with physical disabilities. These buses may be equipped with one or a combination of features, including a hydraulic lift, that allow easier access for passengers with limited mobility or those confined to wheelchairs **(Figure 9.32)**. Hydraulic lifts raise passengers in wheelchairs from curb height to assist them onto the bus and lower them back to curb height when they wish to exit. The lift may be located at the front, middle, or rear of the vehicle and may have its own access point. By operating a control next to the door, the bus driver converts the stairway into a lift. When the control is operated, the stairs fold out into a lift platform. From that position, the platform may be lowered or raised.

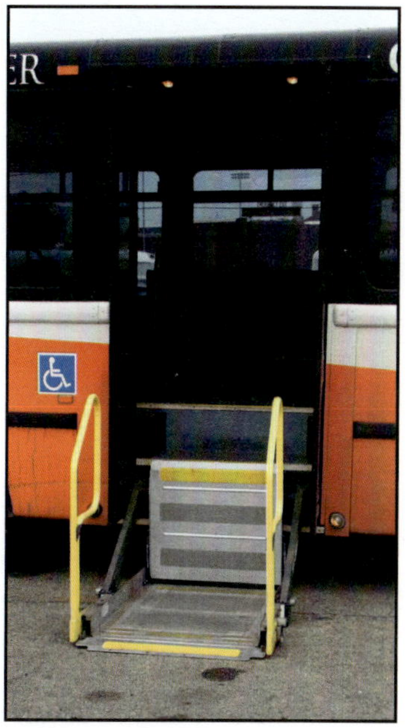

Bus Battery Systems

Bus battery systems vary based on the classification of bus. The following types of bus battery systems will be described in this section:

- School bus batteries
- Transit bus batteries
- Commercial bus batteries

Figure 9.32 A hydraulic lift system on a transit bus.

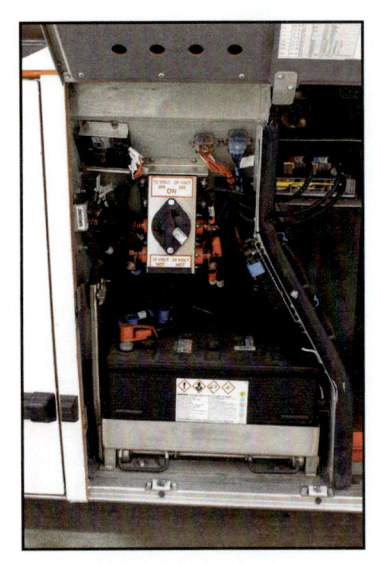

Figure 9.33 The battery compartment on a transit bus.

School Bus Batteries
On type A and some type B buses, the batteries are usually located in the engine compartment. On most type B, C, and D buses, the batteries are typically located in a separate compartment on the driver's side of the vehicle. A bus equipped with an electric lift may have a separate battery for the lift. This battery is usually located in a separate compartment on the driver's side of the vehicle. Disconnecting the lift battery will not interrupt power to the engine.

Transit Bus Batteries
The low voltage (12V and 24V) battery banks on nearly all transit buses are located in a compartment on the driver's side of the vehicle, just forward of the rear wheels **(Figure 9.33)**. For ease of access, the batteries are grouped together on a tray that can be pulled out when the battery door is open. Most transit buses are also equipped with a battery shutoff switch located in the battery compartment. Power from the batteries can be interrupted by simply moving this switch to the OFF position.

Commercial Bus Batteries
The location of the batteries on commercial motor coaches varies depending on the manufacturer of the bus. Many are found just aft of the front wheel on the passenger side of the bus.

Regardless of the location of the batteries, all manufacturers place an electrical disconnect switch in the battery compartment. **(Figure 9.34)**. This switch will either be directly above or below the batteries. Electrical service to the bus's 24-volt systems, such as air conditioning, can be interrupted via this switch. In some cases, interior emergency lights will still have power even though the battery switch is off.

To de-energize emergency systems, rescuers will need to disconnect or cut the battery cables. When isolating the battery, disconnect the negative terminal first.

Bus Electrical Systems
In buses, rescuers can use a number of different methods to interrupt the electrical power supply. They can operate the battery shutoff switch located in the battery compartment, disconnect the battery cables, or cut the cables. The following text addresses the most common battery locations for most buses. Rescuers should anticipate variations in battery location.

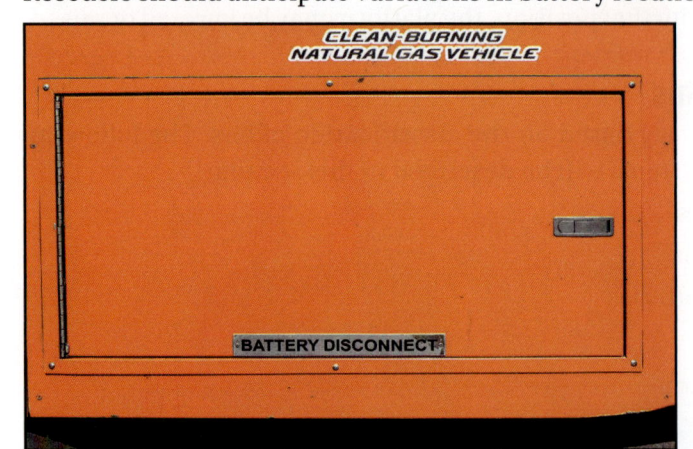

Figure 9.34 The battery shut off switch is clearly labeled on this bus.

Batteries on Type A and B school buses are usually located in the engine compartment. Buses with electric lifts may have a separate battery for the lift. This battery is usually located in a separate compartment on the driver's side of the vehicle. Disconnecting the lift battery will not interrupt power to the engine.

On Type C and D school buses, the batteries are either under the hood or in a separate compartment on the driver's side of the bus. Rescuers may need a hex key or Allen wrench to unlatch the compartment door. The required key is usually inside the school bus near the driver's area.

The battery banks of nearly all transit buses are on the driver's side of the vehicle, just forward of the rear wheels. Most transit buses have battery shut-off switches in the battery compartment. Interrupt power from the batteries by moving this switch to the OFF position. If the bus does not have a battery shutoff witch, access the batteries by pulling out the tray on which the batteries are grouped.

The location of the batteries on commercial motor coaches varies depending on the manufacturer. Many are found behind the front wheel on the passenger side of the bus. Regardless of the batteries' location, all manufacturers place an electrical disconnect switch in the battery compartment. This switch will either be directly above or below the batteries. Electrical service to the bus's 24-volt systems, such as air-conditioning, can be interrupted by operating this switch. In some cases, interior emergency lights will still have power even though the battery switch is off. To de-energize emergency lights, disconnect or cut the battery cables.

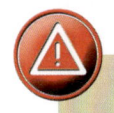

Bus Shutdown Operations

If a bus's engine is still running, rescuers should shut it off prior to disconnecting or disabling the batteries. Rescuers should attempt to turn the ignition key or push the ignition system to the OFF position. On buses equipped with an alternate fuel system, such as LPG or propane, shutting off the fuel system main supply valve will also stop the engine.

Some buses may have engine stop switches located on the driver's console, usually to the left of the driver's seat. A stop switch is also located in the rear engine compartment. It should be clearly marked and is usually found in the top left or right corner of the compartment. The stop button may have either an on/off position or it may be a push button that has to be depressed until the engine comes to a complete stop.

While the bus engine runs, carbon dioxide, halons, or halon replacement agents can be discharged into the air intake located at the rear corner of the vehicle. Air intakes may be located on either or both sides of the vehicle. If rescuers are unable to stop a running engine, they should discharge the extinguishing agent into the air intake screen area, aiming the main stream of it inward and toward the front of the vehicle. Because this method is dangerous, it is to be used ONLY if all other attempts to stop the engine have failed.

Bus Fuel Systems

Modern buses run on a variety of fuels. These fuel sources include the following:

- Gasoline and diesel
- CNG, LPG, and LNG
- Hydrogen fuel cells
- Hybrid electric
- Electricity

Gasoline and Diesel

Most school bus fuel systems use either gasoline or diesel fuel **(Figure 9.35)**. Nearly all transit and commercial buses are powered by diesel fuel, although some are powered by a mixture of diesel fuel and kerosene. Fuel tanks on type A and B school buses are commonly in the rear of the vehicle. The fuel tank(s) on school buses, transit buses, and commercial buses may be as large as 180 gallons (720 L). In type C and D school buses, as well as most transit and commercial buses, the fuel tank is located in the midship portion of the bus or slightly ahead of midship, just behind the front wheels. The fuel filler is usually located on the passenger side, just behind the front wheels, although some commercial buses may be equipped with fillers on both sides of the vehicle.

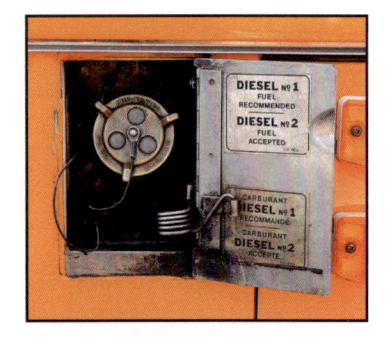

Figure 9.35 Diesel fuel is commonly used to power all types of buses.

CNG, LPG, and LNG

Many transit buses are powered by engines using alternative fuels — those other than gasoline or diesel. Most larger transit vehicles are powered by CNG while more of the smaller buses may use LPG or LNG. CNG is stored in a gaseous state at high pressure (approximately 3,600 psi [25 000 kPa]), while LNG is stored onboard as a purified and condensed liquid. LNG must be stored in a double-walled, vacuum-insulated pressure vessel. These cylinders may be mounted to the roof of the bus, or can be located on the frame underneath the skirting of the bus saddle tanks **(Figure 9.36)**.

Buses may indicate the presence of an alternative fuel system with decals or other signs on the exterior of the vehicle indicating the type of fuel in use **(Figure 9.37)**. Otherwise, the presence of a fuel filler and main supply valve at some point on the lower half of the vehicle body may be the only indication. In any case, the fuel filler and main supply valve will be located at the same point, and this point should be relatively easy to access because it is where the filler hose connects.

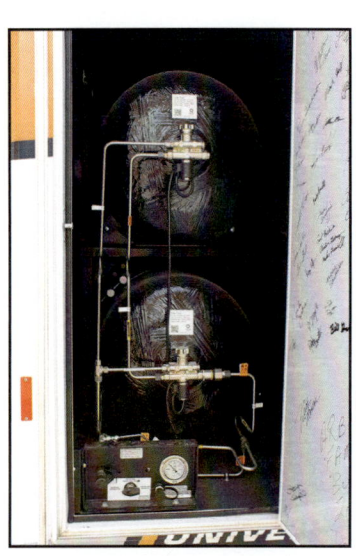

Figure 9.36 Many buses use alternative fuels such as CNG.

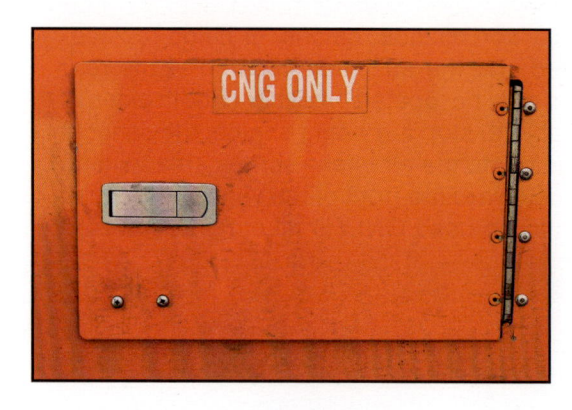

Figure 9.37 This CNG label is clearly seen on a bus.

Alternative fuels behave differently when released into the atmosphere because of their differing vapor densities. CNG and LNG are lighter than air, so they will rise when released, perhaps filling the passenger compartment. LPG is heavier than air, so it will fall when released and will collect in depressions and other low areas. In all cases, at the point of optimum fuel/air mixture, these are both highly flammable gases and represent significant safety hazards.

Hydrogen Fuel Cells

Hydrogen fuel celled vehicles typically have the same components as all other hybrids; they just have a different source of electricity. Hydrogen fuel cells generate electricity through a chemical reaction between stored hydrogen and the oxygen from the atmosphere, which propels the vehicle and re-charges the high voltage batteries. Fuel cells are typically found where the internal combustion engine would be located on non-hybrid vehicles. Each cell usually produces about 0.7 volts of DC current with most vehicles having enough cells to generate approximately 600 volts of DC electricity. The size of the total fuel cell depends on the size, weight, and the amount of current needed to propel the electric motor of the vehicle.

Hydrogen must be stored on the vehicle. Most vehicles store it on the roof in aluminum tanks that are wrapped in carbon fiber, much like modern self-contained breathing apparatus (SCBA) cylinders. Each tank stores the hydrogen at approximately 5,000 psi (35 000 kPa). Pressure regulators reduce the highly pressurized hydrogen from 5,000 psi down to 80-100 psi (35 000 down to 560-700 kPa) for use by the fuel cell. When buses using this or any other alternative fuel are introduced into an area, the rescue personnel in that jurisdiction should familiarize themselves with the fuels and their characteristics.

Hybrid Electric Buses

Numerous cities in the United States and around the world use hybrid propulsion systems for transit buses to reduce hydrocarbon fuel consumption and improve air quality in these locations.

These systems contain a vehicle propulsion system (a diesel- or gasoline-powered internal combustion engine), a battery system to store electricity, and an electric motor. The electric motor often runs the bus on level terrain or in tunnels while the internal combustion engine provides power on surface streets and when climbing grades.

Similar to passenger vehicles, hybrid buses have both high- and low- voltage battery systems. The low-voltage batteries are usually 12V or 24V systems, depending upon the ancillary power needs of the particular vehicle, such as lights and instrumentation. The location of these low voltage batteries varies. The high voltage batteries store power to drive the electric motor and are recharged through regenerative braking, similar to passenger vehicles. These batteries can store up to 800V of DC electricity and can be in multiple locations. These electrical systems most often have a service disconnect and some, although not all, have emergency shutdown switches. The high voltage system may hold a charge for up to thirty minutes after shutdown.

There are two primary hybrid propulsion system configurations: series and parallel. In the series configuration, the internal combustion engine runs a generator that provides power for the battery and electric motor. In the parallel configuration, the electric motor and the internal combustion engine are both connected to the vehicle's transmission to individually or simultaneously propel the vehicle. Some hybrid buses are equipped with a larger, secondary battery storage system that can be recharged at night from the local electrical grid.

Hybrid buses physically resemble conventional buses and most construction features are similar. However, hybrid bus construction includes the battery storage system, electrical motor, and the wiring to connect them. Extrication personnel must be cautious while isolating the power supplies on these vehicles because of the high voltage carried in these systems.

Electric Buses

Some local transit buses are powered by electricity supplied from either a high voltage battery system or from overhead wiring through a rooftop apparatus called a **pantograph**. Electric buses do not utilize an internal combustion engine and operate either by an external charging system or exclusively through electricity generated in the overhead wires **(Figure 9.38)**. Electric buses with high voltage batteries typically store them on the top of the bus, but storage locations may differ with various manufacturers.

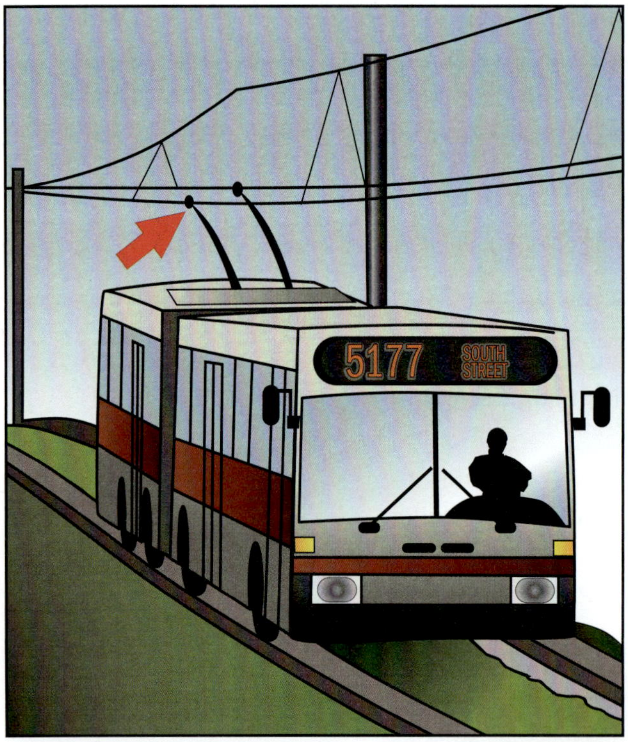

> **Pantograph** — Mechanical linkage device which maintains electrical contact with a contact wire and transfers power from the wire to the traction unit of electric buses, locomotives, and trams.

There are three different types of external charging systems. The Level 1 system uses a 120V AC charging port on the exterior of the vehicle and can take many hours to recharge a system. Although these charging ports are not in a standardized location, they are typically in a location that is easily reached from ground level. Level 2 charging systems use a 240V AC and take much less time to recharge. Level 3 charging systems utilize two types of inductive charging mechanisms strategically located at stop points along the route. The driver either aligns the bus with an overhead drop-down charging mechanism or comes to stop on top of charging mats or charging plates, which continually charge the bus at each public transit station

Bus Suspension Systems

Similar to medium and heavy trucks, most buses have a conventional heavy-duty suspension (leaf and/or coil springs) system. These systems are a vital component of ensuring the safety and comfort of everyone on board. Bus suspension systems available today have been designed to improve vehicle handling and stability and to absorb road shock for optimal driver and passenger comfort.

Figure 9.38 Some buses are powered by electricity that is supplied from overhead wires through a pantograph.

Many buses are also equipped with air suspension systems. These systems replace conventional metal springs with compact rubber air bags that are somewhat similar to a bellows. Air suspension systems often adjust to changing load conditions and improve ride quality. Each axle has air-suspension bags — two or four on each axle, depending on the system used. An on-board compressor maintains the air pressure within the bags as high as 120 psi (840 kPa). Depending upon the load of the vehicle and the condition of the road, the

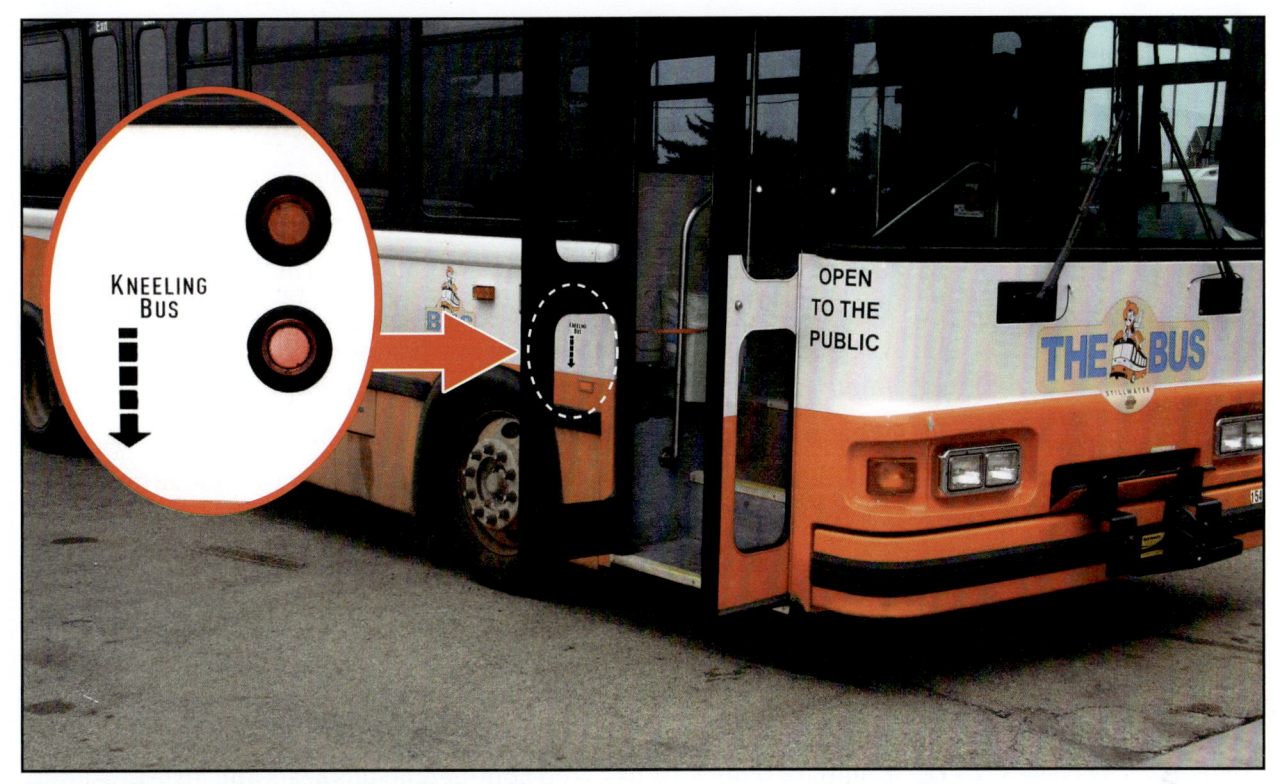

Figure 9.39 A transit bus in the "kneeling" position.

pressure within each bag automatically increases or decreases to maintain the vehicle in a level state. If the pressure in an air suspension bag is lost because of damage to the bag or its associated piping, the bus chassis can suddenly drop several inches without warning.

Another feature allows the front end of the bus to be lowered to curb level, often referred to as **kneeling**, so that a passenger is not required to step as high up to get into the bus. **(Figure 9.39).** By controlling the air in the suspension system bellows, the driver can lower the level of the step from its normal height of about 12 inches (300 mm) down to about 6 inches (150 mm). Stay clear of an unsupported bus with an air suspension system. If the air suspension system fails, anyone underneath would be crushed.

Kneeling — Ability of some buses to lower the front end of the bus to curb level for ease of passenger boarding.

WARNING!
Never put any part of your body beneath an unstabilized bus with an air suspension system.

Chapter Review

1. What characteristics define a truck as a medium or heavy truck?
2. What are some types of medium and heavy trucks?
3. What types of cabs are found in medium and heavy trucks?
4. What types of trailers are rescuers likely to encounter at vehicle incidents?
5. What types of materials are used in the construction of medium and heavy truck components?
6. What systems in medium and heavy trucks should rescuers should be familiar with in order to operate safely on scene?
7. What is the purpose of the fifth wheel on medium and heavy trucks?
8. How do the four types of school buses found in North America differ from each another?
9. What are some of the differences in the design, use, and operation of transit, commercial and specialty buses?
10. What are the various types and functions of bus doors?
11. How is the construction and operation of windows different in school, transit and commercial buses?
12. Compare school, transit, and commercial bus seats and aisles.
13. What construction components may be found in school, transit and commercial buses?
14. Where are batteries located in different types of buses, and how are they accessed?
15. How can rescuers interrupt the electrical power supply to a bus?
16. List the types of fuel systems found on buses.
17. What hazards are associated with bus suspension systems?

Discussion Questions

1. What types of medium and heavy trucks are you likely to encounter in your jurisdiction?
2. What types of buses are you likely to encounter in your jurisdiction?
3. What are the main differences between the construction of medium and heavy trucks and the construction of smaller passenger vehicles?

Commercial/Heavy Vehicle Stabilization Operations

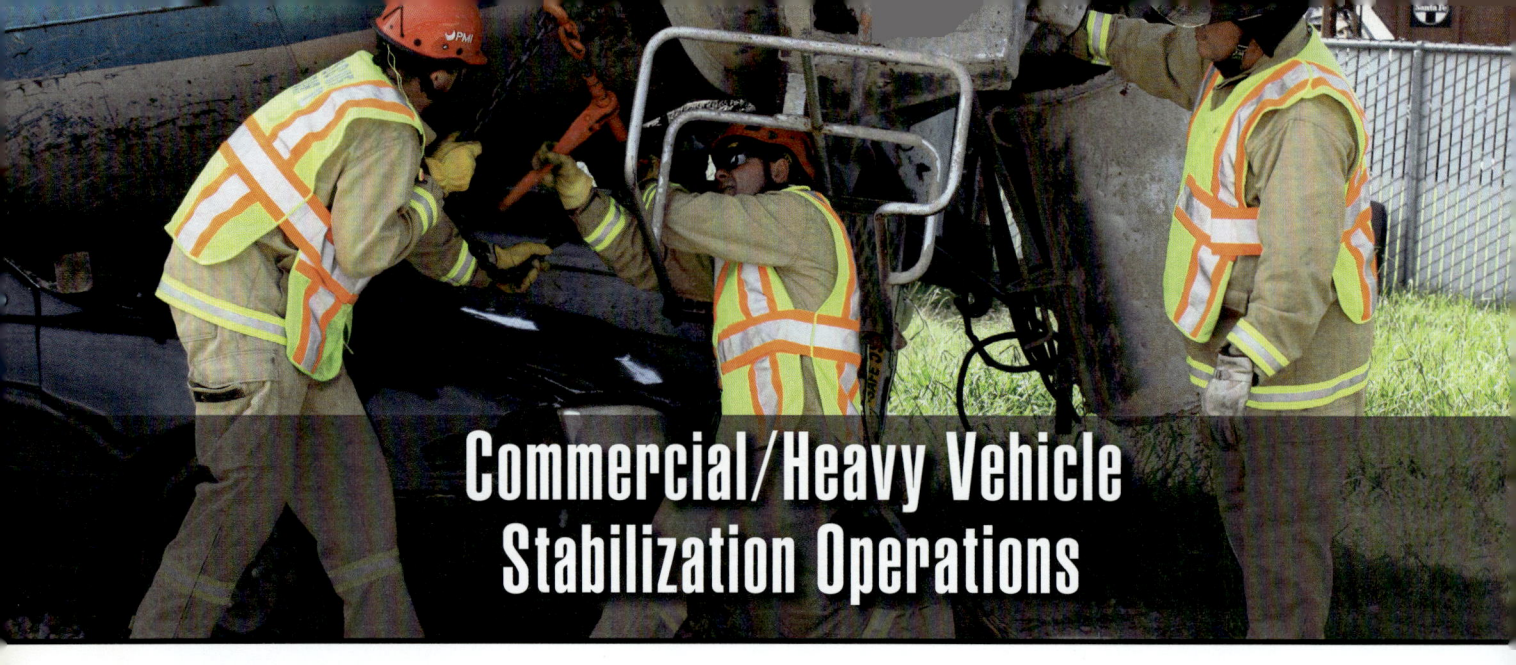

Chapter Contents

Operations Level Stabilization:
    Review **383**
Commercial/Heavy Vehicle Stabilization
    Considerations **385**
    Medium and Heavy Truck Stabilization 385
    Bus Stabilization 389
Chapter Review **394**
Discussion Questions **394**
Skill Sheets **395**

chapter 10

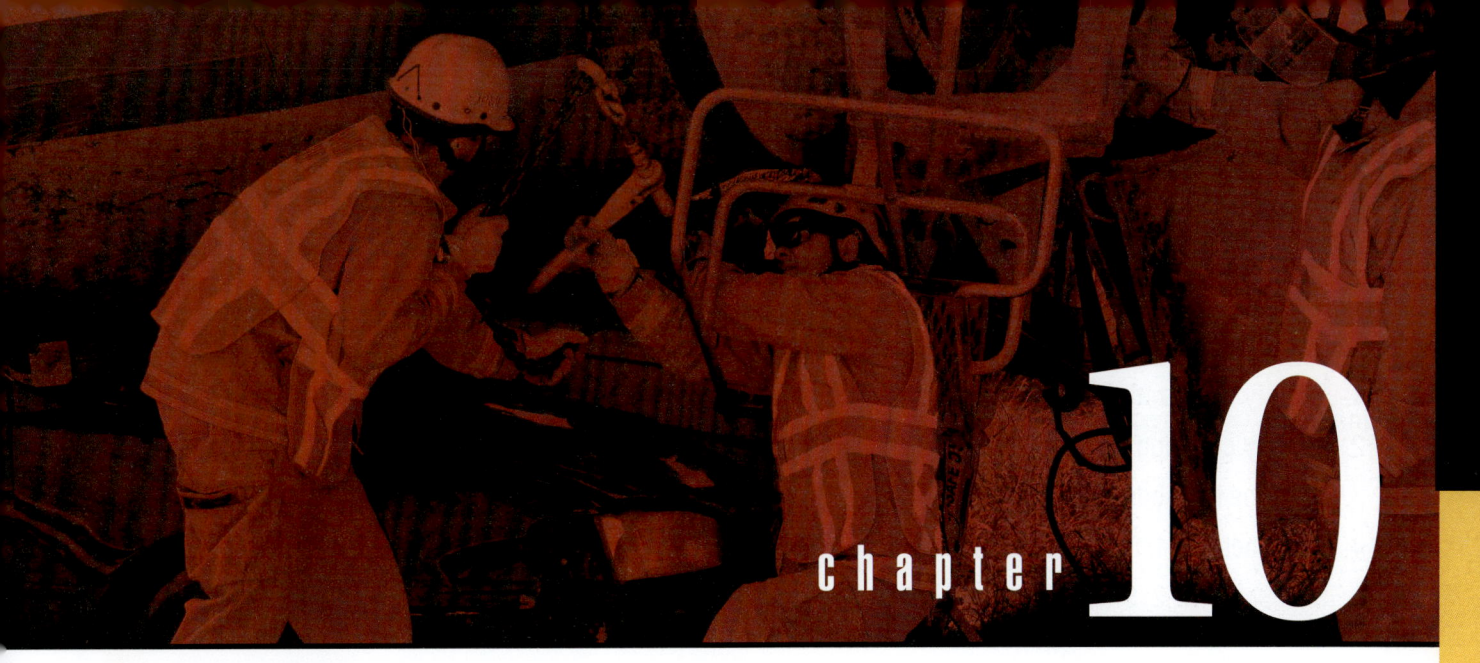

Key Terms

Bombproof Anchor Point	389
Four-point Box Crib	386
Jack Plate	391
Kingpin	387
Leaf Spring Suspension	390
Pikepole	385

JPRs addressed in this chapter

This chapter provides information that addresses the following job performance requirements of NFPA 1006, *Standard for Technical Rescuer Professional Qualifications (2017)*.

8.3.2

8.3.5

Commercial/Heavy Vehicle Stabilization Operations

Learning Objectives

1. Identify stabilization considerations that are common to both passenger and commercial/heavy vehicles.
2. Identify common stabilization points and surfaces for commercial/heavy vehicles.
3. Describe methods used to stabilize commercial/heavy vehicles.
4. Skill Sheet 10-1: Stabilize a wheel-resting commercial/heavy vehicle using cribbing.
5. Skill Sheet 10-2: Stabilize a side-resting commercial/heavy vehicle using struts (opposite side independent).

Chapter 10
Commercial/Heavy Vehicle Stabilization Operations

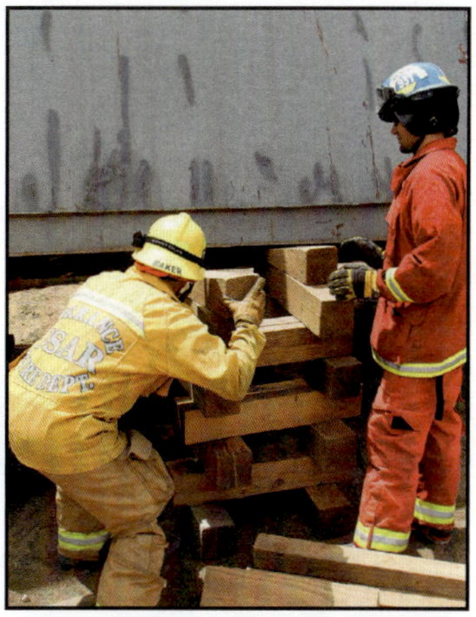

Rescuers may have to perform stabilization operations on commercial/heavy vehicles. These operations may include stabilization of medium and heavy trucks and buses. **Skill Sheet 10-1** lists the steps for stabilizing a wheel-resting commercial/heavy vehicle using cribbing. **Skill Sheet 10-2** lists the steps for stabilizing a side-resting commercial/heavy vehicle using struts. Rescuers can perform these skills on a medium or heavy truck, a bus, or any other type of commercial/heavy vehicle. Rescuers should follow AHJ policies and procedures for commercial/heavy vehicle stabilization operations.

Operations Level Stabilization: Review

The information in this chapter is intended to build upon knowledge and skills learned at the Operations level. The tools and equipment used to stabilize passenger vehicles may also be used to stabilize commercial/heavy vehicles. Stabilization tools include the following:

- Wheel Chocks
- Cribbing Materials
- Pneumatic Lifting Bags and Cushions **(Figure 10.1)**
- Jacks
- Levers
- Hitches
- Chains **(Figure 10.2)**
- Wire Rope
- Synthetic Slings
- Rigging **(Figure 10.3, p. 384)**
- Struts
- Recovery Vehicles **(Figure 10.4, p. 384)**

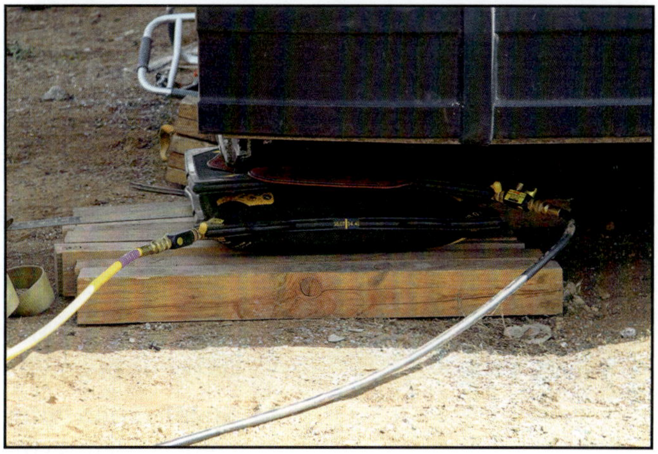

Figure 10.1 Pnuematic lifting bags are used to stabilize heavy vehicles.

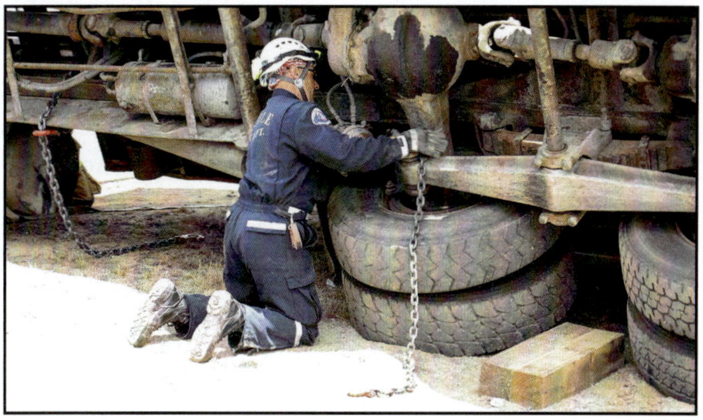

Figure 10.2 An example of how chains are used to stabilize a commercial truck.

Section D • Chapter 10 – Commercial/Heavy Vehicles Stabilization Operations   383

Figure 10.3 Rigging is used to stabilize a commercial truck.

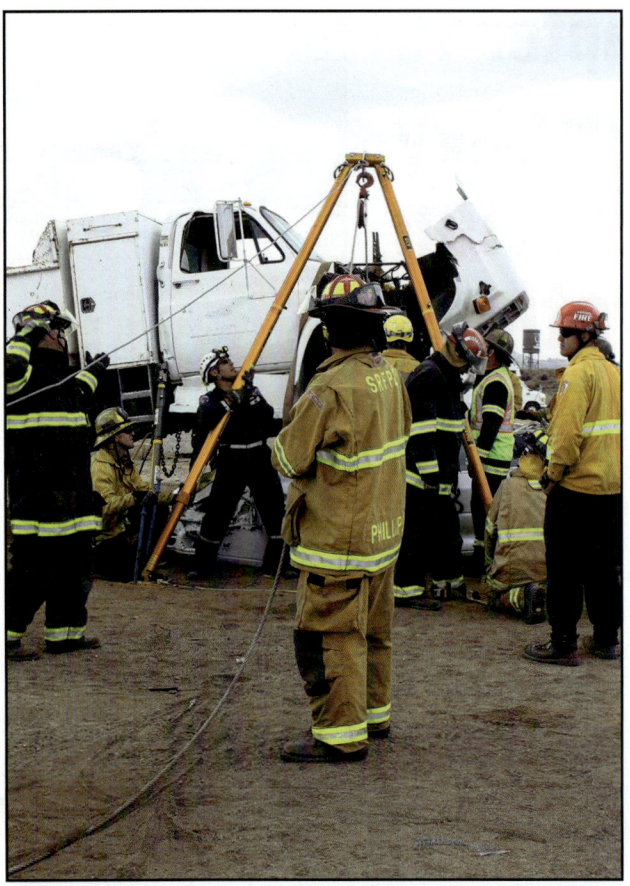

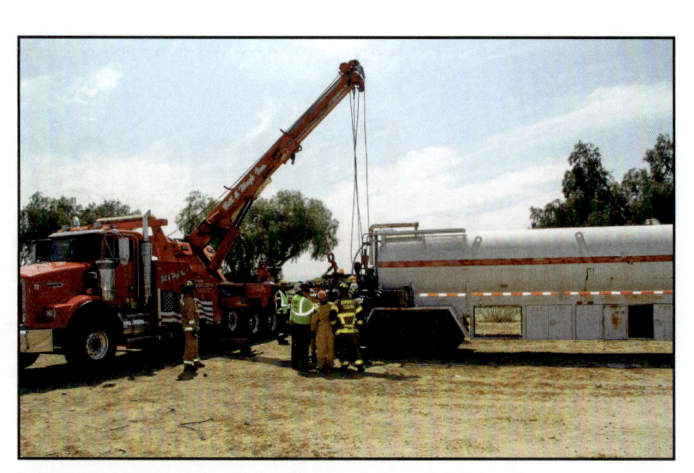

Figure 10.4 An example of a recovery vehicle.

In addition, information on stabilization considerations is similar to those used when stabilizing passenger vehicles. Those considerations are summarized as follows:

- **Mechanism of Movement** — Concept of how an object moves based upon its center of gravity and position.

- **Stabilization Points and Surfaces/Terrain** — Stabilization points on heavy vehicles may be in different locations, but serve the same purposes. Types of terrain for stabilization are the same and may include concrete, asphalt, dirt, sand, or sod. However, many commercial vehicles equip each axle with a piece of tubing welded on the axle near each wheel; rescuers can use these locations for stabilization. In addition, some commercial vehicles have specially designed jack plates and engine supports that rescuers may use as contact points for cribbing or jacks. A later section of this chapter discusses these points of contact in more detail.

- **Lifting** — Lifting techniques are similar to those used on passenger vehicles; however, commercial/heavy vehicles are much heavier than passenger vehicles which makes lifting operations more difficult **(Figure 10.5)**.

- **Maintaining Vehicle Stability** — Just as with passenger vehicles, commercial/heavy vehicles should remain stable throughout extrication operations. Ongoing size-up is critical to maintaining commercial/heavy vehicle stability.

Rescuers should never place any part of themselves under any portion of an unsupported vehicle. They should push cribbing into position using another piece of cribbing, a **pike pole**, or some similar device. Jacks should be equipped with handles that allow rescuers to operate them from outside the perimeter of the vehicle.

The remainder of this chapter focuses on stabilization considerations that are particular to commercial/heavy vehicles. For further review of general techniques, see Chapter 7, Passenger Vehicle Stabilization Operations.

Commercial/Heavy Vehicle Stabilization Considerations

Rescuers must consider the significant weight of commercial/heavy vehicles when attempting to stabilize them. These larger and heavier vehicles will require stabilization tools and equipment with higher capacities. Rescuers must calculate the load they need to stabilize before beginning stabilization operations. Although all commercial/heavy vehicles are manufactured differently, rescuers can use some general guidelines when calculating a load. Rescuers can estimate approximately 20,000 pounds (10 000 kg) for each drive axle. Rescuers can also estimate the weight of the steering axle (front axle) based on the profile of the tires. For thin- or slim-profile tires, rescuers can estimate 10,000 pounds (6 000 kg). For "balloon," wide-profile tires, rescuers can estimate 25,000 pounds (12 500 kg). Rescuers can add the steering and drive axle weights together to safely estimate the total load of the commercial/heavy vehicle.

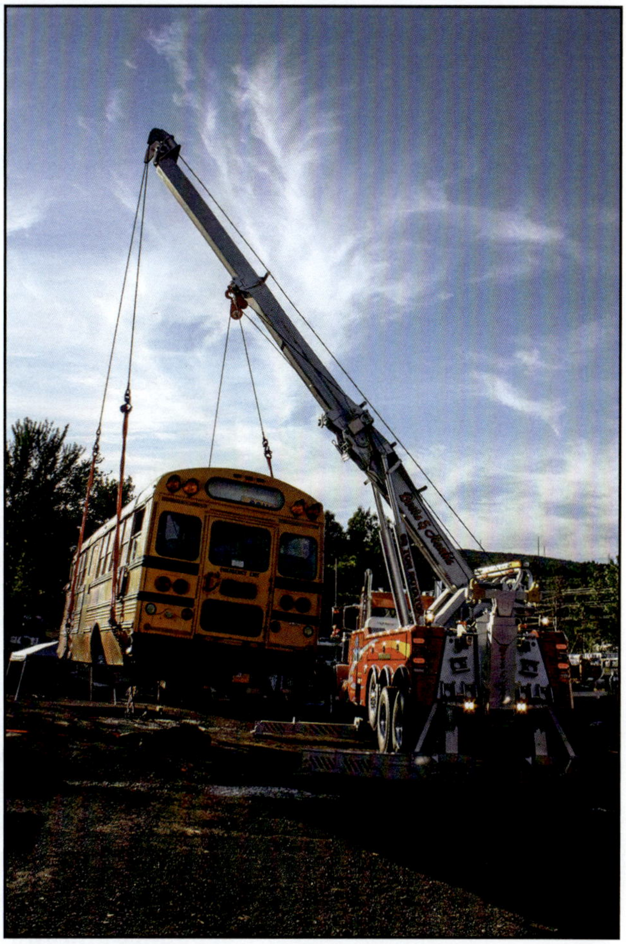

Figure 10.5 Lifting commercial/heavy vehicles requires specialized recovery vehicles.

Pike Pole — Sharp prong and hook of steel, on a wood, metal, fiberglass, or plastic handle of varying length, used for pulling, dragging, and probing.

The exact weight will vary depending on the type of vehicle. To find an exact gross vehicle weight rating (GVWR) of a commercial/heavy vehicle, rescuers should to look on the vehicle for that information. The GVWR will include the weight of the vehicle itself plus fuel, passengers, cargo, and trailer tongue weight.

Rescuers should know the capacities of their tools and equipment prior to attempting any stabilization operations. If rescuers figure weight calculations incorrectly or use stabilization tools and equipment beyond their rated capacities, the equipment will fail and the load will become unstable.

Medium and Heavy Truck Stabilization

Before rescue personnel enter the cab or sleeper of a crashed truck, they must stabilize the truck. To stabilize the truck, rescuers should create a sufficient number of points of contact between the truck and a stable surface, such as the ground or the pavement **(Figure 10.6, p. 386)**. The techniques employed to stabilize a medium or heavy truck will vary depending upon the position in which the vehicle is found and the ratings of the equipment to be used. The following sections discuss the stabilization techniques used for a medium or heavy truck that is wheel resting, side resting, roof resting, and in other positions.

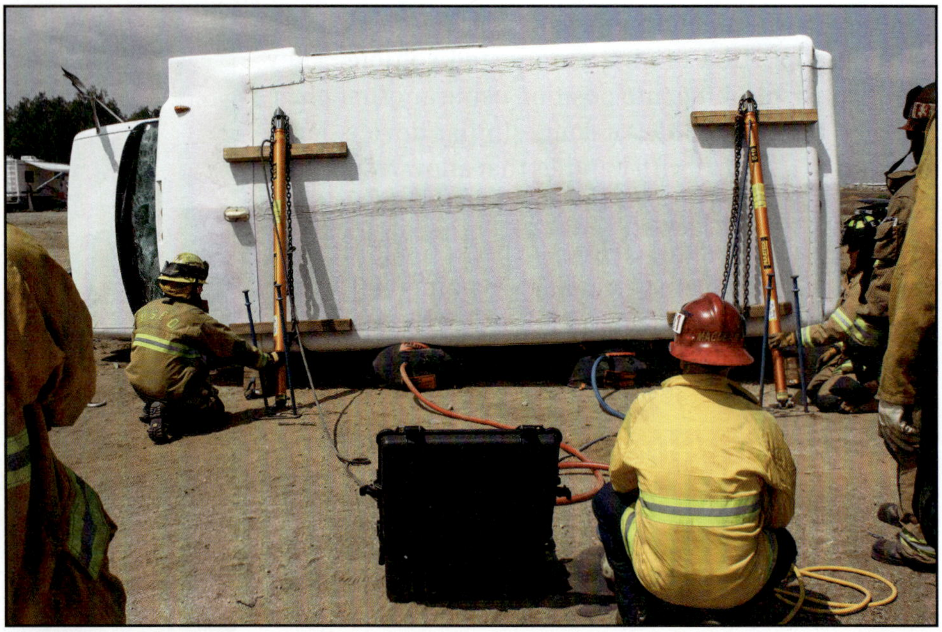

Figure 10.6 Rescuers using heavy duty struts to stabilize a side-resting commercial truck.

Wheel-Resting Truck Stabilization

The majority of trucks involved in collisions will be found wheel-resting. These trucks will not necessarily be stable. Inflated tires allow a certain amount of movement, especially laterally. Also, the vehicle's suspension system will allow the vehicle's chassis to move in various directions. Even these small amounts of bounce and sway could aggravate a trapped victim's injuries.

There are major differences between stabilizing a car or pickup truck and a medium or heavy truck. First, the distance between the road surface and the bottom of the chassis is significantly greater in medium or heavy trucks than in other vehicles. This makes the truck's center of gravity significantly higher than that of other vehicles. Second, medium and heavy trucks generally weigh much more than the smaller vehicles.

In some cases, rescuers will need to install a **four-point box crib** under the front portion of the vehicle's frame and both sides of the truck frame **(Figure 10.7)**. Rescuers should use large wheel chocks, such as those carried on fire apparatus, to prevent the vehicle from rolling forward or backward (initial stabilization). On cab-over units, rescuers should secure the cab with rope, webbing, or chains to prevent it from tilting forward unexpectedly during extrication operations.

Other truck cabs, mounted on air suspension systems (air-ride cab), allow movement of the cab independent of the chassis. Rescuers should marry the two components together to attempt to minimize this movement. To marry the cab to the frame, rescuers should fill the voids of the cab with cribbing and secure the cab to the frame with a tensioning device. Once rescuers have taken these measures, rescuers will have established enough stability to begin the victim assessment phase of the operation.

Rescue personnel should also secure and stabilize anything attached to the truck. At commercial/heavy vehicle incidents, rescuers must not overlook the trailer attached to the tractor. The trailer is often loaded with a variety of cargo

Four-Point Box Crib — Cribbing constructed with four points that is made to look like a box.

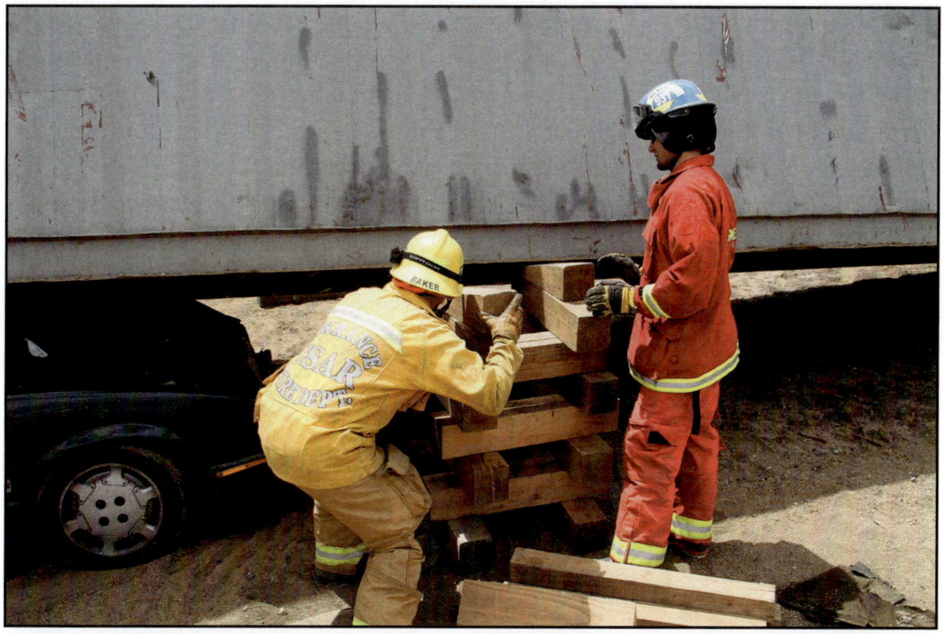

Figure 10.7 Rescuers constructing a box crib under a heavy truck to maintain stability.

that can significantly increase the weight of the trailer. Rescuers should chock the wheels of the trailer, confirm that the **kingpin** is locked, and lower the landing gear to stabilize the trailer. Rescuers must give careful consideration to stay within the working load limits of the stabilization equipment they use.

Kingpin — Attaching pin on a semitrailer that connects with pivots within the lower coupler of a truck tractor or converter dolly while coupling the two units together.

Disconnecting Glad Hands

In vehicle accidents involving a wheel-resting heavy vehicle, such as a tractor trailer, rescuers must consider applying the air-brake system as an added means of vehicle stabilization. A major portion of this process involves disconnecting the air system from the tractor to the trailer. Rescuers can disconnect the glad hand connection between the tractor and trailer to disconnect the air system. The spring brakes will engage after rescuers disconnect the air-brake system and release air from the system. The spring brakes will lock the brakes when the pressure falls below 20-40 psi (140-280 kPa).

Rescuers should only disconnect glad hands after completing initial stabilization and once the area is deemed safe for rescuers to approach the glad hand connections. To disconnect the glad hands, rescuers should turn the connection approximately 90 degrees and pull the connections apart. Some trailers provide a dummy connection to attach the glad hand to in order to avoid system contamination, in instances requiring extrication this should not be a main concern for the rescuer.

Side-Resting Truck Stabilization

A medium or heavy truck on its side can sometimes be easier to stabilize than other smaller vehicles because the weight and shape of these trucks often make them relatively stable when they come to rest. However, a truck on its side may behave differently if it is fully loaded than it would if it were empty.

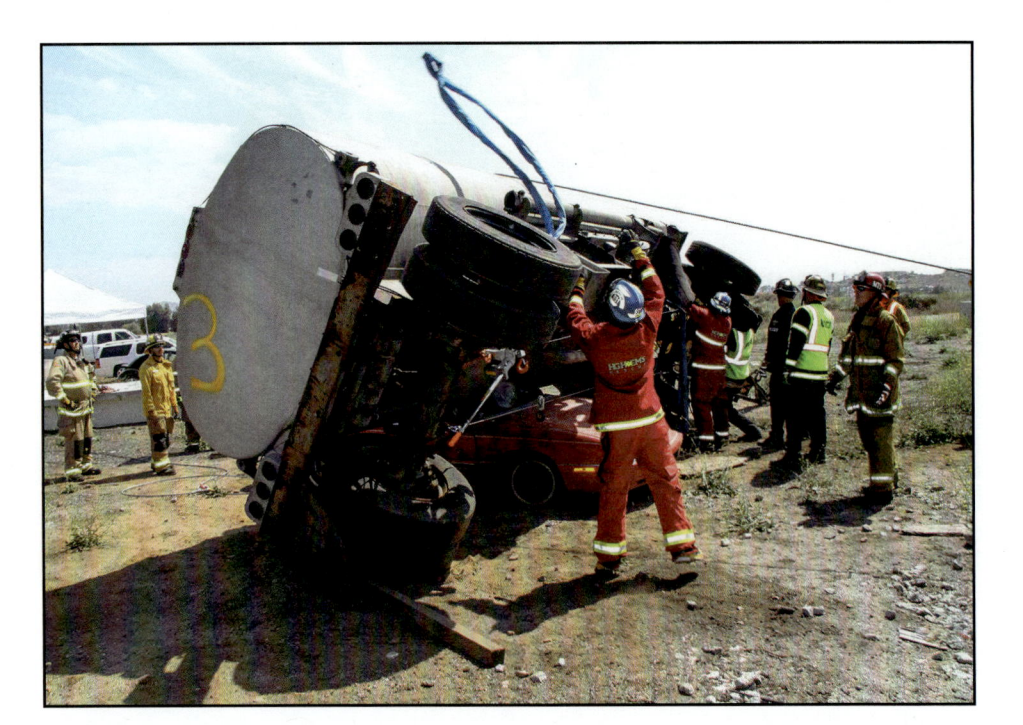

Figure 10.8 Rescuers securing a side-resting heavy truck with rope and webbing.

In the case of a tractor/trailer, the tractor and trailer have different centers of gravity. Therefore, if someone uncouples the tractor from the trailer, the tractor may suddenly shift back toward the wheel-resting position while the trailer remains on its side.

To stabilize a side-resting truck, rescuers should install cribbing or other supports at the cab's door posts. Rescuers may need to invert step chocks before sliding them under the vehicle because of the roundness of the cab's roof edge. Depending upon the truck's stability after this, rescuers may need to crib the underside of the truck to prevent any possibility of it rolling back onto its wheels. Rescuers can also secure the truck with rope, chain, or webbing to prevent it from rolling back onto its wheels **(Figure 10.8)**.

Roof-Resting Truck Stabilization

A truck on its roof may present more stabilization challenges than one on its side. The rounded roofs of most truck cabs offer few if any positive purchase points. However, inverted step chocks installed at the door posts and box cribbing installed under the front will often suffice. In some cases, rescuers may need to crib the truck's bed to prevent the truck from rocking. Depending upon the situation, it may be practical to stabilize these trucks with ropes, chains, or webbing.

Stabilization of Trucks in Other Positions

Stabilizing trucks found in positions other than those already described will test the ingenuity of rescue personnel. Regardless of the technique used, rescuers must emphasize safety. While speed and efficiency are highly desirable, the security and effectiveness of the stabilization measures are far more important. A rapidly installed crib that fails is far worse than one that takes longer to install but holds the load.

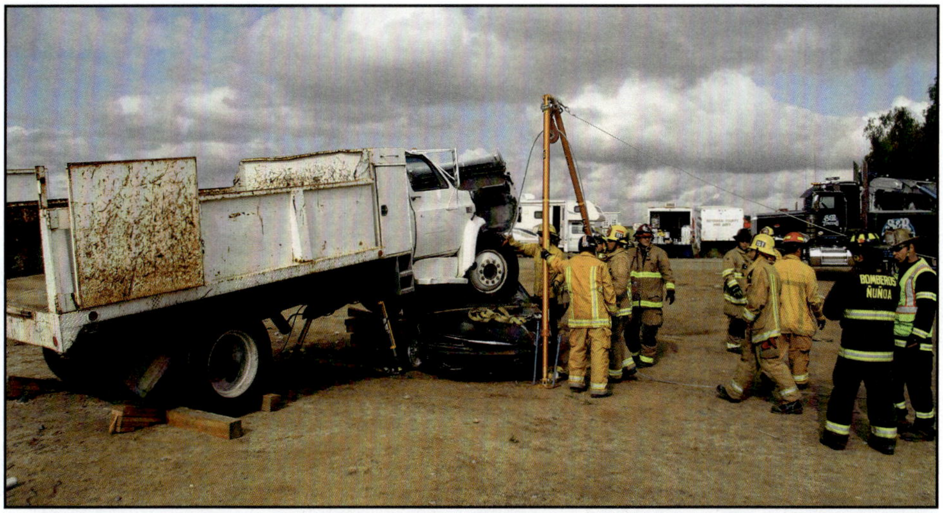

Figure 10.9 Rescuers use rigging to prevent movement of a commercial truck.

When deciding how to stabilize a truck that rests in an unusual position, rescue personnel should consider the vehicle's center of gravity, mass, cargo, as well as the capabilities of their equipment. These basic physical principles will dictate how a truck may move when rescuers manipulate or remove its components during extrication operations. If a truck stops on a steep slope or hangs over the edge of a bridge or cliff, rescuers can use cribbing and/or rigging to offset the forces of gravity and secure the vehicle in place **(Figure 10.9)**. If the vehicle is wedged under another vehicle or other object, rescuers should attempt to limit if not eliminate the vehicle's reaction when they remove the overlying object. As discussed in previous text, rescuers may need to attach two vehicles or objects together to make extrication safer. The situation will dictate how rescuers should accomplish this. Given the size of these trucks, extrication personnel may have to call for secondary or outside sources to secure and stabilize these trucks such as tow trucks, commercial riggers, and even cranes.

Bus Stabilization

As with other vehicle incidents, rescuers should stabilize buses before attempting to reach victims. The following sections discuss stabilizing wheel-resting, side-resting, roof-resting, and alternatively-positioned buses.

Wheel-Resting Bus Stabilization

Stabilizing a wheel-resting bus should prevent it from moving in the most likely directions — horizontally and vertically. Chocking the wheels usually prevents any bus, regardless of type or size, from moving forward or backward. Whenever possible, rescuers should use wheel chocks, and not pieces of cribbing **(Figure 10.10, p. 390)**. However, if the bus is on a slope — especially if it is in danger of rolling sideways down the slope — it may be necessary to supplement the wheel chocks with a chain, cable, or webbing attached to the bus and a **bombproof anchor point**. Rescuers should only consider an anchor point bombproof if the weight of any object attached to that anchor absolutely will not move the anchor point. Stabilizing a bus horizontally may require a heavy-duty tow truck, a huge boulder, or a large, fully mature tree as an anchor point.

> **Bombproof Anchor Point** — (1) Slang reference to an anchor that is absolutely immovable, such as a huge boulder, a large tree, or a fire engine. (2) Any anchor point capable of withstanding forces in excess of those that might be generated by the rescue operation or even catastrophic failure (and resultant shock load) of a raising or lowering system.

Section D • Chapter 10 – Commercial/Heavy Vehicles Stabilization Operations

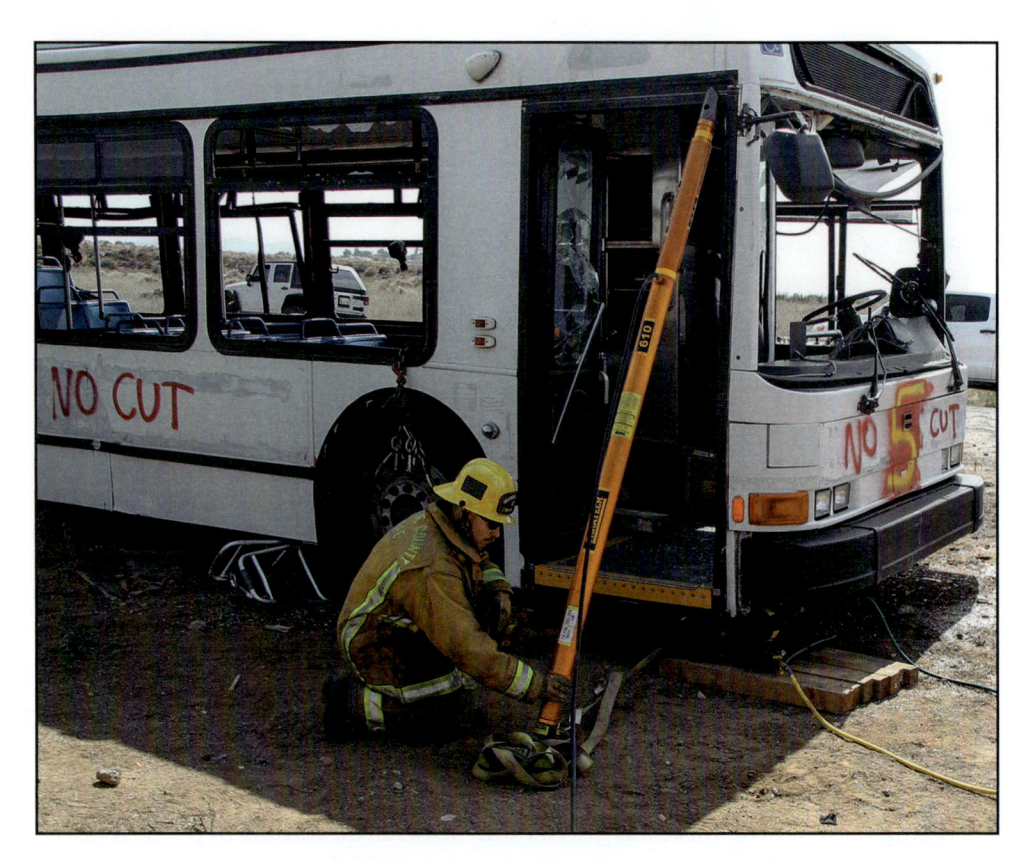

Figure 10.10 A rescuer uses a combination of equipment to stabilize a wheel-resting bus.

Leaf Spring Suspension — Type of suspension system consisting of several long, narrow, layers of elastic metal bracketed together.

In general, vertically stabilizing a school bus requires no different methods than those used to vertically stabilize any other bus. Most school buses built by either integral construction or the body-on-chassis method have conventional heavy-duty suspension — in the form of coil and/or **leaf springs** **(Figure 10.11 A and B)**. Most transit, commercial, and some newer school buses have air suspension systems. These systems replace the conventional metal springs with compact rubber air bags. Each wheel has two air suspension bags, one on each side of the axle. An on-board compressor maintains the air pressure within the bags as high as 120 psi (840 kPa). Depending upon the load of the vehicle and the condition of the road, the pressure within each bag automatically increases or decreases to maintain the bus in a level state. If an air

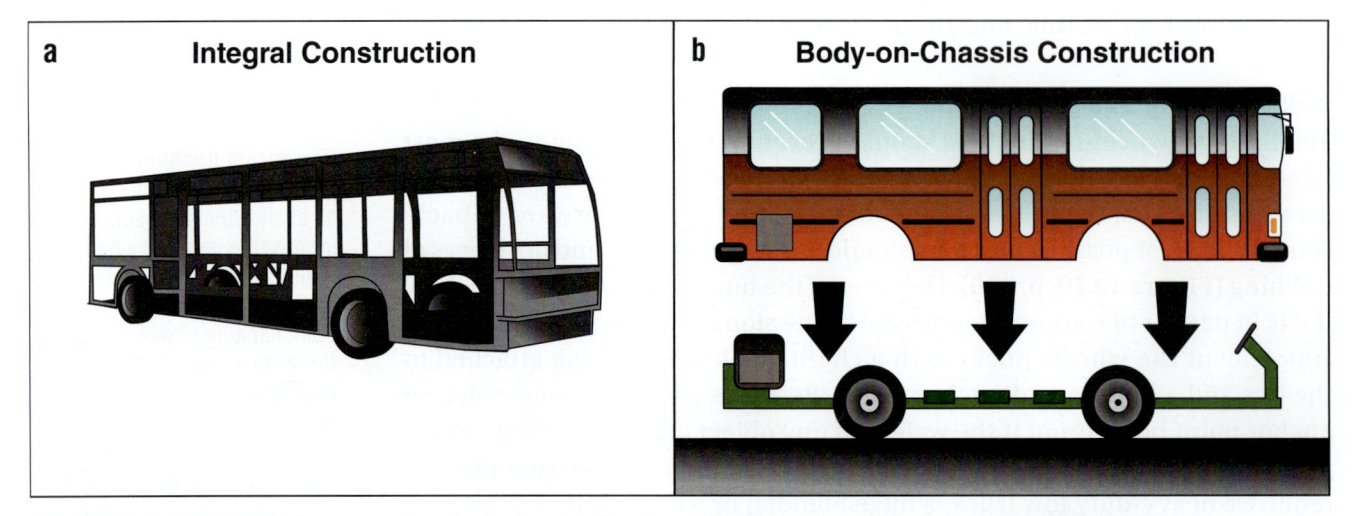

Figure 10.11 a. In integral construction, the body and chassis are built as one unit. **b.** In body-on-chassis, the body and chassis are built separately and then connected together.

suspension bag loses pressure because of damage to the bag or its associated piping, the chassis of the bus can suddenly drop without warning to within 3 to 3½ inches (75 to 90 mm) of the roadway surface.

Some transit and commercial buses have an air inlet valve on the front end. In a controlled environment, this valve allows trained vehicle service technicians to hook the bus to an air compressor or cascade system to re-inflate a collapsed suspension system. Due to the potential for catastrophic failure of the system that could cause further injuries to victims and rescuers, emergency response personnel should not consider reinflating a suspension system.

Unless rescuers are positive that the bus has a mechanical suspension system, they should treat the bus as if it has an air suspension system.

Because most transit and commercial buses do not have a rigid frame, they have specially designed **jack plates** for use as contact points for cribbing or jacks. On transit buses, these plates are located slightly behind each axle, near each wheel. On commercial buses, the jack plates are located under the body between the two rear axles and in back of the front axle. Cribbing may be used on these points, although they are designed more for use with hydraulic jacks. Rescuers should support all four jack plates to completely stabilize the vehicle. If rescuers cannot locate the jack plates on a bus, cribbing the body at any solid frame member can stabilize the vehicle. If possible, rescuers should also crib the middle axle.

> **Jack Plate** — Unattached flat metal plate that is larger in area than the stabilizer foot; placed on the ground beneath the intended resting point of the stabilizer foot, in order to provide better weight distribution. *Also known as* Jack Pad or Stabilizer Pad.

When using cribbing to stabilize a bus, rescuers must use cribbing large enough to hold the weight of the bus. If rescuers use hydraulic jacks to lift the bus, they should use jacks of at least 8-ton capacity. Many bus manufacturers equip each axle with a piece of tubing welded on the axle near each wheel. This tubing accepts the shaft of a jack to prevent the jack from slipping.

In some cases, rescuers can use the engine supports as jack points. However, they should do so only if they have no other alternative and rescuers can access these supports without placing themselves beneath the unsupported bus. Because of their location beneath the bus, using these engine supports as jack points can be dangerous.

WARNING!
Do not place body parts underneath an unstabilized bus.

To stabilize a bus, rescuers should install cribbing and wedges or shims at a sufficient number of points to prevent the bus from settling any further. If they use jacks, they should extend the jacks only to the point where they would begin to lift the bus. Rescuers intend to lift the bus, they should extend the jacks slowly and evenly. As rescuers raise the bus they should add cribbing to minimize the distance the bus will fall should the jack(s) fail. The bus should be raised only as much as necessary to stabilize it — and no more.

NOTE: Lift an inch, crib an inch.

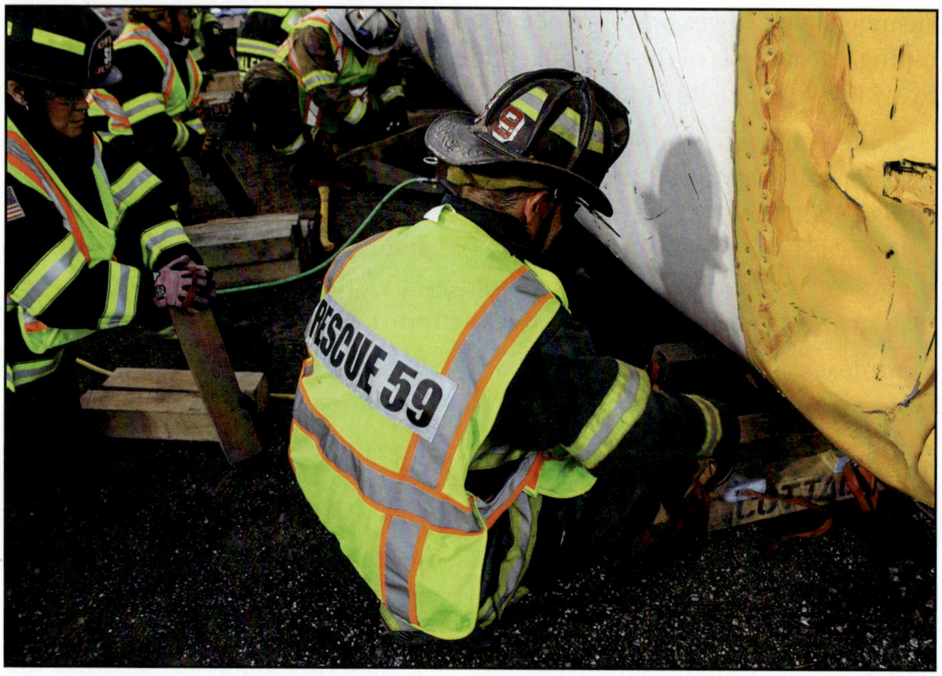

Figure 10.12 Rescuers using cribbing to stabilize a side resting bus.

Side-Resting Bus Stabilization

Depending upon the dynamics of the crash and other variables in the situation, a bus on its side may leak fuel and other flammable fluids. Access to the means of controlling these and other hazards may be difficult if not impossible. The battery compartment may be on the underside of the vehicle. The fuel supply valve on an LPG- or LNG-fueled vehicle may likewise be inaccessible. These situations make the need for fire protection a high priority. Rescuers should provide fire protection with no less than two 1½-inch (38 mm) hoselines with foam capability.

Because the sides of most buses are large flat surfaces, side-resting buses tend to be relatively stable. However, if the crash that caused the bus to roll has drastically altered its original shape, or if it came to rest on an uneven surface, a bus on its side may be unstable.

To stabilize the bus, rescuers should create points of contact between the bus and the surface on which it rests in order to prevent sudden and unexpected movement of the bus in any direction **(Figure 10.12)**. Rescuers usually use cribbing, step chocks, struts, or a combination to achieve this stability. Rescuers may also need to secure the bus to a solid object with chains, cables, or webbing.

Roof-Resting Bus Stabilization

Just as with passenger vehicles, most buses have rounded contours along the junction between their roof and sides. In addition, the roof itself is usually rounded **(Figure 10.13)**. Unless its roof was significantly flattened during the crash, a bus resting upside down on a flat surface will require stabilization via the installation of multiple step chocks or other similar devices along both sides of the bus, and perhaps both ends.

Roof-resting buses may leak even greater amounts of fluid than side-resting buses. Liquid fuels will almost certainly leak from the fuel filter. Engine oil

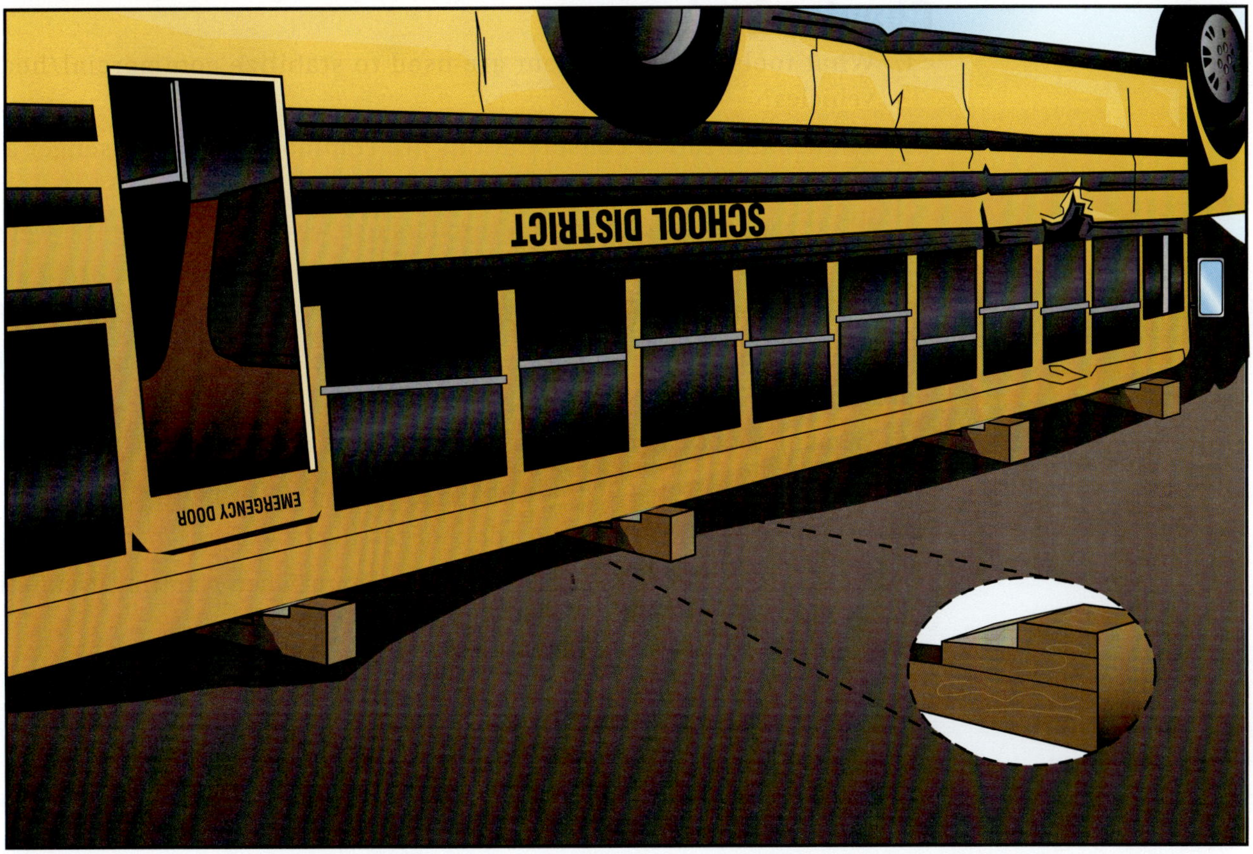

Figure 10.13 This illustration shows how step chocks can be used to stabilize a bus that has overturned onto its roof.

will drain from the crankcase, and battery acid may drain from the batteries. This combination of uncontrolled fluids can drain into electrical components, causing short circuits and increasing the danger of fire ignition. Therefore, fire protection is a high priority.

Stabilization of Buses in Other Positions

Buses rest in any of a variety of positions other than those already described. A bus may be still on its wheels but on such an angle that it is in danger of falling onto its side — or even worse — rolling down a steep hillside. The lives of those trapped inside the bus may depend upon rescuers quickly and efficiently stabilizing the bus. Buses in these unusual situations can tax the ingenuity and resourcefulness of these rescuers. The situation will dictate the means by which rescuers can stabilize the bus **(Figure 10.14)**. Therefore, rescuers must be thoroughly trained in the use and adaptation of all available tools and equipment, both from within the agency and from outside sources.

When a bus loaded with passengers has come to rest in an unusual position, rescuers may have to use a combination of cribbing, jacks, and other devices. They may have to secure the vehicle with chains, cables, or webbing attached to a secure anchor point. Or, they may have to employ tow trucks or cranes to stabilize the vehicle.

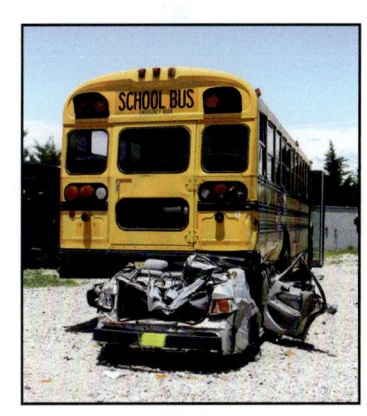

Figure 10.14 Rescuers must be thoroughly trained to properly stabilize a bus resting on top of a passenger car.

Section D • Chapter 10 – Commercial/Heavy Vehicles Stabilization Operations **393**

Chapter Review

1. What tools and equipment are used to stabilize commercial/heavy vehicles?
2. What stabilization considerations are common to both passenger and commercial/heavy vehicles?
3. What general guidelines can rescuers use when calculating the weight of a commercial/heavy vehicle?
4. How can rescuers find a vehicle's exact gross vehicle weight rating (GVWR)?
5. How are commercial/heavy vehicles different than passenger vehicles with regards to stabilization?
6. What methods can rescuers use to stabilize a wheel-resting truck?
7. How does the trailer of a side resting truck affect its stability?
8. What stabilization challenges do roof-resting trucks present for rescuers?
9. What factors should rescuers take into account when planning to stabilize a truck in an unusual position?
10. What methods can rescuers use to stabilize a wheel-resting bus?
11. How should rescuers handle the suspension systems of buses during stabilization operations?
12. Why is establishing fire protection a special priority when stabilizing a side-resting or roof-resting bus?

Discussion Questions

1. What resources for stabilizing commercial/heavy vehicles are available in your jurisdiction?

10-1
Stabilize a wheel-resting commercial/heavy vehicle using cribbing.

SKILL SHEETS

REMINDER: Not all agencies advocate the following practices. The following skill sheets present a snapshot of various procedures utilized during vehicle incident operations. Always follow manufacturer's recommendations and local SOPs. Rescuers must wear full PPE including hand, eye, and respiratory protection. It is recommended that rescuers maintain communication with victims and make them aware of pertinent rescue information.

WARNING: Rescuers must ensure that the vehicle is properly stabilized and the scene is safe.

CAUTION: Rescuers must take necessary precautions to protect themselves and victims from hazards including, but not limited to, glass fragments and dust, jagged metal, SRS gas cylinders, undeployed air bags, and fire hazards. Ensure that the equipment used is appropriate for the commercial/heavy vehicle and load to be stabilized.

NOTE: Monitor equipment throughout the operation and make adjustments as needed.

Step 1: Identify vehicle's construction, condition, and integrity.
Step 2: Identify and calculate the load.
Step 3: Provide initial stabilization.
Step 4: Identify support locations on the vehicle.
Step 5: Verify that the surface under the support locations will support weight of vehicle and equipment. Construct a solid base or use alternative actions to provide base support, if necessary.
Step 6: Position sufficient cribbing material at each support location.
Step 7: Crib the vehicle, allowing the ends of the cribbing pieces to extend at least four inches (100 mm) beyond the individual pieces of the base until the required height has been achieved.
Step 8: Use wedges to provide the maximum amount of contact between the crib and the vehicle.
Step 9: Inspect the vehicle and confirm that it is stabilized. Monitor and maintain the integrity of the cribbing.

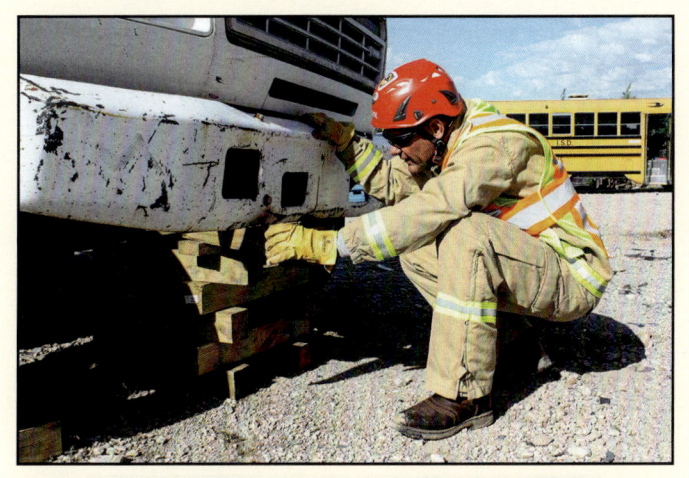

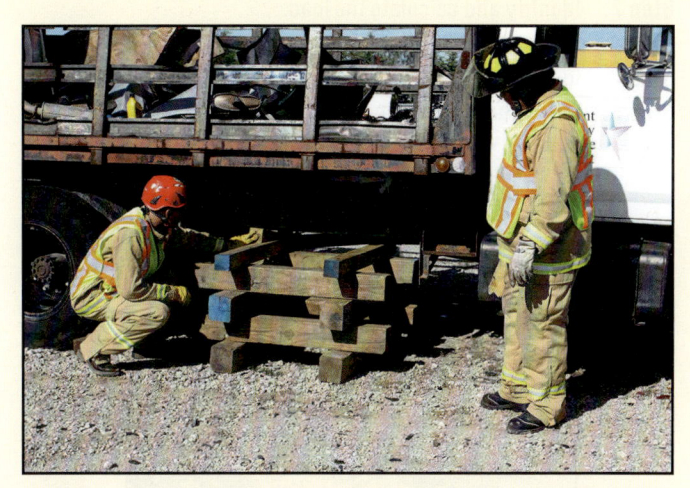

Section D • Chapter 10 – Commercial/Heavy Vehicles Stabilization Operations

SKILL SHEETS

10-2

Stabilize a side-resting commercial/heavy vehicle using struts (opposite side independent).

WARNING: Rescuers must ensure that the vehicle is properly stabilized and the scene is safe.

CAUTION: Rescuers must take necessary precautions to protect themselves and victims from hazards including, but not limited to, glass fragments and dust, jagged metal, SRS gas cylinders, undeployed air bags, and fire hazards.

NOTE: Inspect and maintain all equipment according to local SOPs and manufacturer's guidelines. Monitor equipment throughout the operation and make adjustments as needed.

Step 1: Identify vehicle's construction, condition, and integrity.
Step 2: Identify and calculate the load.
Step 3: Provide initial stabilization.
Step 4: Identify support locations on the vehicle.
Step 5: Verify that the surface under the support locations will support weight of vehicle and equipment. Construct a solid base or use alternative actions to provide base support, if necessary.

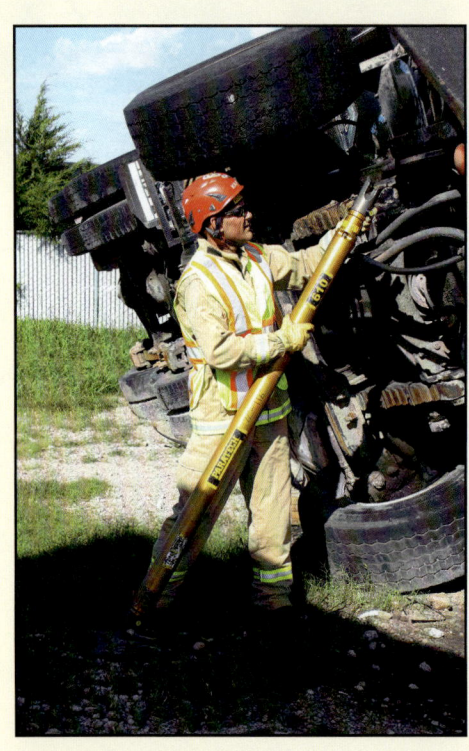

Step 6: Set and engage struts on least stable side of vehicle.

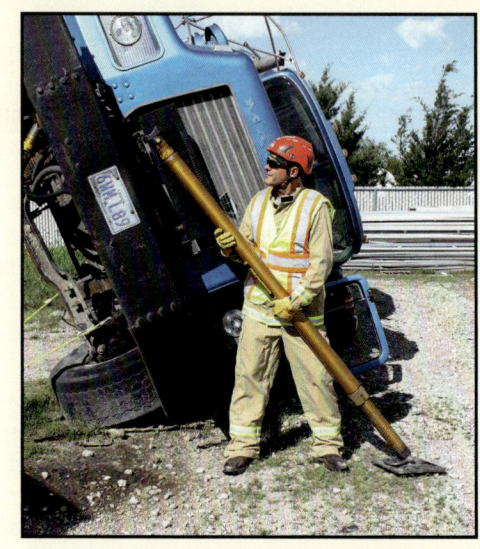

Step 7: Set and engage struts on opposite side of the vehicle.

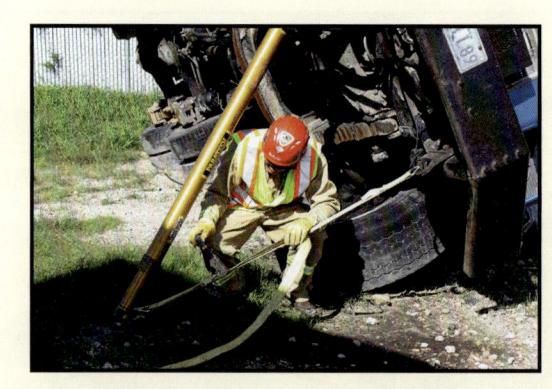

Step 8: Attach base strapping as low as possible.
Step 9: Apply tension to the system.

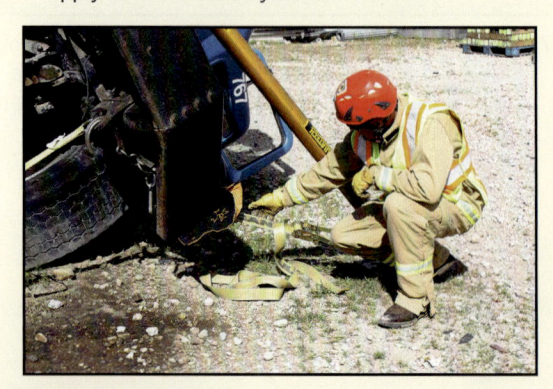

Step 10: Check that straps and tip engagements are tight. Adjust if necessary.
Step 11: Inspect the vehicle and confirm that it is stabilized.

Commercial/Heavy Vehicle Disentanglement

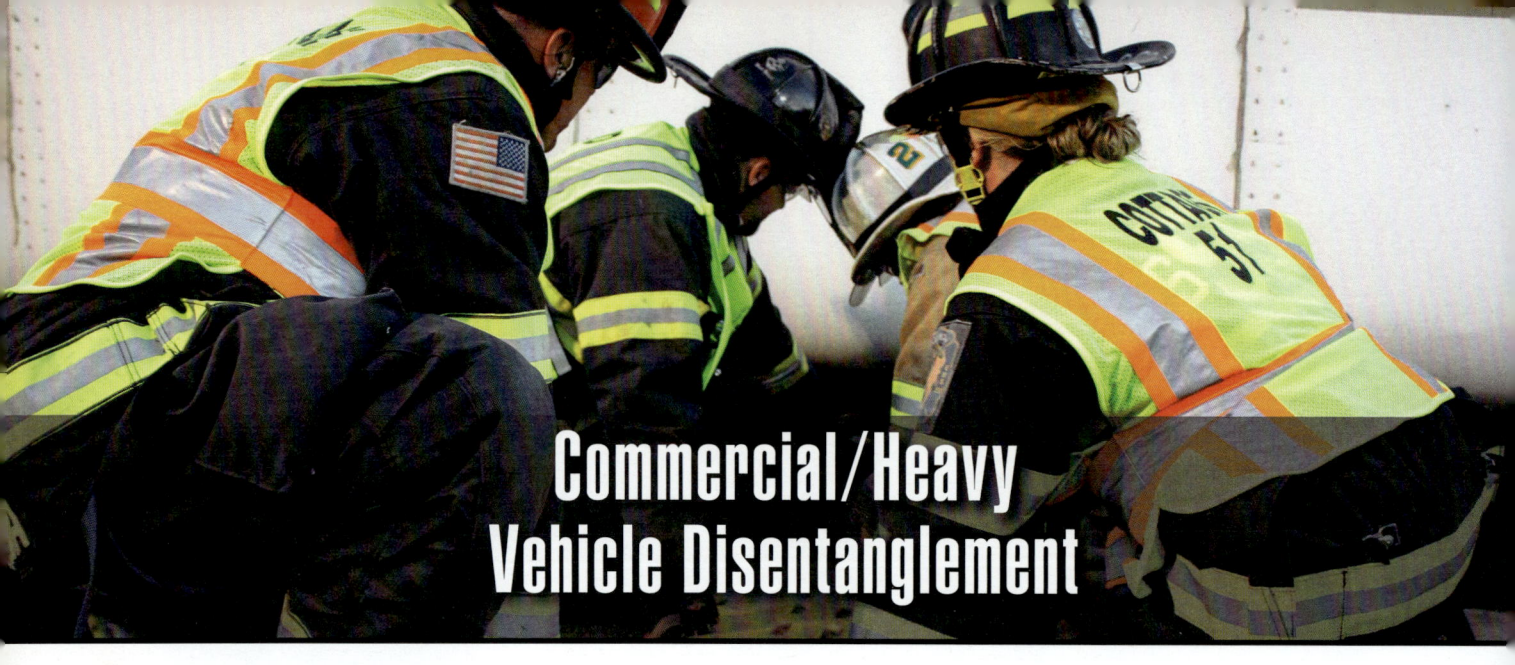

Chapter Contents

Review: Operations Level Disentanglement and Extrication 401

Medium and Heavy Truck Access and Egress Points 401

Medium and Heavy Truck Access and Egress Routes 402

Medium and Heavy Truck Entry Points 402

Medium and Heavy Truck Extrication Operations 403

Techniques for Creating Access and Egress Openings on Medium and Heavy Trucks 404

Techniques for Disentangling Victims from Medium and Heavy Trucks 407

Bus Access and Egress Points 408

Bus Access and Egress Routes 408

Bus Entry Points 409

Bus Extrication Operations 410

Techniques for Creating Access and Egress Openings on Buses 410

Techniques for Disentangling Victims from Buses 418

Chapter Review 422

Discussion Questions 422

Skill Sheets 423

chapter 11

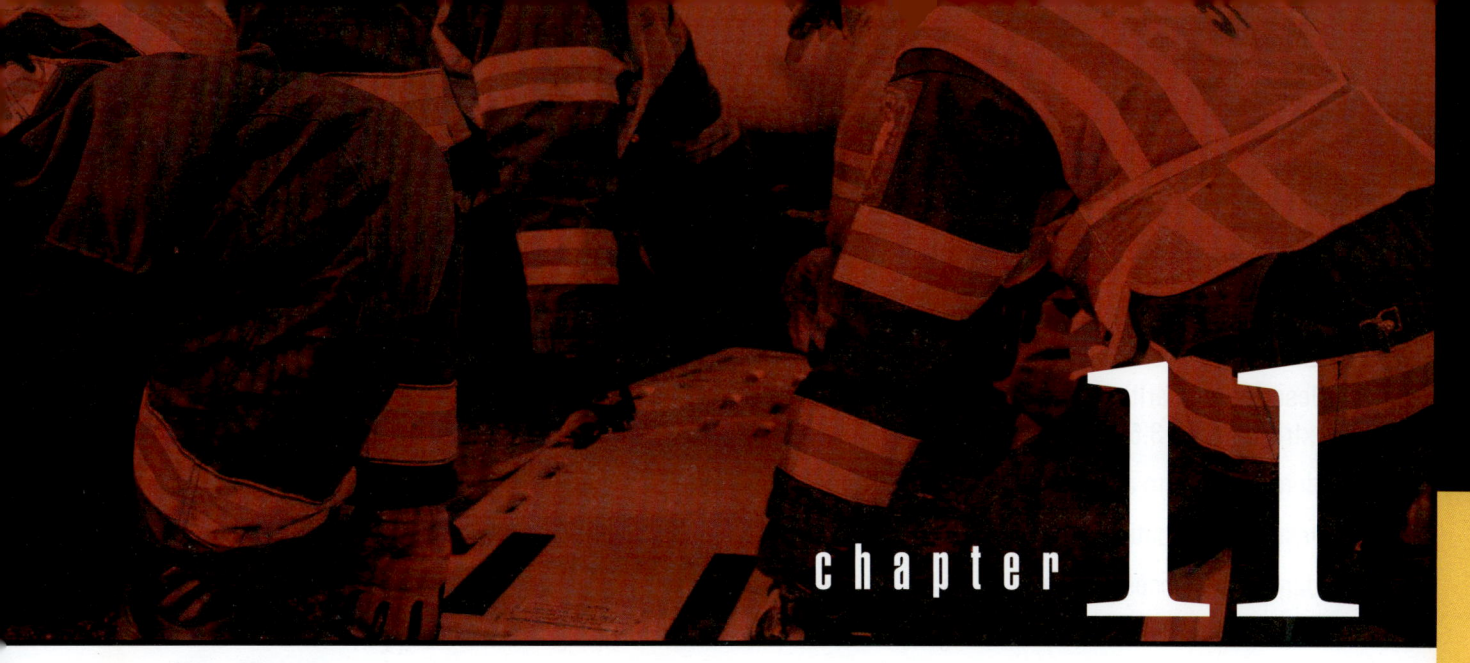

Key Terms

A-Post	407
B-Post	407
Flash Fire	418
Halligan Tool	412
Nader Pin	405
Pneumatic Chisel	416
Reciprocating Saw	417

JPRs addressed in this chapter

This chapter provides information that addresses the following job performance requirements of NFPA 1006, *Standard for Technical Rescuer Professional Qualifications (2017)*.

8.3.3

8.3.4

8.3.5

Commercial/Heavy Vehicle Disentanglement

Learning Objectives

1. Describe similarities between commercial/heavy vehicle and passenger vehicle disentanglement and extrication. [8.3.5]
2. Identify medium and heavy truck access and egress routes. [8.3.3, 8.3.4]
3. Describe extrication and disentanglement methods used on medium and heavy trucks. [8.3.3, 8.3.4, 8.3.5]
4. Identify bus access and egress routes. [8.3.3, 8.3.4]
5. Describe extrication and disentanglement methods uses on buses. [8.3.3, 8.3.4, 8.3.5]
6. Skill Sheet 11-1: Determine commercial/heavy vehicle access and egress points. [8.3.3]
7. Skill Sheet 11-2: Open or remove a commercial/heavy vehicle door. [8.3.4]
8. Skill Sheet 11-3: Create an access opening in the roof or wall of a commercial/heavy vehicle. [8.3.4]
9. Skill Sheet 11-4: Create an access opening utilizing the front door of a bus. [8.3.4]
10. Skill Sheet 11-5: Open or remove the rear door of a bus. [8.3.4]
11. Skill Sheet 11-6: Remove an emergency window of a school bus. [8.3.4]
12. Skill Sheet 11-7: Cut through the side wall of a bus utilizing a window opening. [8.3.4]
13. Skill Sheet 11-8: Create an access opening in the roof of a side-resting bus. [8.3.4]
14. Skill Sheet 11-9: Flap a bus roof. [8.3.4]
15. Skill Sheet 11-10: Create an access opening in the floor of a side-resting bus. [8.3.4]
16. Skill Sheet 11-11: Use high-pressure pneumatic lifting bags to free a victim trapped beneath a side-resting commercial/heavy vehicle. [8.3.5]

Chapter 11
Commercial/Heavy Vehicle Disentanglement

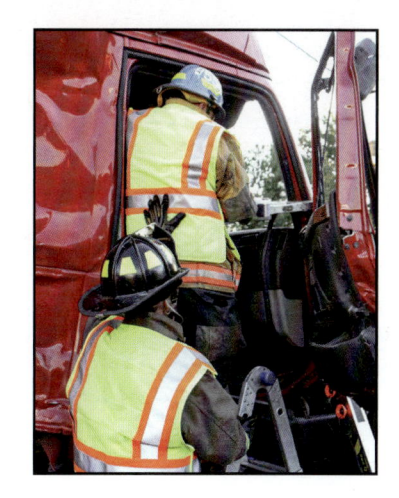

In some incidents, such as when they strike a bridge or each other, commercial/heavy vehicles sustain heavy damage. However, most commercial/heavy vehicles involved in a collision or accident sustain less damage than passenger vehicles.

Rescuers must remember that any extrication or disentanglement procedure may ultimately affect the structural stability of the commercial/heavy vehicle. Removing door posts or other components in order to disentangle and extricate victims from a roof-resting vehicle may weaken the vehicle's structural integrity. Weakened cabs may move suddenly and unexpectedly, perhaps aggravating a victim's injuries. Therefore, rescue personnel must anticipate the consequences of each extrication action. If removing a structural component will weaken or destabilize the vehicle, rescuers must take steps to counteract those effects, or consider another option.

Review: Operations Level Disentanglement and Extrication

Many techniques for disentangling victims from commercial/heavy vehicles are similar or identical to those used on passenger vehicles. The basic factors that rescuers must consider when performing disentanglement are similar enough to follow the same procedures, including:

- Victim Locations
- Victim Entrapment
- Points of Entrapment
- Dynamics of Disentanglement
- Multiple Vehicle Incident — Considerations
- Multiple Vehicle Incident — Operations
- Minimizing Hazards to Victims
- Eliminating Points of Entrapment/Disentanglement

The remainder of this chapter describes disentanglement and extrication considerations that are particular to commercial/heavy vehicles. To review information that applies to passenger vehicles, see Chapter 8, Victim Disentanglement and Passenger Vehicle Extrication.

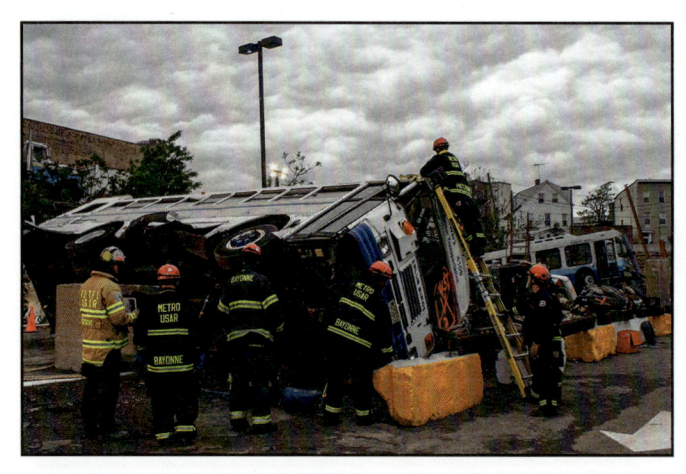

Figure 11.1 Rescuers practicing disentanglement operations on a transit bus. *Courtesy of Ron Jeffers.*

Medium and Heavy Truck Access and Egress Points

When rescuers first respond to a vehicle incident, they do not know the extent of the crash victims' injuries. Rescuers need to access the interior or crashed vehicles so they can access, disentangle, and free victims. Most medium and heavy trucks only have one or two occupants. This section will cover the access and egress routes of a vehicle incident and the entry points of a vehicle.

Medium and Heavy Truck Access and Egress Routes

Rescue personnel must determine how best to gain access to and remove trapped victims from medium and heavy trucks involved in an accident. This may mean deciding between several possible actions, including:

- Removing a door or window
- Removing or penetrating the roof
- Using the wall as an access or egress point

Rescuers must take into account the vehicle's location and position, the number and location of victims, the known and unknown hazards, available tools and equipment, and the skill set of the rescue personnel. Rescuers should make all personnel aware of the influencing factors and the decided-upon access and egress route **(Figure 11.1)**. For example, rescuers may decide that the most effective way to access a trapped victim is to remove the windshield. Then, they should focus all efforts on coordinating the flow of personnel, tools and equipment, and any victims to support the operation.

> **CAUTION**
> When accessing and egressing vehicles, personnel should watch out for sharp objects such as broken glass or jagged metals. They should identify these objects, cover them, and/or remove them from the vehicle.

Because of their height, medium and heavy trucks may necessitate working from platforms. Door locks, hinges, and victims can be up to 12 feet (4 m) above ground level. Rescuers may use pickup trucks/utility vehicles as quickly accessible platforms. If available, a flatbed truck (roll back) may provide a large, stable working platform with the weight capacity for multiple rescuers and equipment. If rescuers cannot access a vehicle or a wrecker, they can use commercially available rescuer platforms, or they can build a platform using cribbing, long timbers, and/or folding ladders **(Figure 11.2)**. To build a platform, rescuers should first build two crib boxes 4 to 6 feet (1 to 2 m) apart and to the height required to access the vehicle. Rescuers can use resources such as long timbers, ladders, or backboards to bridge the two crib boxes and create a solid work platform.

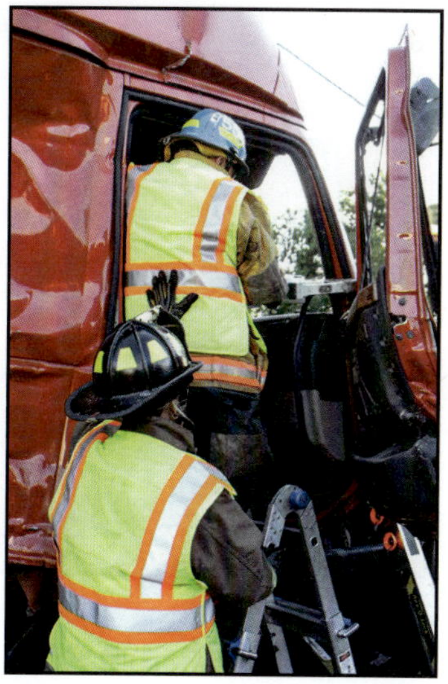

> **CAUTION**
> Do not operate from an unstable or unsafe platform. Falling off the platform may cause injury.

Figure 11.2 Ladders may be used to access heavy vehicles.

Medium and Heavy Truck Entry Points

Once rescuers have stabilized a truck, they should gain access to the interior of the cab. There are a number of access and egress points on medium and heavy trucks. Rescuers may use existing entry points (door or window), or may need to create them (roof or floor panel). These access and egress points include:

- **Doors** — Rescuers should use the door handle to try to open the door to determine whether the door is unlocked, locked, or inoperable. In many cases, the doors are either locked, jammed, or both. If the door opens, rescuers should hold the door handle in the open position to prevent the door from latching again if it closes when released. If operating the exterior or interior door handle does not open the door, it sometimes helps to operate both handles simultaneously. Doors often form a part of the vehicle's structural integrity, and under some circumstances opening the door may compromise the vehicle's structural integrity. The specific situation will determine whether rescuers need to remove the doors, open them, or leave them in place **(Figure 11.3, p. 404)**.

- **Windows** — If the doors are locked or jammed, rescuers may need to remove the side windows to allow access to the door locks and handles. Depending upon the specific situation, rescuers may or may not need to remove the vehicle's windshield.

- **Roofs** — When victims are trapped inside a side-resting heavy/commercial vehicle, rescuers may open the door on the top side of the vehicle to gain access. However, removing all or part of the vehicle's roof allows more room to care for and remove victims.

- **Floor panels** — While rescuers may make access through the floor, they should use such access as a last resort. The cab floor and underlying structures are usually made of heavy-gauge material. Manufacturers also bolt components to the floor such as seats, cabinets, and other cab components. These components may limit the amount of room rescuers have to work. Rescuers will need tools capable of cutting through the heavy floor structure and will need to carefully monitor the victim's location. **Skill Sheet 11-1** provides practice determining commercial/heavy vehicle access and egress points

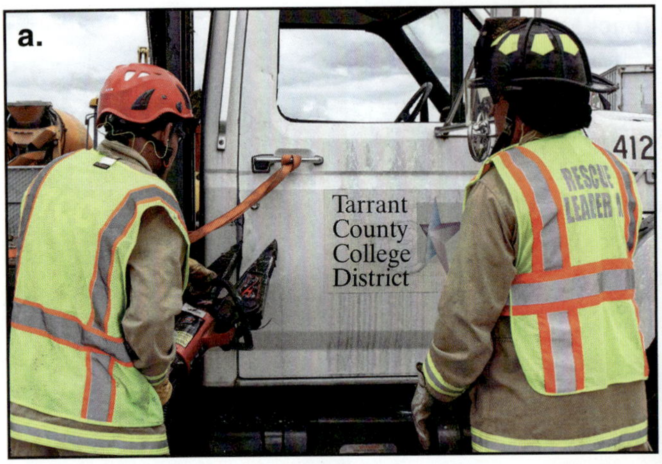

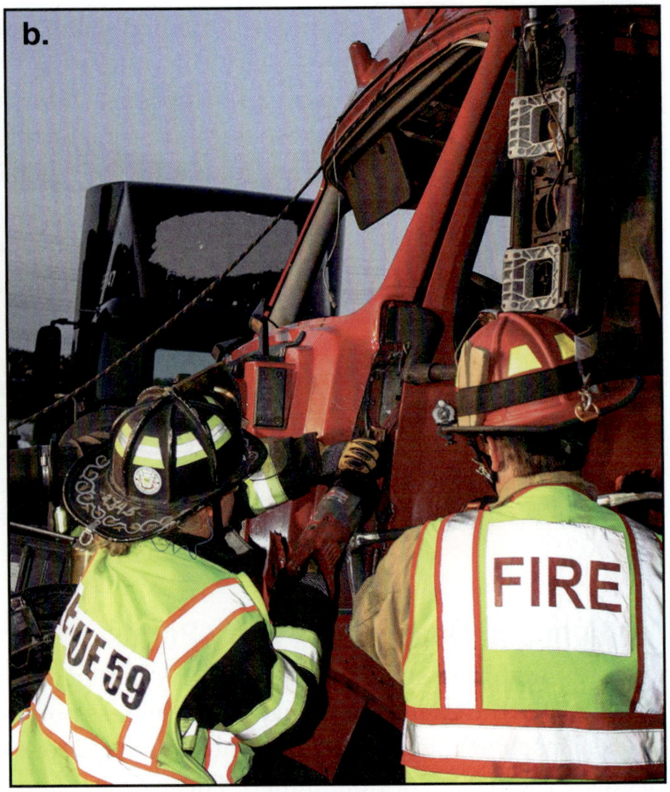

Figure 11.3 a. Rescuers using spreaders to remove a heavy vehicle door. **b.** Rescuers using a power saw to remove a heavy vehicle door.

Medium and Heavy Truck Extrication Operations

Once they stabilize the medium or heavy truck, rescuers can begin extrication operations. Rescuers should use the most appropriate extrication technique to extricate a victim. They should choose a technique based on a number of factors, such as the position of the vehicle and the location of any victims.

NOTE: Rescuers can best follow the instructions for gaining access to the interior of medium and heavy trucks described in this chapter if they use the tools as described in Chapter 4, Tools and Equipment.

NOTE: Refer to Chapter 5 for information on victim care. In the extrication techniques that follow, it is assumed that rescuers provide victim care at the same time as extrication operations, if possible.

Techniques for Creating Access and Egress Openings on Medium and Heavy Trucks

This section will cover the following techniques for creating access and egress openings on medium and heavy trucks:

- Medium and heavy truck door access and egress
- Medium and heavy truck window access and egress
- Medium and heavy truck roof access and egress
- Medium and heavy truck wall access and egress

Medium and Heavy Truck Door Access and Egress

Manufacturers may mount medium and heavy truck doors with conventional automotive or piano style hinges. They may construct the door panels of steel, aluminum, or composite materials. Heavy truck doors usually do not contain collision beams.

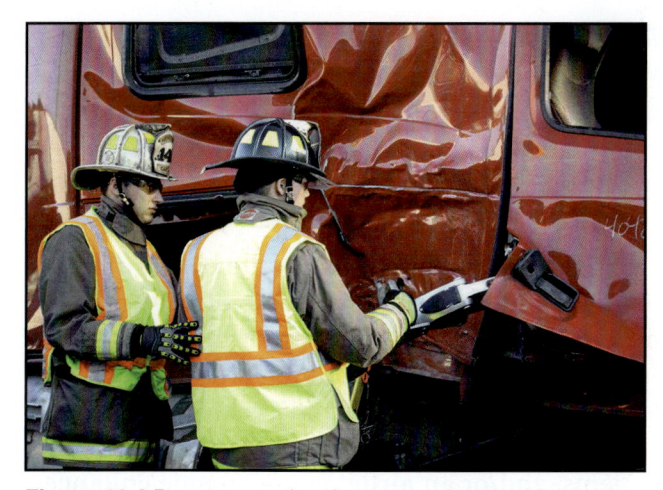

Figure 11.4 Door access involves removing the Nader pin or other latching mechanisms.

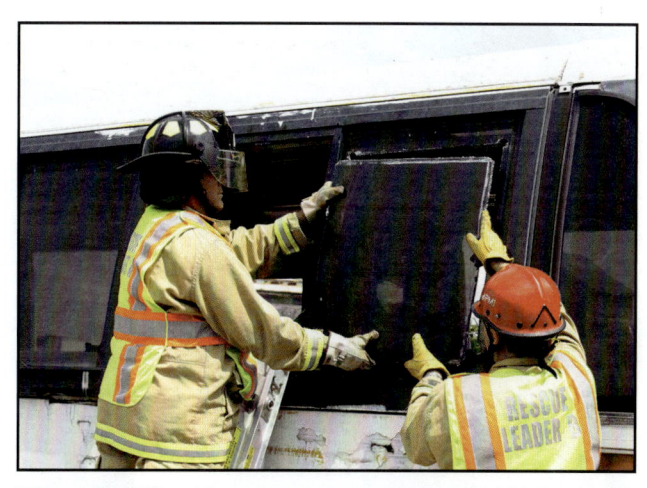

Figure 11.5 Breaking glass on a commercial vehicle should be done with caution to avoid injuring passengers.

Rescuers may opt to attack exposed door hinges. Rescuers can cut or disassemble these hinges, choosing the quickest method as dictated by the situation. If the door has a piano-style hinge, rescuers may need to remove the retaining bolts instead of attempting to cut the hinge off. Freeing a door from a latching mechanism may require repositioning the tool or the angle of the tool several times to get the best purchase to overcome the **Nader pin** or other latching mechanism **(Figure 11.4)**. Parts of the door may tear away without releasing the door from the retaining point.

NOTE: Skill Sheet 11-2 describes the steps for opening or removing a commercial/heavy vehicle door.

> **Nader Pin** — Bolt on a vehicle's door frame that the door latches onto in order to close.

Medium and Heavy Truck Window Access and Egress

Rescuers may use a window to access and egress a medium and heavy truck. The windshield is usually mounted with a gasket (seal) that is somewhat different than those used for passenger vehicle windshields, although rescuers will use basically the same removal methods. On some medium and heavy trucks, rescuers may have to remove a center post between dual-front windshields. To remove this post, rescuers should cut the upper and lower portions of the post and remove the middle section. Because side and rear windows are typically tempered glass, rescuers can remove them with the same techniques as they use with passenger vehicles **(Figure 11.5)**. If rescuers need to break a window to access a victim, they should choose a window as far away from the victim as possible, and protect the victim from glass dust and chips.

CAUTION
Rescuers should wear full PPE, including eye protection, when creating window access and egress openings.

Section D • Chapter 11 – Commercial/Heavy Vehicle Disentanglement

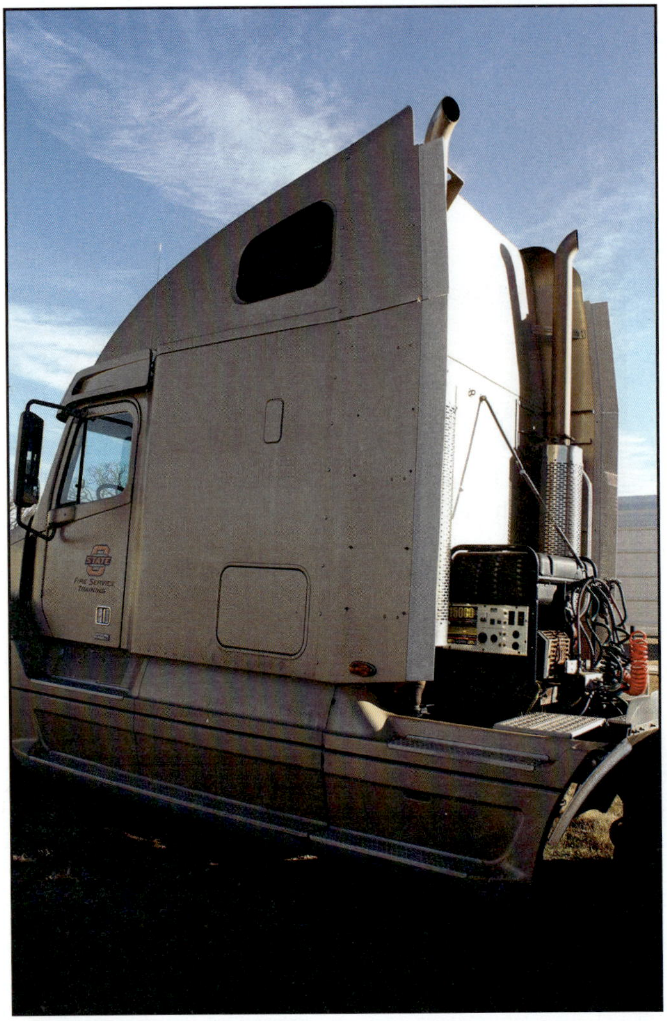

Figure 11.6 An airfoil on a truck roof can hinder cutting operations.

Medium and Heavy Truck Roof Access and Egress

When rescuers encounter a medium or heavy truck they may choose roof removal as the best option for creating a clear opening through which they can extricate the victims — provided they can do so without compromising the vehicle's stability.

If rescuers cannot maintain the truck's stability if they flap down or remove the roof, then rescuers may choose to cut through the roof and leave the roof frame intact. Rescuers should carefully select the location in which they cut into a vehicle's roof. Items such as global positioning systems, air conditioning systems, and/or an airfoil (aerodynamic enhancer) may hinder the cutting operations. After selecting a cutting location, rescuers should use a cutting tool to cut around the edge of the roof and remove the sheet metal and any cross members **(Figure 11.6)**. This will create a relatively large opening through which rescuers can extricate victims. However, compared to roof removal, cutting through the roof takes considerably longer. **Skill Sheet 11-3** lists the steps for creating a roof access opening in the roof or wall of a commercial/heavy vehicle.

Medium and Heavy Truck Wall Access and Egress

Creating wall access and egress involves using cutting tools to flap or remove the sides or rear panel of a vehicle **(Figure 11.7)**. Rescuers should carefully select the cutting area before performing this operation to avoid exposing any hazards or complicating the operation. Rescuers should cut the outer skin away, cut the inner support structures, and then pull or cut away any interior cladding, insulation, cabinets, and other components to allow access to victims. Rescuers should not remove more material than necessary because doing so could jeopardize the vehicle's structural integrity.

NOTE: Rescuers can initially tunnel through the sleeper cab to gain access to the victim and to provide care. Rescuers should expect to find a variety of personal items in the sleeper cab.

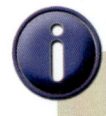

Third Door Conversion

Third door conversion involves using cutting tools to flap the side panel of a vehicle. Rescuers may need to use this technique in a truck collision if the sleeper area is an extension of the cab and not a separate compartment. In this case, rescuers should flap the sidewall of the cab aft of the door rearward.

Techniques for Disentangling Victims from Medium and Heavy Trucks

Due to the large size and height of medium and heavy trucks, disentanglement is not as common as it is on passenger vehicles. However, at some extrication incidents, after creating an access opening, rescuers will have to disentangle a victim. Regardless of the trapped victims' locations within the truck, rescuers must disentangle any victims in a way that will not aggravate the victims' injuries.

If a victim is entrapped within the truck due to a crushed or compressed cab, rescuers may have to enlarge the cab's opening as a means of disentanglement. Rescuers can use extension rams to perform this operation. To enlarge an opening, rescuers should place the extension rams between two points, such as an **A-post** and **B-post**, and extend the ram to the desired opening size. This process may take multiple extension ram sizes as the opening gets larger. Rescuers can use this disentanglement technique to move a door or window frame, the dashboard (when entrapping a victim), or some other cab access point. If necessary, rescuers should consider making relief cuts to allow for appropriate displacement of the structural components. This may require rescuers to expose the engine compartment and make relief cuts on the supports located inside.

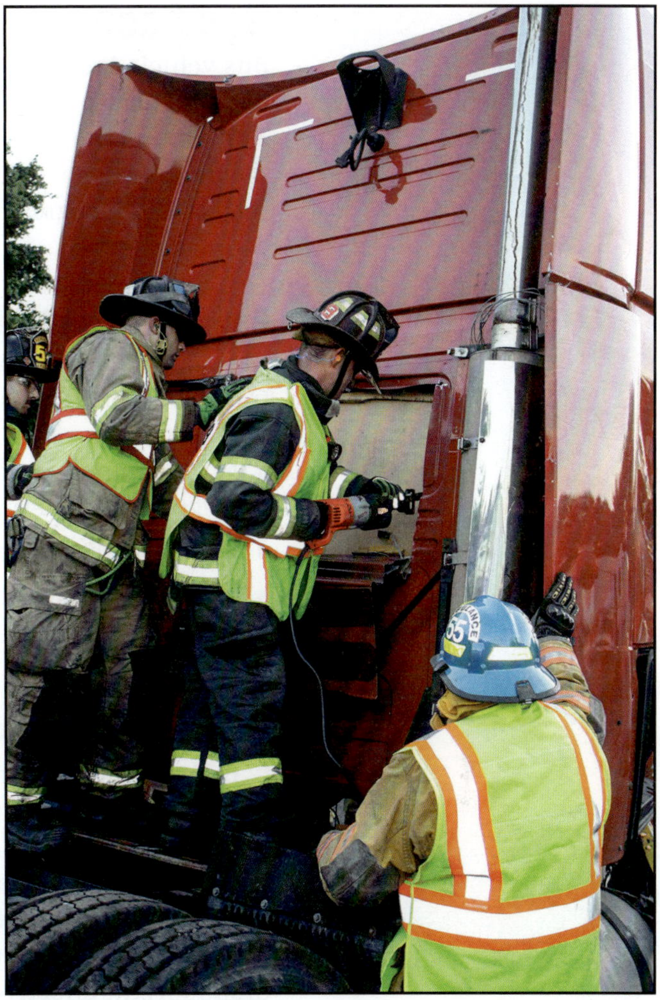

Part of disentangling a victim may require rescuers to move a steering wheel or steering column. To perform this disentanglement technique, rescuers should use an extension ram to move the wheel or column an appropriate distance. This technique involves placing the extension ram between the vehicle's floor and the wheel or column, extending the ram, and elevating the wheel/column up and away from the victim. Rescuers could also use spreaders with tip attachments and chains to pull the steering column up and off an entrapped victim.

A heavy or medium truck's pedals can entrap the feet of drivers. The techniques for cutting and displacing pedals on passenger vehicles are similar to the techniques for medium and heavy trucks. Chapter 8, Victim Disentanglement and Extrication describes the techniques for cutting and displacing pedals.

Rescuers also use the disentanglement technique of displacing a vehicle's seats. On rigid seats, rescuers may use extension rams or spreaders to move the seats away from any victims. On trucks with air-ride seats, rescuers should release the air from the seat prior to attempting displacement. Once they have dispelled the air, rescuers may use extension rams or spreaders to push or pull the seat material and construction components away from the victim.

Figure 11.7 Rescuers removing the rear panel of a truck for an access/egress point.

A-Post — Front post area of a vehicle where the door is connected to the body.

B-Post — Post between the front and rear doors on a four-door vehicle, or the door-handle-end post on a two-door car.

Bus Access and Egress Points

Bus vehicle incidents will likely involve multiple victims. Some buses can carry up to 90 passengers. Rescuers will have to gain access to the interior of a bus in order to provide the bus with a means of access and egress. At these incidents, rescuers must coordinate bus access and egress as well as identify the access and egress points that rescuers will use throughout the bus extrication operations.

Bus Access and Egress Routes

Rescue personnel must determine how best to gain access to and remove trapped victims from buses involved in an accident. Buses will likely contain a large number of victims with varying degrees of injuries, which will create a victim removal problem. When determining the most appropriate access and egress route, rescuers should consider the following:

- Vehicle's location and position
- Number and location(s) of victims
- Hazards
- Available tools and equipment
- Skill set of available rescue personnel

Bus extrication operations may offer more than one access and egress route. For example, rescuers may use both the front door and rear emergency exit door to expedite bus evacuation. Rescuers may need to clear less injured victims out of access ways prior to moving other, possibly more seriously injured victims. Whatever the determined access and egress route, all personnel should coordinate the flow of personnel, tools and equipment, and especially victims to support the effectiveness of the operation. Rescuers may have to minimize any panic that slow egress operations may instill in victims.

> **CAUTION**
> When accessing and egressing vehicles, personnel should watch out for sharp objects such as broken glass or jagged metals. Rescuers should identify, cover, and/or remove these objects from the vehicle.

Rescuers should continue to coordinate the flow of victims once they egress from the bus. These victims will likely need medical care and supervision, so rescuers should make efforts to provide for their needs.

Like medium and heavy trucks, buses are taller than most passenger vehicles and may necessitate working from platforms or ladders **(Figure 11.8)**. If necessary, rescuers should also use a platform to help with access or egress. Rescuers should take care when working on a platform and handling/assisting victims with egress.

> **CAUTION**
> Do not operate from an unstable or unsafe platform. Falling off the platform may cause injury.

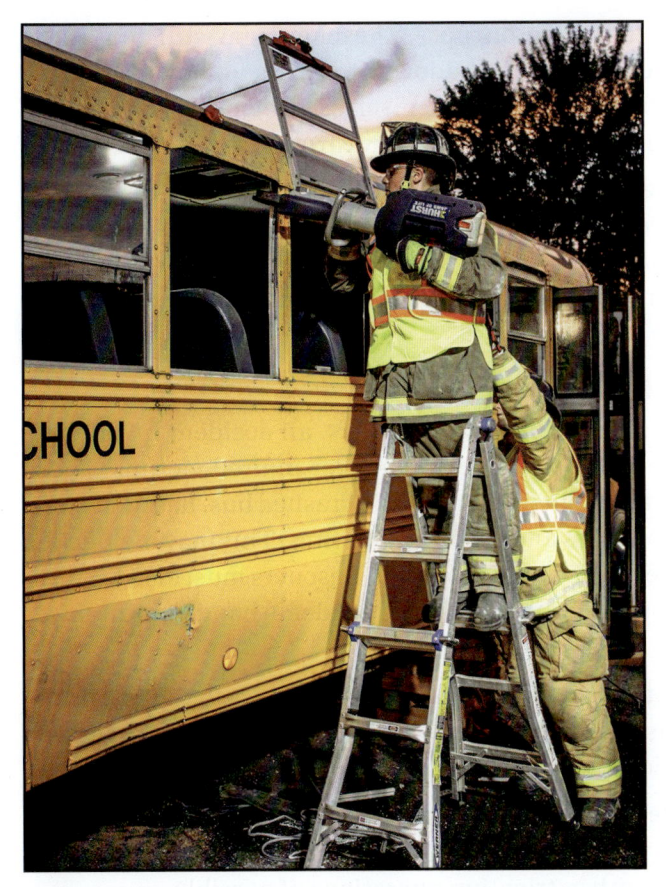

Figure 11.8 Rescuers use ladders to access school bus windows.

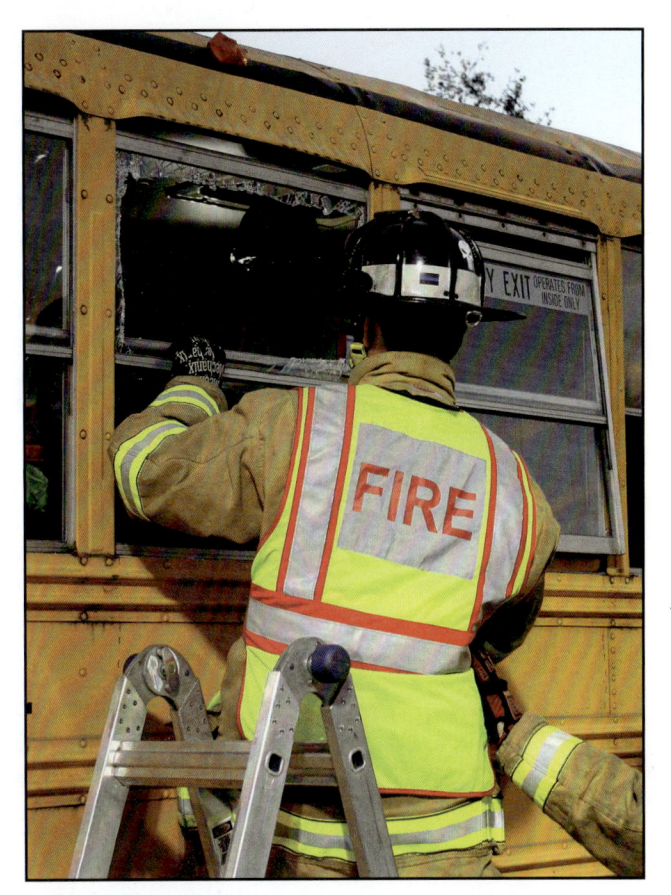

Figure 11.9 School bus windows can be used to gain access into a school bus.

Bus Entry Points

In any extrication incident involving a bus, the access and egress points include the following:

- **Doors** — Rescuers should first attempt to open doors in the way that doors were designed to operate. Most front doors on buses operate only from the inside, while rear emergency doors operate from both the inside and outside. Rarely are all doors inoperable following a collision.

- **Windows** — Rescuers can use the windshield and side and rear windows as access points for gaining entry into a bus **(Figure 11.9)**.

- **Sidewalls** — When the bus has remained upright but rescuers cannot use the front and rear exits, rescuers can use the sidewalls as an access point. If rescuers have the proper equipment, they can cut a large hole that will provide maximum access to the passenger area.

- **Rear walls** — Rescuers may need to remove part of the rear wall of the bus if the rear door does not provide a large enough opening to remove immobilized victims.

- **Roofs** — When a bus lands on its side, the front door may be useless. It will either be under the bus, making it inaccessible, or it will be on top, making

Section D • Chapter 11 – Commercial/Heavy Vehicle Disentanglement **409** it difficult to use for evacuation purposes. Rescuers may still access the interior through the rear emergency door or windshield; however, these openings may not be sufficient or may themselves be blocked. Any of these situations may require rescuers to make entry through the roof.

- **Floor panels** — Rescuers should only consider gaining access through the floor of a bus as a last resort. Any attempt to breach this area will require a considerable amount of time because of the many layers of materials that manufacturers combine to construct the floor.

Bus Extrication Operations

Because buses carry a large number of passengers, an accident involving a bus may result in a large number of trapped and/or injured victims. These victims may be trapped inside, outside, or under a crashed bus. Rescuers must determine the best way to access and egress the victims. This may include the extrication techniques described in this section. Rescuers must also take immediate actions to request additional resources in order to handle the multiple victims.

NOTE: To best follow the instructions for gaining access to the interior of buses as described in this chapter, rescuers should use the tools as described in Chapter 4, Tools and Equipment.

NOTE: Refer to Chapter 5 for information on victim care. In the extrication techniques that follow, it is assumed that if possible, rescuers will provide victim care concurrently with extrication operations, if possible.

Techniques for Creating Access and Egress Openings on Buses

This section will cover the following techniques for creating openings on buses:

- Creating openings through bus doors
- Creating openings through bus windows
- Creating openings through bus sidewalls
- Creating openings through bus rear walls
- Creating openings through bus roofs
- Creating openings through bus floor panels

NOTE: Refer to Chapter 10 for information on bus anatomy and hazards.

NOTE: Several of the skills in this section are listed as specific to buses, rescuers may also apply them to other types of commercial/heavy vehicles. Always follow local SOPs.

Stair Removal

Rescuers may use hydraulic cutters in combination with reciprocating saws or pneumatic tools to cut the entrance steps from a bus. Because of the materials involved in the construction of the steps, this process can take a long time.

> **WARNING!**
> Before cutting into a bus, rescuers should be aware of the hazards on the roof, floor, and wall panels. For example, fuel lines are located on the vehicle's undercarriage.

Creating Openings through Bus Doors

If possible, rescuers can use doors to create access and egress openings on a bus. However, depending on the operability and location of the door, rescuers may have to vary their approach.

Operable front doors. Entry may be somewhat difficult if the front door is the operable door but closed. However, passengers may open the door from the inside.

On buses so equipped, could use the emergency opening button located below the center of the windshield to open the door. Some newer buses have this button located on the exterior of the A-post in front of the door. On other buses, rescuers can quickly create an avenue of access to the center pivot arm control and operate the door in the normal manner in one of the following two ways:

- Remove the windshield so that a rescuer can reach through the opening and manually operate the control.

- Reach in through the driver's side window with a pike pole to operate the control **(Figure 11.10)**.

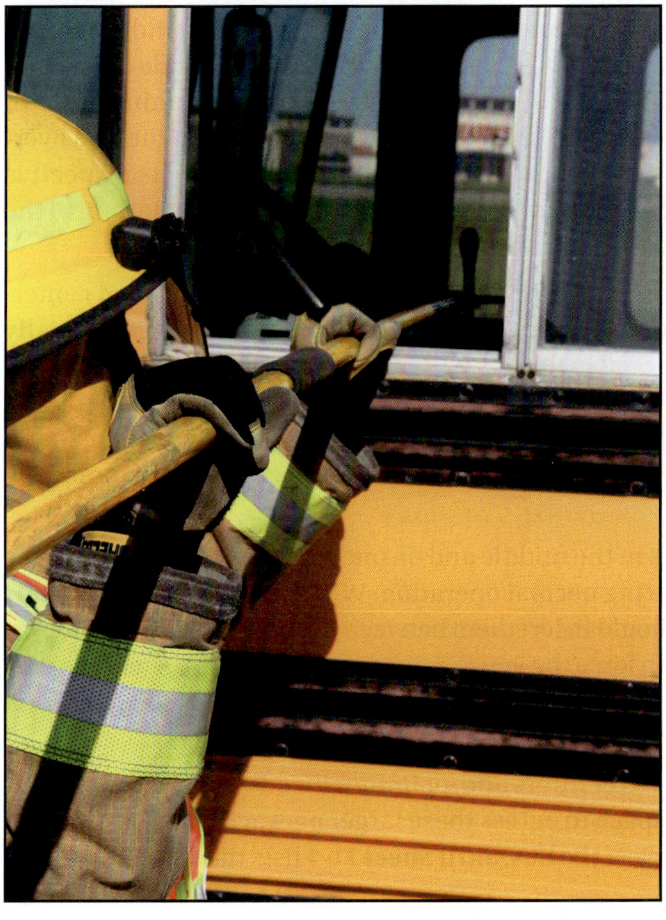

Figure 11.10 A rescuer using a pike pole to operate the manual door opening pivot arm control.

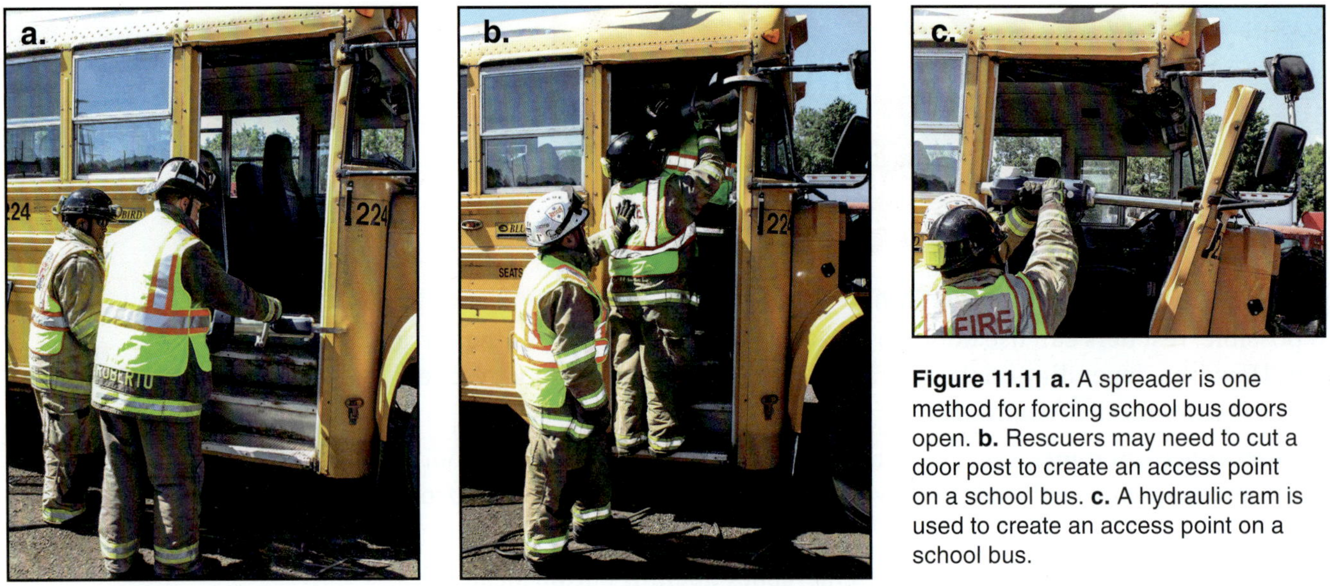

Figure 11.11 a. A spreader is one method for forcing school bus doors open. **b.** Rescuers may need to cut a door post to create an access point on a school bus. **c.** A hydraulic ram is used to create an access point on a school bus.

If the bus has an alternate method to operate the door, such as an air-actuated control mechanism, rescuers can reach in through the driver's side window and operate the main switch. This switch is usually located to the left of the driver's instrument console. Buses will also have a backup emergency release mechanism in the stairwell just inside the door. The readily identifiable release button or switch permits the airlock device to release the door. Then, rescue personnel can manually move the door through its normal path of travel.

Inoperable front doors. If rescuers need to force the doors, they may use a spreading tool **(Figure 11.11 a and b and c)**. First, rescuers should locate the hinges to identify the type of door. If there are hinges on either side of the door and an overlapping rubber seal in the middle, it is a center-opening door. To open this type of door, rescuers can insert a spreader between the two overlapping seals about halfway up the door and force each half to its respective side. Rescuers may need to repeat this procedure at the top and bottom of the door to maximize the size of the opening.

Rescuers can also cut apart, disconnect, or disassemble a jammed center-opening door. To remove the door, rescuers may break the hinges (usually piano hinges) that connect it to the bus. To break the hinges, rescuers can drive the wedge end of a **Halligan tool** into the hinge area with a sledgehammer. This will usually fracture the hinge, enabling rescuers to remove the door. Rescuers will also have to cut or detach the pivot control arm to completely remove the door.

If the door has hinges in the middle and on one side, it will open toward the side with the hinges during normal operation. When using spreaders on this type of door, rescuers should insert them between the non-hinged side and the frame. Rescuers can then force the entire door toward the hinged side. Depending on the circumstances, rescuers may need to completely remove the door.

Because of the narrowness of the front door area on some older buses, rescuers may need to maneuver litters and/or immobilized victims through that area. To allow enough space to egress these larger packages, rescuers should widen the front door area of the bus. **Skill Sheet 11-4** lists the steps to perform this operation.

Halligan Tool — Prying tool with a claw at one end and a spike or point at a right angle to a wedge at the other end. *Also known as* Hooligan Tool.

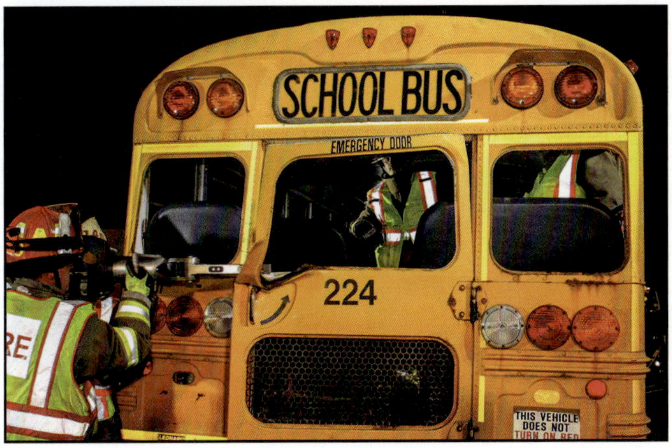

Figure 11.12 Rescuers using a spreading tool to open the rear door of a school bus.

Rear doors. Rescuers may need to force open and use the rear emergency exit door for access following a rear-end collision. One or three latch points hold the rear exit door secure. The main latch is at the edge of the door near the control handle. The other two latches, if present, are at the top and bottom of the door, locking into the bus body and the floor assembly. To force this type of door open, rescuers may insert a prying or spreading tool between the door and the frame and separate the two **(Figure 11.12)**.

Inserting a spreading tool on the hinged side of the door and operating it to rip the hinges off the frame will remove the door. If rescuers do not have a spreading tool, they can also disassemble, disconnect, or cut apart the rear door with a variety of other rescue tools.

One reason that rescuers have more difficulty removing a rear door than removing other doors is that the rear door is normally higher above the roadway surface. Rescuers will have to stand on something, such as a platform, to effectively operate the rescue tool.

Sometimes opening or removing the rear door still does not provide a large enough opening to remove immobilized victims. In these cases, rescuers may need to remove part of the rear wall of the bus.

NOTE: Skill Sheet 11-5 provides the steps to open and remove a rear bus door.

Creating Openings through Bus Windows

Rescuers should familiarize themselves with the various bus windows and how to use them for access and egress openings. Many of these windows open and close, and victims can use them as a means of egress in the event of an emergency. One window in particular, the emergency window, offers a larger egress opening for bus passengers. If the passengers cannot open the emergency window, rescuers should be able to open the window from the exterior of the bus using appropriate extrication techniques. **Skill Sheet 11-6** lists the steps for removing the emergency window in a school bus. Rescuers should also familiarize themselves with the procedures to access a bus's windshield and side window.

Windshield access. Rescuers can enter through the windshield when the front exit is unusable or the bus has come to rest on its side. Removing the windshield will give rescuers quick access to the interior of the bus and will also provide a route for removing victims **(Figure 11.13, p. 414)**.

Section D • Chapter 11 – Commercial/Heavy Vehicle Disentanglement

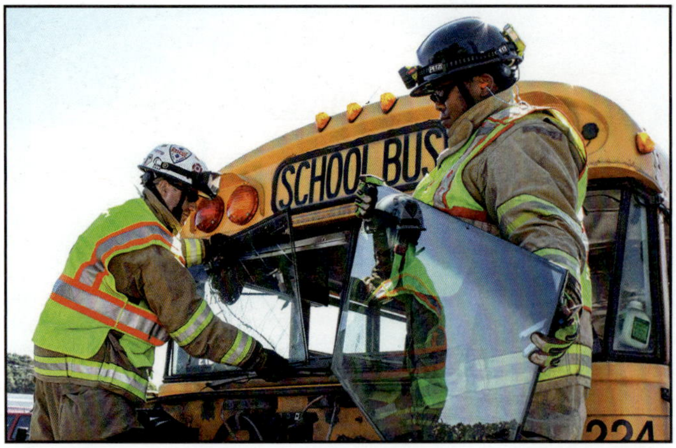

Figure 11.13 Removing the windshield of a school bus provides an escape route for passengers.

Unlike passenger vehicle windshields, manufacturers often divide bus windshields into two or more parts, which may be separated by posts. Manufacturers mount bus windshields with somewhat different gaskets than those used for passenger vehicle windshields, although rescuers can use basically the same removal methods. To remove a bus windshield, rescuers should cut and remove the rubber mounting gasket.

Once rescuers remove the gasket, a rescuer should next remove each piece of the windshield. If no rescuer is inside the bus, rescuers can sometimes reach through the gasket gap with the end of a baling hook and gently pull the glass toward them. If a rescuer is already inside the bus, the rescuer can push gently on the glass to loosen it enough that the rescuers on the outside can remove it. After they remove the glass rescuers can remove the center windshield post to provide a full-width opening through which they can work.

NOTE: Rescuers can remove rear windows in a similar manner; however, it is preferable to use the rear exit door or completely cut away the rear walls whenever possible. **Skill Sheet 11-6** shows how to remove an emergency window of a school bus.

Side window access. Gaining access through the side windows may be difficult for two reasons: They are small, and they may be 6 to 8 feet (2 to 2.5 m) above ground level. Rescuers should work from elevated platforms. If rescuers do not have a platform and cannot build one, rescuers may work from ladders, which will make it more difficult to handle tools and victims.

Even with the latching systems found on many transit and commercial buses, rescuers can pry the side windows open from the outside with a rescue tool. Many buses have a small access hatch that rescuers can reach through to open a window from the inside. This hatch is usually level with the bottom of the last window on the passenger side of the bus. On commercial buses, it is located directly outside the restroom. The rescuer will need to stand on a ladder or other object to reach this hatch. Once they open the hatch, rescuers can reach in and operate the window latch to open the window. Then, rescuers can enter and open more windows as necessary.

Most school buses have side windows that only slide down part way. They provide an opening of about 9 x 22 inches (225 mm by 550 mm), which is too small to be useful. Therefore, rescuers will need to enlarge the window opening. To double the size of the window opening, rescuers should break the glass and remove the aluminum frame from the opening. Rescuers can use almost any cutting tool to cut away the soft aluminum window frame.

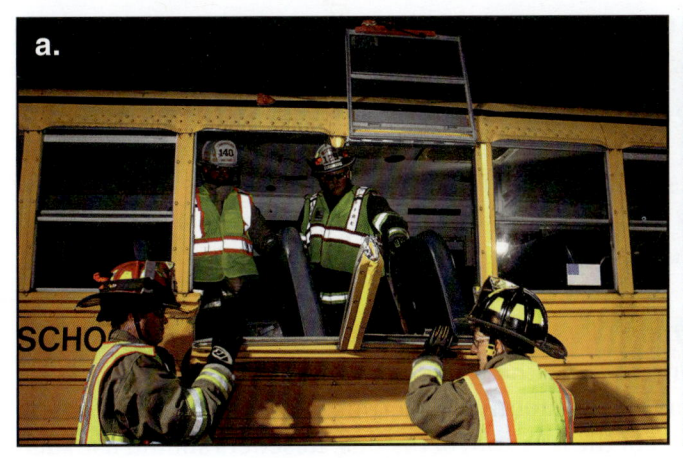

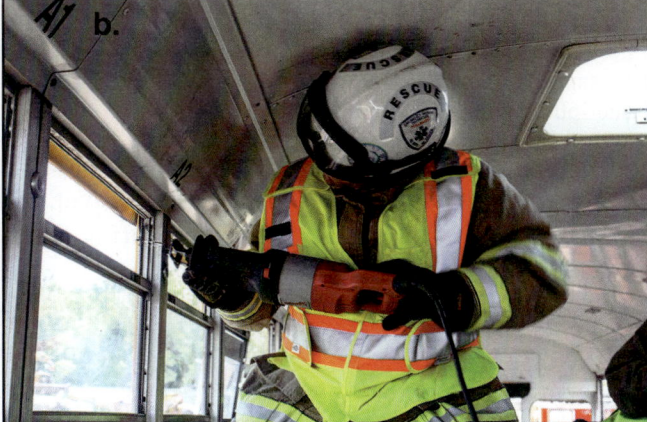

Figure 11.14 a. To enlarge the opening around an emergency exit window, rescuers can remove the post between windows. **b.** A rescuer removing the window from inside the school bus.

If a window is too small for extrication purposes, rescuers can remove two adjacent windows, the post between them, and the same section of sidewall to enlarge the opening **(Figure 11.14 a and b)**. If necessary, rescuers can remove more windows and cut the posts. However, removing too many posts may compromise the structural integrity of the bus.

Creating Openings through Bus Sidewalls

Forcible entry through the side of a bus will require considerable work to cut a usable opening. Prior to performing any cutting operations, rescuers should use the horizontal coping on the exterior sidewall as a guide to identify the seat and floor levels on the bus. The heaviest beams in bus construction are located on the floor, where the seats bolt to the wall, and above and below the windows.

Rescuers should remove the seats before opening a sidewall. If time allows, rescuers can unbolt the seats from the floor **(Figure 11.15)**. If not, rescuers can cut the steel tube seat frame with any number of cutting tools. Cutting the legs or supports may leave sharp stubs, which rescuers should cover to prevent additional injuries.

Once rescuers have cleared the seats away and removed the windows and posts, they may begin cutting on the sidewall. To accomplish this, rescuers could use a reciprocating saw with a 6-inch (150 mm) metal cutting blade. This combination will cut through any of the structural components found in the sidewall of the bus.

Figure 11.15 Rescuers can remove bus seats before opening a sidewall.

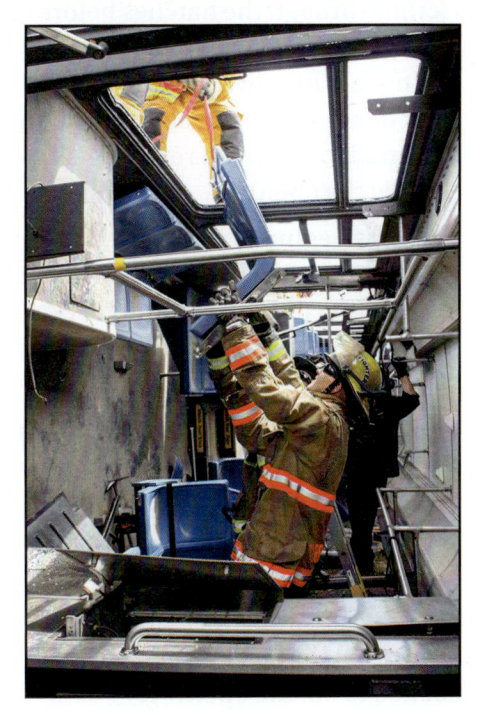

Section D • Chapter 11 – Commercial/Heavy Vehicle Disentanglement

> **Pneumatic Chisel** — Tool designed to operate at air pressures between 100 and 150 psi (700 kPa and 1 050 kPa); during periods of normal consumption, it will use about 4 to 5 cubic feet (113 L to 142 L) of air per minute. It is useful for extrication work. *Also known as* Air Chisel, Impact Hammer, or Pneumatic Hammer.

NOTE: Skill Sheet 11-7 provides the steps to cut through the sidewall of a bus utilizing a window opening.

Rescuers could also use a **pneumatic chisel** to pop the rivets or welds that hold the sheets of the sidewall and to remove entire sheets of metal. Once they remove the sheets, rescuers can cut the individual beams on the side of the bus. However, this method is considerably slower and noisier than using a reciprocating saw and rescuers should only use it as a last resort.

Creating Openings through Bus Rear Walls

Sometimes opening or removing the rear door still does not provide a large enough opening to remove immobilized victims. In these cases, rescuers may need to remove part of the rear wall of the bus. Rescuers should use such natural openings as windows or doors to begin cuts and make purchase points. For example, prior to cutting the center upper part of the center two pillars, rescuers should remove the rear glass to create a natural. A rescuer can then use a suitable tool to cut along the bottom edge of both side panels of the rear of the bus. Next, rescuers should cut the outer two pillars on the outside edge from the window edge, allowing the door and both rear sides of the bus to open up for a full rear access or egress point. Removal of one or two rows of the rear seats will allow greater access to the interior of the bus.

If a school bus comes to rest on its side with the hinge side up, the weight of the rear door may make it difficult for occupants to push it open. Rescuers should first try to open the door using the handle. Once they open the door, rescuers must secure it in the open position. If time permits, rescuers should remove the door. Rescuers should try to remove the rear wall of a side-resting bus. This eliminates the need to step over the wall every time someone goes through the exit.

Creating Openings through Bus Roofs

If the bus has roof escape hatches, rescuers should first attempt to remove victims through the hatches before cutting the roof. Rescuers can easily force these hatches from the outside. They can pry most off with any standard prying tool or power spreading tool. However, these hatches only provide a clear opening of up to about 2 square feet (200 000 square mm). They may be too small to allow the removal of immobilized victims, requiring rescuers to enlarge the opening.

Before beginning to cut, rescuers must determine the best location for the roof opening. They should consider the location of the victims inside the bus, the position of the bus, and the type and amount of damage to the bus. Each situation will dictate the best location for rescuers to cut.

Cutting an opening in the roof of the bus can sometimes be difficult and time consuming. The roof is composed of two layers of sheet metal with supports, insulation, and wiring sandwiched between them. However, the overall benefits can easily justify the time involved. Cutting an opening in the roof can provide rescuers with access to the interior of the bus **(Figure 11.16)**.

While rescuers can use an air chisel if it is the only tool available, it is not ideal. Because an air chisel can only cut one layer of metal at a time, rescuers have to cut the layers one at a time. This virtually doubles the amount of time needed to cut the opening.

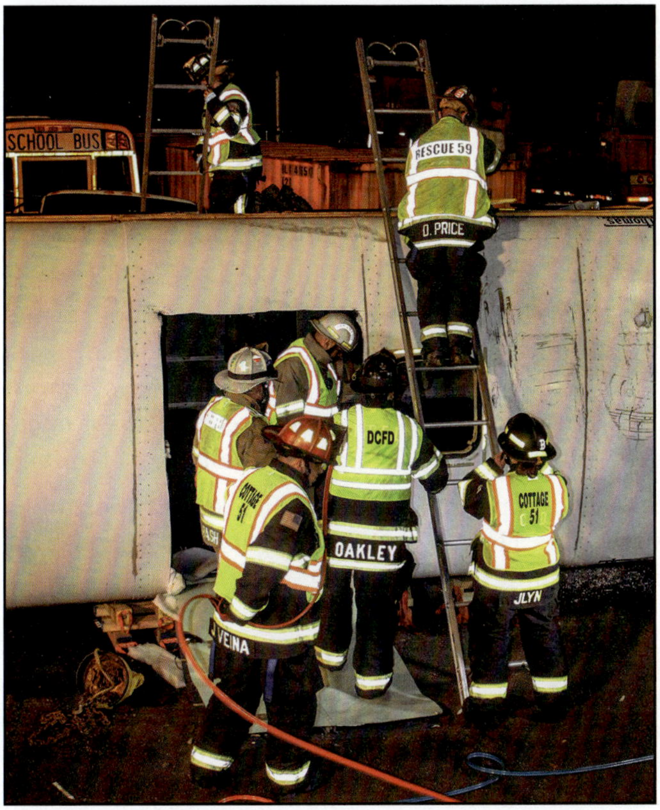

Figure 11.16 A large opening in the bus roof can provide rescuers with access to the interior of the bus.

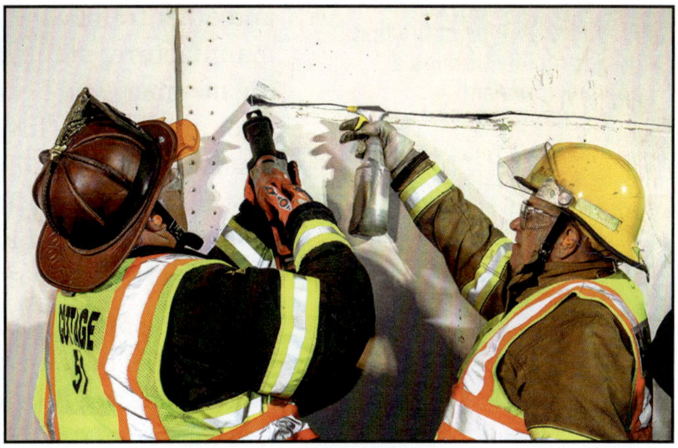

Figure 11.17 This rescue crew is creating an opening in the roof of a school bus with a reciprocating saw. Soap and water is used to lubricate and cool the blade during cutting.

Rescuers can use a reciprocating saw with at least a 6-inch (150 mm) blade to cut roof panels **(Figure 11.17)**. The **reciprocating saw** will produce a smooth cut through all layers of material at one time, and with little chance of igniting any flammable vapors in the area.

When an occupied bus has come to rest on its side, the occupants will be come to rest on the bottom side. Their general condition will depend upon the event that caused the bus to roll over and whether it slowly rolled onto its side or if it rolled over several times and came to rest on its side. In either case, access from either end of the bus will be difficult because the center aisle will be horizontal and movement within the bus will involve climbing over each row of seats. Therefore, rescuers may find it more efficient to cut a large opening in the roof of the bus near its middle. Such an opening reduces the distance that occupants need to travel in order to escape and that rescuers need to travel to reach trapped victims.

NOTE: For procedures on creating an access opening on the roof of a side-resting bus, refer to **Skill Sheet 11-8**.

Sometimes rescuers will need to access the interior through the front of the bus. In these cases, rescuers may need to flap a portion of the roof backward. While this procedure is possible with the proper equipment, it will be difficult. **Skill Sheet 11-9** lists the steps for flapping a bus roof.

Creating Openings through Bus Floor Panels

Bus floors consist of a heavy frame to support the entire bus, plus sheet metal, plywood, and a vinyl or rubber floor covering. Manufacturers often place beams

> **Reciprocating Saw —** Electric saw that uses a short, straight blade that moves back and forth.

Flash Fire — Type of fire that spreads rapidly through a vapor environment.

and other framework as close as 9 inches (225 mm) apart. Depending on the manufacturer of the bus, only every third or fourth beam is a solid, supporting member. The beams in between are only welded to the underside of the floor and provide little support or hindrance to rescue operations. Because rescuers will likely only attempt through-the-floor access on side-resting or roof-resting buses, the fuel tank, which is mounted under the vehicle, will be inverted and probably leaking fuel near the cutting area. This makes the risk of a **flash fire** high.

Because of the massive understructure associated with transit buses and commercial buses, access through the undercarriage and floor is a difficult and tedious job. When a storage area is located between the bottom of the bus and the actual underside of the floor, rescuers must first cut an access opening through the storage area floor and then through the main floor of the bus.

Operations to create an access opening in a bus floor are time consuming and rescuers should use them as a last resort. **Skill Sheet 11-10** provides the steps for creating an access opening in a bus floor.

Techniques for Disentangling Victims from Buses

Upon accessing victims in a vehicle, rescuers may find that some entrapped victims require disentanglement. This section will cover the following:

- Bus driver's seat disentanglement
- Bus steering wheel disentanglement
- Bus interior features (seats and partitions) disentanglement
- Other bus disentanglement considerations

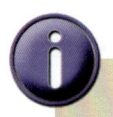

> **Motor Coaches**
>
> As mentioned in Chapter 10, Medium/Heavy Vehicles Stabilization Operations, some commercial buses have been converted into mobile living quarters and/or offices. Entertainers on tour and others whose jobs require them to relocate frequently may use these buses as campers or mobile living quarters. Rescuers can usually distinguish these vehicles from commercial buses by their blacked-out windows and sometimes ornate signage on the vehicle's exterior. The interior layout of some of these vehicles will vary considerably from that of standard motor coaches. Some of these vehicles may have fully equipped galleys for meal preparation and may carry one or more LPG tanks for cooking and for heating water. All of these alterations can complicate the disentanglement and extrication processes.

Bus Driver Seat Disentanglement

Pneumatically controlled seats may automatically reposition the seat due to changes in weight or pressure. The seat's automatic adjustment can hold the driver against the steering wheel and make him or her appear trapped. Operating the seat adjustment control may release enough air to lower the seat and free the driver.

If lowering the seat does not free the driver, or if rescuers do not have the option to lower or otherwise move the seat, rescuers should attempt other disentanglement options. Rescuers can cut the steering wheel spokes or ring to free the driver. Rescuers can also unbolt the seat from the floor and move the seat. Rescuers may need to remove the partition behind the driver's seat to create enough room to lay the driver's seat back.

Bus Steering Wheel Disentanglement

A bus involved in a front- or rear-end collision often remains in an upright position. In front-end collisions, the steering wheel sometimes traps the driver. Bus drivers often must tilt the steering wheel down into their laps when they take the driver's seat. In the event of a collision, the wheel in this lowered position traps the driver even before any impact. After impact, the driver usually cannot move the steering wheel into its original position and, therefore, cannot get out of the driver's seat.

Rescuers may want to pull the steering column and steering wheel up and away from the driver, as they do in passenger vehicle extrication. This technique is not recommended. Just as in a passenger vehicle, tilting the steering wheel or cutting the steering wheel ring puts the driver at less risk of injury from the end of the steering column pivoting into his or her torso. In many cases, rescuers can tilt the steering wheel toward the windshield to free the driver. A bridge system can be set up in front of the dash, and a hook or chain assembly used to lift the steering column up and off of the driver. In some older buses, rescuers may need to cut the brace between the steering column and the front wall of the bus. Otherwise, rescuers may need to cut the steering wheel's spokes or ring.

The steering wheel on a bus is constructed from a hardened steel ring molded inside a covering of rubber or plastic. The quickest method of freeing the victim is to cut away the bottom half of the steering ring. While rescuers can use a hacksaw or reciprocating saw to cut the ring, they should use a cutter. Often, cutting the ring will free the driver, thus eliminating the need for further action.

Bus Interior Features (Seats and Partitions) Disentanglement

Rescuers may need to move or remove interior features of the bus to facilitate removal of victims. The narrow aisles in buses create a limited working space. Most litters and backboards will not fit in the aisle and rescuers will have to place them on the top of the seat cushions or across the tops of the seat backs. Seat frames are easily bent during a collision and can entrap a victim.

Deciding whether to simply move a seat or to remove it will depend on the position of the victim and the rescuers' need for operating space. In many cases, rescuers will need to remove the seat and get it out of the way. Rescuers may use a winch, come-along, or power-spreader to pull the seats from their moorings. Rescuers should not remove a seat if any victims are still trapped close to the seat being pulled because the seat may suddenly dislodge and aggravate their injuries.

CAUTION
Use of power tools in close proximity to victims increases the chances that extrication operations will result in further victim injuries.

There are several good methods for removing seats. Rescuers could use a power spreader to dislodge the legs connected to the floor and then break the seat-to-wall connection. Rescuers could also cut the legs of the seats. The legs are made of tubular steel and rescuers can cut them with power cutters. Rescuers should cut the legs as close to the floor as possible and tape or cover the sharp stubs with duct tape. If victims are in close proximity, rescuers may have to use hand tools to remove seat mounting hardware.

Many school buses have partitions in front of the first row of seats, on either side of the aisle. These dividers are usually made only of thin sheet metal attached to a tubular steel frame. Manufacturers connect the divider unit to the bus in a manner similar to the seats. Rescuers can remove these partitions in the same manner as a seat.

Likewise, most of the objects inside transit or commercial buses are either seats or partitions. Rescuers bolt both of these assemblies to the floor. They may also connect partitions to the ceiling. If rescuers need to remove either of these objects, they can unbolt them and remove them from the bus. If rescuers cannot unbolt them, they can cut most with any number of cutting tools. Manufacturers generally construct legs or supports from easily cut tubular steel. Cutting these legs or supports will leave behind sharp stubs. Rescuers should cover them as described earlier.

Commercial buses also have overhead storage bins. If rescuers need to remove them to facilitate extricating immobilized victims, rescuers may need to cut or chop them out. Any type of saw or air chisel will work. If rescuers do not have a saw, they may use a crash axe or standard fire axe. Rescuers should use caution when chopping inside a bus as the space is confined and the potential for striking oneself or another person is high. They should use short, controlled strokes. To reduce the slip and fall hazard for those working inside the bus, rescuers should remove debris as soon as it is cut or chopped away.

Additional Bus Disentanglement Considerations

Even though most bus passengers do not wear seat belts, the likelihood of them being ejected in a rollover is relatively low. However, bus rollovers may still result in passengers being trapped beneath the vehicle when it comes to rest **(Figure 11.18)**. There are two primary methods for removing a person trapped beneath a bus. First, if the bus rests on soft ground, rescuers may dig the victim out. Rescuers may need to lift the bus off the victim. Rescuers may use any one of a number of lifting tools to perform the actual lifting Regardless of the tool used, the method for performing the rescue will be the same.

The rescue device best suited to perform this operation is the pneumatic lifting bag. **Skill Sheet 11-11** lists the steps for using pneumatic lifting bags to free a victim trapped beneath a commercial/heavy vehicle. Rescuers must utilize a capturing device (cribbing or struts) as the vehicle's lift progresses so that the vehicle does not fall back onto the victim in the event of an equipment failure. If using cribbing as a capturing device, rescuers may have to use wedges to maximize contact between the cribbing and the vehicle because many vehicles have curved edges where the roof meets the sidewall.

If they do not have pneumatic lifting bags, rescuers can use hydraulic jacks to lift a bus. When lifting on soft ground, rescuers will need to place a board

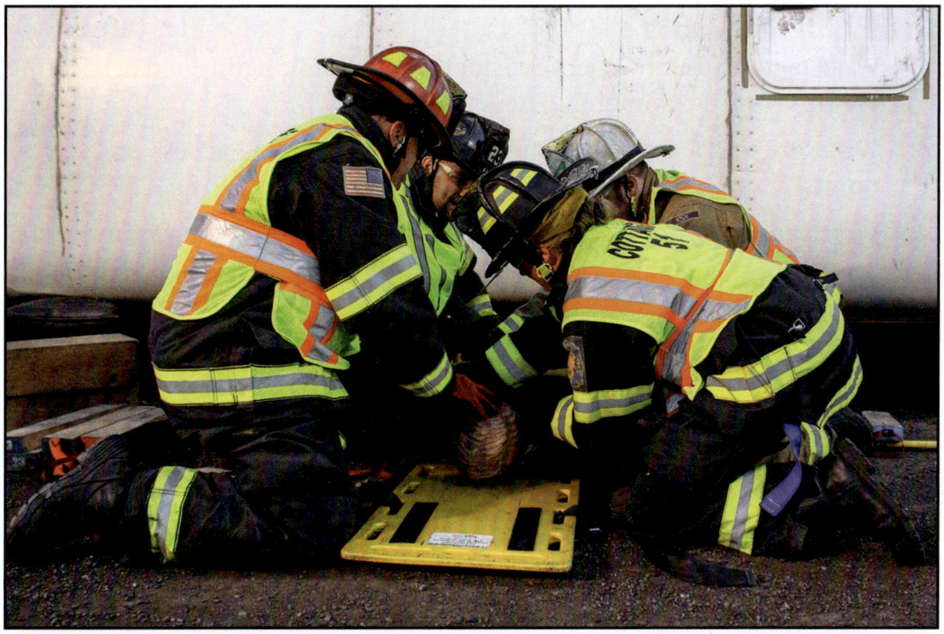

Figure 11.18 Rescuers work as a team to remove passengers trapped under a bus.

beneath the base of the jack. Because of the overall height of most jacks, rescuers may need to dig a hole beneath the intended lifting area in order to place the jack. Once rescuers position a jack, one rescuer can operate it while the other rescuers concentrate on building the box crib or adjusting the chocks.

Rescuers could also use a heavy wrecker. These wreckers have long booms and the necessary straps to lift a bus or large vehicle quickly and safely. Personnel using a wrecker must be well trained with the equipment before participating in a life safety situation. The IC should assign a rescuer to the wrecker operator to ensure proper communications during the extrication.

When an occupied bus has come to rest on its roof, the occupants will be concentrated on the ceiling because that is now the lowest point. If the bus rolled over several times, there can be significant distortion of the seats, partitions, and other interior features. The dynamics creating this distortion can result in many occupant injuries and entrapments.

Unlike a bus on its side, one on its roof can allow easier movement within the bus — if the roof did not collapse in the rollover. If the roof still has its structural integrity, removing the windshield and the rear and side windows will allow uninjured passengers to crawl out and rescuers to crawl in. Ultimately, rescuers may need to remove portions of a sidewall and to remove seats and other features to facilitate movement inside the bus.

Removing too much of the sidewall may weaken the side of the bus and allow the bus to collapse. If rescuers must remove a large area of the wall must be removed, the bus may require additional stabilization.

Chapter Review

1. What factors must rescuers consider when disentangling and extricating victims from a commercial/heavy vehicle?
2. What are four common commercial/heavy vehicle access and egress points?
3. Why should rescuers use the vehicle floor as a last resort for victim access?
4. What techniques can be used to create access openings through the doors of medium and heavy trucks?
5. How can rescuers remove windows in medium and heavy trucks?
6. What items installed on or in a medium or heavy truck's roof can complicate cutting operations?
7. What is one method of enlarging an opening in a medium or heavy truck in order to disentangle victims?
8. How does the likelihood of multiple victims affect operations when creating access openings on a bus?
9. What parts of a bus can serve as access openings?
10. What methods can be used to create access openings through bus doors?
11. How can rescuers create access openings using bus windows?
12. What methods can be used to create openings in the rear wall of a bus?
13. What hazards should rescuers be aware of when creating openings in the floor of a bus?
14. What methods can be used to disentangle a bus driver from the steering wheel or column?
15. What interior bus features may need to be removed in order to facilitate victim extrication?

Discussion Questions

1. Compare and contrast the resource needs and operational considerations of an incident involving two passenger vehicles with an incident involving a bus full of passengers and a heavy commercial truck.
2. Why is it critical for rescuers to adequately train and prepare for incidents involving commercial/heavy vehicles?

11-1
Determine commercial/heavy vehicle access and egress points.

SKILL SHEETS

REMINDER: Not all agencies advocate the following practices. The following skill sheets present a snapshot of various procedures utilized during vehicle incident operations. Always follow manufacturer's recommendations and local SOPs. Rescuers must wear full PPE including hand, eye, and respiratory protection. It is recommended that rescuers maintain communication with victims and make them aware of pertinent rescue information.

Directions: Read each scenario and study the accompanying diagram. Complete the steps below for each scenario.

NOTE: There may be multiple access locations and methods for each scenario. Refer to local SOPs to determine the method used in your jurisdiction.

Step 1: Identify probable victim locations and points of entrapment.

Step 2: Determine the appropriate locations for rescuer and equipment access and for victim removal.
  a. Factor in time constraints and available resources.
  b. Ensure that vehicle stability will not be compromised.

Step 3: Assess the impact that the vehicle's stability and position will have on the victim(s) and on rescue operations.

Step 4: Describe the safety precautions that must be taken before extrication can begin.

Step 5: Describe the method of stabilization that will be used.

Scenario 1
You are in charge of the rescue teams dispatched to the scene of a single-vehicle incident involving a heavy truck. The driver lost control and the truck came to rest on its side. The driver is trapped and injured. There are no other occupants in the truck.

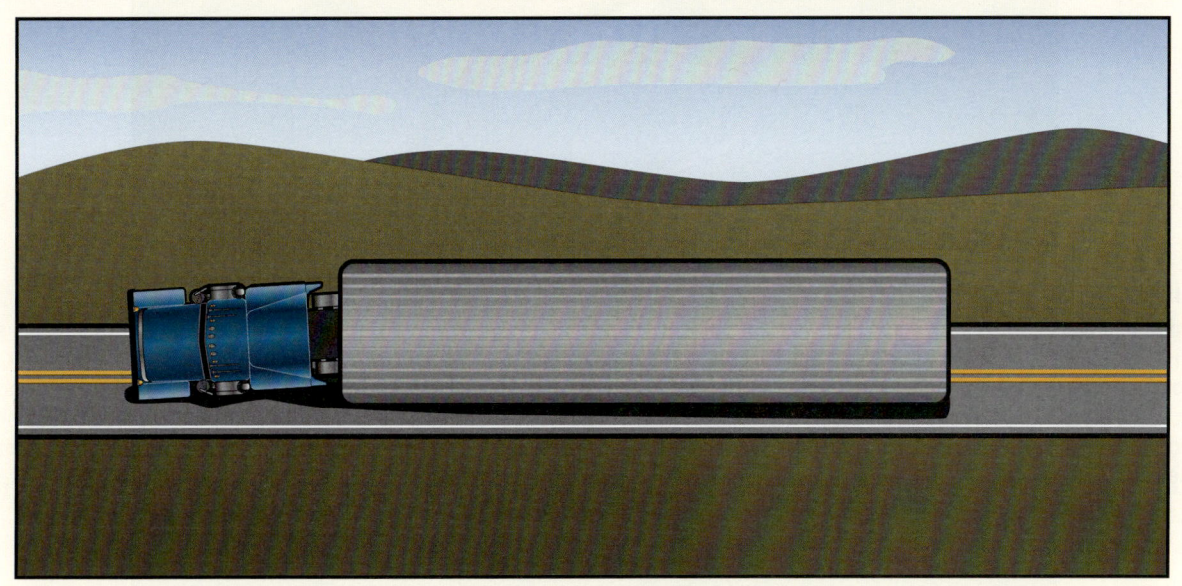

Section D • Chapter 11 – Commercial/Heavy Vehicle Disentanglement

SKILL SHEETS

11-1
Determine commercial/heavy vehicle access and egress points.

Scenario 2
You arrive at the scene of a school bus accident. The front end of the bus is wheel-resting in a ditch that is several feet (meters) deep. The rear of the bus is in the air, but is accessible from the road. This specific bus model does not have any side emergency exit doors, and the front door is blocked by debris. The driver is trapped. Some of the other occupants were able to exit the vehicle on their own, but ten passengers require extrication.

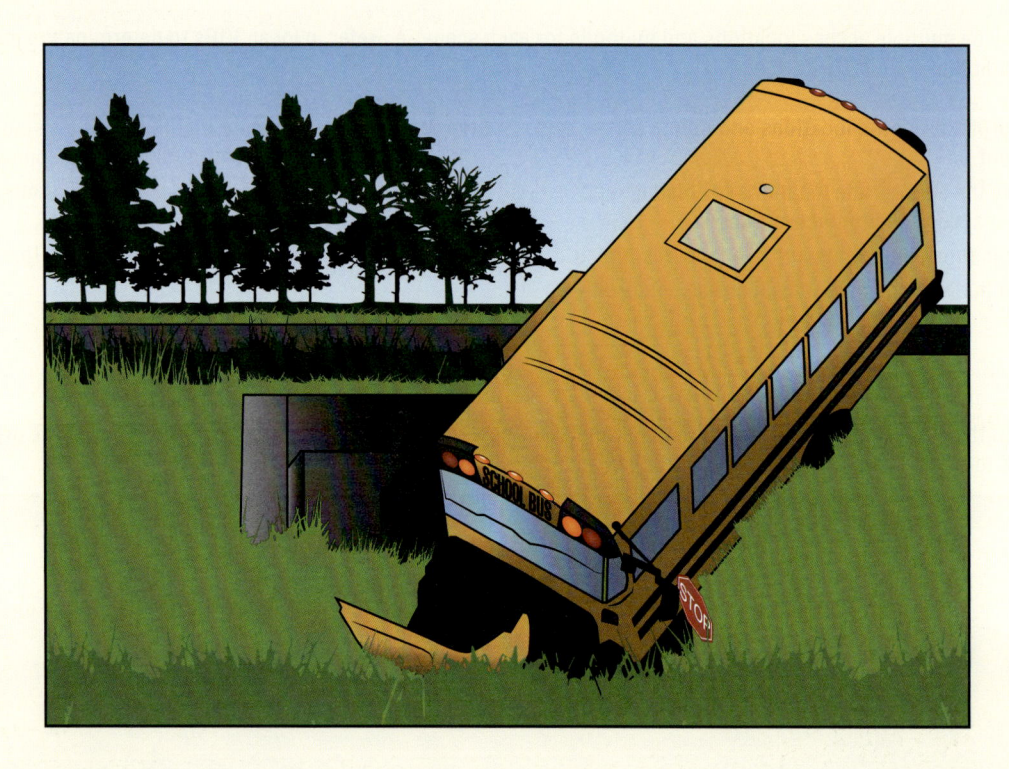

Scenario 3
You respond to an incident on a two-lane highway just outside of town. A medium truck was driving in the right lane when it was struck on the driver's side by a two-door sports car. The car is wedged beneath the truck at approximately a 30 degree angle. The driver, who is the only occupant of the truck, is inaccessible through the driver's door, but the passenger side door can be opened. The only occupant of the car is the driver. The driver's side door of the car is operable. The front and rear windows, as well as the passenger side door, are in poor condition or otherwise obstructed by the truck. The area on the passenger side of the truck is a grassy shoulder which appears safe for rescuer use.

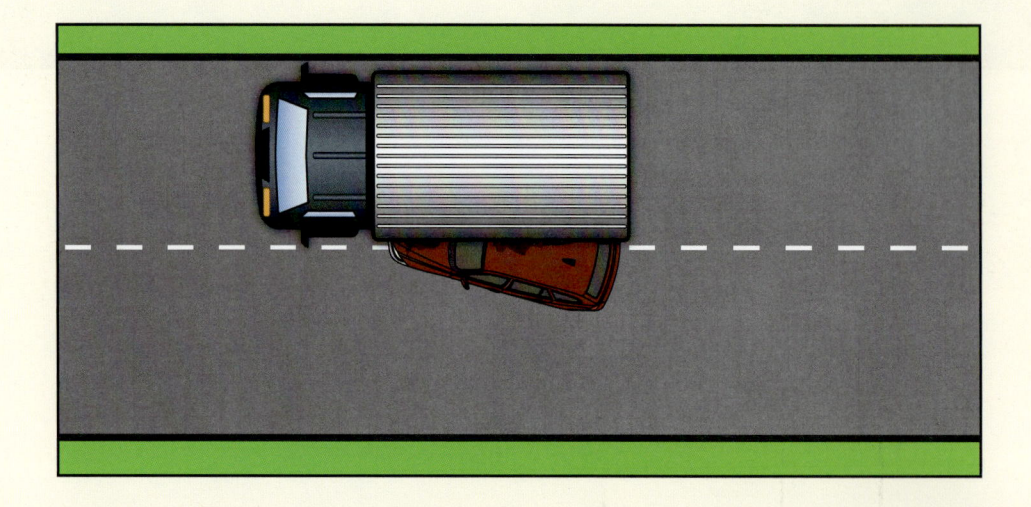

11-2
Open or remove a commercial/heavy vehicle door.

WARNING: Rescuers must ensure that the vehicle is properly stabilized and the scene is safe.

CAUTION: Rescuers must take necessary precautions to protect themselves and victims from hazards including, but not limited to glass fragments and dust, jagged metal, SRS gas cylinders, undeployed airbags, and fire hazards.

Hydraulic Rescue Tools

NOTE: This method is for use on doors with automotive style hinges rather than piano hinges.

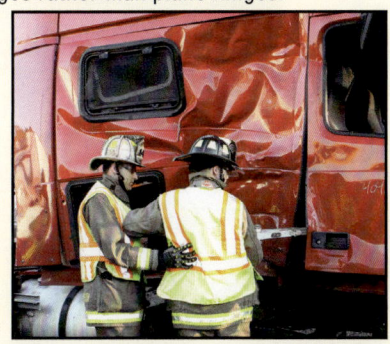

Step 1: Create a purchase point at or slightly above the door handle.
Step 2: Insert the spreader tips in such a position that they will push the door outward and toward the ground.
Step 3: Maintain control of the door.

CAUTION: Never use personnel to maintain control of the door with their body. Instead, a rope, chain, strap, or tubular webbing should be used to tether the door.

Step 4: Open the spreader arms until the door opens.
Step 5: Insert the spreader tips slightly above the first hinge in a position so that they will push the door down and away from the vehicle.
Step 6: Open the spreaders until the hinge side fails or can be cut.
Step 7: Remove the door.

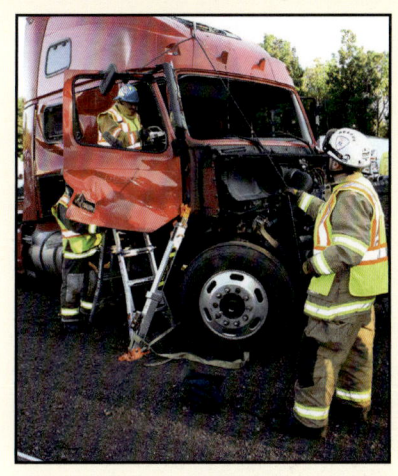

Pneumatic or Reciprocating Rescue Tools

Step 1: Create a purchase point at the top or bottom of the hinges.
Step 2: Insert the tip of the tool.
Step 3: Maintain control of the door.
Step 4: Cut through the hinges.
Step 5: Create a purchase point near the latching mechanism.
Step 6: Insert the tip of the tool.
Step 7: Cut through the latching mechanism.
Step 8: Remove the door.

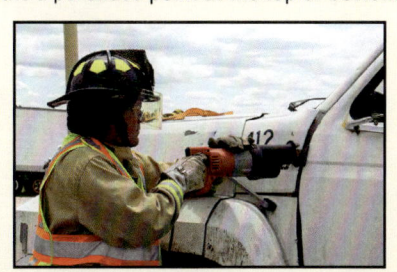

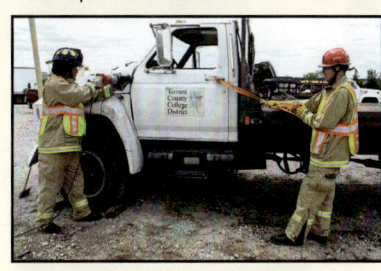

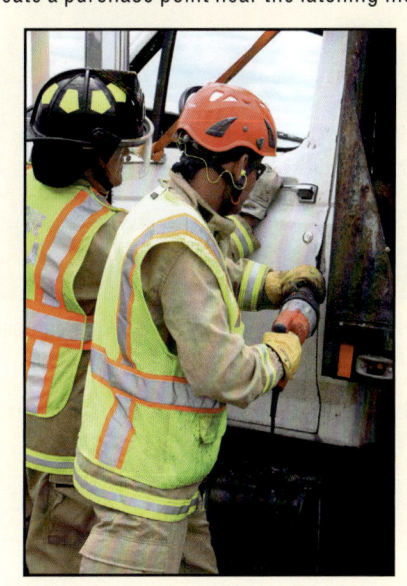

Section D • Chapter 11 – Commercial/Heavy Vehicle Disentanglement

SKILL SHEETS

11-3 Create an access opening in the roof or wall of a commercial/heavy vehicle.

WARNING: Rescuers must ensure that the vehicle is properly stabilized and the scene is safe.

CAUTION: Rescuers must take necessary precautions to protect themselves and victims from hazards including, but not limited to glass fragments and dust, jagged metal, SRS gas cylinders, undeployed airbags, and fire hazards.

NOTE: This skill may be used to create an access opening in the roof, side wall, or rear wall, depending on orientation and available access and egress routes. The size of the access opening will vary by incident.

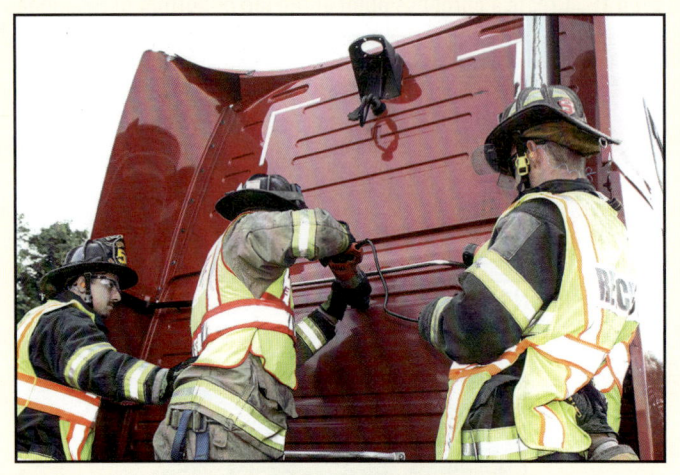

Step 1: Cut the outer skin away from the area to be opened.

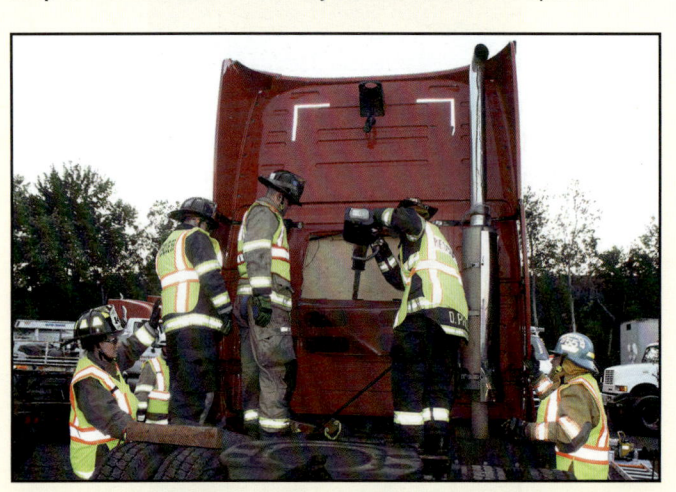

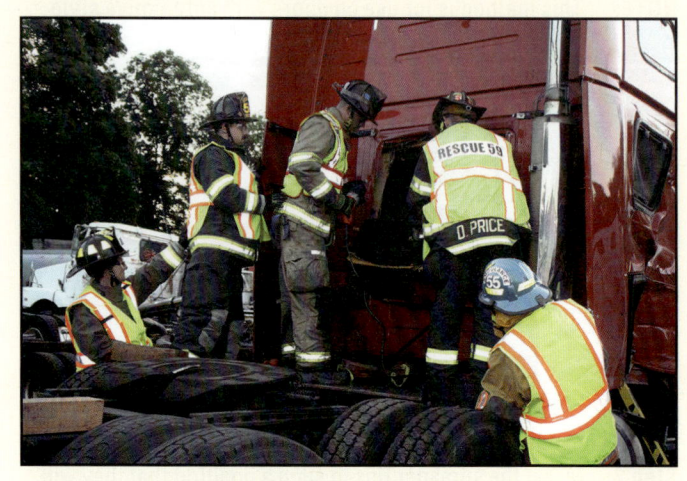

Step 3: Pull or cut away interior headliner, insulation, and other obstructions to allow access to victim.

Step 2: Cut inner support structures to create an opening large enough to access and remove the victim.

CAUTION: Removing more material than necessary could jeopardize the vehicle's structural integrity.

11-4
Create an access opening utilizing the front door of a bus.

WARNING: Rescuers must ensure that the vehicle is properly stabilized and the scene is safe.

CAUTION: Rescuers must take necessary precautions to protect themselves and victims from hazards including, but not limited to glass fragments and dust, jagged metal, SRS gas cylinders, undeployed airbags, and fire hazards.

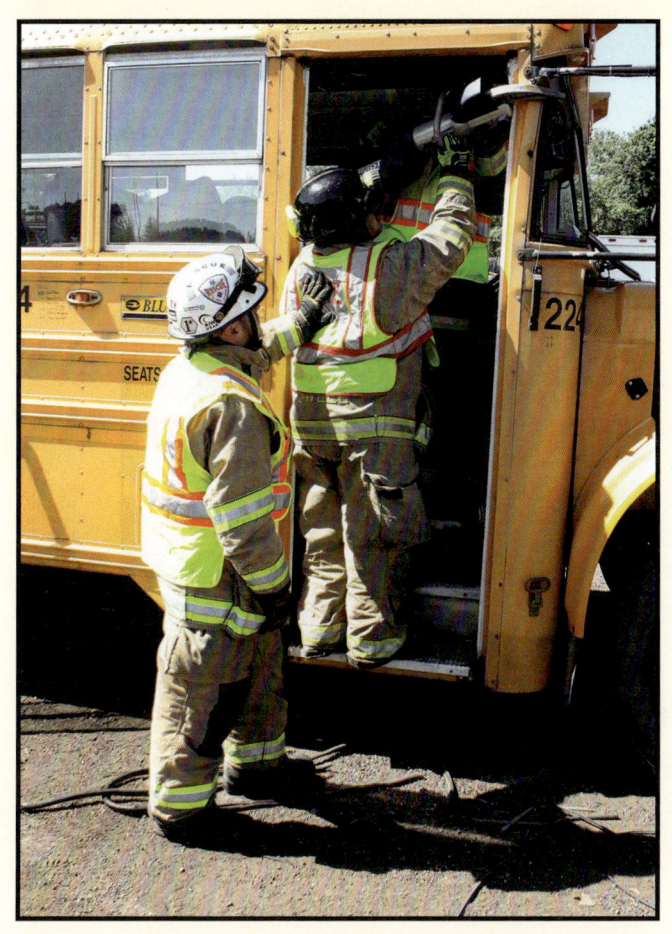

Step 1: Cut through the A-post at the top of the windshield opening.

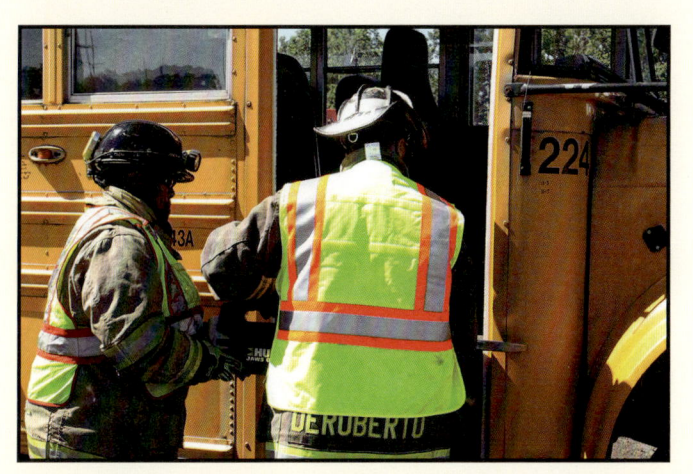

Step 2: Make a relief cut in the bottom of the A-post at floor level.

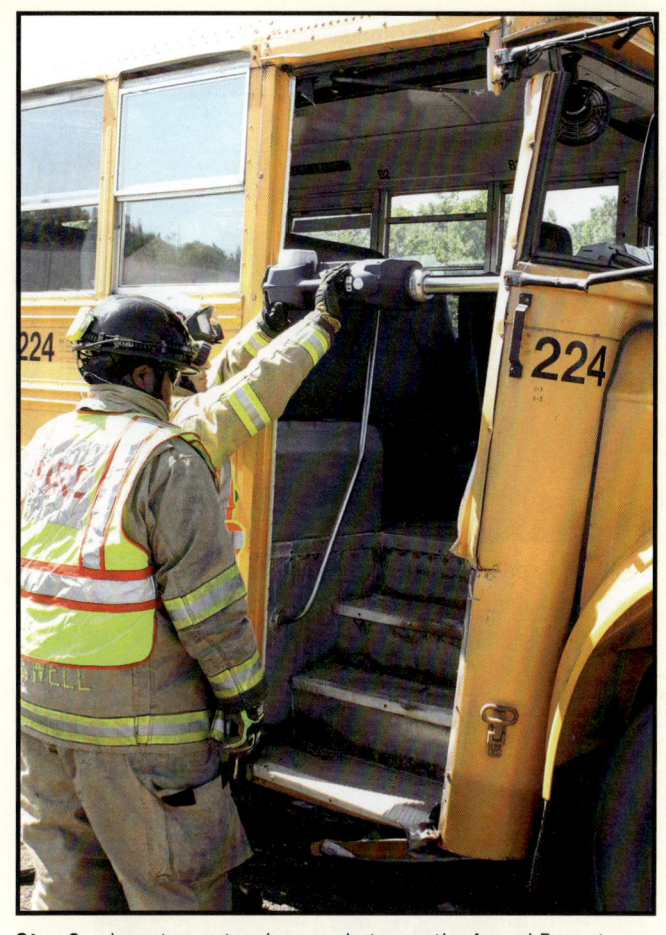

Step 3: Insert an extension ram between the A- and B-posts, parallel to the ground at the top of the dashboard level.

Step 4: Extend the ram to push the front wall forward.

Section D • Chapter 11 – Commercial/Heavy Vehicle Disentanglement 427

SKILL SHEETS

11-5
Open or remove the rear door of a bus.

> **WARNING:** Rescuers must ensure that the vehicle is properly stabilized and the scene is safe.

> **CAUTION:** Rescuers must take necessary precautions to protect themselves and victims from hazards including, but not limited to glass fragments and dust, jagged metal, SRS gas cylinders, undeployed airbags, and fire hazards.

Step 1: Insert a prying or spreading tool between the door and the frame at the latch.

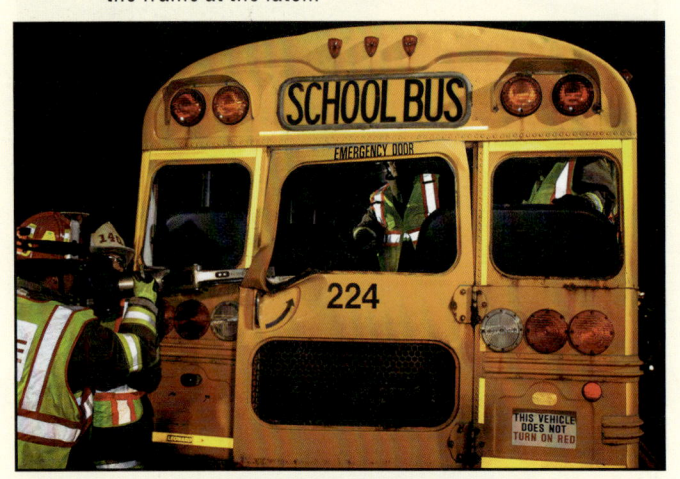

Step 2: Pry or separate the door and frame.

Step 3: Open the door or proceed with total removal.

NOTE: If the door will not be removed, secure it open with straps or webbing.

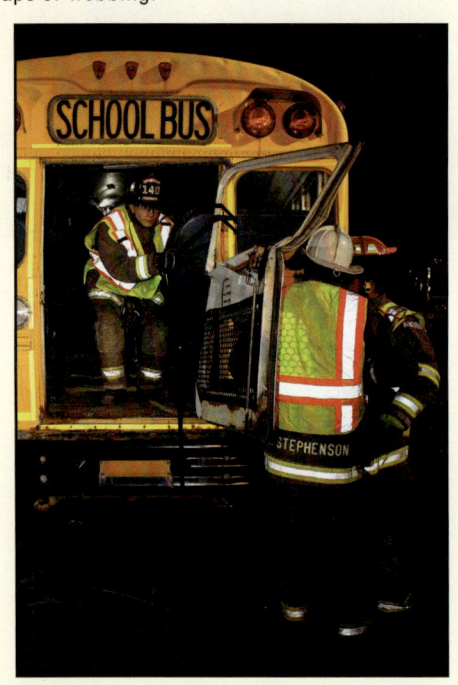

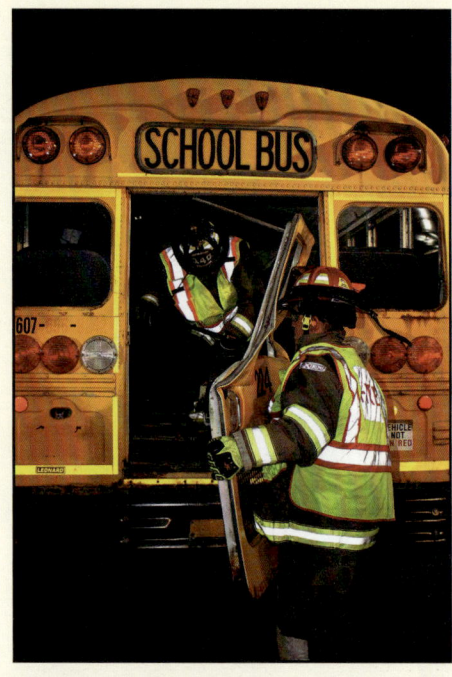

Step 5: Remove the door.

Step 4: Remove, cut, or displace the door hinges.

428 Section D • Chapter 11 – Commercial/Heavy Vehicle Disentanglement

11-6
Remove an emergency window of a school bus.

WARNING: Rescuers must ensure that the vehicle is properly stabilized and the scene is safe.

CAUTION: Rescuers must take necessary precautions to protect themselves and victims from hazards including, but not limited to glass fragments and dust, jagged metal, SRS gas cylinders, undeployed airbags, and fire hazards.

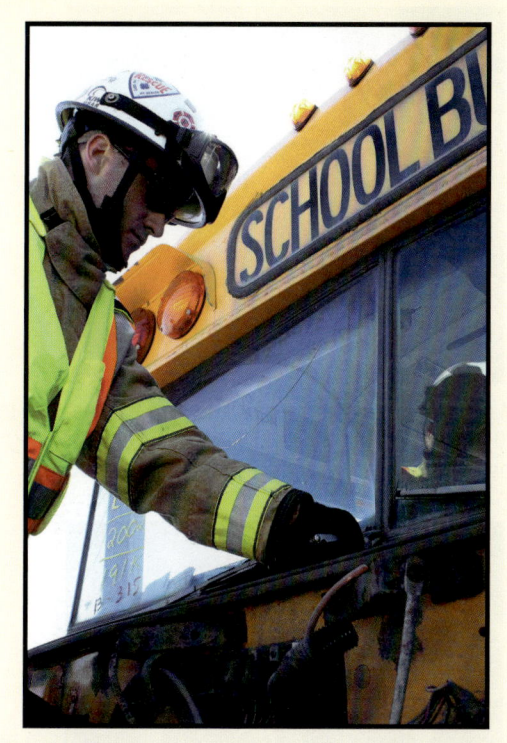

Step 1: Insert the tool under the middle bead of the gasket.

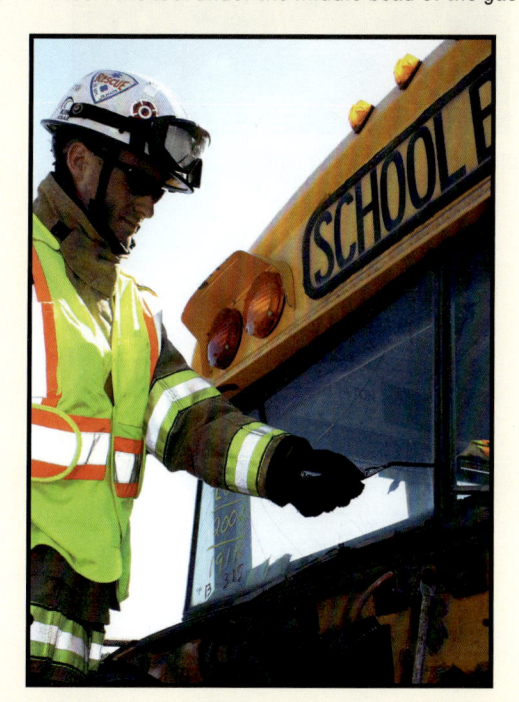

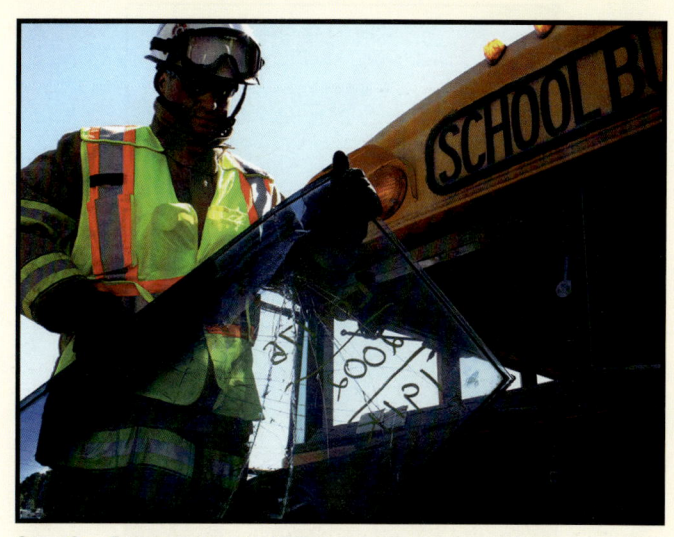

Step 3: Remove the window.

Step 2: Pull the middle bead of the gasket completely out from around the window.

Section D • Chapter 11 – Commercial/Heavy Vehicle Disentanglement

SKILL SHEETS

11-7
Cut through the side wall of a bus utilizing a window opening.

WARNING: Rescuers must ensure that the vehicle is properly stabilized and the scene is safe.

CAUTION: Rescuers must take necessary precautions to protect themselves and victims from hazards including, but not limited to glass fragments and dust, jagged metal, SRS gas cylinders, undeployed airbags, and fire hazards.

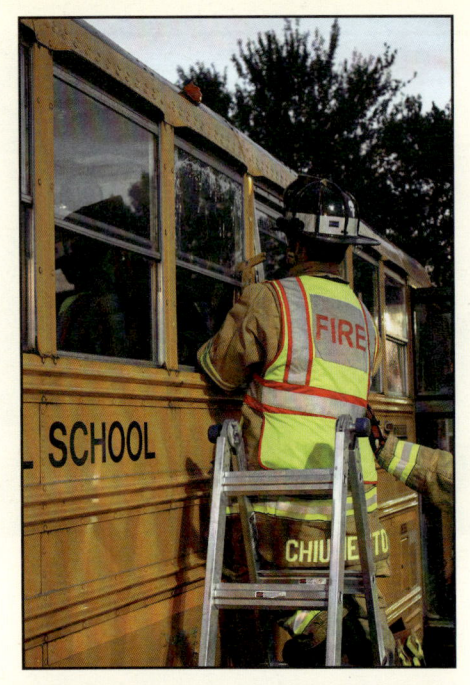

Step 1: Remove glass and cut away the window frame.

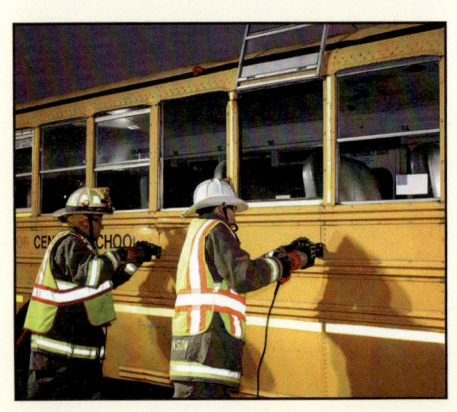

Step 2: Make vertical cuts straight down from two window posts, extending only as far as necessary to allow sufficient access.

CAUTION: Do not cut into the heating and coolant line that may run just above the floor, which commonly runs on the driver's side.

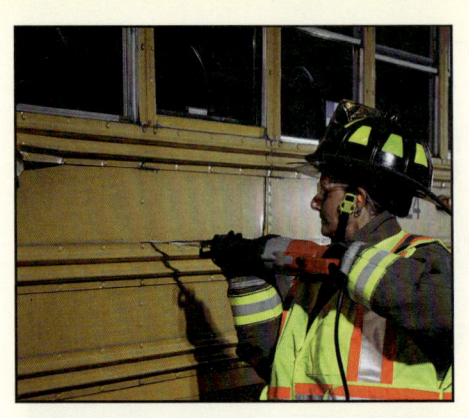

Step 3: Make short horizontal relief cuts, 1 to 2 inches (25 to 50 mm) long from the end of each vertical side cut toward the center of the portion to be laid down.

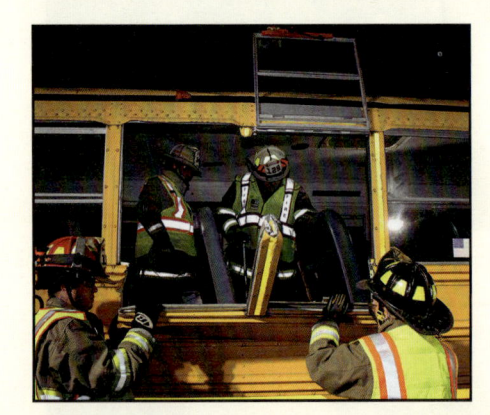

Step 4: Fold the wall section down.

430 Section D • Chapter 11 – Commercial/Heavy Vehicle Disentanglement

11-8
Create an access opening in the roof of a side-resting bus.

WARNING: Rescuers must ensure that the vehicle is properly stabilized and the scene is safe.

CAUTION: Rescuers must take necessary precautions to protect themselves and victims from hazards including, but not limited to glass fragments and dust, jagged metal, SRS gas cylinders, undeployed airbags, and fire hazards.

NOTE: This procedure is specifically for cutting an access opening in the roof of a school bus. The same procedure can be used with transit and commercial buses, except that commercial buses have overhead storage bins along each outside wall. To avoid these bins, rescuers must cut access openings as near the centerline of the roof as possible.

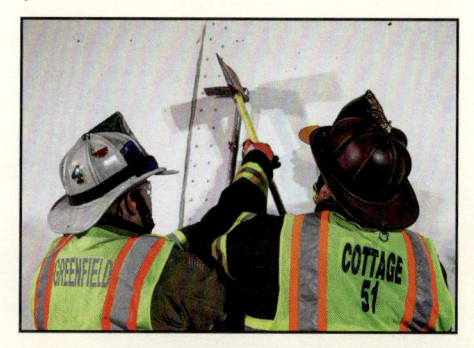

Step 1: Create a purchase point near a row of rivets with either a pick-head axe or the point of a Halligan tool.

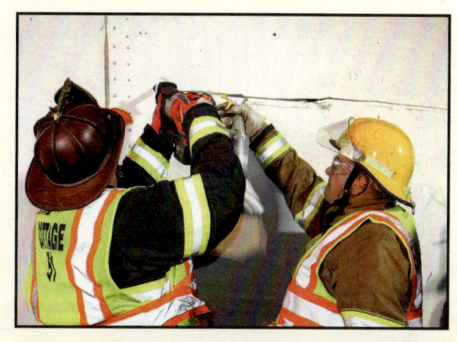

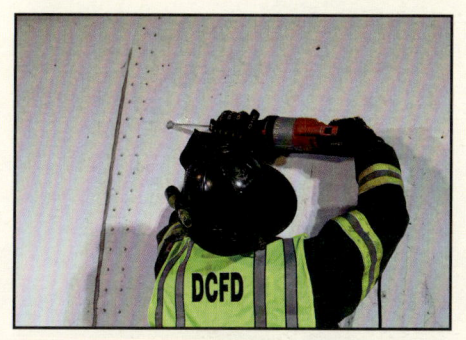

Step 2: Insert the saw blade into the hole.

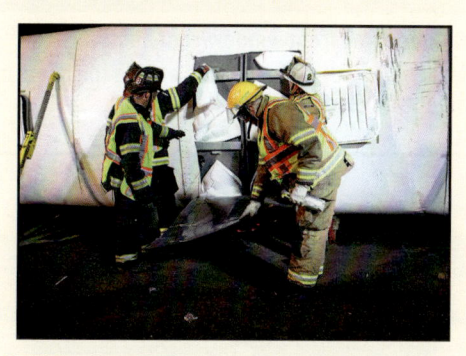

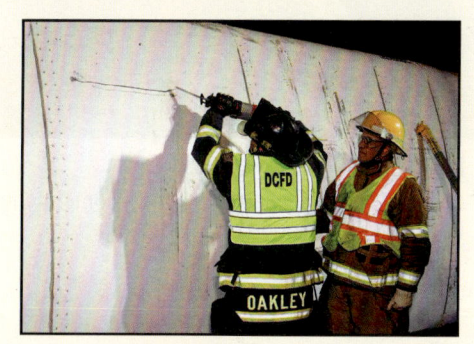

Step 3: Make a horizontal cut across one row of rivets, stopping short of the second row.

Step 4: Make a vertical cut from each end of the horizontal cut down to ground level.

Step 5: Fold the flap of roof down to the ground.

SKILL SHEETS

11-9
Flap a bus roof.

WARNING: Rescuers must ensure that the vehicle is properly stabilized and the scene is safe.

CAUTION: Rescuers must take necessary precautions to protect themselves and victims from hazards including, but not limited to glass fragments and dust, jagged metal, SRS gas cylinders, undeployed airbags, and fire hazards.

Step 1: Remove the windshield.

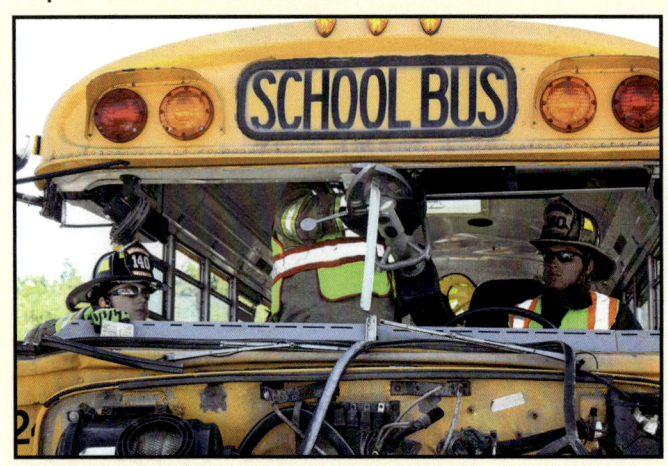

Step 2: Cut the three front window/roof posts.
Step 3: Make relief cuts into the roof behind the posts of the area to be displaced.

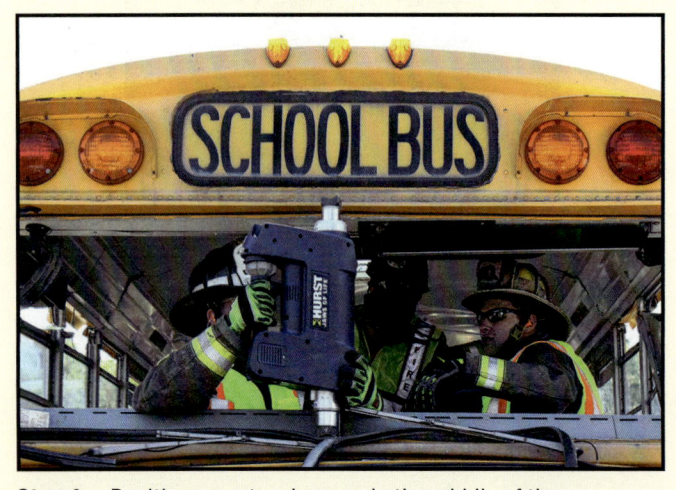

Step 4: Position an extension ram in the middle of the windshield opening.

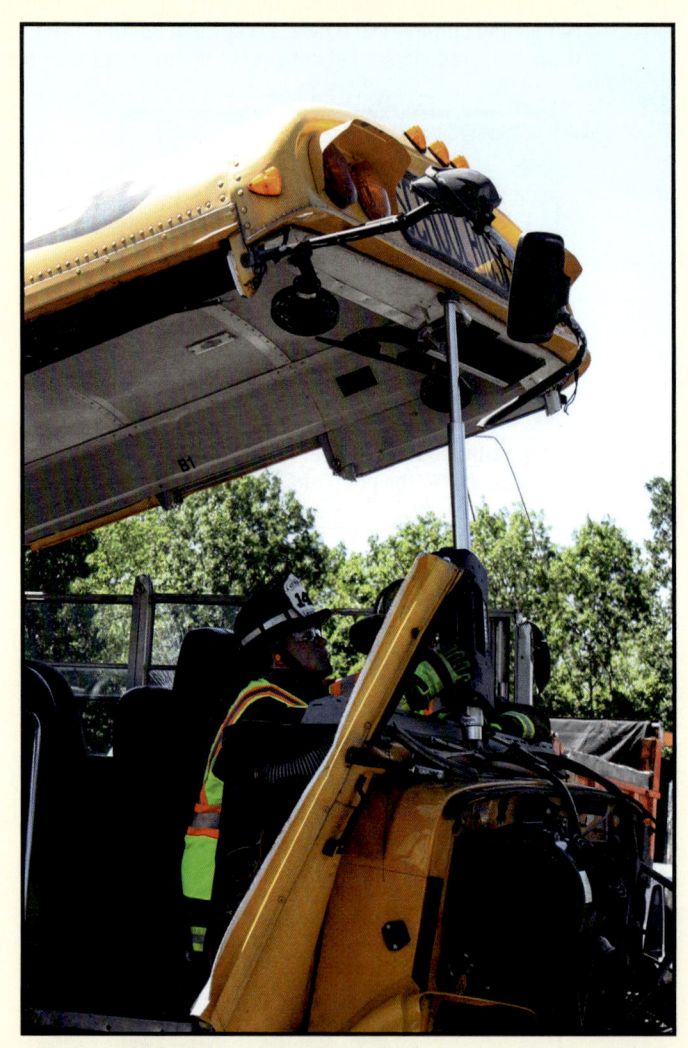

Step 5: Push the roof up.
NOTE: As an alternative, chains and chain come-alongs can be used to pull the roof up.

432   Section D • Chapter 11 – Commercial/Heavy Vehicle Disentanglement

11-10
Create an access opening in the floor of a side-resting bus.

> **WARNING:** Rescuers must ensure that the vehicle is properly stabilized and the scene is safe.

> **CAUTION:** Rescuers must take necessary precautions to protect themselves and victims from hazards including, but not limited to glass fragments and dust, jagged metal, SRS gas cylinders, undeployed airbags, and fire hazards.

Step 1: Identify the two adjacent main supporting beams between which the opening will be made.

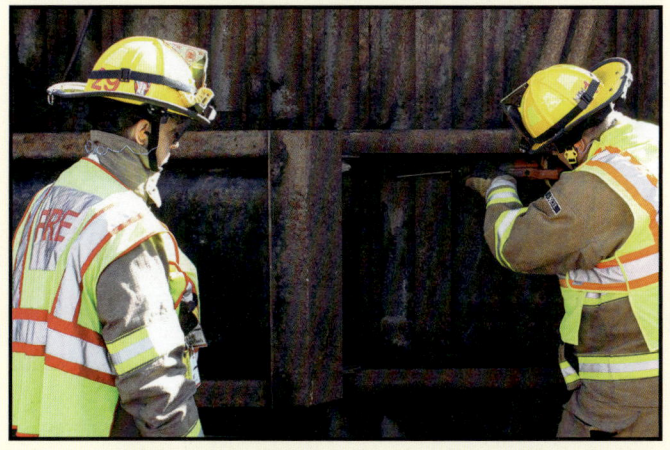

Step 2: Make two cuts in the end of each of the non-supporting beams that lie between the main supporting beams.
  a. Make the first cut at the end of each beam.
  b. Make a second cut at least 3 inches (75 mm) inside the first cut.

Step 3: Knock out the section of beam between the cuts.

Step 4: Create a purchase point in the floor of the bus.

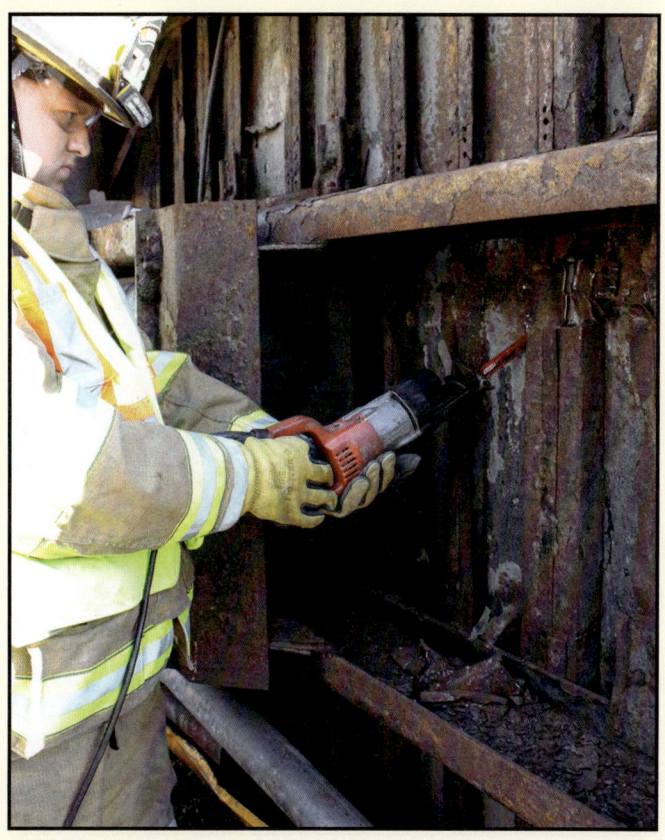

Step 5: Insert the saw blade into the purchase point and cut the floor on three sides.

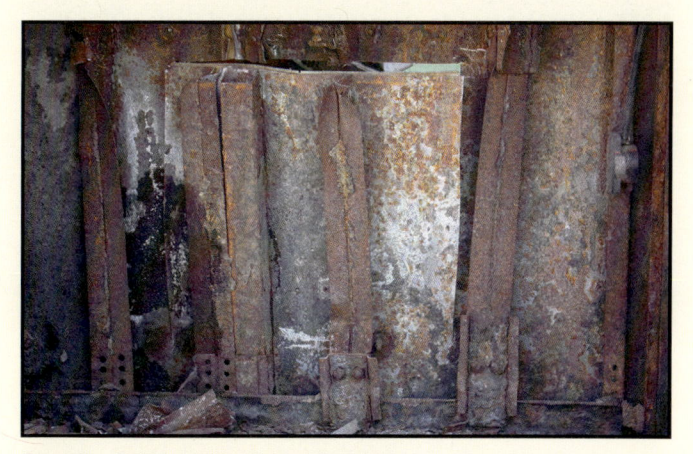

Step 6: Fold back the flap of flooring.

Section D • Chapter 11 – Commercial/Heavy Vehicle Disentanglement

SKILL SHEETS

11-11
Use high-pressure pneumatic lifting bags to free a victim trapped beneath a side-resting commercial/heavy vehicle.

WARNING: Rescuers must ensure that the vehicle is properly stabilized and the scene is safe.

CAUTION: Rescuers must take necessary precautions to protect themselves and victims from hazards including, but not limited to glass fragments and dust, jagged metal, SRS gas cylinders, undeployed airbags, and fire hazards.

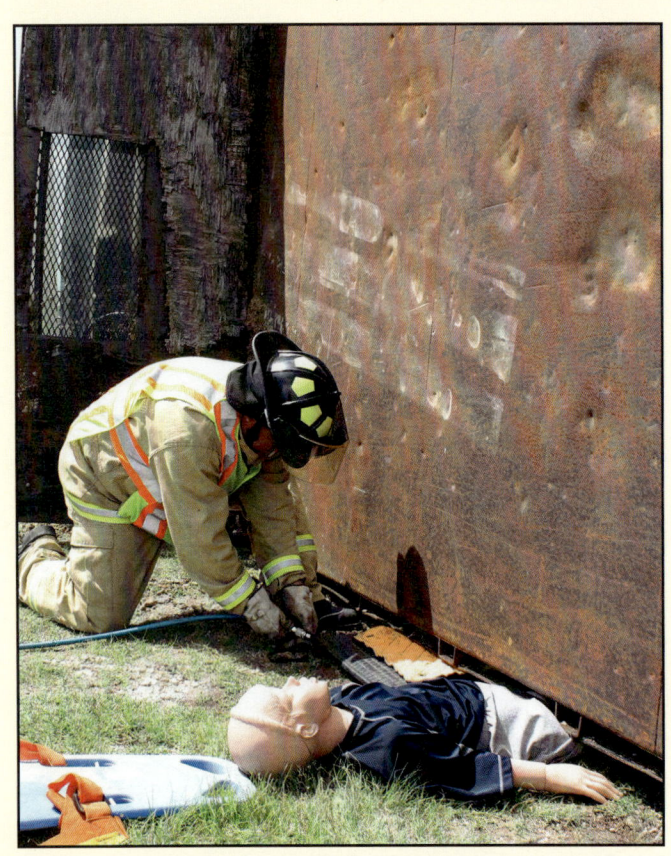

Step 1: Insert at least one pneumatic lifting bag beneath the vehicle on each side of the victim. Center the middle of each bag beneath a roof truss support.

NOTE: Truss supports are marked by rows of rivets across the roof structure.

Step 2: Place cribbing or struts on either side of the victim.

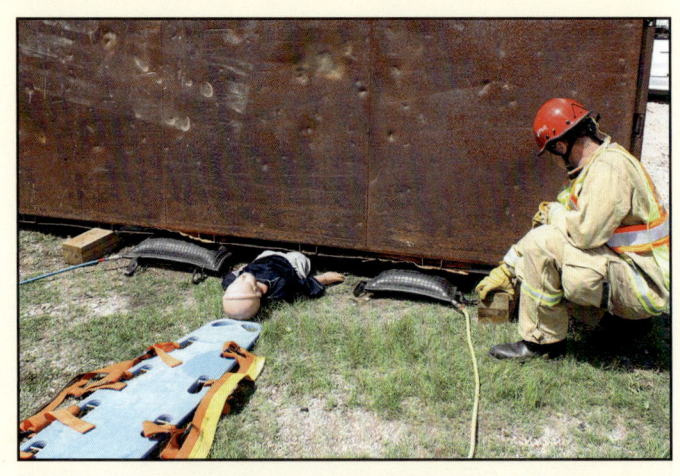

Step 3: Operate the lifting bags until there is sufficient access to the victim. Adjust the capturing devices to maintain capture as the lift progresses.

Step 4: Monitor and maintain the integrity of the capturing devices.

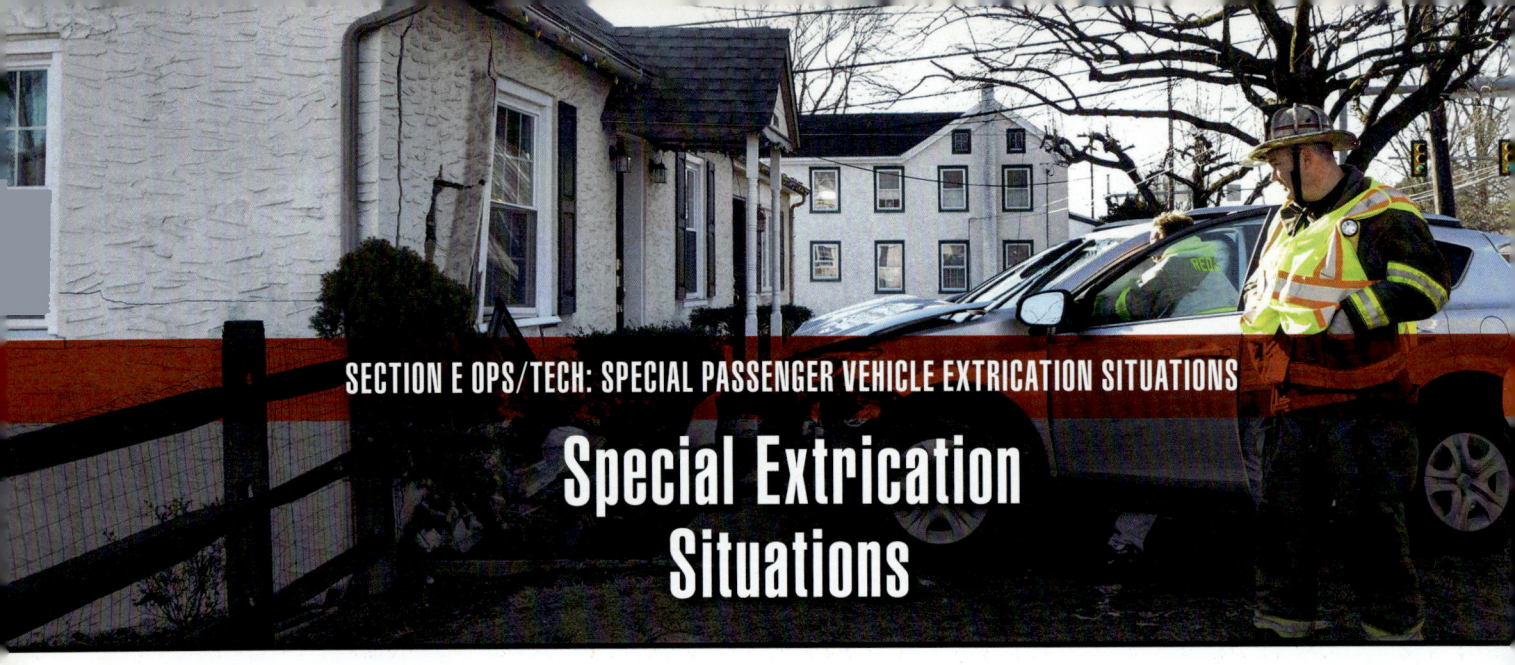

SECTION E OPS/TECH: SPECIAL PASSENGER VEHICLE EXTRICATION SITUATIONS

Special Extrication Situations

Courtesy of Bob Esposito.

Chapter Contents

Vehicles in a Structure 440	**Railcars** 464
Vehicles in a Structure — Considerations 440	Types of Railcars 464
Vehicles in a Structure — Operations 441	Railcar Anatomy, Construction, and Features 469
Vehicles in Water 442	Railcar Incident Size-Up 475
Vehicles in Water — Considerations 442	Railcar Hazards 476
Vehicles in Water — Operations 443	Railcar Stabilization 477
Hanging Vehicles 444	Railcar Access and Egress 479
Hanging Vehicles — Considerations 444	Railcar Extrication Situations 483
Hanging Vehicles — Operations 445	**Chapter Review** 486
Recreational Vehicles (RVs) 446	**Discussion Questions** 487
RV Considerations 446	
RV Operations 447	
Industrial and Agricultural Vehicles 447	
Types of Industrial and Agricultural Vehicles 447	
Industrial and Agricultural Vehicle Anatomy, Construction, and Features 453	
Industrial and Agricultural Incident Size-Up 457	
Industrial and Agricultural Vehicle Hazards 459	
Industrial and Agricultural Vehicle Stabilization 459	
Industrial and Agricultural Vehicle Extrication 461	

436 Section E • Chapter 12 – Special Extrication Situations

chapter 12

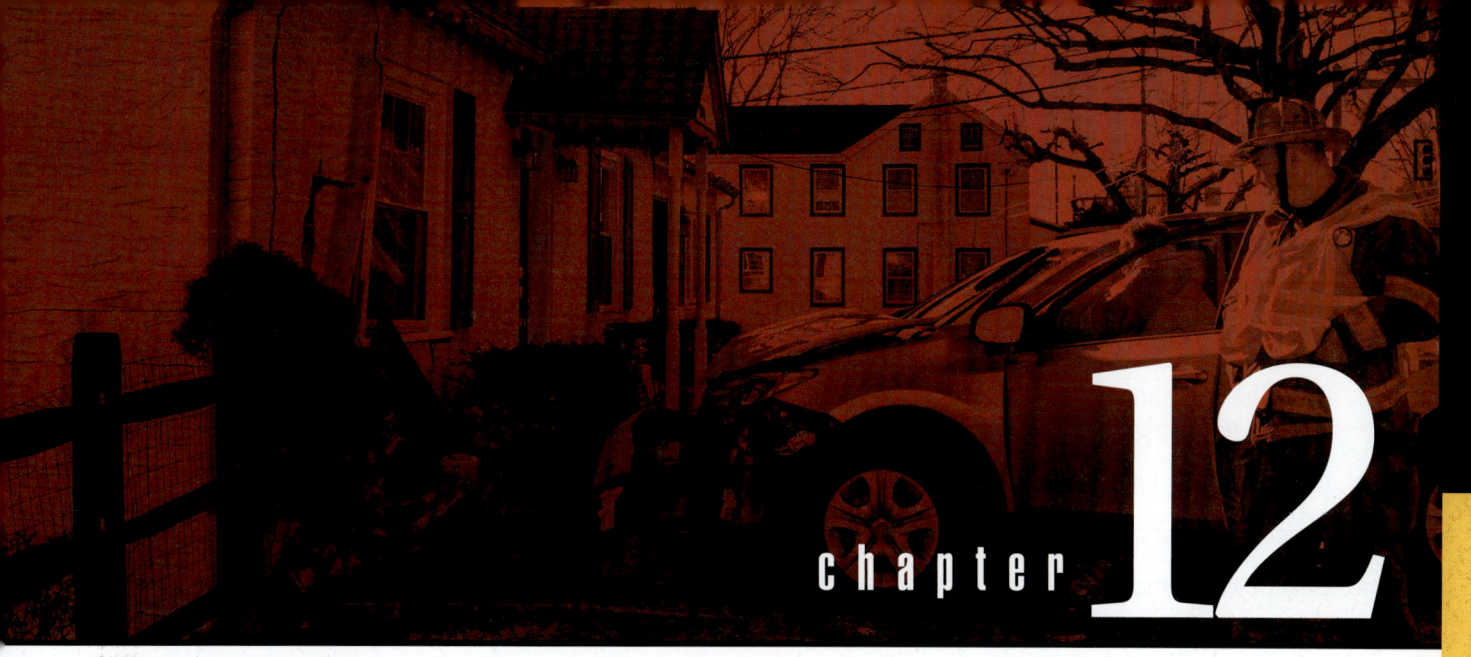

Key Terms

Berm 480	Pantograph 466
Catenary system 466	Self-Contained Underwater
Consist 464	Breathing Apparatus 443
Lexan® 470	Shoring 440

JPRs addressed in this chapter

This chapter provides information that addresses the following job performance requirements of NFPA 1006, *Standard for Technical Rescuer Professional Qualifications (2017)*.

8.2.3	8.3.4
8.2.7	8.3.5
8.3.3	

Section E • Chapter 12 – Special Extrication Situations

Special Extrication Situations

Learning Objectives

1. Describe operations involving a vehicle that has crashed into a structure. [8.2.3, 8.2.5, 8.2.6, 8.2.7, 8.3.1, 8.3.2, 8.3.3, 8.3.4, 8.3.5]
2. Describe operations involving a vehicle in water. [8.2.3, 8.2.5, 8.2.6, 8.2.7, 8.3.1, 8.3.2, 8.3.3, 8.3.4, 8.3.5]
3. Describe operations involving a hanging vehicle. [8.2.3, 8.2.5, 8.2.6, 8.2.7, 8.3.1, 8.3.2, 8.3.3, 8.3.4, 8.3.5]
4. Describe operations involving recreational vehicles. [8.3.1, 8.3.2, 8.3.3, 8.3.4, 8.3.5]
5. Describe operations involving industrial and agricultural vehicles. [8.3.1, 8.3.2, 8.3.3, 8.3.4, 8.3.5, 8.3.6]
6. Describe operations involving railcars. [8.3.1, 8.3.2, 8.3.3, 8.3.4, 8.3.5, 8.3.6]

Chapter 12
Special Extrication Situations

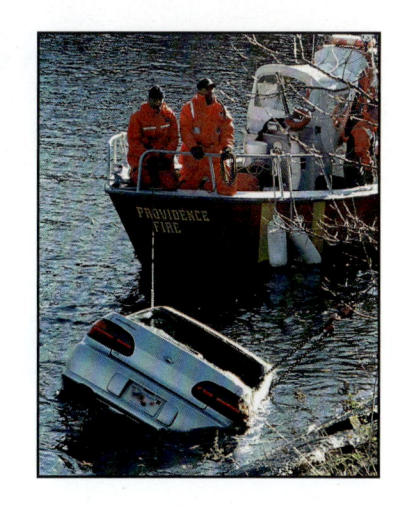

This chapter focuses on special extrication situations. Some firefighters and other rescue personnel handle special extrication situations almost daily, while others seldom handle them. Those who deal with special extrication situations often become adept at handling them. However, even these rescuers risk growing complacent and overconfident. It is imperative that rescuers conduct adequate pre-incident planning and that agencies provide rescuers with the appropriate level of training and equipment. Pre-incident planning should identify where to locate and how to obtain resources within and outside the agency that agencies might need during special extrication situations.

Any number of factors can cause special complications at a vehicle incident:

- Environment in which the incident occurred
- Number of vehicles involved
- Number of trapped victims
- Presence of fire or the potential for fire or explosions
- Presence of a large quantity of hazardous materials
- Unfamiliarity with the vehicles involved
- Size of vehicles involved

The first-arriving personnel at a special incident must be able to recognize that the situation is not routine, is beyond the capabilities of the responding rescue resources, and that a technical rescue team or other specialized resources should be called. Answering the following questions will aid rescuers in recognizing a non-routine situation:

- How many vehicles are involved, and what is their condition?
- Did the vehicle crash into a structure? If so, what are the conditions of the structure and the vehicle? **(Figure 12.1, p. 440)**
- Did the vehicle come to rest in a body of water? Is the vehicle underwater?
- Are multiple vehicles involved? What types of vehicles are involved, and what are their conditions?
- Will rescuers need heavy wrecker/recovery trucks? Will they need cranes, barges, or other specialized resources to handle this incident?

After answering questions about the scene and discovering that the incident qualifies as a special situation, rescuers must apply the information to an ac-

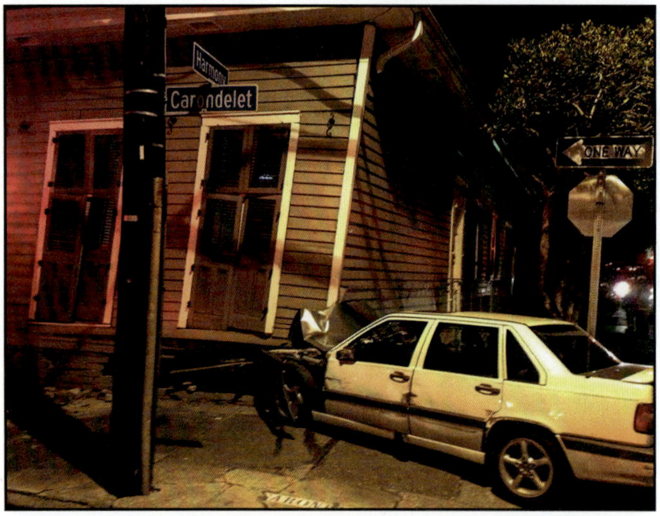

Figure 12.1 Rescuers need to determine the condition of both the vehicle and the structure if a vehicle is embedded in a structure. *Courtesy of Ron Jeffers.*

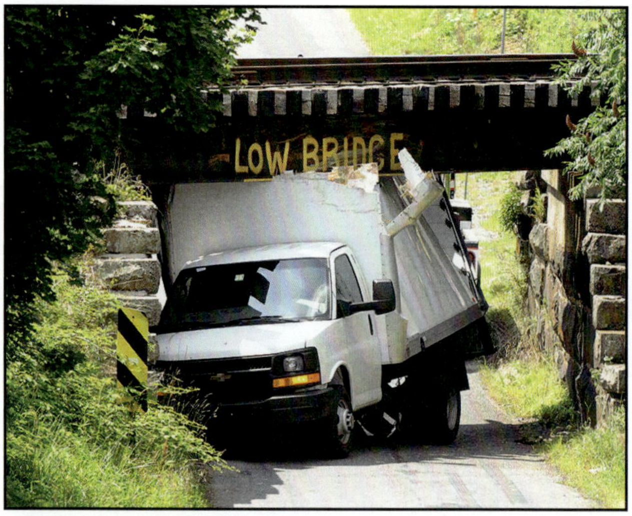

Figure 12.2 Rescuers must first check the integrity of the concrete bridge to make sure it is stable before attempting to remove the vehicle. *Courtesy of Bob Esposito.*

tion plan. This chapter discusses several special situations with an emphasis on helping rescuers meet the challenges of the situation. For purposes of this manual, special extrication situations involve any of the following:

- Vehicles in a structure
- Vehicles in water
- Hanging vehicles
- Recreational vehicles (RVs)
- Industrial and agricultural vehicles
- Railcars

Vehicles in a Structure

When faced with a vehicle in a structure, rescuers must first check the condition of the structure, then the condition of the vehicles. Vehicles hold a minimal amount of people compared to that of a structure. A failed structure could lead to the deaths of more people than a failed vehicle. In this context, the term structure refers to any stationary man-made object into which a vehicle has crashed **(Figure 12.2)**. The object could be a building, bridge abutment, or tunnel.

Vehicles in a Structure — Considerations

Rescuers must assess the integrity of the structure along with the other items normally associated with the assessment of a vehicle incident. Rescuers should first ask: Has the structure been damaged to the point that a collapse is likely? If the answer is yes, a structural collapse rescue team or other qualified personnel should start **shoring** the structure. While waiting for the structural collapse team to arrive, on-scene personnel should establish and maintain control of the scene, and perform any other duties that would not require them to enter the collapse danger zone. Rescuers should request the response of the local

Shoring — General term used for lengths of timber, screw jacks, hydraulic and pneumatic jacks, and other devices that can be used as temporary support for formwork or structural components or used to hold sheeting against trench walls. Individual supports are called shores, cross braces, and struts. Commonly used in conjunction with cribbing.

building department whenever structural stability is in question. Once they have shored the structure, rescuers should begin the process of assessing the condition of the vehicle.

Before stabilizing the vehicle, rescuers should conduct an assessment of the trapped victim(s). Depending upon the type of vehicle and the type of structure, this assessment may take time and may present difficulties. Rescuers should assess how the victims are entrapped and what rescuers will need to extricate them. During this assessment, rescuers should consider the following questions:

- Are victims trapped because the structure into which the vehicle crashed will not allow rescuers or victims to open the vehicle's doors?
- Did some part of the vehicle collapse around the victims and entrap them?
- Do rescuers need special tools, equipment, or other resources to free the victim?

If the assessment cannot adequately be performed in place, rescuers may have to consider the cost/benefit of pulling the vehicle out of the structure. Since removal could be risky for any trapped victims, it should be considered only in the most extreme situations.

Vehicles in a Structure — Operations

Once structural collapse is no longer a risk, rescue personnel can begin to stabilize the vehicle. Given adequate space in which to operate, rescuers should use the skills as described in Chapter 7 or Chapter 10 to stabilize a vehicle.

If the shoring needed to stabilize the building restricts the operating space around the vehicle, making it impossible for rescuers to stabilize the vehicle, rescuers must consider the cost/benefit of pulling the vehicle from the building **(Figure 12.3)**. As mentioned earlier, moving the vehicle before stabilizing the occupant can be risky. Therefore, rescuers should only consider this option in the most extreme situations.

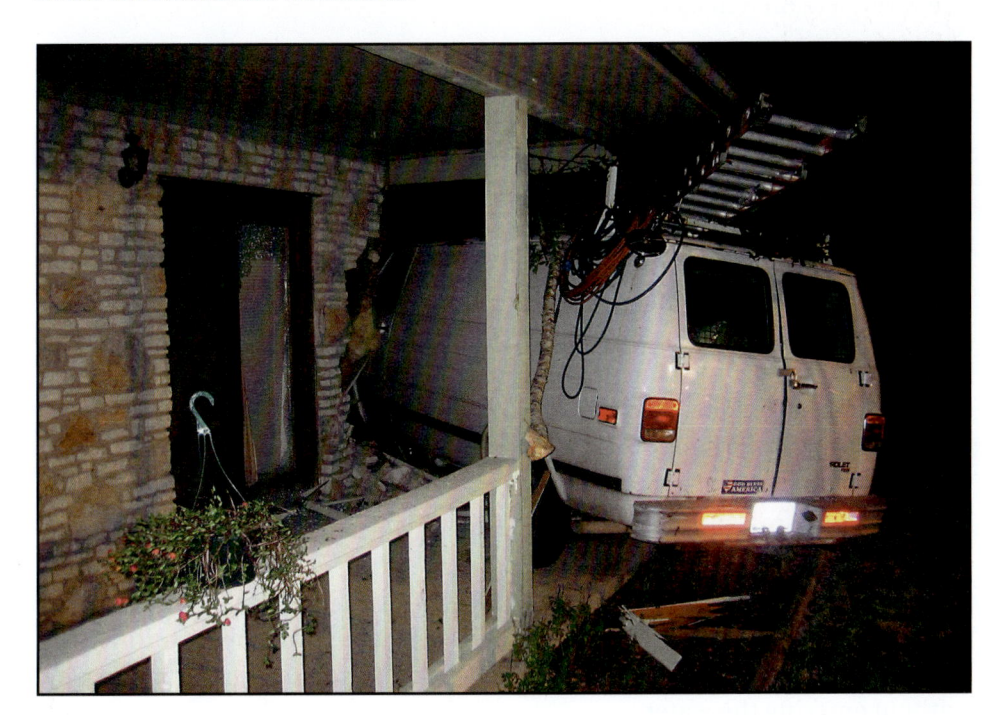

Figure 12.3 When vehicles collide with buildings, rescuers must take into account the stability of a structure as well as vehicle extrication procedures. *Courtesy of Buda (TX) Fire Department.*

Once rescuers have stabilized the structure and the vehicle, they can use extrication tools and techniques to gain access into the vehicle. However, if the vehicle is inside a building, rescuers may have limited operating space and extrication personnel must avoid disturbing or dislodging any of the shoring that supports the structure. Extrication personnel should consider ventilation and atmospheric monitoring when operating inside a structure using gas-powered equipment.

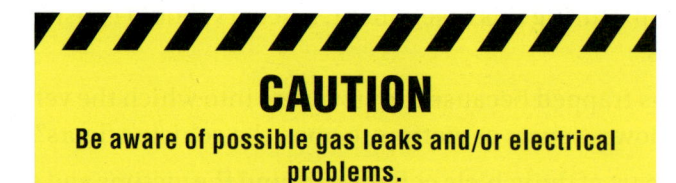

> **CAUTION**
> Be aware of possible gas leaks and/or electrical problems.

Space limitations and other environmental challenges may also affect the disentanglement and extrication processes. Rescuers may need to package victims so that they can manipulate the receiving device (litter, cot, backboard) that holds the victims in a variety of ways (even vertically) to avoid the shoring used to stabilize the building. Rescuers must remain careful not to disturb or dislodge the structural shoring.

NOTE: Chapter 5 describes victim packaging techniques.

Vehicles in Water

Vehicles sometimes leave the roadway and come to rest in a body of water, such as a river or lake. A submerged vehicle would have its passenger compartment totally under the water, while a partially submerged vehicle would have a portion of the passenger compartment above the water. Rescuers should determine the submersion of a vehicle based on the bottom of the waterway. Partially submerged vehicles may be floating, only to become submerged. Rescuing victims from a floating vehicle can be one of the most hazardous scenarios a team will face.

Vehicles in Water — Considerations

If a vehicle comes to rest into a body of water, rescue personnel should ask: Can rescue personnel perform extrication operations without having to enter the water? If the answer is no, trained personnel wearing appropriate PPE and personal flotation devices (PFDs) should conduct the rescue. On-scene personnel should establish and maintain control of the scene, and perform any other tasks that would not require them to enter the water. If the agency has one or more rescue boats, personnel trained in boat-based rescue operations can perform those tasks that they can accomplish from the boat. If the vehicle fell from a great height into the water, or if the vehicle and its occupants have been submerged for more than an hour, the operation is almost certainly a body recovery and not a rescue.

The overall situation — the type of vehicle, the nature of the body of water, how much of the vehicle is above the surface of the water, and the vehicle's orientation — can affect the process of assessing the vehicle's condition **(Fig 12.4)**. Much of the vehicle damage may be hidden below the waterline. The vehicle may be entirely submerged, making damage assessment impossible without entering the water.

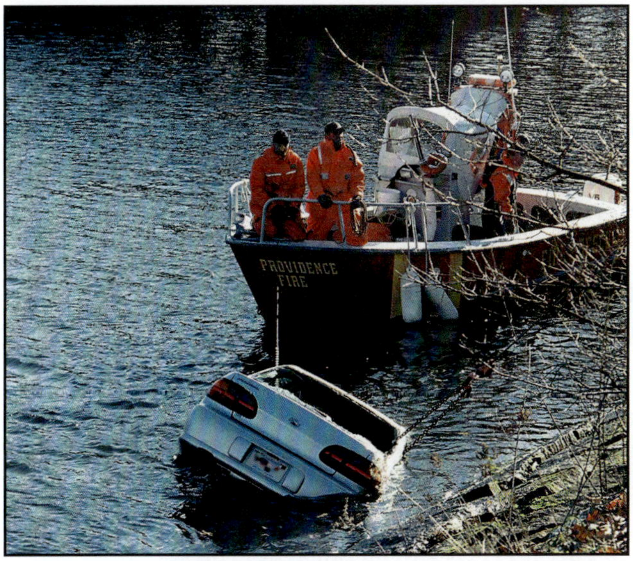

Figure 12.4 It can be difficult to stabilize vehicles that enter deep water. *Courtesy of Michael Porowshi.*

Depending upon how much of the vehicle is visible above the water, it may be possible to see into the vehicle and determine the number of victims and their condition. In other cases, rescuers may only be able to establish the presence of victims inside the vehicle. Rescuers may have to delay a more thorough assessment of victims' conditions until they have pulled the vehicle from the water and stabilized it. Rescuers should call a properly trained and equipped dive rescue team at the first indication that a vehicle is in a body of water.

Vehicles in Water — Operations

In most cases, there is little that anyone can do to stabilize a vehicle that is immersed in water except secure the vehicle to the shore with rope, chain, cable, or webbing attached to a secure anchor point. Rescuers may face the major challenge of preventing the vehicle from sinking to the bottom or floating downstream. Depending upon the vehicle's position and the amount of the vehicle above the water's surface, rescuers may need to pull the vehicle from the water before attempting any other extrication activities.

There is a remote possibility that the occupants of a submerged could use a pocket of air trapped inside the vehicle passenger compartment to survive. A dive rescue team may provide vehicle occupants with spare **Self-Contained Underwater Breathing Apparatus (SCUBA)** devices in the event the vehicle fills with water. If rescuers attempt to cut through the roof or to remove the rear window, any trapped air can escape and may allow the vehicle to sink and possibly drown the occupants.

> **Self-Contained Underwater Breathing Apparatus (SCUBA)** — Protective breathing apparatus designed to be used underwater by divers to allow the exploration of underwater environments. *Also known as* SCUBA gear *or* underwater breathing gear.

CAUTION
Creating openings in a submerged vehicle may allow air trapped in the vehicle to escape.

Only rescuers trained in water rescue should attempt the disentanglement and extrication of victims trapped in submerged vehicles. Once rescuers have pulled the vehicle from the water, they can use the same extrication processes as in any other vehicle incident with that type of vehicle, with the following exceptions:

- Electrically powered extrication tools and equipment must be used only where contact with water is not likely.
- Rescuers must secure the vehicle with a rope, chain, cable, or webbing attached to a secure anchor point to prevent rescue operations from causing the vehicle to roll back into the water.

WARNING!
Swift water and steep underwater terrain create extreme danger to rescuers attempting to reach occupants of a submerged vehicle — especially one that has not been secured against further movement.

Hanging Vehicles

A hanging vehicle incident is one in which a vehicle has crashed through a guardrail on a bridge, highway overpass, cliff, or an embankment and has come to rest with the cab or passenger compartment no longer in contact with any surface. In this type of incident, rescuers should try to prevent rescue personnel, victims, or the occupied portion of the vehicle, from falling.

Hanging Vehicles — Considerations

When responding to hanging vehicle incidents, rescuers should first ask: Can the trapped victims be reached from below with standard fire service ground ladders or aerial devices? If not, then rescuers should call a technical rescue team to rig the necessary rope rescue systems in order to access the victims. While waiting for the technical rescue team, on-scene personnel should establish and maintain control of the scene. During scene assessment, and until the vehicle can be stabilized, rescuers must keep everyone — rescue personnel and all others — out of the area directly below the hanging vehicle. In addition, on-scene personnel can take any safe and appropriate actions to stabilize the vehicle as long as those actions do not endanger entrapped victims or rescuers. If all or part of the vehicle moves or drops before it has been stabilized, it could seriously harm anyone below it **(Figure 12.5)**.

Rescuers should also control vehicular traffic near the scene. Personnel should stop traffic in both directions and detour it around the scene at a sufficient distance to ensure that traffic-generated vibration will not affect the stability of the hanging vehicle.

Getting close enough to assess the damage to a vehicle that is hanging from a high point may be dangerous. The vehicle may be ready to plunge downward or the location from which the vehicle is hanging may be in danger of collapsing. Rescuers may have to stand some distance away and use binoculars to assess the damage to the vehicle. Rescuers may face similar challenges assessing victims, and may have to do so from a distance.

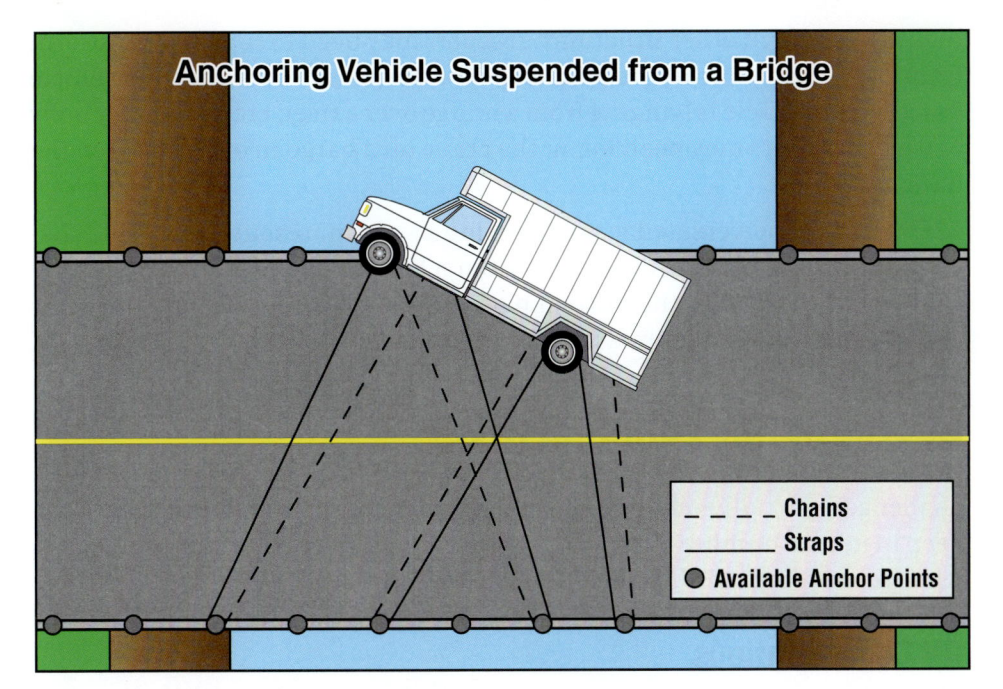

Figure 12.5 A hanging vehicle must be anchored to prevent further movement.

Determining how to remove the trapped victims from their precarious situation will influence the decisions about what tools and techniques rescuers should use to accomplish that. If rescue personnel will have to work from scaffolding or some other platform — perhaps one suspended from a crane boom — they should select only the appropriate types of tools and equipment for those conditions. In most cases, these should be fully portable and self-contained. Tools that require cords and hoses connected to power units mounted on rescue vehicles may not be safe and effective to use to extricate victims from hanging vehicles.

Hanging Vehicles — Operations

Stabilizing a hanging vehicle may be the most challenging of any vehicle stabilization situation. The height of the vehicle above the ground (or water) can make this one of the most dangerous situations for rescuers and trapped victims. When devising a plan to stabilize the vehicle rescuers must consider the following:

- Type and weight of vehicle involved
- Height above the surface
- Likelihood of the vehicle falling

Rescuers may need to secure the vehicle to anchor points with as many ropes, chains, or pieces of webbing as they can safely and quickly apply in order to provide initial stabilization. Depending upon the specific circumstances, rescuers may need to stabilize the hanging portion of the vehicle with a sling suspended from the boom of a crane or heavy recovery vehicle.

Reaching the hanging part of the vehicle may present as many difficulties as gaining access into it. Once they have reached the hanging part, rescuers must create a stable platform so they have a safe place from which to work. Under some circumstances, such as a vehicle hanging from a highway overpass, rescuers may be able to work from an aerial device positioned on the highway below. In other situations, rescuers may need to suspend a platform from the boom of a crane positioned below the point from which the vehicle hangs. If the vehicle is hanging from a bridge over a river, creek, or other body of water, rescuers may need to put the crane on a barge in order to reach the hanging vehicle.

Once they have created a safe working platform, rescuers may find disentangling and extricating victims from a hanging vehicle to be relatively routine. In addition to the normal packaging used for extrication, rescuers should provide each victim with fall protection.

Recreational Vehicles (RVs)

Incidents involving recreational vehicles (RVs) may present rescuers with challenges, partially due to their shape and construction. Rescuers should keep in mind a number of special considerations and operations procedures when responding to RV incidents.

RV Considerations

RV incidents may put rescue personnel and others at greater risk if a liquefied petroleum gas (LPG) or other fuel tank or associated piping has been damaged and is leaking. Under these circumstances, on-scene personnel should establish and maintain control of the scene, and perform any other duties that would not require them to enter the hot zone until the flammability hazard has been mitigated **(Figure 12.6 a and b)**.

Assessing the damage to RVs involved in collisions may pose fewer challenges than assessing other types of vehicles, unless the RV is in a hazardous environment. The structures of most RVs make them highly susceptible to damage but relatively easy to access. Most RVs are constructed on a chassis with a rigid frame and are built more like mobile homes than highway vehicles.

Motor homes and travel trailers normally have a small number of occupants compared to some other vehicles, but this may not be true in some incidents. If the RV was parked when struck by another vehicle, there could be several victims in the RV as well as in the other vehicle.

Because of the relatively lightweight construction of most RVs, rescuers will

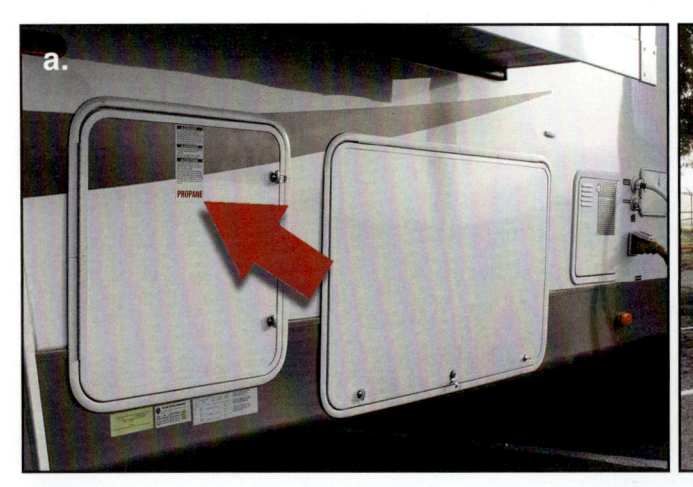

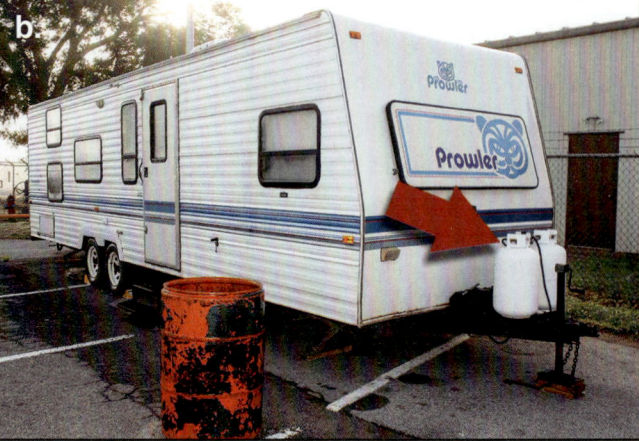

Figure 12.6 a. Fuel tanks on an RV are flammable. This RV stores them in a designated compartment. **b.** This RV stores them outside.

likely only require basic extrication tools and equipment. However, rescuers cannot make this assumption due to ever-changing vehicle construction technology, and the possibility that owners made alterations to their vehicles.

RV Operations

Stabilizing an RV may be more like stabilizing a bus than stabilizing any other type of vehicle. Whether or not rescuers use techniques for stabilizing a passenger vehicle or stabilizing a bus will depend upon the size of the RV.

Gaining entry to an RV is often easy because of the RV's lightweight construction. However, rescuers should not view the ease of entry as an excuse to ignore safety rules. RVs have hazards associated with them that rescuers will not encounter with other types of vehicles.

Depending upon the type of RV involved and other variables in the particular incident, disentangling and extricating victims from these vehicles may be relatively simple or quite challenging. In a collision, the furnishings and other contents of the RV may turn its interior into a mess. This mass of material can make disentangling and extricating the victims much more difficult. Rescuers may even face difficulties verifying that they have located all the victims.

If an RV leaves the roadway and rolls over several times before coming to rest at the bottom of a steep slope, the vehicle may disintegrate as it tumbles, leaving a trail of objects and occupants on the hillside. However, if the steepness of the slope requires more than low-angle rescue, responders should call in a technical rescue team to extricate the victims. Otherwise, extricating victims from RVs requires the same techniques and equipment described in previous chapters.

Industrial and Agricultural Vehicles

Rescuers will often encounter industrial and agricultural vehicle incidents. This section will cover the following topics:

- Types of industrial and agricultural vehicles
- Industrial and agricultural vehicle anatomy, construction, and features
- Industrial and agricultural vehicle hazards
- Industrial and agricultural vehicle stabilization
- Industrial and agricultural vehicle extrication

Types of Industrial and Agricultural Vehicles

Industrial and agricultural vehicles have a wide variety of shapes and sizes. They range from small farm tractors to huge earthmovers used in construction and mining **(Figure 12.7, p. 448)**. Manufacturers constantly introduce new types of vehicles and improved models of existing vehicles. Some of them are modern versions of vehicles that have existed for many decades. Others are new because the tasks they have been designed to perform did not exist before. Industrial vehicles are used in warehouses, as well as in building and highway construction site work. The massive size, extreme weight, and heavy-duty construction of these vehicles provide additional challenges to extrication operations **(Figure 12.8, p. 448)**.

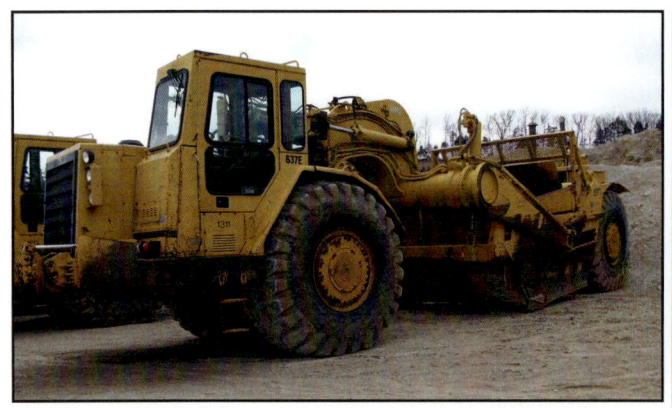

Figure 12.7 An example of an articulating earthmover. *Courtesy of Alan Braun, University of Missouri Fire Institute Training.*

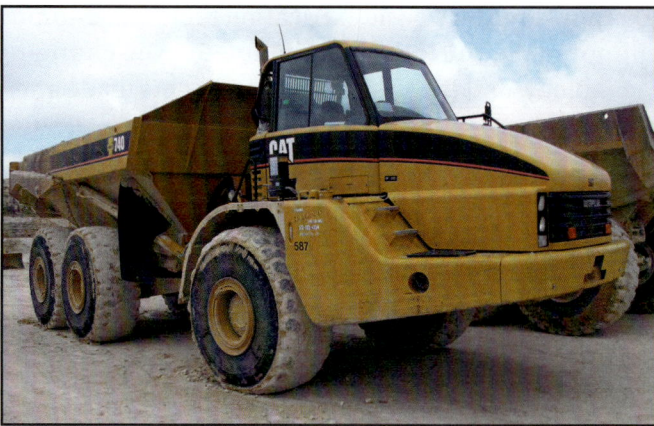

Figure 12.8 Oversize dump trucks are frequently used in strip mining operations. *Courtesy of Alan Braun, University of Missouri Fire Institute Training.*

Rescue personnel must gain familiarity with the types of industrial and agricultural vehicles in their communities, the construction of these vehicles, and how to perform extrication procedures for each type of vehicle. Many extrication tools cannot cut the materials used in the construction of these vehicles, so rescuers may need to disassemble the vehicles. This section will further describe the following types of industrial and agricultural vehicles:

- Tractors
- Harvesters
- Graders
- Booms
- Cranes
- Forklifts

> **CAUTION**
> Emergency responders should be aware that these types of vehicles may contain hazardous materials. Personnel should take proper precautions when dealing with these hazards.

Tractors

Tractors are used in a variety of industrial and agricultural settings that range from airports and construction sites to farms, ranches, and highways. Like other types of vehicles, tractors come in many different sizes and configurations. There are two broad classes of off-road tractors: wheeled tractors and tracked vehicles. Tractors incorporate a number of attachments and/or implements for various purposes.

Wheeled tractors. Typical wheeled tractors have large rear wheels (normally up to 50 inches [1 250 mm]) and smaller front wheels (normally up to 38 inches [950 mm]), with rubber tires. Depending upon the specific use, the front wheels may be set the same distance apart as the rear wheels or they may be closer together. Some wheeled tractors are two-wheel drive and others are all-wheel

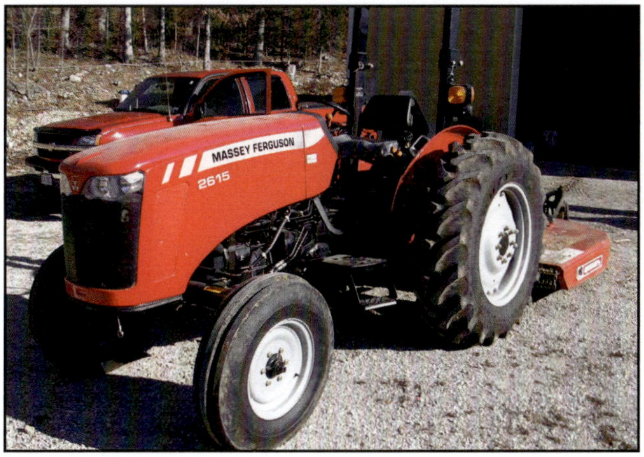

Figure 12.9 A wheel-based agricultural tractor. *Courtesy of Alan Braun, University of Missouri Fire Institute Training.*

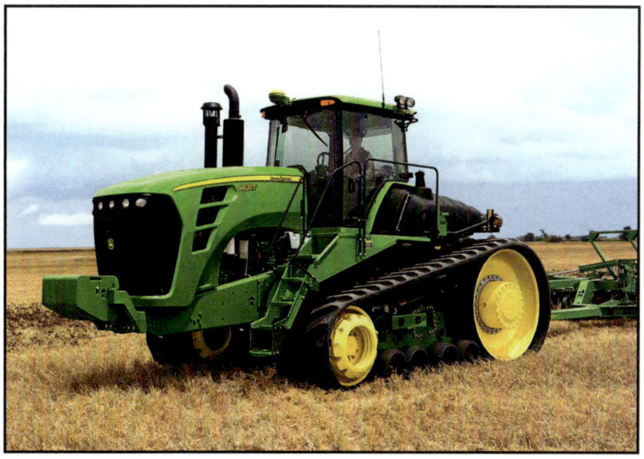

Figure 12.10 A crawler-type tractor with rubber tracks. *Courtesy of John Deere.*

drive, often referred to as manual front wheel drive (MFWD). On some two-wheel drive tractors, the rear tires have traction treads and the front tires are grooved for lateral purchase; however, some may be found with turf or industrial type tires **(Figure 12.9)**.

The front and rear tires on all-wheel drive tractors have heavy traction treads. Because these tractors are relatively light in weight and are often used to pull heavy loads, large cast-iron weights are sometimes bolted to the wheels, and/or the tires are filled to approximately 90 percent with a solution of calcium chloride or ethylene glycol and water to improve traction. In other cases, tractors are equipped with multiple front and/or rear wheels for the same purpose.

Regardless of their configuration, all individual wheeled tractors tend to have a high profile that makes them more prone to rolling over than other types of vehicles. Their relatively narrow track (horizontal distance from 60 to 100 inches [1 500 to 2 500 mm] between wheels on the same axle) and their high ground clearance make them susceptible to lateral rollovers. The Occupational Safety and Health Administration (OSHA) requires that manufacturers equip all wheeled tractors manufactured after October 1976 with seat belts and roll bars, officially known as rollover protection systems (ROPS).

On flat, level ground, individually wheeled tractors have a center of gravity along their centerline roughly halfway between their front and rear axles. When a wheeled tractor travels on a hillside, its center of gravity shifts toward the downhill wheels. If the downhill wheels drop into a depression or the uphill wheels hit a slight bump, or both, the tractor may roll over laterally. Likewise, if a wheeled tractor climbs a steep slope, its center of gravity shifts to the rear axle. If the front wheels hit a large enough bump while the rear wheels are in a depression, it can cause the front wheels to leave the ground and the front end to rotate around the rear axle, with the unit coming to rest upside down — perhaps pinning the operator beneath it. To reduce this possibility, manufacturers equip some wheeled tractors with up to 1,400 pounds (700 kg) of cast iron weights attached to the front of their chassis.

Tracked vehicles. Steel or rubber tracks, rather than wheels, provide the locomotion for some tractors. These tractors are generally larger and heavier than most wheeled tractors, have a wider track, and a lower profile. Therefore, tracked vehicles are less susceptible to rollover than wheeled tractors **(Figure 12.10)**.

Attachments and implements. Tractors accommodate a wide variety of attachments and implements. Attachments are those auxiliary appliances that are attached to the chassis of the tractor. Attachments can affect a tractor's stability and sometimes result in tractor rollovers. Examples of attachments include:

- Front-end loaders
- Back hoes
- Scraper blades

Implements are those appliances that are temporarily attached to and usually towed or carried by the tractor. Typical farm implements include the following:

- Planters
- Manure spreaders
- Chemical spraying rigs
- Hay rakes
- Balers

Tractors can be configured to accomplish numerous tasks. Wheeled tractors may have a scraper blade on the front or rear for snow removal and light-duty grading. Tracked vehicles may have massive steel blades on their front ends for heavy-duty grading and excavation **(Figure 12.11)**. Some tracked vehicles also have attachments on the rear of the vehicle such as huge rippers or trenching attachments.

Tracked vehicles are sometimes used at airports, especially during inclement weather, to tow aircraft from one point to another. These vehicles are often equipped with rubber tracks or rubber pads on steel tracks to avoid damaging the taxiway surface.

Harvesters

Sometimes called combines, harvesters are wide, stable vehicles that have a relatively low center of gravity **(Figure 12.12)**. Despite their design, these vehicles can still roll over if given a sufficiently steep slope and enough lateral force. Many harvesters discharge grain into a truck or trailer following the harvester.

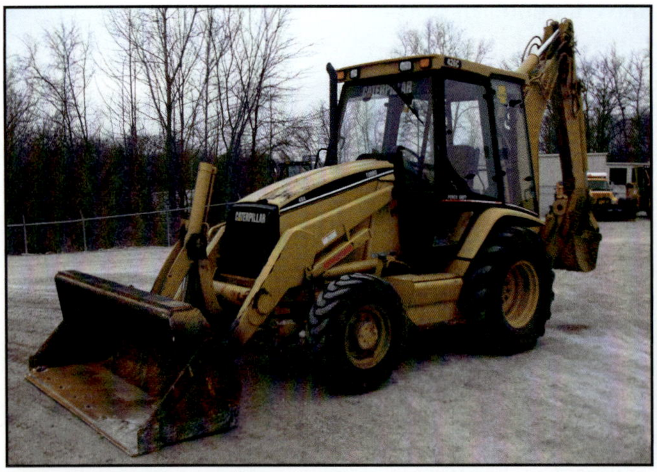

Figure 12.11 This tractor is equipped with a front-end loader and backhoe attachments. *Courtesy of Alan Braun, University of Missouri Fire and Rescue Training Institute.*

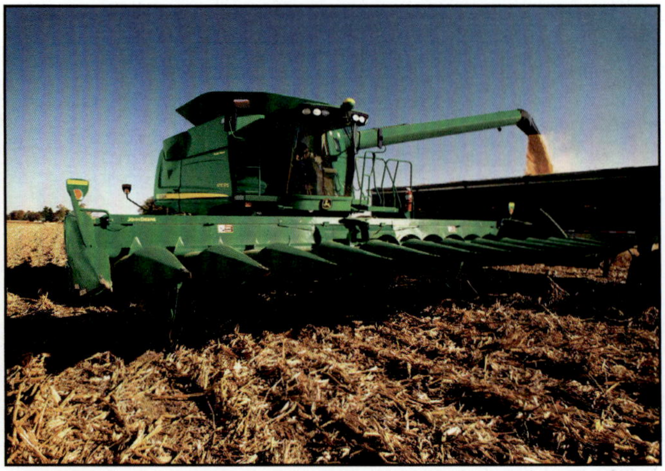

Figure 12.12 A harvester or combine. *Courtesy of John Deere.*

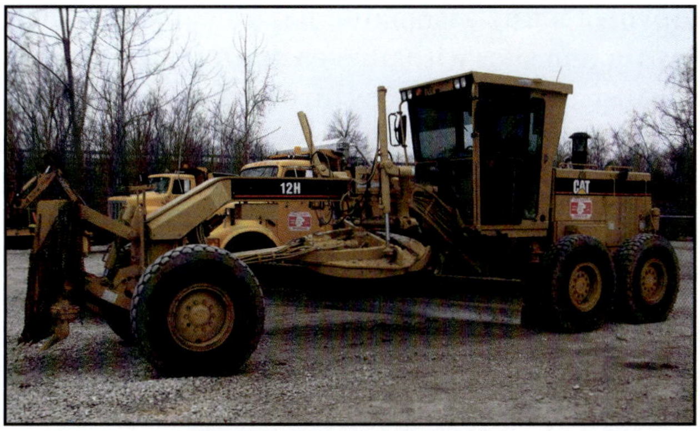

Figure 12.13 A standard grader or maintainer. *Courtesy of Alan Braun, University of Missouri Fire and Rescue Training Institute.*

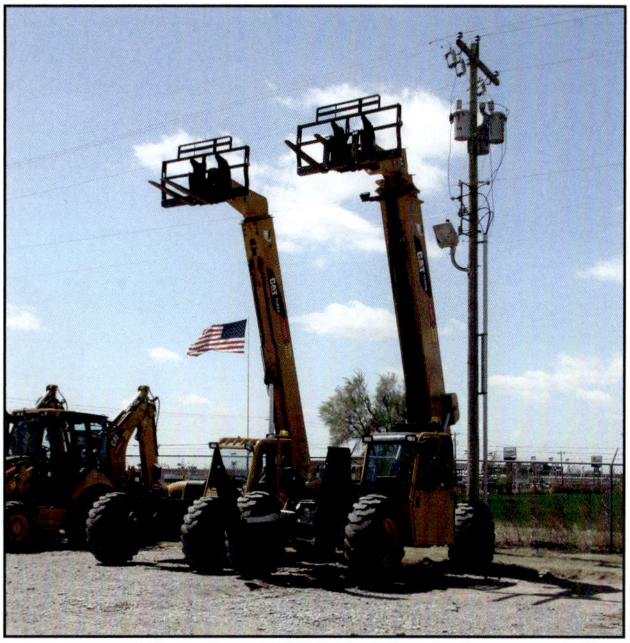

Figure 12.14 The difference between a boom and forklift is that a boom can lift materials higher.

Farm workers who enter the truck bed or trailer to manipulate the material inside can become trapped in the grain and suffocate if not extricated in time.

Some harvesters use an enclosed auger to discharge the grain into a following vehicle. Many farm workers have had an extremity pulled into these augers when their clothing became entangled in the mechanism. Disentanglement in these cases most often involves disassembly of the drive chains, gears, or belts before entry. Some units are operated by flowing hydraulics. When rescuers encounter hydraulic lines, they should first address the end farthest from the victim.

Graders

Graders, also called maintainers, are road maintenance vehicles that rescuers may find on unsurfaced roads or at highway construction sites **(Figure 12.13)**. Despite the ability to laterally tilt their front wheels, given enough lateral force, graders can roll over when operated on a sufficiently steep slope. Their enclosed cabs are similar to those on tractors and other industrial or agricultural vehicles. These vehicles may have a movable scraper blade mid-mounted with ripper teeth on the blade or attached to the front or rear end.

Booms

Booms are some of the most versatile single-purpose vehicles **(Figure 12.14)**. They consist of a vehicle-mounted boom that can telescope more than 40 feet (12 m) and lift from 7,000 to 10,000 pounds (3 500 to 5 000 kg). The end of the boom may be fitted with forks for lifting material on pallets, a platform or basket similar to those on fire service aerial devices, or a bucket such as those on front-end loaders. Many of these vehicles have all-wheel steering in addition to all-wheel drive. Some have fully enclosed cabs similar to those described in the section on forklifts.

Incidents with booms involve many associated hazards. Booms often operate on unsurfaced construction sites with uneven and/or unstable soil, which can cause the boom to turn over. Booms may turn over when the boom is fully extended vertically – especially in a strong crosswind. Booms, like fire department aerial devices, create a potential hazard when they are operated in close proximity to power lines. If the vehicle contacts the power lines, it may become charged.

> **WARNING!**
> Personnel should be aware of overhead hazards such as power lines when working around booms in the elevated position. The vehicle may become electrically charged if it comes in contact with a power line.

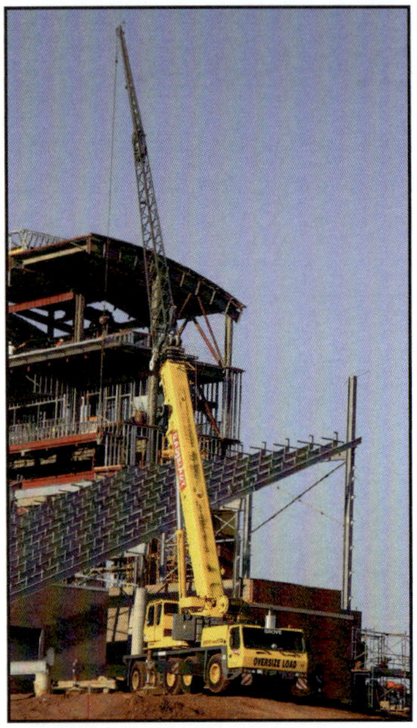

Cranes

These massive vehicles may have large pneumatic tires and can be driven from site to site, or they may be crawlers that must be transported from site to site on lowboy trailers **(Figure 12.15)**. Regardless of their means of locomotion, cranes are subject to the same hazards as booms.

Forklifts

The OSHA regulations in 29 CFR 1910.178 refer to forklifts as powered industrial trucks. They are also known as lift trucks or fork trucks. Forklifts lift heavy objects and transport them over short distances **(Figure 12.16)**. They are found in working environments such as warehouses, lumberyards, and construction sites. Urban search and rescue teams use forklifts in structural collapse incidents. While lifting capacity varies with the manufacturer and the model of the vehicle, most forklifts can lift from 2,000 to 80,000 pounds (1 000 kg to 40 000 kg).

Some forklifts operate on rechargeable lead-acid batteries of 24, 36, or 48 volts. Others have internal combustion engines that operate on gasoline, diesel, or liquefied petroleum gas (LPG) **(Figure 12.17)**. Some have dual fuel systems that can operate on both gasoline and LPG.

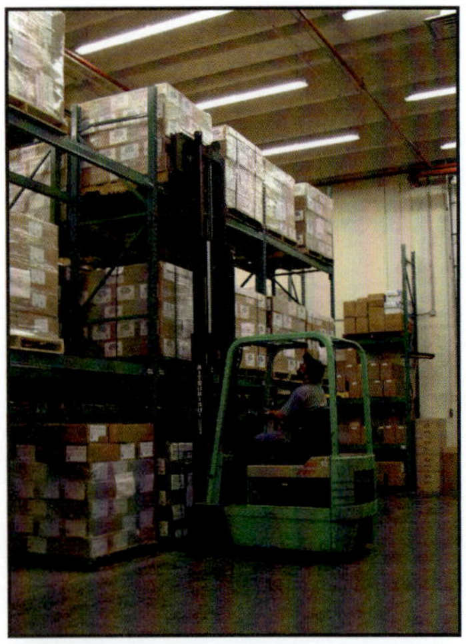

Figure 12.15 A wheel-based crane at a construction site.

Figure 12.16 Forklifts are useful in lifting and moving products and materials.

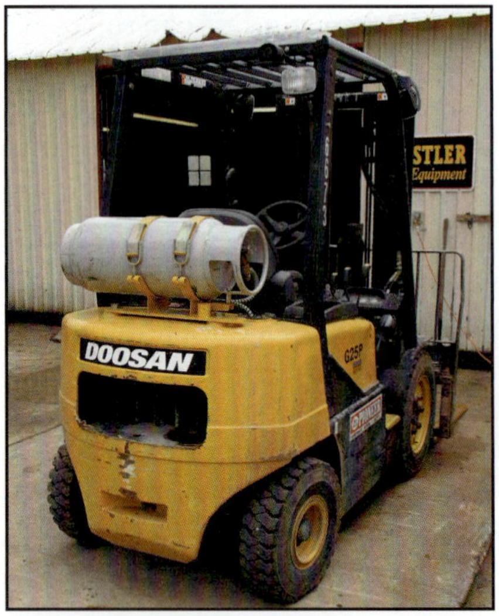

Figure 12.17 The compressed gas fuel tank on a forklift.

Most forklifts have two broad lifting forks, approximately 4 feet (1 m) long. The forks can move laterally to adjust to the width of a particular load. Some forklifts have more specialized lifting devices for lifting unique loads. The lifting device is attached to a horizontal cross beam that can be elevated or lowered on rollers that travel in a pair of vertical tracks, called the mast. Operators can deflect these masts from five to seven degrees from vertical to increase control of the load. Some masts telescope, which increases the vertical lift range. They may also have a side shift feature to move the load laterally. Forklifts equipped with a four-stage telescoping mast have a vertical lift range of up to 30 feet (9 m). The higher the lift, the greater the chance of the unit falling over because of the increase in leverage at the top of the lift mechanism. As with fire department aerial devices, operators should avoid extending the units close to power line, due to the danger of the mast or the load coming into contact with the power lines.

The design of each forklift chassis varies with the manufacturer and the intended purpose of the vehicle. All chassis have a relatively low profile and are made of heavy materials such as cast iron and steel. Some forklifts weigh as little as 2,000 pounds (1000 kg) while others weigh as much as 36,000 pounds (18 000 kg). The bulk of the weight of a forklift chassis is concentrated at the end opposite the lift mechanism to act as a counterweight. Some forklifts have additional counterweights added to the end of the chassis. Many forklifts, especially those operated in warehouses and other areas with concrete floors, have small solid rubber tires mounted on 12 to 21 inch (300 mm to 525 mm) wheels. Forklifts intended for outdoor use generally have either pneumatic tires or cushion tires. All of these design features intend to increase the stability of these vehicles.

All forklifts have some form of overhead operator protection system designed to deflect falling objects. Most are heavy-gauge wire screen or a steel grille over a steel frame. Forklifts that routinely operate outdoors sometimes have a fully enclosed cab. The enclosure usually consists of the standard operator protection system enclosed with Plexiglas® panels or window panes and a laminated safety glass windshield.

CAUTION
Use extra care when cribbing, locking out, or stabilizing an elevated load.

Industrial and Agricultural Vehicle Anatomy, Construction, and Features

Rescue personnel should learn as much as possible about the anatomy, construction, and features of the industrial and agricultural vehicles in their jurisdiction. This section will discuss the following as they relate to industrial and agricultural vehicles:

- Drivetrain
- Operational controls
- Tracked vehicles
- Vehicle Tires

- Articulating and telescoping vehicles
- Industrial and agricultural vehicles fuel systems
- Industrial and agricultural vehicles brake systems
- Industrial and agricultural vehicles auxiliary power sources
- Industrial and agricultural vehicles rollover protection systems
- Jacks

Drivetrain

Industrial and agricultural vehicles primarily have two different types of drivetrains: two-wheel drive and all-wheel drive. This section will further describe these drivetrains.

Two-wheel drive vehicles. Many wheeled tractors and similar vehicles have two-wheel drivetrains. In most of these vehicles, the driving wheels are at the rear of the vehicle and the steering wheels are at the front. Most forklifts have the opposite configuration. The front wheels do the driving and the rear wheels do the steering. Regardless of which wheels provide locomotion, poor traction makes two-wheel drive vehicles prone to rollovers on hillsides and other slopes. A two-wheel drive vehicle attempting to move diagonally up and across a slope may begin to slide sideways and then downslope. A vehicle that hits an obstruction while moving diagonally up a slope may roll over.

All-wheel drive vehicles. Four-wheel and/or all-wheel drive vehicles better handle situations involving poor traction and steep slopes. Some of these vehicles have all-wheel steering. All-wheel vehicle operators often have a false sense of invulnerability due to the capability and maneuverability of their vehicle. This mindset can cause the operator to take imprudent risks, sometimes resulting in a rollover.

Operational Controls

Industrial and agricultural vehicles employ a variety of control devices. While some vehicles use a steering wheel, others may use hydraulics or a clutch-brake system. Many modern tracked vehicles use a joystick control to steer the vehicle. Some of these steer, some increase a vehicle's stability, and still others power or control auxiliary devices. On some equipment, a global positioning satellite (GPS) system may be used to guide the equipment without input from the operator.

Tracked Vehicles

Often, manually operated levers or joysticks apply or release a separate brake for each track to control the direction of travel for tracked vehicles. Some tracked vehicles exert a ground pressure of as little as 2.5 psi (17.5 kPa) because the tracks spread the weight of the vehicle. They are often used in extreme environments so are still vulnerable to rollovers. Their size and weight can make extrication from rolled over tracked vehicles much more difficult than with most wheeled tractors.

Vehicle Tires
Manufacturers may equip industrial and agricultural vehicles with pneumatic or solid rubber tires, with tread designs selected according to the vehicle's use and the environment in which it works. Small and large vehicles may have pneumatic tires. Massive earthmoving vehicles used in mining and heavy construction also feature pneumatic tires. To improve the traction of drive wheels with large pneumatic tires, it is common practice to fill the tires to about ninety percent with water or some other inert fluid such as antifreeze and then inflate the tires to their normal operating pressure with air.

Some forklifts and similar vehicles have cushion tires. These solid rubber tires that look like the pneumatic tires used on automobiles and light trucks. Cushion tires lack valve stems.

Other solid rubber tires on forklifts are quite obvious. They generally are smaller in diameter than either cushion or pneumatic tires, and they usually have no treads.

Articulating and Telescoping Vehicles
The most common articulating vehicles are large earthmovers and large tractors. Earthmovers are very stable because of their huge wheels and low center of gravity. However, given a steep enough slope, unstable soil, or sufficient lateral force, earthmovers can roll over. Other examples of articulating vehicles include:

- All-wheel drive farm tractors
- Log skidders
- Large front-end loaders
- Rough-terrain forklifts
- Large dump trucks

Telescoping vehicles include beams and cranes that are capable of lifting heavy loads.

Industrial and Agricultural Vehicle Fuel Systems
Industrial and agricultural vehicles may operate on a variety of fuels. Many of the largest and heaviest vehicles operate on diesel fuel and carry up to 100 gallons (400 L) in their tanks. Other industrial and agricultural vehicles operate using gasoline and/or LPG, such as propane. Still others operate on CNG. Some forklifts and other vehicles use electricity from banks of rechargeable wet-cell batteries.

Vehicles that operate on liquid or gaseous fuels add the danger of fire to the other hazards associated with collisions, rollovers, and other vehicle incidents. Rescuers should give careful consideration to the possibility of fuel tank failure due to the lightweight materials that make up some fuel systems. Sudden failure of these fuel systems could release large amounts of fuels that would potentially surround personnel in the immediate vicinity.

Industrial and Agricultural Vehicle Brake Systems
Manufacturers typically mount brakes on industrial and agricultural vehicles inside the rear axle. Most of these vehicles do not have front brakes. The rear brakes can be operated independently or locked together with a bar mounted

to the pedals. Using them independently allows the operator to turn a tractor in a short distance. Tracked vehicles use brakes for changing direction (steering). When the operator of one of these vehicles wants to turn left, he or she pulls a lever or steps on a pedal that applies a brake to the left track, slowing or stopping it. Since the left track at least momentarily moves slower that the right track, the vehicle veers to the left. The greater the difference in the speed of the right and left tracks, the faster and more abrupt the turn. A fully applied brake to one track or the other will cause the vehicle to spin around a fixed point.

Industrial and Agricultural Vehicle Auxiliary Power Sources

To increase versatility, some tractors and similar vehicles have one or more auxiliary power sources. They may have power take-off systems (PTOs) to operate implements such as portable grain augers or conveyor belts. They may have hydraulic pumps they can use to raise or lower farm implements such as plows or mowers. In addition, many tractors are equipped with pneumatic and additional electrical resources to supply any needed ancillary equipment. As with any power source, if the proper guards are not in place or if the operators fail to exercise appropriate caution when using the devices, parts of the operator's clothing can become entangled in the mechanism and this can pull the operator into the machinery.

> **Controlling PTO Power**
>
> After stabilizing a tractor or farm machine, one must first disengage the PTO and then shut off the tractor engine (power supply). This will allow for the rescuer to control and stabilize any stored energy in the PTO. Remember that any power supply to the tractor can be transferred to the implement or attachment. Personnel should remember that shutting off the tractor engine does not always stop the implement or attachment from operating.

> **CAUTION**
> Rescuers should ensure that they do not accidentally re-engage live PTO systems.

Industrial and Agricultural Vehicle Rollover Protection Systems

OSHA requires a ROPS on industrial and agricultural vehicles, except those in which the operator stands. Even in vehicles not covered by the OSHA regulations, manufacturers often install ROPS for liability reasons. Sometimes the operator's insurance carrier requires ROPS. The owner will commonly remove or alter these systems to reduce the height of the vehicle.

Jacks

Also called stabilizers or outriggers, these hydraulically operated devices extend from both sides of an equipped vehicle. They are similar to the stabilizing jacks on a fire department aerial device. As the name implies, these devices stabilize a tractor or other vehicle that is operating an attachment such as a backhoe or a boom. When applied, stabilizing jacks normally lift the vehicle's wheels off the ground, and the jacks bear the full weight of the vehicle.

These jacks make the vehicle stable unless something goes wrong. If one or more of the jacks suddenly loses hydraulic pressure, the vehicle can lurch to one side. If the vehicle were positioned across a slope and the downslope jacks failed, the vehicle could easily topple over. Also, if the ground under the jacks on one side of the vehicle collapses into an excavation, the vehicle may roll over.

Industrial and Agricultural Incident Size-Up

Rescuers should systematically conduct the size-up of a vehicle incident involving an industrial or agricultural vehicle including assessments of the following:

- Overall scene
- Vehicles involved
- Trapped victims
- Extrication requirements of the particular incident

  Initial size-up should answer the following questions:

- Is the incident location clearly known and readily accessible, or will rescue personnel have to search for the scene?
- Is the trapped operator the only person at the scene who is familiar with the operation of the machine, or will rescuers need a farm advisor or other expert?
- Are additional medical resources needed such as medevac air transport or specialized trauma teams?
- As the rescuers near the scene, they should consider the following questions to identify other problems:
  — Is smoke (especially that with an unusual color) or steam rising from the scene?
  — Will fire protection be an even higher priority because of a known flammability hazard?
  — Will rescuers need large-scale foam-making capability?
  — Will rescuers need a hazardous materials team because of a known release or a high potential for the release of a pesticide or other IDLH (immediately dangerous to life or health) substance?
  — Will rescuers need to request any additional resources to control and mitigate the known and potential hazards involved in this incident?
- What hazards are involved? To identify potential hazards, the IC must ask the following questions:
  — What type of load is the vehicle carrying?
  — What are the load's contents?
  — How are these arranged?
  — Are the materials (packages in a crate or liquid within a tank) visible?
  — How will the load affect the vehicle during the rescue operation?
  — Is the load stable or will rescuers need to secure and remove it in order to perform the rescue safely?

  NOTE: As always, rescuers should continue size-up throughout the incident.

In industrial and agricultural settings, the load the vehicle carries may contain hazardous materials. The load may have placards or other identification decals on them; however, in a farm setting the contents of tanks may not be readily apparent. Farmers and private individuals are not required to placard individual tank loads of product. Many of these products, such as anhydrous ammonia, fungicides, and pesticides, are hazardous to emergency responders and victims. Many of these materials will form a hazard once they come in contact with each other. Often these chemicals and/or materials are packaged separately, but transported together.

Most incidents involving industrial and agricultural vehicles will have only one occupant in each vehicle. Rescuers must still consider the possibility that several persons may have been riding in the vehicle. The size and weight of these vehicles may make extricating one victim more challenging and time consuming than extricating several victims from more conventional vehicles. Rescuers should look for victims to determine their number, location, and medical conditions. During this process rescuers should pay special attention to crush injuries. Even though an industrial or agricultural vehicle may seem stable in its present position, rescuers must attempt to assess the trapped victims without causing additional movement to the vehicle — especially the cab.

Some industrial equipment will require specialized tools beyond those rescue vehicles normally carry. Rescuers should consider using plant resources or local dealers for the tools and equipment they would need in such instances. Agencies should collect contact numbers, including after hours contacts, for these resources during the preincident planning process.

Key points to consider when attempting a tractor rollover rescue include:

- Fire is a threat in an overturn situation if there is spilled fuel present. Ideally, a 1½-inch (38 mm) hoseline should be available throughout the rescue, at a minimum, ABC-type extinguishers should be present.

- Before using thermal cutting equipment to free a victim, consider using alternative methods that are less likely to increase the possibility of ignition.

- Shut off the tractor engine. Rescuers should always stop a running tractor engine. Rescuers should stabilize the vehicle to ensure that the engine stays off because even if the tractor engine is not running, movement of the rear wheels can start the engine.

- If the ground is soft, it may be possible to dig the victim out from under the tractor.

- As with other vehicle incidents, rescuers should stabilize the machine to prevent it from tipping and causing more injuries.

- Lifting the tractor is the best way to deal with rollovers of large, modern tractors. A second tractor or a tow truck may be needed to perform the lift. If a tractor must be rolled away from the victim, rescuers must use load capture to minimize settling of the lower side.

- As the tractor is raised, add cribbing for proper stability.

- Hydraulic jacks can be used to lift smaller tractors. Crib the axle on both sides to prevent the tractor from rocking onto the victim.

- Lifting bags can be used to raise an overturned tractor **(Fig 12.18)**.

- Bags are more stable if they are stacked alternately with the cribbing.

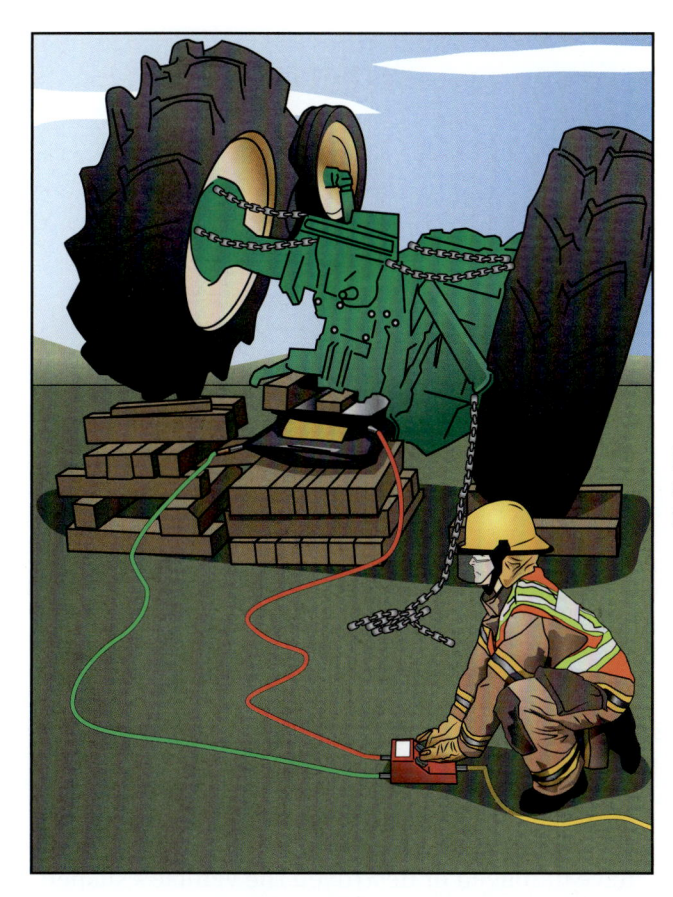

Figure 12.18 A lifting bag system being used to lift a tractor.

Industrial and Agricultural Vehicle Hazards

Just as with passenger and commercial/heavy vehicles, rescuers must shut down the engine and isolate the electrical system. Stabilize pneumatic system components if the air will be released in order to prevent movement of the air-operated implement or equipment. If necessary, disconnect the air supply and shut it down at the farthest point from the victim in an effort to reduce injury. Leave pneumatic systems intact if they have no bearing on the extrication outcome.

In agricultural settings, the load the vehicle carries may contain hazardous materials. The load may have placards or other identification decals; however, in a farm setting rescuers may not be able to easily identify the contents of tanks. Farmers and private individuals are not required to placard individual tank loads of product. Many of these products, such as anhydrous ammonia, fungicides, and pesticides, are hazardous to rescuers and victims. Many of these materials are safe until they come in contact with another material. Often these chemicals and/or materials are packaged separately but transported together. Emergency responders should consider these risks when responding to emergencies in these settings.

Industrial and Agricultural Vehicle Stabilization

Like any other vehicle involved in an extrication, rescuers must stabilize an industrial or agricultural vehicle before rescue personnel can enter to assess, stabilize, package, and disentangle trapped victims. As with other types of vehicles, the techniques and equipment used to stabilize an industrial or agricultural vehicle may vary depending upon how the vehicle came to rest —wheel-resting, side-resting, roof-resting, or in some other position.

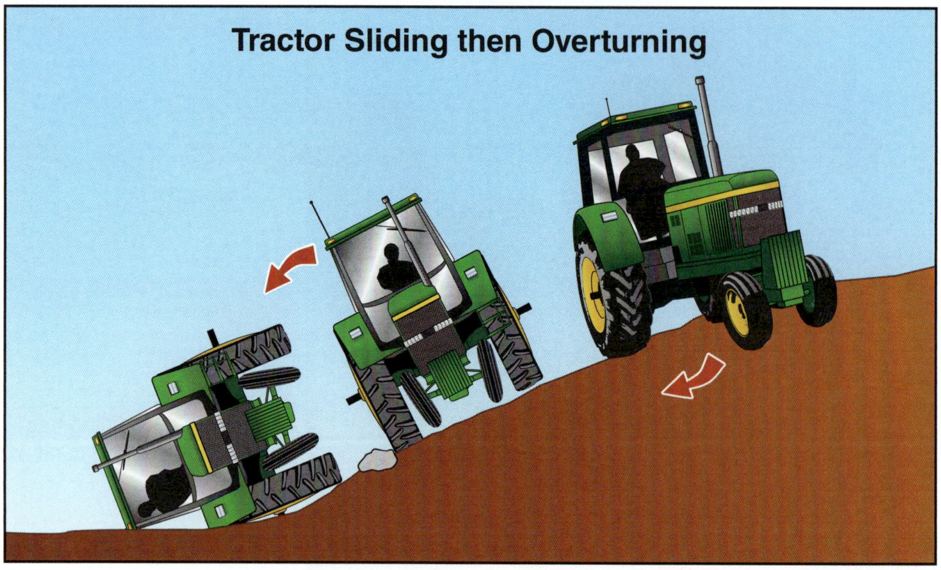

Figure 12.19 Two-wheel drive tractors can slide sideways and roll over if they strike an obstacle while trying to travel over a slope.

Stabilization of Wheel-Resting Industrial and Agricultural Vehicles

When an industrial or agricultural vehicle is wheel-resting following a destructive event, it is likely to be stable vertically because of the extremely heavy suspension, or absence of suspension, on many of these vehicles. However, the destructive event may have damaged or destroyed the vehicle's suspension system (if any), so rescuers should still apply vertical stabilization. Both vertical and horizontal stabilization may involve the usual equipment and techniques, such as cribbing and struts, installed at the appropriate points. Rescuers may need wheel chocks and/or webbing and chains to provide horizontal stability. How and where rescuers apply these techniques will depend on the specifics of the situation.

Stabilization of Side-Resting Industrial and Agricultural Vehicles

Just as with heavy trucks, industrial or agricultural vehicles may seem stable if they have rolled onto their sides. However, if the vehicle has come to rest on a slope or on unstable soil, it may suddenly and unexpectedly rolling over. To create a safe working environment for rescue personnel, rescuers may need to first secure the vehicle from the top with webbing and/or chains attached to a secure anchor point **(Figure 12.19)**. Then, with that antiroll protection in place, rescuers can install shoring on the underside of the vehicle.

Stabilization of Roof-Resting Industrial and Agricultural Vehicles

Because many industrial and agricultural vehicles do not have roofs, the vehicle may rest on a roll bar or on its fenders **(Figure 12.20)**. Regardless of what part of the vehicle supports the rest of it, in this position it is likely to be unstable. Because the vehicle's center of gravity is relatively high in this position, it is imperative that it be effectively stabilized as soon as possible.

Stabilizing an upside-down industrial or agricultural vehicle may involve installing cribbing, shoring, and/or struts at various points. Wheeled tractors and similar vehicles may require box cribbing under the rear axle, one stack on each side between the differential and the wheel. Other types of vehicles

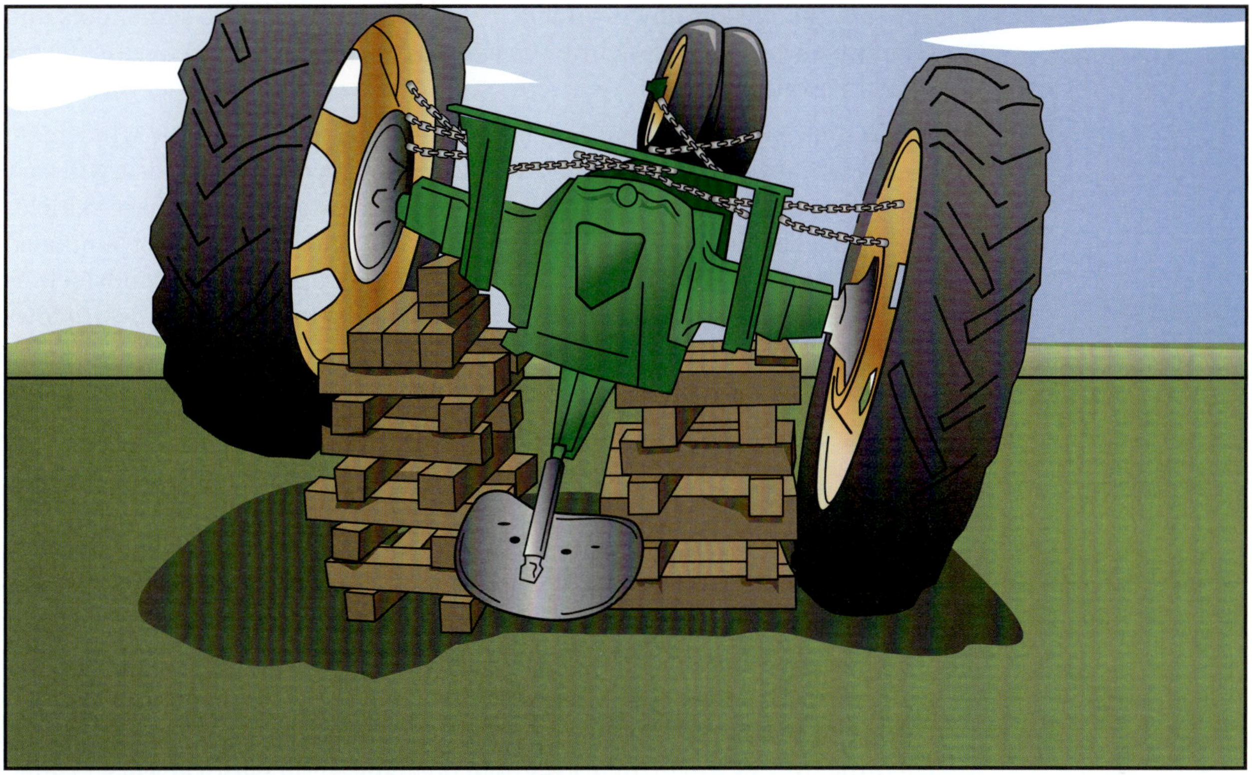

Figure 12.20 Using cribbing to stabilize an overturned tractor.

may require more elaborate cribbing depending upon the situation. Because of the unusually heavy weight of many of these vehicles, rescuers may need to build solid cribbing stacks or use larger dimension lumber to provide adequate support.

Stabilization of Industrial and Agricultural Vehicles in Other Positions

Industrial and agricultural vehicles may come to rest at odd angles and in precarious positions. These unusual angles can dictate the use of extraordinarily long shoring or that rescuers stabilize the vehicle from the top side with webbing and/or chains or cables. If rescuers use long timber they may have to construct a stabilization system similar to those used to shore weakened building walls. It is important to calculate the weight of the vehicle and utilize a stabilization system that will support the determined load. As always, rescuers should try to create as many points of contact between the vehicle and a stable surface as needed to stabilize the vehicle.

Industrial and Agricultural Vehicle Extrication

When performing extrication on industrial and agricultural vehicles, rescuers should consider the following:

- Industrial and agricultural vehicle access
- Industrial and agricultural vehicle extrication tactics
- PTO incidents

Industrial and Agricultural Vehicle Access

Once they have stabilized an industrial or agricultural vehicle, crews can safely work on gaining access into the vehicle's cab. Unless the cab is crushed beneath the upside-down vehicle, rescuers should use the same tools and techniques to gain access into the cab are as those they use to gain access into other vehicles.

Window entry. The tools and techniques used to remove the windshield and/or windows from the cab of an industrial or agricultural vehicle will vary depending upon the materials used in the windows. Some of these vehicles have Plexiglas® in the side and rear windows, with tempered glass or laminated safety glass in the windshield. Others have tempered glass in the windshield as well as in the side and rear windows. Some manufacturers mount the windows in rubber frames. Other windows are held in place with industrial adhesive. Still others are bolted to steel hinges or brackets attached to the frame of the cab and have steel safety bars or screens mounted to them.

Door entry. The cabs of most industrial and agricultural vehicles have outward swinging doors with a window that may or may not open. Those that open may slide horizontally or swing open, either partially or fully. Because the cabs of these vehicles are usually 4 feet (1.2 m) or more above the ground, the door latches are located near the bottom of the door panel.

If the door is jammed and must be removed, rescuers can cut off the exposed hinge pins on the outside of the cab with a rotary saw equipped with a metal-cutting blade or with a cutting torch. Once rescuers cut through the hinges are cut through, they can lift or pry the door off manually or with a power spreader.

Roof entry. If rescuers have no other route of entry into the cab of an industrial or agricultural vehicle, then they can attempt to enter through the roof. However since the roof panel is part of the ROPS, it is made of substantial material — usually steel — which can make entry through the roof a slow process. Some roof panels gain strength from stamped-in contours, which rescuers can cut through with most standard extrication tools. Some manufacturers use fiberglass or plastic roof panels for access to equipment (such as heating, air conditioning and computer modules) housed under them. These roofs will be easier to penetrate. Depending upon the manufacturer, some vehicles may have one or more steel cross members under the panel. Rescuers will have to cut these cross members to remove the roof.

Floor entry. Rescuers may need to enter through the floor to remove the victim. Manufacturers equip some vehicles with a floor hatch for this purpose. However, due to the methods of construction, floor access is often virtually impossible.

Industrial and Agricultural Vehicle Extrication Tactics

The goal during the process of extricating the operator of an industrial or agricultural vehicle is to remove the vehicle from the victim without causing further injury. Likewise, if a victim is caught in a piece of machinery, rescuers must remove the machinery from around the victim.

Disentanglement. Because the vehicle's cab usually provides the vehicle's rollover protection system (ROPS), the strength of the structure can make freeing the operator extremely challenging **(Figure 12.21)**. Cutting or removing any part of an intact ROPS system may cause the vehicle to fall, injuring the victim and rescuers. Rescuers should cut any part of a ROPS only when necessary. When rescuers have applied sufficient force to deform these structural

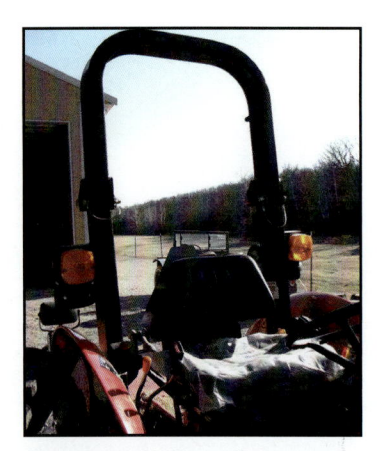

Figure 12.21 The rollover protection system (ROPS) on a tractor. *Courtesy of Alan Braun, University of Missouri Fire and Rescue Training Institute.*

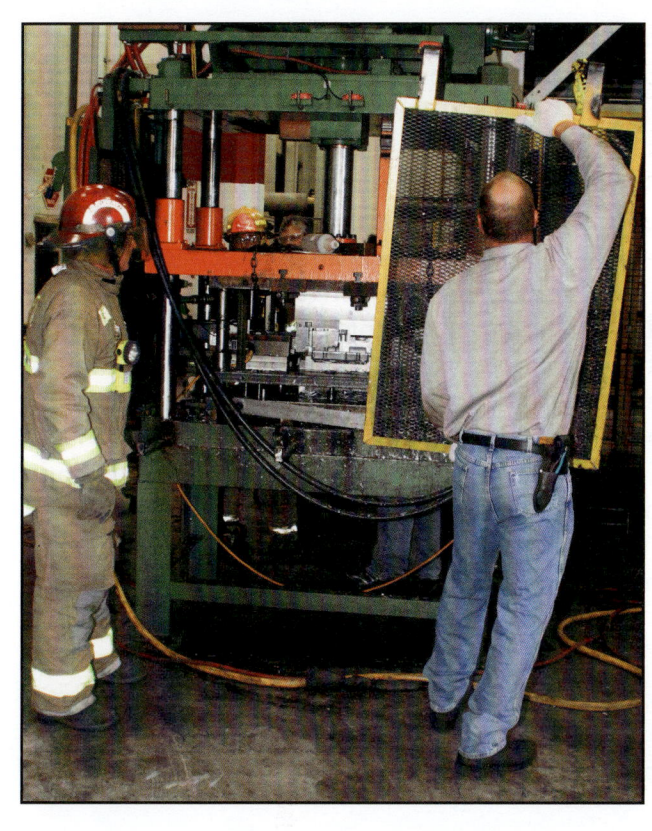

Figure 12.22 Machinery maintenance personnel can prove helpful in disassembling machinery components.

components and entrap the operator, rescuers may have to apply an equal amount of force to disentangle the victim. Otherwise, rescuers may have to dismantle the cab or ROPS. Rescuers most often need power spreaders, cutters, and extension rams.

If the victim is pinned under the cab or caught in some piece of machinery, the specifics of the situation will dictate the tools and techniques used. Whether caught in a conveyor chain, an auger, or in some other piece of equipment, rescuers must dismantle the equipment to free the victim **(Figure 12.22)**.

Victim removal. Removing an injured victim from inside the wrecked cab of an industrial or agricultural vehicle can be difficult because of the limited working room within the cab. There may only be enough room for one rescuer to enter the cab of the vehicle to assess, treat, stabilize, and package the patient for removal. In this situation, it may be faster (and less traumatic for the patient) to simply dismantle the cab before attempting extrication.

> **CAUTION**
> Cutting or removing part of an intact ROPS may cause unanticipated movement or sudden failure.

> **WARNING!**
> Unless it is deemed safe to do so by a subject matter expert, never reverse the machinery in an attempt to free the victim.

Section E • Chapter 12 – Special Extrication Situations

Power Take Off (PTO) Incidents

PTO shafts transmit power from a tractor or other power source to an implement. The two speeds commonly used with PTO shafts are 540 and 1,000 rpm. PTO shafts can wrap 424 feet (138 m) of rope in one minute at 540 rpm. At 1,000 rpm, a shaft can wrap 785 feet (239 m) of rope in one minute. This means a 540 rpm shaft can wrap a victim's extremity nine times a second, while a 1,000 rpm shaft can wrap a victim's extremity sixteen times a second. PTO shaft injuries range from minor lacerations to complete body dismemberment. PTO entanglement injuries can produce different injury patterns depending on the type of clothing the victim is wearing. Victims may have first and/or second degree burns, even if the PTO strips only the clothing from their body. Nylon and other synthetics tend to cut into skin and muscle tissue of a victim rather than rub across it. PTO shafts can grind away skin, muscles, tendons, and break bones when an unshielded PTO shaft entangles a victim. The tools required to rotate the PTO shaft backward may not be readily available and the victim may occupy the space required to disassemble the shaft.

Railcars

Rescuers may encounter railcar incidents. This section will cover the following topics:

- Types of railcars
- Railcar anatomy, construction, and features
- Railcar hazards
- Railcar stabilization
- Railcar extrication
- Railcar extrication situations

Types of Railcars

Trains use many different types of railcars. In the United States, the word **consist** is a document that identifies a group of railcars that make up a train. Passenger trains will have one or more locomotives, baggage cars, and passenger cars in the consist. Freight trains are composed of one or more locomotives and a string of freight cars. On freight trains, the only cars likely to contain victims are the locomotives, whereas passenger trains will likely have a high life hazard due to a significant number of crew and passengers **(Figure 12.23)**.

Rescue personnel who serve in areas where rail travel is common should familiarize themselves with the various types of railroad equipment common to their area. This section presents only general information about railcars. These railcars include the following:

- Locomotives
- Passenger cars
- Baggage cars
- Freight cars
- Material handling cars
- Lounge/food service cars

> **Consist** — Rail shipping paper that contains a list of cars in the train by order; indicates the cars that contain hazardous materials. Some railroads include information on emergency operations for the hazardous materials on board with the consist. *Also known as* Train Consist.

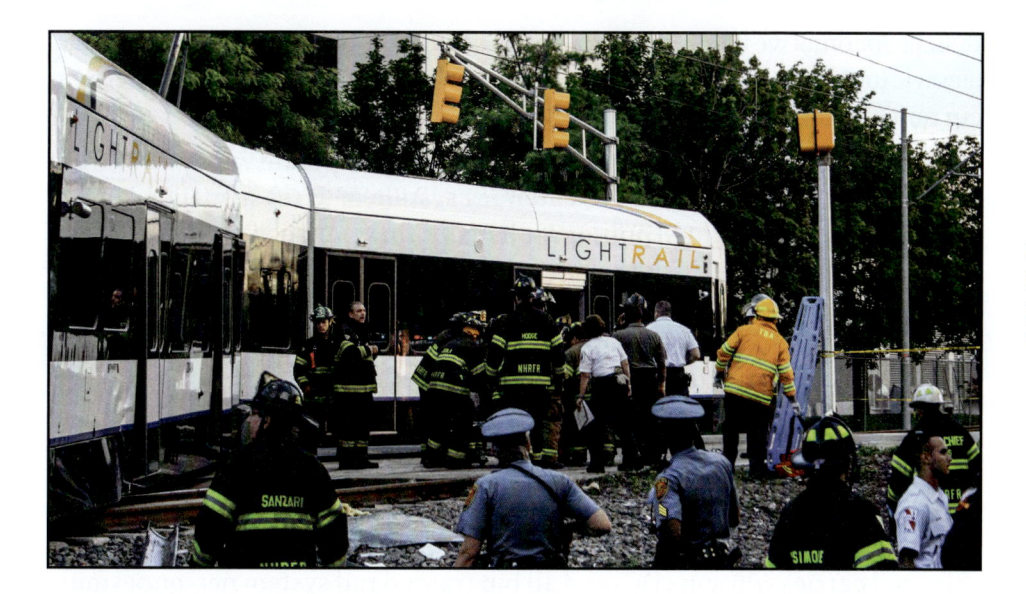

Figure 12.23 Rescuers need to check each section in a passenger train for possible victims. *Courtesy of Ron Jeffers.*

Locomotives

Locomotives are the engine for the train. Locomotives differ in how they are powered and how they are employed. The most common types of locomotives are:

- Diesel and diesel/electric locomotives
- Electric locomotives
- Steam locomotives

Diesel and diesel/electric locomotives. Some locomotives are powered by diesel engines only. Most of the locomotives in North America use a combination of diesel and electric power. Diesel engines operate onboard generators that power electric motors on each axle to drive the wheels. In addition to those used in main line operations, terminals and shop areas use many of these locomotives as switching engines.

Diesel/electric locomotives can weigh from 130 to 175 tons (120 to 160 T), develop as much as 4,250 horsepower, and carry between 1,800 to 2,200 gallons (7 200 to 8 800 L) of diesel fuel inside or under the locomotive **(Figure 12.24)**. Locomotives have a top speed of up to 125 mph (200 km/h). The volume of combustible diesel fuel carried by such locomotives present one type of hazard found during train incidents.

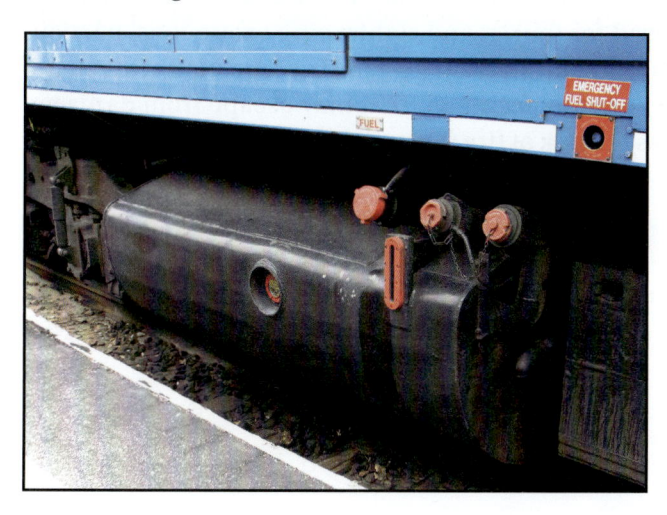

Figure 12.24 The fuel tanks on a diesel/electric locomotive. *Courtesy of Rich Mahaney.*

Section E • Chapter 12 – Special Extrication Situations   **465**

Catenary System — A series of overhead wires used to transmit electrical power to buses, locomotives, and trams at a distance from the energy supply point.

Pantograph — Need a definition

Each locomotive truck has two electric drive motors. While running, diesel/electric locomotives generate both high-and low-voltage AC and DC electrical current for train operation.

Electric locomotives. Most electric locomotives operate with power from a 12,000 volt AC to 25,000 volt AC **catenary system** of wires suspended above the tracks. A roof-mounted **pantograph** maintains contact with the overhead wires to provide power to the locomotive. The systems of electric locomotives have high voltage and present a danger of electrocution. These locomotives weigh as much as 100 tons (90 T), develop as much as 7,000 horsepower, and have a top speed of up to 150 mph (240 km/h).

NOTE: Both catenary systems and pantographs are discussed in greater detail later in this chapter.

Some trains have all-electric locomotives operated by power from an electrically charged third rail between or adjacent to the regular rails. This enclosed third rail carries 600 volts DC, and all but trained rail system personnel must avoid it.

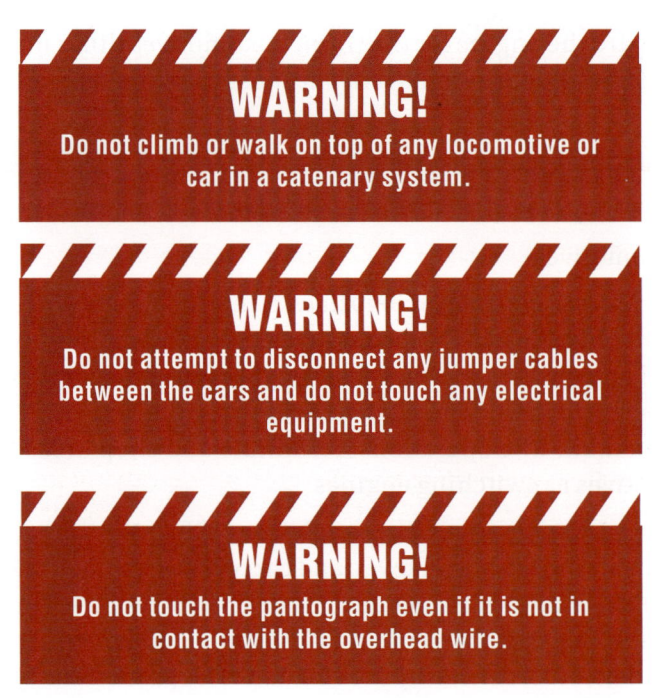

WARNING!
Do not climb or walk on top of any locomotive or car in a catenary system.

WARNING!
Do not attempt to disconnect any jumper cables between the cars and do not touch any electrical equipment.

WARNING!
Do not touch the pantograph even if it is not in contact with the overhead wire.

Steam locomotives. While rare, some areas still use steam locomotives. These locomotives are used for tourist and sightseeing excursions, particularly in Colorado, California, and Arizona. Hazards associated with steam locomotives include the potential for steam that may escape from damaged piping or boilers as well as the risk of fire from the unit used to heat the boiler **(Figure 12.25)**.

Passenger Cars
Rail systems operate a variety of passenger cars, such as:

- Coach cars
- Coach dome cars
- High-level cars
- Sleeping cars

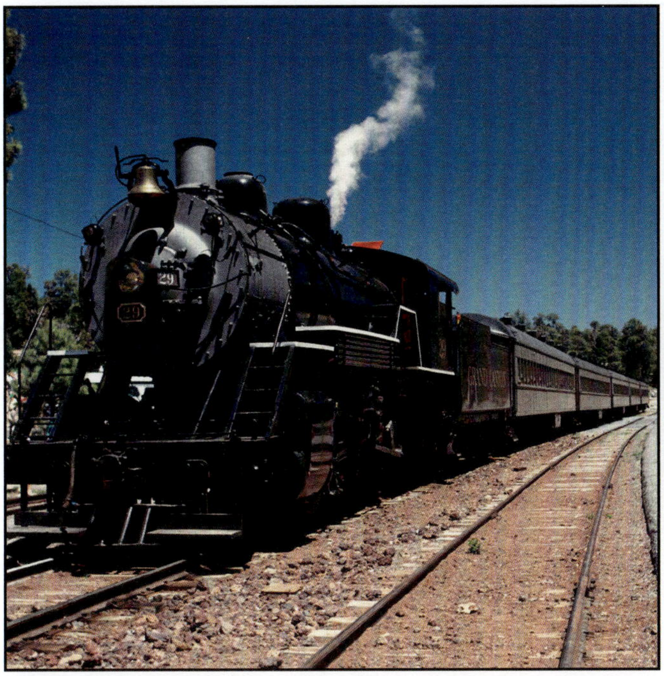

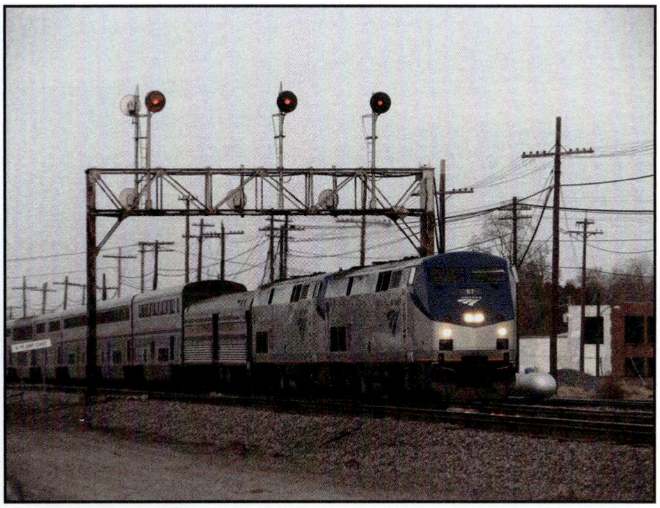

Figure 12.26 A common passenger train. *Courtesy of Rich Mahaney.*

Figure 12.25 A steam engine used for sightseeing excursions. *Courtesy of Bill Accord.*

These passenger cars provide seating space for between 44 and 85 passengers, depending on the layout of the cars **(Figure 12.26).** High-level cars provide two levels of passenger space. Some coach cars also provide crew sleeping space. The 85-passenger coaches have seating facilities for passengers with disabilities. These coaches are usually the last in the consist, and some contain secondary controls that allow conductors to operate the train in reverse from the last car without turning the train around.

Sleeper cars provide passengers with seating room and sleeping accommodations. Some sleepers also provide day time private rooms for first-class passengers. These cars are normally located either toward the front or rear of the train.

Passengers and crew members may be present in passenger cars during train operation. Rescuers should check all sleeping/bedroom, seating, and toilet areas for victims during rescue operations **(Figure 12.27).**

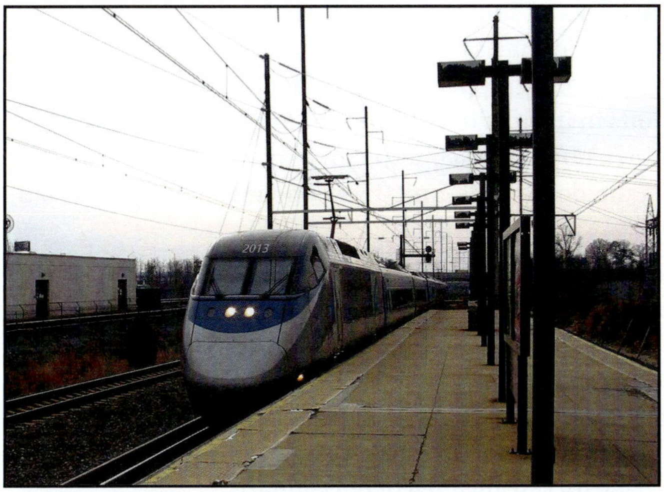

Figure 12.27 A high-speed passenger train. *Courtesy of Rich Mahaney.*

Section E • Chapter 12 – Special Extrication Situations **467**

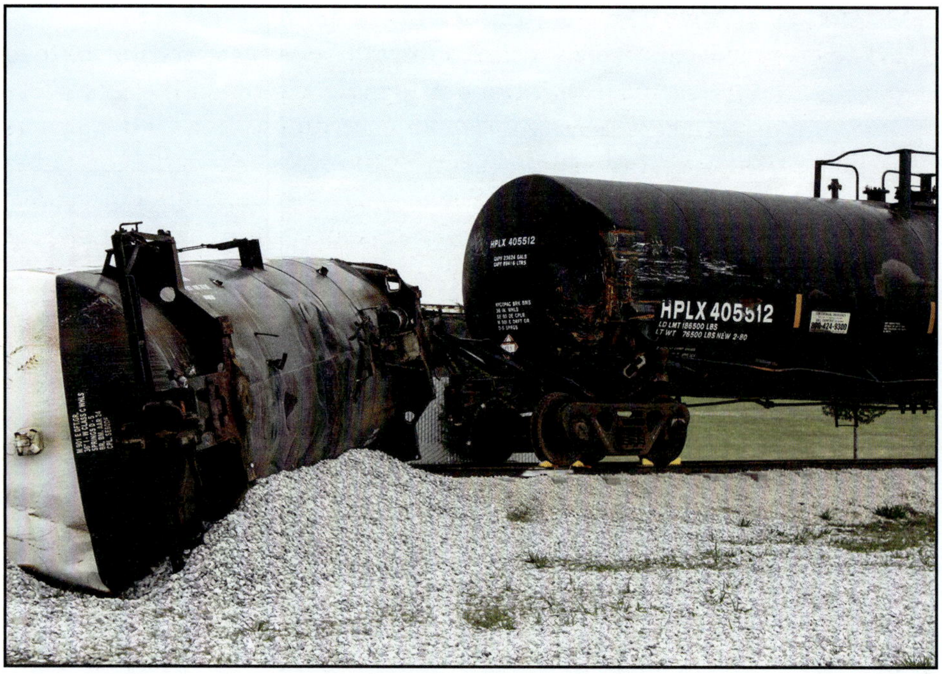

Figure 12.28 A freight train accident scene.

Baggage Cars

The baggage car transports passenger baggage. Some coach/baggage cars provide upper level coach space for passengers and space on a lower level for transporting baggage. These cars are normally located directly behind the locomotive at the front of the consist. An assistant conductor may be present in the car during train operation. Therefore, it is essential that rescuers check all areas of the car for crew members during rescue operations.

Freight Cars

Freight cars include flat cars, box cars, hopper cars, tank cars, and a number of other specialized cars. In addition to hauling lumber, steel, and similar products, flatcars also carry semitrailers and huge intermodal shipping containers. Freight cars do not carry passengers, meaning rescue personnel should only have to conduct extrication operations on a freight car if it has come to rest on top of an occupied passenger vehicle or railroad passenger car.

The contents of freight cars and shipping containers can greatly complicate any incident. A derailed tank car that is leaking a flammable, corrosive, or toxic liquid threatens rescue personnel, trapped victims, and the environment. Even if the load is not hazardous in itself, if tons of lumber or thousands of boxes or other containers are strewn about the scene, it can make all phases of the operation much more difficult, dangerous, and time consuming **(Figure 12.28)**.

Material Handling Cars

Material handling cars are essentially standard boxcars used for carrying baggage and mail. They are usually located directly behind the locomotive or at the end of the consist. In addition to having side doors only, these cars have plug doors that operators must pull outward before sliding laterally. Material handling cars are usually unoccupied during train operation, but rescuers must check these cars to verify the absence of passengers.

Lounge/Food Service Cars

Also known as club cars or dining cars, lounge/food service cars provide food and beverage service and entertainment to passengers aboard trains. Some lounge/food service cars include an upper level dining area for passengers as well as a food preparation area in the lower level of the same car. Other configurations also provide limited passenger coach space. Full-dome lounge cars provide food and beverage service for passengers and crew members, as well as a panoramic view. These cars are normally located in the center of the consist. Passengers and crew members may be present in these areas during train operation. Rescuers should check all dining, bar, and food storage areas for passengers and crew members during rescue operations.

Railcar Anatomy, Construction, and Features

Regardless of what types of railcars are involved in an incident, they all have similar anatomy, construction, and features, such as the following:

- Railcar doors
- Railcar windows
- Railcar floors
- Railcar walls and roofs
- Railcar trucks
- Railcar brakes
- Railcar electrical systems
- Catenary systems
- Third-rail systems
- Roadbeds

Railcar Doors

All railroad passenger cars have end doors **(Figure 12.29)**. These doors either swing inward or slide sideways to open. Most sliding doors are power assisted, either electrically or electro-pneumatically. In case of power failure, they easily slide open manually. Car end doors are not locked during train operation and function normally while the train is in motion.

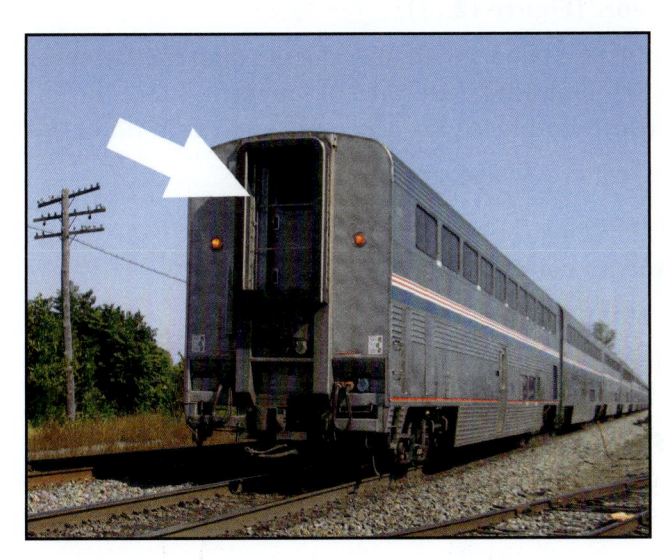

Figure 12.29 An example of an end door on a passenger railcar. *Courtesy of Rich Mahaney.*

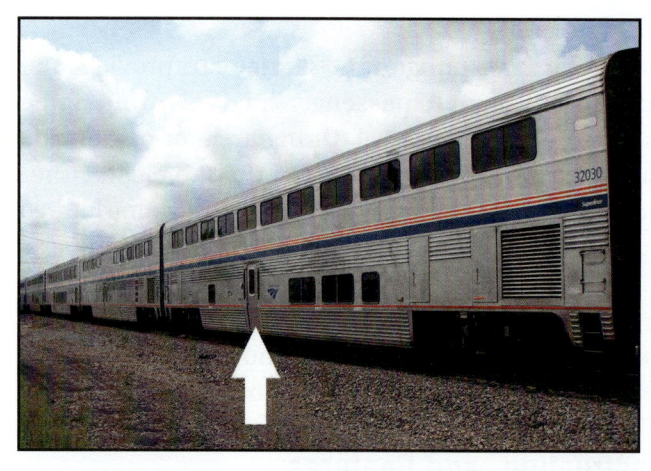

Figure 12.30 A side entry door on a passenger railcar. *Courtesy of Rich Mahaney.*

Some passenger cars also have side-entry doors located at both ends of each car **(Figure 12.30)**. These pocket doors slide sideways into the car body to open. Other passenger cars have inward-swinging side-entry doors located in the center of the car. Because these doors are closed and automatically locked during train operation, rescuers may have to force entry through them following a collision and/or derailment.

Railcar Windows

Railroad passenger cars have windows along the full length of both sides of the car. Some have an upper and lower row, and they may be any of several different styles. Manufacturers use two different window pane materials: **Lexan®** plastic and tempered glass. The type of pane used will vary on different types of cars.

Each car usually has at least four of these window exits (two on each side) and some have more. These windows have double panes — the outer pane is either Lexan® or tempered glass, but the inner pane is always Lexan®.

Railcar Floors

Rescuers may need to gain entry through a railcar floor if a car comes to rest on its side or roof. The floor framing is usually constructed of tubular steel or aluminum attached to the railcar frame. Most passenger railcar floors are composed of ply-metal (plywood and metal, usually aluminum) panels that are attached to the framework **(Figure 12.31)**.

Manufacturers usually insulate floors with fiberglass insulation and cover them with carpet and resilient matting materials. Rescuers may face the following obstructions when attempting to gain access through a car floor:

- Utility lines such as gas, water, sewage, and electric
- Train brake system air lines
- Heating, ventilation, and air conditioning (HVAC) units
- Water and waste water storage tanks
- Electrical generators attached to the underside of a car

Railcar Walls and Roofs

Most railcars have exterior skins made of 3/32-inch (2 mm) stainless steel. Other cars have an aluminum skin. In many cases, the wall construction consists

> **Lexan®** — Polycarbonate plastic used for windows; has one-half the weight of an equivalent-sized piece of glass, yet is 30 times stronger than safety glass and 250 times stronger than ordinary glass. It cannot be broken using standard forcible entry techniques.

Train Floor Construction

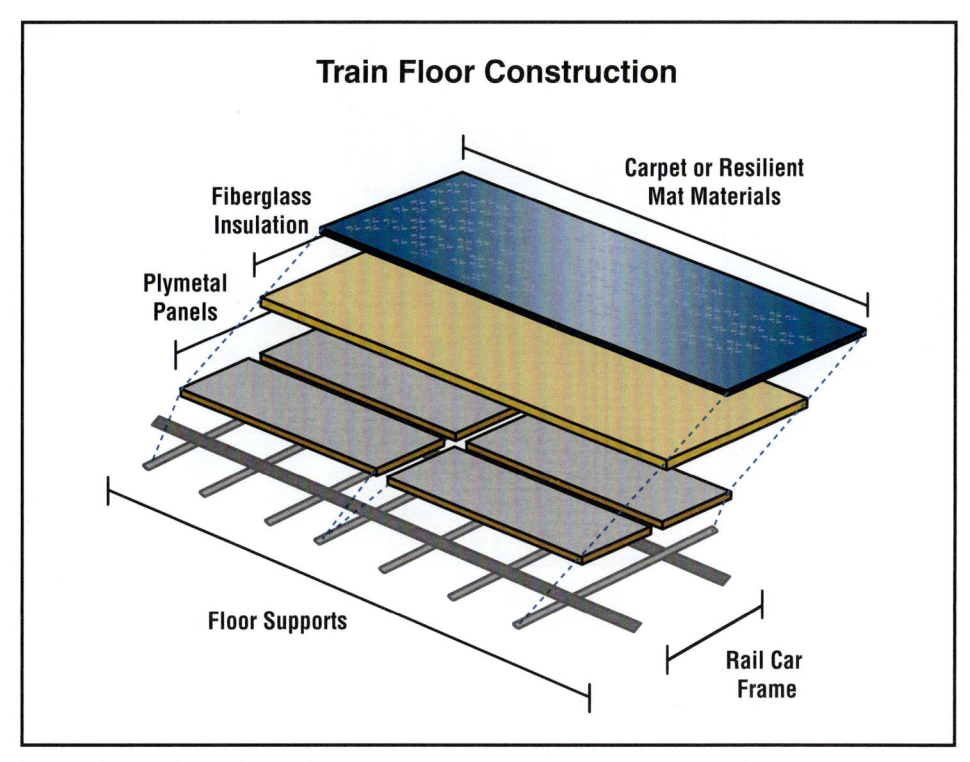

Figure 12.31 Examples of the components used to construct railcar floors.

of steel framing members and plywood sandwiched between two sheets of stainless steel or aluminum. Manufacturers place heavy-duty framing members 12 to 24 inches (300 to 600 mm) on center in the walls, floors, and roof structure. They may also cover roofs with a thin fiberglass skin. Locomotive walls are made from three eigth inch (9 mm) thick steel; the roof is made from one eighth inch (3 mm) steel.

Railcar Trucks

Trucks, also called railroad trucks, are the assemblies to which a railcar's wheel axles are attached. Trucks are constructed of cast steel and can weigh up to 7 tons (6 T). These assemblies are made up of the wheels, suspension, and braking system.

Railcar Brakes

Firefighters and other rescue personnel need to be familiar with the operation of the hand brakes on freight cars. On level tracks, applying the hand brake may be all rescuers need to do to stabilize a car. Braking systems are operated by air pressure up to 140 psi (980 kPa). Rescuers should not attempt to disconnect the airlines prior to shutting off the air supply at the knuckle on the end of the car, as serious injury or death may result.

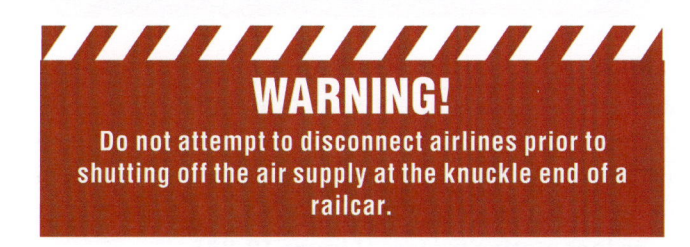

WARNING!
Do not attempt to disconnect airlines prior to shutting off the air supply at the knuckle end of a railcar.

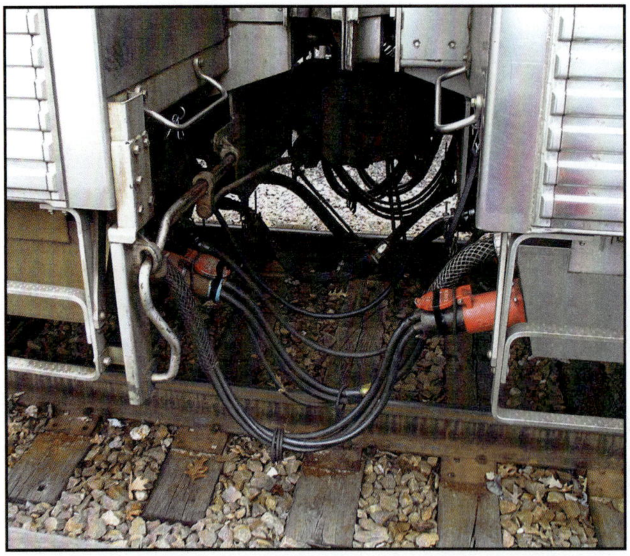

Figure 12.32 Electrical power jumper cable between railcars. *Courtesy of Rich Mahaney.*

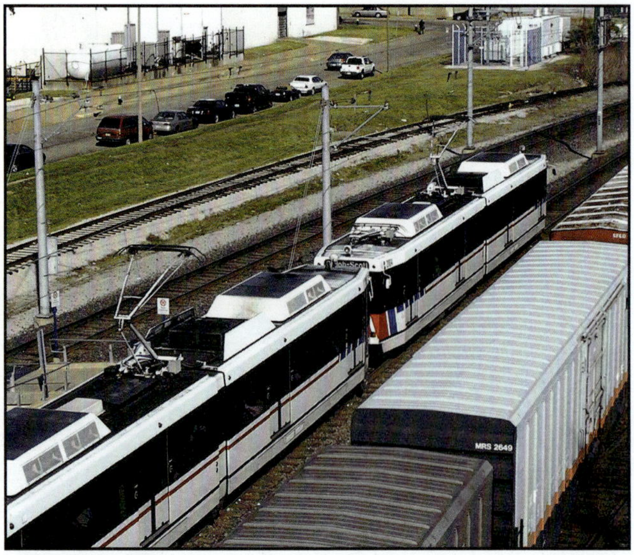

Figure 12.33 A catenary wire system and roof-mounted pantograph on an electric powered rail system. *Courtesy of Bill Accord.*

Railcar Electrical Systems

All railcars are equipped with 480-volt electrical circuits charged by power from the locomotive, commonly called head-end power. An overhead catenary system, a third rail, or diesel generators aboard the locomotive may supply the power. Jumper cables connected between each car supply power to the individual cars **(Figure 12.32)**. Rescue personnel should not remove or attempt to remove these cables. Only trained passenger rail system crew members can safely perform the following actions:

- De-energize head-end power
- Lower locomotive pantographs
- Disengage third-rail shoes
- Ground electrical equipment when required
- Remove or install power cables

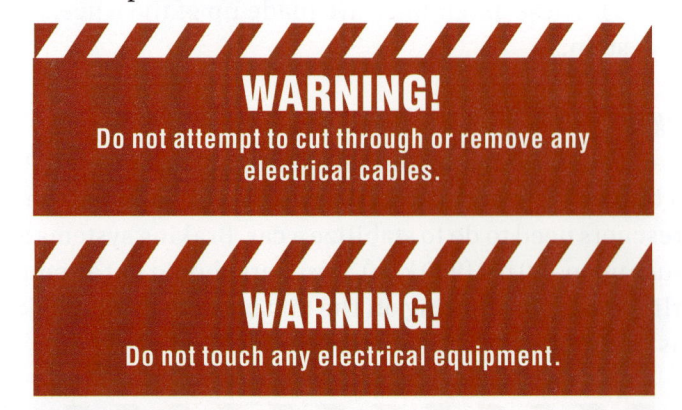

WARNING!
Do not attempt to cut through or remove any electrical cables.

WARNING!
Do not touch any electrical equipment.

Catenary Systems

The overhead **catenary system** consists of longitudinal wires and cables suspended from poles that hold an electrically charged trolley wire in a firm position above the track. The **pantograph** mounted on top of the locomotive maintains contact with the trolley wires to conduct 12,000 volts to 25,000 volts AC, 25 Hz, to the locomotive motors **(Figure 12.33)**.

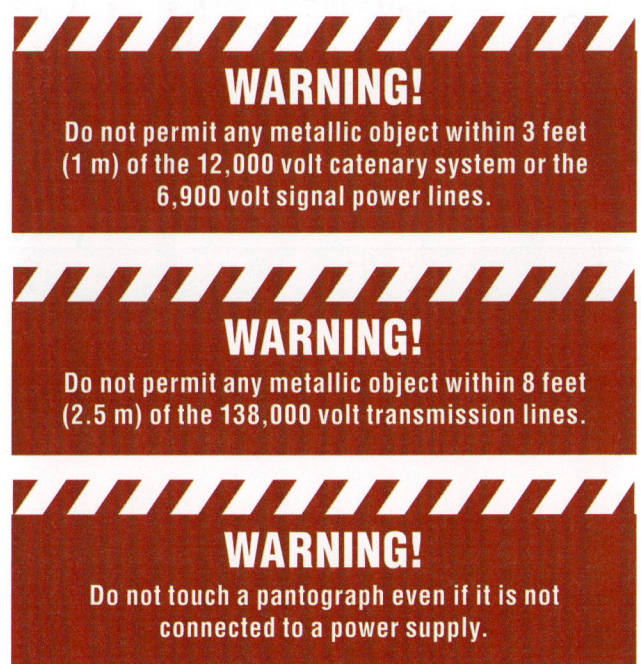

Catenary poles are 14-inch (350 mm) square steel H-sections weighing 84 pounds per foot (12.5 kg/m). They range in height from 70 to 170 feet (20 to 50 m). At the top of each pole is a ground wire located approximately 9 feet (3 m) above the transmission conductors. The ground wire is a return for the propulsion current and protects the transmission line from lightning strikes. Approximately 3 feet (1 m) down from the ground wire are the transmission cross arms, 18 feet (5.5 m) across, and held level by sag rods. Below these cross arms are two transmission lines energized at 138,000 volts.

On one side of the pole is a signal power line energized at 6,900 volts, 100 Hz. The signal line is a transmission line between substations to locations along the right-of-way **(Figure 12.34, p. 474)**. There, it is transformed into various voltages to feed signals, track circuits, and other equipment.

The trolley wires above the tracks are supported between the body span by three units of 10-inch (250 mm) disk-type insulators. Immediately below the insulators is a longitudinal messenger wire. Below this is an auxiliary messenger wire supported by bronze hanger rods. Below the auxiliary wire is the contact or trolley wire, supported from the auxiliary messenger by clips spaced 15 feet (4.5 m) apart. All wires and hardware of the catenary system are energized at a very high voltage, for example 12,000 volts.

Substations on the system are spaced 8 to 10 miles (13 to 16 km) apart. These substations contain power control apparatus for the catenary system, the signal power line, and the transmission line. Firefighters and other rescue personnel should not enter these facilities unless accompanied by qualified rail systems employees.

Under no circumstances should any object contact these wires. Materials such as wood, rope, and clothing that might be considered nonconductive at low voltages are not safe for use in close proximity to high-voltage wires. These materials conduct electricity at higher voltages.

NOTE: Rescuers should follow minimum space requirements for the protection zone or space to keep electricity from arcing into an object at a specific voltage.

> **WARNING!**
> Do not permit any metallic object within 3 feet (1 m) of the 12,000 volt catenary system or the 6,900 volt signal power lines.

> **WARNING!**
> Do not permit any metallic object within 8 feet (2.5 m) of the 138,000 volt transmission lines.

> **WARNING!**
> Do not touch a pantograph even if it is not connected to a power supply.

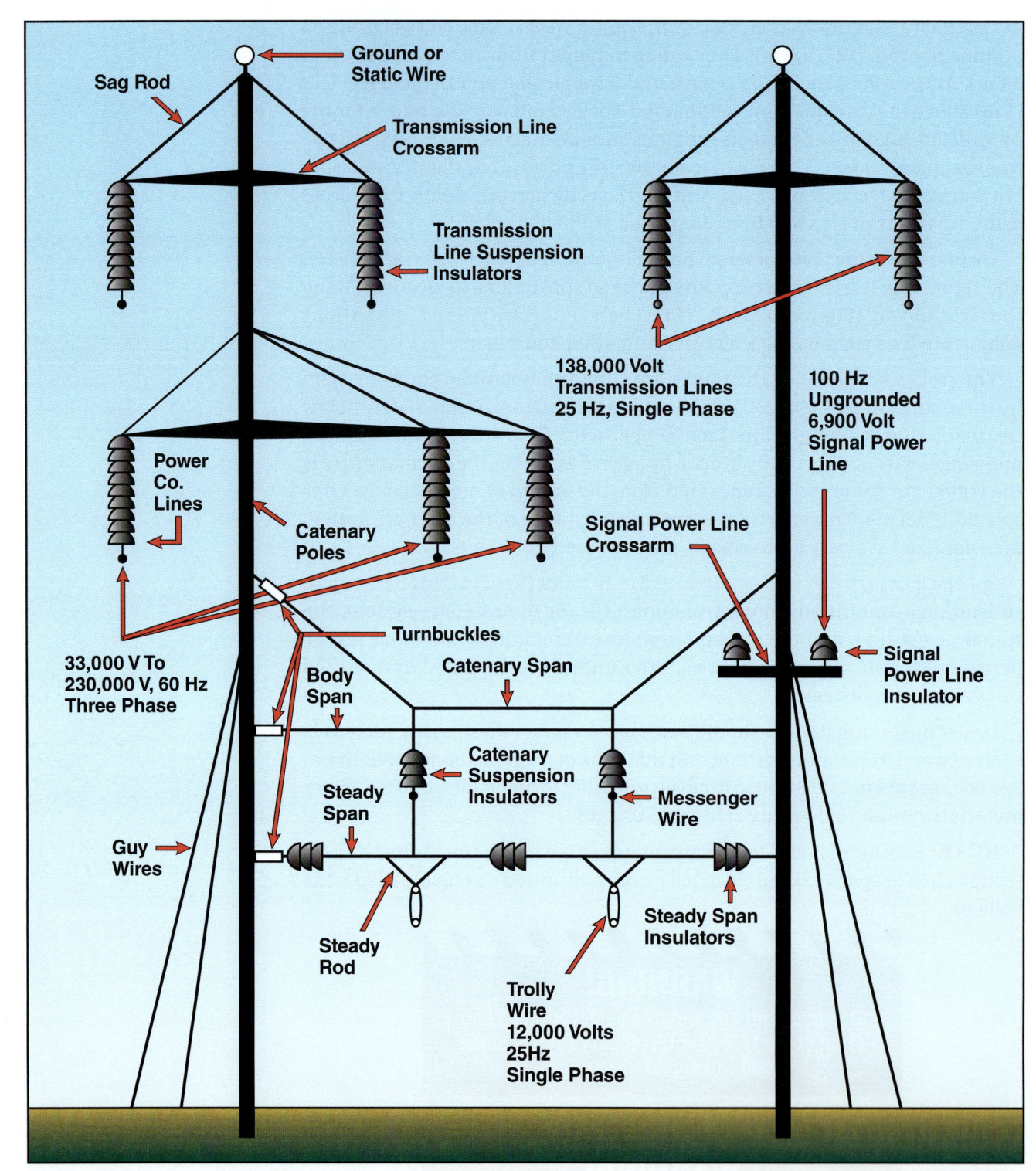

Figure 12.34 Catenary poles and wires.

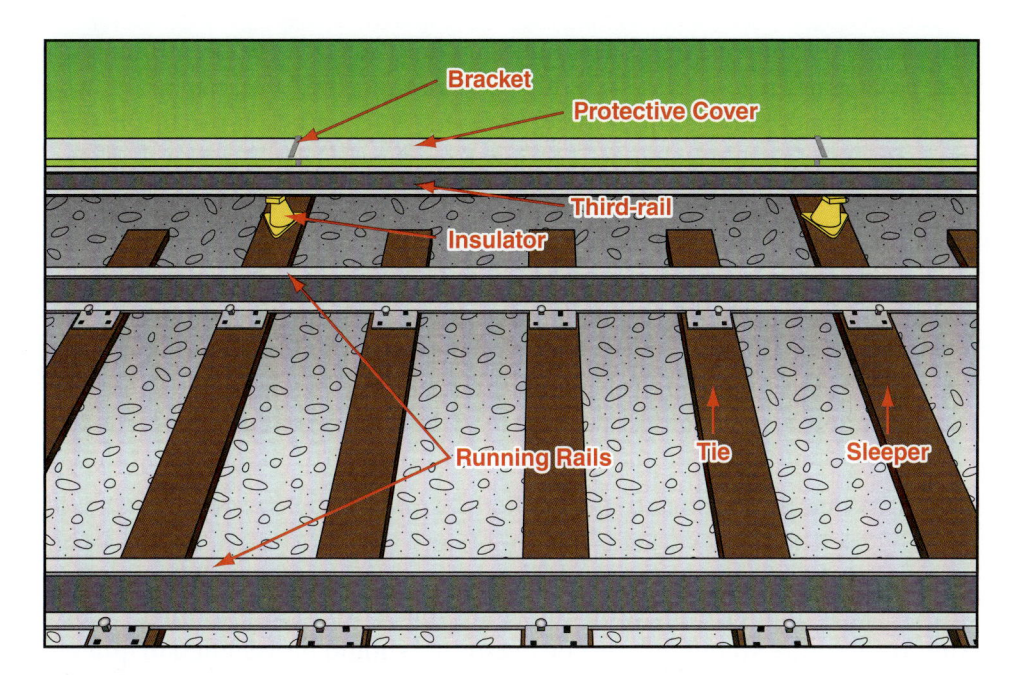

Figure 12.35 A third-rail electric system.

Third-Rail Systems

Third-rail electrical-power distribution systems generally distribute 600-volt DC current. The third rail is usually located slightly above and to the side of the two regular rails on which the train's wheels run. No one should touch a third rail or its protective cover **(Figure 12.35)**.

Roadbeds

Although some percentage of all roadbeds are at grade level, especially in switching yards and loading/unloading areas, much of their length is not. The rails and crossties are set atop a berm that allows the roadbed to be more-or-less level throughout its length. To discourage the growth of vegetation along the roadbed, and thereby reduce the risk of fires, the spaces between the cross ties and down both sides of the berm are covered with coarse gravel **(Figure 12.36)**.

The steeply sloped sides of the roadbed embankment and the loose gravel make traction and footing difficult. Therefore, gaining access and stabilizing crashed vehicles may present rescuers with far more difficulties than other locations. The slope of the embankment and the lack of traction may make it difficult to position rescue vehicles close to the scene. It may be necessary to lay ground ladders on the slopes of the berm to provide secure footing for rescue personnel.

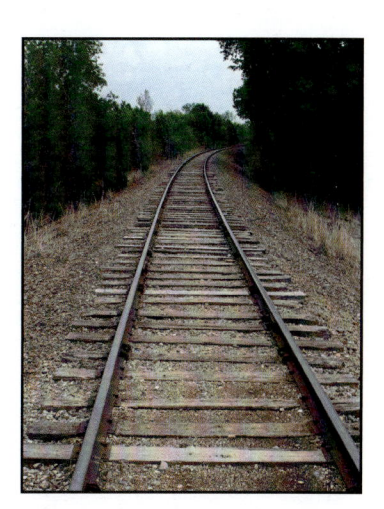

Figure 12.36 A common railroad bed

Railcar Incident Size-Up

As with any other type of vehicle incident, rescuers should assess (size up) train incidents in a systematic way. First, they should assess the scene, followed by an assessment of the vehicles involved. Then, rescuers should assess the victims and the extrication requirements for that particular incident. As always, size-up continues throughout the incident.

Once on scene, the first responders must determine if a legitimate emergency exists. If so, the ranking responder should assume command of the incident and begin a more thorough assessment of the vehicles involved. As with other types of vehicle incidents, the incident commander (IC) must try to determine the number of vehicles involved and their conditions. In the derailment of a long passenger train, scene assessment can be daunting. With railcars resting at various angles and positions along both sides of the track, it can be difficult to see the entire scene from one location. How the cars came to rest — wheel-resting, side-resting, roof-resting — will dictate how much and what types of cribbing materials rescuers will need.

Diesel/electric locomotives can carry up to 2,200 gallons (8 800 L) of diesel fuel in tanks located inside the locomotive or underneath it. Fuel shutoff devices (clearly marked FUEL SHUT OFF) are located on each side of the locomotive body side rails and on the firewall of the cab behind the engineer. To shut off the fuel supply to the engine, push and hold the emergency fuel shutoff device for 8 to 10 seconds. The engine will stop running within about one minute.

In situations presenting a high likelihood of mass casualties, rescuers should prioritize setting up for triage, treatment, and transportation. Before stabilizing train cars, rescuers should question any passengers who have escaped the wreckage about the location and condition of others still trapped inside. After the cars are stabilized, rescue personnel should be assigned to quickly but thoroughly search all cars and triage the passengers trapped inside. The number and condition of the victims may indicate a need for additional and varied medical transport units and resources.

Based on the specifics of the crash — the number of cars involved and their conditions and the number of trapped victims and their conditions — rescuers must determine how much and what types of extrication resources they will need. Assessment questions should include:

- Are there a sufficient number of power spreaders, cutters, and similar equipment available on scene?
- Is there a need for cutting torches, plasma cutters, or burning bars?
- Is there a need for additional personnel to allow more tasks to be performed at the same time or for crew relief if the incident becomes protracted?
- Is there a need for a full rehabilitation unit if the incident becomes protracted?

For incidents involving passenger trains, rescuers will need to triage patients carefully to determine who requires immediate medical treatment and who can wait for treatment. These triage efforts will assist in determining medical transportation requirements. The rescue agency should establish a standard operating procedure (SOP) for train incident triage during preincident planning.

The IC should consider contacting the railroad company dispatcher to stop other rail traffic from entering the area. In areas not controlled with signals or dispatchers, the IC should place flare flaggers up to two miles away on either side of the incident. These flaggers should swing the flare from side-to-side in an arc at arm's length. Engineers will stop the train upon seeing this signal.

Railcar Hazards

The primary hazard associated with electric locomotives is the high voltage involved in such systems and the danger of electrocution. Most operate with power from a 12,000 to 25,000 volt AC catenary system of wires suspended above the tracks. A roof-mounted pantograph maintains contact with the overhead wires to provide power to the locomotive.

> **WARNING!**
> Do not touch the pantograph even if it is not in contact with the overhead wire.

The catenary system can present a significant electrical hazard to rescuers. The pantograph on top of each car conducts electrical power from the overhead wires to the car. When an electrical hazard does exist, qualified personnel can press the "Pantograph Down" button in the locomotive control cab and ground the locomotive to disconnect the overhead power supply **(Figure 12.37)**. Rail system crew members usually do this before emergency responders arrive. If it has not been done, rescuers should see that properly qualified personnel do it.

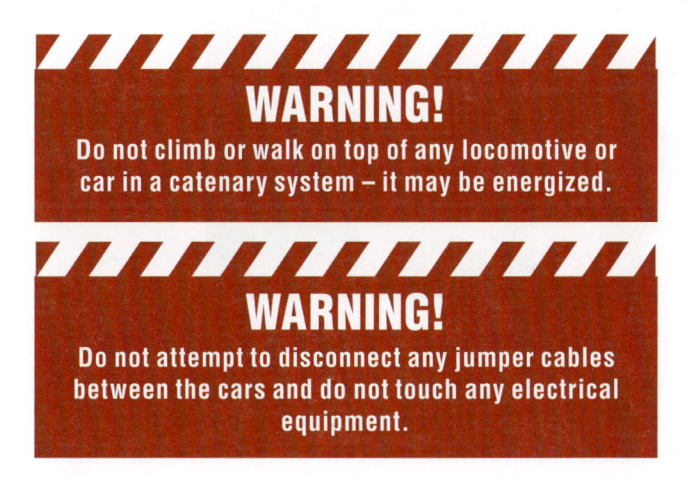

> **WARNING!**
> Do not climb or walk on top of any locomotive or car in a catenary system – it may be energized.

> **WARNING!**
> Do not attempt to disconnect any jumper cables between the cars and do not touch any electrical equipment.

If there is no obvious electrical hazard following a collision and/or derailment on a catenary line, the overhead power should not be disconnected. Electrical power will provide for lighting and electric door operation.

Power from an electrically charged third rail between or adjacent to the regular rails operates some all-electric locomotives. This enclosed third rail carries 600 volts DC, and all but trained personnel must avoid it. Third-rail systems require a different isolation approach. These highly specialized systems typically require the appropriate power director/dispatcher or other specialty personnel to de-energize. These systems also have installed emergency switch boxes, but only personnel from those agencies having direct authority from the local train authority should use them.

As stated earlier, some sightseeing and tourist adventures still use steam locomotives. Hazards associated with steam locomotives include the potential for hot steam that may escape from damaged piping or boiler as well as the risk of fire from the unit used to heat the boiler.

Railcar Stabilization

Railcars are generally stable because of their substantial size and weight. However, following a collision and/or derailment, some of the cars may have come to rest in unstable positions. Rescuers may need to stabilize the cars to protect trapped and injured victims and to provide a safe working environment for rescue personnel. Because much of the equipment used to stabilize

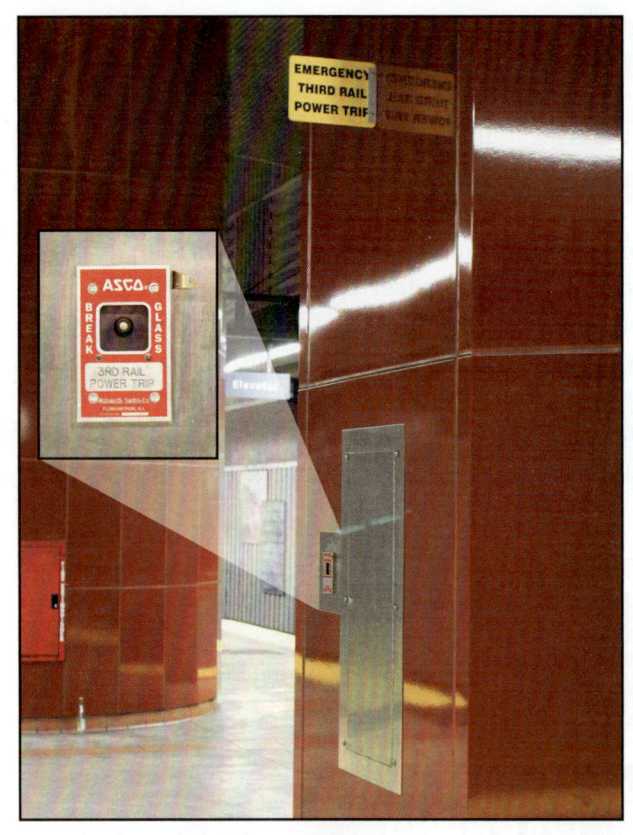

Figure 12.37 An example of an emergency power shut off system switch for a third-rail electrical system. *Courtesy of Robert J. Tremberth*

highway vehicles will be of limited value when trying to stabilize these massive vehicles, determining how to stabilize railcars can be a tremendous challenge. However, the survival of both the trapped victims and rescue personnel depends upon rescuers performing this critical operation quickly and effectively. Normal cribbing will not have sufficient size or strength to handle railroad emergencies. If railroad ties are available at the scene, they may be used as cribbing for stabilization **(Figure 12.38)**.

Stabilizing Wheel-Resting Railcars

Because the majority of the weight of most railcars is concentrated in the lower third of their structure, wheel-resting railcars that are still on the tracks are relatively stable. If a car is still wheel-resting but off the tracks and subject to sliding or rolling down the side of the roadbed embankment, then it may

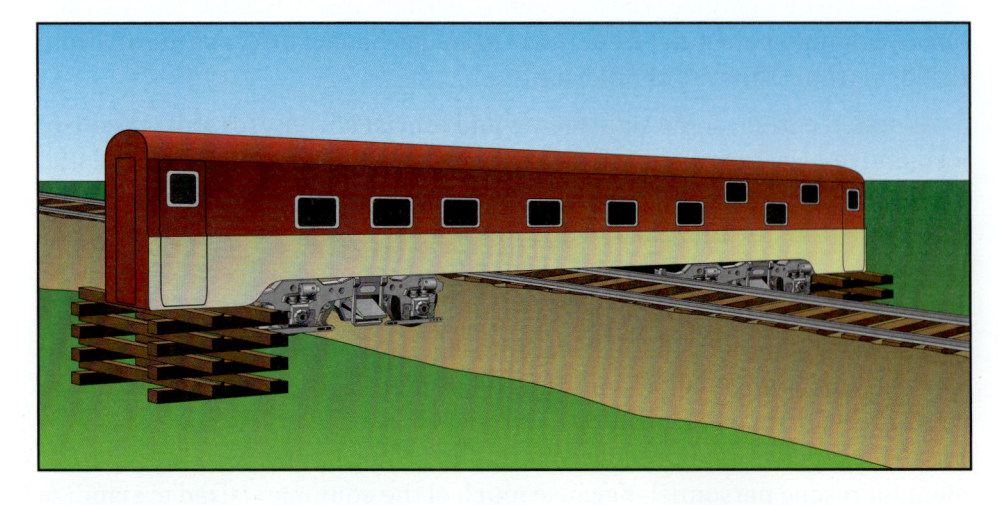

Figure 12.38 Railroad ties can be used by rescuers to construct cribbing to stabilize railcars.

478   Section E • Chapter 12 – Special Extrication Situations require extensive stabilization. Rescuers should apply the railcar's brake to limit movement of the car.

Stabilizing Side-Resting Railcars
Unless affected by slope or similar environmental influences, a railcar on its side is stable. The shape, size, and weight of most railcars make it unlikely that they will move suddenly when resting on their sides on a stable and level surface.

However, if the car is resting on mud, snow, or unstable soil, rescue personnel must exercise caution. Under these conditions, the car may suddenly roll back upright without warning. To reduce this possibility, rescuers should stabilize the car with shoring from the underside.

Stabilizing Roof-Resting Railcars
Because a railcar is top heavy when resting on its roof, this position can be unstable. Unless its movement is limited by an adjacent embankment and/or leaning against other railcars, a car on its roof may suddenly roll to one side or the other. Rescuers should secure the car with webbing, chains, or heavy ropes, before allowing personnel close enough to install cribbing along both sides.

Stabilizing Railcars in Other Positions
The inertial forces involved in many train derailments leave railcars resting in a zigzag pattern, with the forward cars stacked upon each other. Stabilizing several cars at the same time can be difficult. Only the specific situation can dictate which car rescuers should stabilize first and how they should accomplish that stabilization. As mentioned earlier, rescuers may need to stabilize cars to prevent them from sliding or rolling down a steep embankment or into a body of water. Cars that have overridden other cars may need to be stabilized to prevent them from sliding or falling off the cars beneath them. Unlike highway vehicle incidents, the time that rescuers would be need to install a sufficient amount of rigging and heavy shoring to stabilize these railcars may eliminate this as an option. Instead, if heavy construction vehicles are available, they can place their bucket, blade, or articulating arm against the sides of the cars to provide temporary stabilization.

Railcar Access and Egress
When performing extrication on railcars, rescuers should consider the following:
- Railcar access
- Height considerations
- Locomotive entry
- Passenger car door entry
- Passenger car window entry
- Passenger car roof/wall entry
- Interior door locks/latches
- Lounge/food service car entry
- Baggage car entry
- Material handling car entry

Railcar Access

Once rescuer personnel have stabilized the railcars, they can enter the cars for search and rescue. Because of the relative ease of access and egress, using a railcar's doors is better than using the windows for extricating victims. Even if a railcar is on its side or on its roof, the door openings will still allow the easiest passage into and out of the car. If all doorways are blocked, then rescuers will have to remove the victims through the windows. As a last resort, rescuers can remove victims through openings cut in the walls or roof of the car. The following sections describe these entry points in some detail.

Height Considerations

The height of the roadbed above grade, the steepness of the sides of the **berm**, and the poor footing afforded by the loose gravel covering the berm, may force rescue personnel to lay ground ladders on the sides of the berm just to reach the roadbed. Where a paved road parallels the railroad, it may allow rescuers to position an aerial device on the roadway to allow the use of the main ladder or articulating boom to reach the roadbed. Once on the roadbed, rescuers may need ladders to reach the doors and windows of the railcars.

Even when the roadbed is at grade, the height of the railcar doors and windows may require rescue personnel to use their ingenuity to create stable working platforms for extrication operations. If immediately available, rescuers can erect conventional aluminum scaffolding beside a railcar and move it along from car to car as needed. Rescuers can use wooden planks between two stepladders as a makeshift scaffold. A flatbed truck or a fire engine positioned beside a railcar can provide a relatively large, stable platform from which to work, and rescuers can move it from car to car as needed. If railcars are stacked rescuers may need ground ladders and/or aerial devices to reach the necessary access points.

Locomotive Entry

Most locomotive cabs have two doors on each side. Some models have an additional door in the nose. To open almost all locomotive cab doors, turn the door latch and push inward. These doors are not locked during train operation, so rescue personnel should not need to force entry following a collision and/or derailment.

Because the cab doors on most locomotives are too narrow to accommodate many standard rescue boards, rescuers may need to remove the locomotive windshield or side windows and pass injured crew members out through the opening. Side door and sliding cab windows are single panes of either Lexan® or tempered glass that slide sideways to open and are not usually locked. Some locomotive windshields are single-pane, laminated safety glass; others are Lexan®. The windshield is over one half-inch (12.5 mm) thick and is held in place by a heavy frame system. It is time consuming and labor intensive to remove. If rescuers cannot gain through the side windows, they should remove any windshield protector and then remove the windshield. If rescuers cannot make entry through the windows or doors, they should use the one eighth inch (3 mm) steel roof as the next option.

Berm — Outside or downhill side of a ditch or trench; a mound or wall of earth.

Passenger Car Door Entry

All railroad passenger cars have end doors, and some have side-entry vestibule doors. Rescuers should first attempt to enter through these doors. The following sections provide more detailed information about exterior entry doors on passenger cars.

Passenger coach end doors. Passenger coach end doors normally remain unlocked during train operation and will likely remain so following a collision or derailment. If not, the majority have manually operated latches. Some end doors have push plates or bars marked "PUSH TO OPEN" or "PRESS." These push plates activate an electric or electro-pneumatic power assist opening device. If this device is not operable, the door can be opened manually by either pushing it inward or sliding it sideways. Power-assisted end doors have power cut-out switches on both sides of the door, permitting door operation during malfunctions and emergencies. Rescuers may unlock lockable end door latches with a standard railcar coach key obtainable from a crew member.

Passenger car side-entry doors. Some passenger coaches, sleepers, and lounge/food service cars also have side-entry vestibule doors. Some of these doors are manually operated and pneumatically locked. These doors are automatically locked by an inflatable weather seal that releases when the door handle is pulled, opening the latch. If the seals do not deflate, open the ceiling panel directly above the door on the public address system locker side, and open the door seal cut-out valve. This allows the manual opening of both doors in that vestibule.

Other side-entry doors are electrically actuated and locked. To open them, rescuers should obtain a standard railcar coach key from a crew member. If electrical power is still on to the door circuits, the door will slide open. If the power is off, grasp the outside door indentation and push it sideways. To open these doors from the inside, rescuers or passenger may pull down on the door lock handle located in a ceiling recess above the door. To open the door, slide it sideways.

Some side-entry doors may be opened from outside the car by opening the door seal cut-out valve located under the car adjacent to the door. Preferably, a trained railcar crew member should perform this function to ensure that nearby air brake lines remain operative.

While many side-entry vestibule doors slide sideways to open, the side-entry doors on some other cars swing inward to open. These doors are closed and latched during train operation. When unlatched, the door can be opened manually. If the door is jammed, open the door window using the latch handle in the frame.

Passenger Car Window Entry

While most passenger coaches have relatively small side windows measuring 29½ inches wide by 16½ inches high (737 mm by 412 mm), the Talgo coaches have larger side windows that measure 63 inches wide by 39 inches high (1.6 by 1 m). With the glass completely removed, these windows offer adequate clearance for most backboards and litters.

As described earlier in this chapter, railcar window openings are covered with either tempered glass or Lexan®, or both. Since tempered glass is designed to fracture into many small pieces when broken, rescuers and victims may suffer minor scratches and small cuts from contact with these small pieces of glass. To break tempered glass, strike a bottom corner of the pane with a pointed object, such as the pick end of an axe. To break smaller panes, press a spring-loaded center punch into the bottom corner of the window pane.

Lexan® will not break when struck with a forcible entry tool. In fact, the tool will bounce off the Lexan®, which can injure the rescuer or others nearby. Rescuers will need to remove the entire pane or to cut through it with a power saw.

Window panes are removable from the outside in a manner similar to those used for over-the-road trucks. Rescuers can remove emergency exit windows from outside of the car. To identify the emergency windows, look for a plate with the removal instructions located next to each emergency exit window. These plates are also located at the ends of each car.

Passenger Car Roof/Wall Entry

As described in the section on railcar anatomy, the construction of railroad passenger cars is similar to but much heavier than that used in the construction of buses. The exterior walls are generally reinforced stainless steel designed to resist impact forces. This type of construction resists forcible entry, and rescuers should attempt forcible entry only if they have no other means of access. Breaching the walls of a railroad passenger car will almost certainly require the use of oxyacetylene cutting torches and/or other exothermic cutting devices.

Unlike buses and heavy trucks, the roof of a railroad passenger car is made of the same gauge material as the walls. Therefore, forcible entry through this area is unlikely to produce positive results.

Interior Door Locks/Latches

Once inside a rail passenger car, rescue personnel will find a variety of locking and latching mechanisms on interior doors. Most are similar to those found in industrial settings and their operation is obvious from their construction. Mechanical locks may require a standard railroad car coach key obtainable from a train crew member. This section covers only those locks and latches unique to trains or those whose functions may not be immediately apparent.

Toilet door latches. The toilet room latch is similar on most models of cars. When the "Occupied" display is showing, rescuers should assume that someone is inside. To open the door, rescuers should insert a screwdriver or similar object into the oval opening in the slide bolt and move the bolt to the left. The door will unlock and open inward. Rescuers may use standard railroad car coach keys to unlock toilet doors on other models.

Sleeping car bedroom door latches. To open some sleeping car bedroom doors, remove the two Phillips head cover plate screws exposing the key way. Open the lock using a standard coach key.

Sleeping car intercommunicating door latches. These doors are generally locked and unlocked by one of three different slide bar devices. Rescuers should use the following instructions to open each different type of slide bar latch:

- Slide bar #1: use the standard railroad car coach key.

- Slide bar #2: use the slide mechanism on one side of the bedroom divide.
- Slide bar #3: use the slide mechanism on the other side of the bedroom divider.

Sleeping car room door latches. All sleeping car rooms lock from the inside. To open locked doors from the outside, remove the two slotted screws on the outside door handle. The pin inside the door is attached to the outside cover plate. When the plate is removed, the latch drops, allowing the door to slide open.

Lounge/Food Service Car Entry

Rescuers should attempt entry into lounge cars through their side-entry vestibule doors. If they do not succeed, they should try the end doors. Diner and buffet cars do not have side-entry doors, so rescuers should use the end doors. The kitchen and bar loading doors are locked during train operation, so rescuers should make entry through other doors or windows. If rescuers cannot enter through the door, they should enter through the emergency exit windows.

Baggage Car Entry

Enter baggage cars through the sliding side doors or through the end doors. The side doors are usually locked during train operation. They feature a slide-type lock a few inches above the floor of the car. The end doors will usually not be locked if a crew member is inside the car. If rescuers cannot enter through the end doors and the side doors are locked, rescuers can enter through the windows in the side doors. The door window panes consist of a single pane of Lexan® that can be removed using the procedure described.

Material Handling Car Entry

Material handling cars have plug doors that must extend clear of the door opening before sliding sideways. The door automatically extends outward when the lever handle or wheel is operated. These doors are normally closed and locked during train operation, so rescuers will have to use forcible entry following a collision and/or derailment. Rescuers should enter through the side doors. If the doors are jammed, rescuers will have to use a rescue saw or power-spreading equipment to forcibly open them.

Railcar Extrication Situations

Vehicle incidents that occur in tunnels, on elevated railways, on railroad bridges, and in similar high-hazard environments will present technical rescue problems that are beyond the scope of this manual. However, there are still numerous special situations with which firefighters and other emergency responders must be prepared to deal. These include the following:

- Disentanglement/tunneling
- Loading platform incidents
- Train/highway vehicle collisions
- Train/pedestrian collisions
- Trams

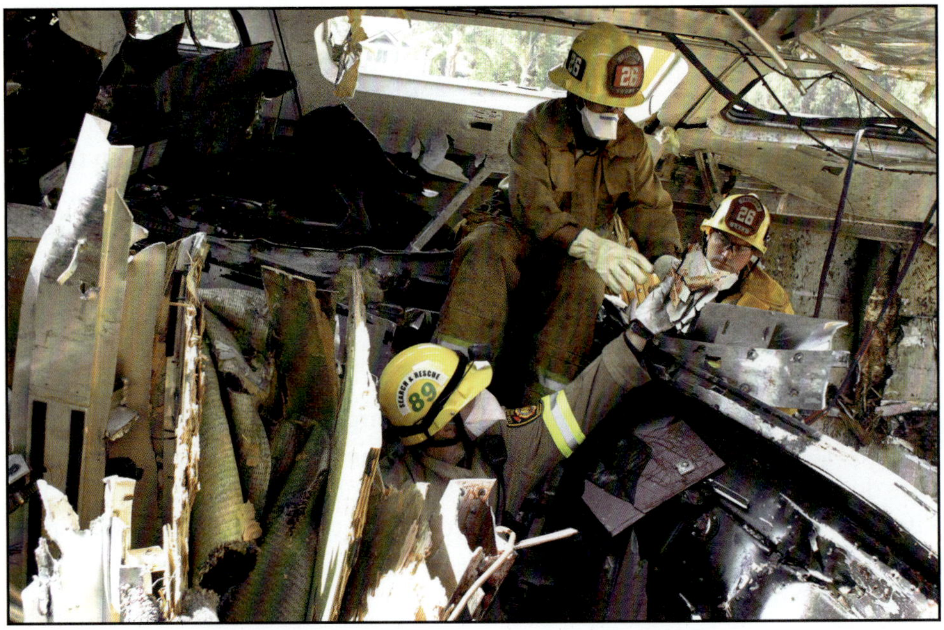

Figure 12.39 The interior of a railcar following a train collision. *Courtesy of Los Angeles Fire Department*.

Disentanglement/Tunneling

The tremendous inertial forces involved in many train wrecks can cause significant damage to railcars. These forces can rearrange the cars' interior configurations and entrap passengers and crew members. The heavy-gauge material composing these vehicles makes the entrapment that much more complete. The same problems involved in disentangling victims trapped in buses are involved in freeing those in railcars but made more difficult by the heavy construction **(Figure 12.39)**.

Because of the mass of railroad passenger cars, when they are stacked one upon the other, it may be necessary for rescue personnel to tunnel through the wreckage in much the same way that rescuers tunnel through rubble and debris following structural collapse. Many of the same tunneling techniques can be used. Before rescue personnel are allowed to work beneath heavy overhanging objects — heavily damaged railcars or parts thereof — these objects must be stabilized. Box cribbing may be sufficient in some cases, but rescuers may need heavy timber shoring or hydraulic/pneumatic shoring.

Loading Platform Incidents

These incidents most often involve one or more individuals who have left the platform and are on the roadbed. They may be in close proximity to a third rail, lying on tracks used by high-speed commuter trains, or under a standing railcar. In most cases, railway personnel will be on the scene when rescue personnel arrive. In these cases, a unified command made up of the first-arriving responder(s) and a railway representative is most appropriate. This will allow the incident action plan (IAP) to accurately reflect the expertise, capabilities, and limitations of both agencies and will most likely make the IAP realistic, safe, and effective.

NOTE: Refer to Chapter 3 to review descriptions of the Incident Action Plan.

If rescue personnel arrive on the scene before railway personnel, they should notify the railway operator of the situation. They should ask the operator to shut down all train traffic coming to the area and to send emergency response personnel. Rescue personnel should avoid the third rail (if present), cordon off the area, and deny entry to all but authorized personnel. Depending upon the specifics of the situation, rescue personnel may be able to take effective action to rescue the victims prior to the arrival of railway personnel. However, they should only initiate these actions if they have a reasonable expectation of success and they do not involve unnecessary risk for rescue personnel.

Train/Highway Vehicle Collisions

Motorists who have their car windows rolled up, music playing at high volume, and who may be distracted, may not hear a train approaching an ungated crossing. All too often, a motorist misjudges the speed of a train approaching a crossing and attempts to cross the tracks before the train arrives. These and other similar scenarios can produce tragic results. Trains have the right of way.

There are two basic types of train/highway vehicle collision incidents: those where the train is derailed and those where it is not. Those that involve train derailment can be complex, especially if there are victims trapped in both the highway vehicle and the railcars. This type of incident lends itself to a command structure with multiple area commands governing divisions or groups.

Even if the train does not derail, the situation surrounding the derailment could be complex. For example, a collision between a train and a highway vehicle carrying hazardous materials can create a complex incident, especially if it occurs in a densely populated area. A locomotive colliding with a loaded bus or with a truck loaded with farm workers can create mass casualty incidents that will severely tax the resources of many small agencies. Also, these incidents may occur at relatively remote rural crossings many miles from the nearest trauma center or fully staffed emergency medical facility. Victims will require efficient on-scene triage, treatment, and transportation.

Train/Pedestrian Collisions

These incidents occur in every locality that has active rail lines. Pedestrians put themselves in the path of an oncoming train for a wide variety of reasons. Some motorists attempt to dash across the tracks before the train passes. Others, under the influence of alcohol or drugs, may fall asleep on the tracks or fall and knock themselves unconscious. Others do so in an attempt to commit suicide.

Unless all or part of the victim is in or under the railcar, it is technically not a vehicle incident but merely a medical trauma call that occurred on railroad property. However, if it is a vehicle incident involving a train, rescuers should use any available resources to save the victim's life and to remove the victim from further harm. Working closely with on-scene railway personnel will increase the victim's chances of survival.

Trams

Like other classes of transportation vehicles, trams come in a wide variety of sizes and configurations. They range from individual railcars powered by diesel engines or electric motors to cable-drawn vehicles such as the famous San Francisco cable cars. There are also cable-drawn trams that travel at a steep angle on rails set against a mountainside and some that are suspended from a cable high above the ground. How incidents involving these vehicles are handled, and who handles them, will vary depending upon the specific situation and on local protocols.

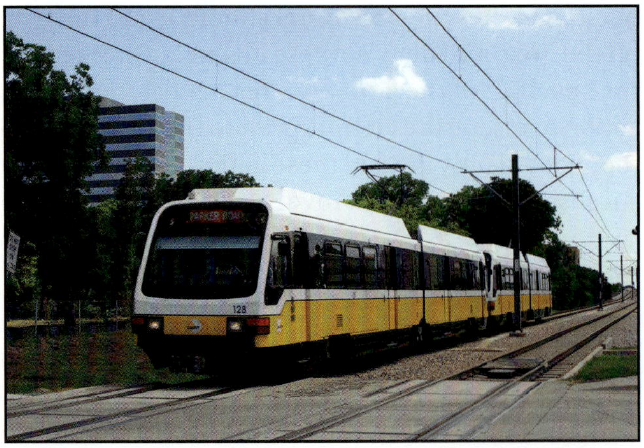

Figure 12.40 A larger tram.
Courtesy of Ed Chapman.

Many trams are like buses or street cars that travel on rails **(Figure 12.40)**. Extrication operations in them can be handled much the same way as extrication from buses, as described in Chapter 11. When dealing with electrically powered trams, rescue personnel should follow the same safety precautions as those described earlier in this chapter. Vehicle incidents involving trams that travel either on elevated tracks or suspended by an overhead cable — essentially those that are beyond the reach of fire department ground ladders or aerial devices — can prove challenging. Subject to the dictates of local protocols, technical rescue teams trained and equipped to operate in these environments should handle these incidents.

Chapter Review

1. What challenges may arise when rescuers must free victims trapped in a vehicle that has crashed into a structure?
2. What should rescuers do once they determine that a vehicle is underwater?
3. What factors must be considered when determining how to stabilize a hanging vehicle?
4. What special challenges do RVs pose to rescuers?
5. What types of tractors may rescuers encounter?
6. What features of industrial and agricultural vehicles make them susceptible to rollovers?
7. What types of fuels do industrial and agricultural vehicles use?
8. How can rescuers minimize hazards at an incident involving industrial or agricultural vehicles?
9. What types of stabilization must be applied to wheel-resting, side-resting, and roof-resting industrial or agricultural vehicles?
10. What factors must be considered during the size-up of an incident involving industrial or agricultural vehicles?
11. What techniques can be used to gain access to victims in industrial and agricultural vehicles?
12. What difficulties do industrial and agricultural vehicles pose to rescuers when disentangling and extricating victims?

13. How does railcar construction impact rescue operations?
14. What questions should rescuers ask when conducting size-up at a railcar incident?
15. What hazards are rescuers likely to encounter at railcar incidents?
16. How can rescuers stabilize railcars?
17. What methods can rescuers use to gain access to victims trapped in a railcar?
18. What actions can rescuers take to extricate victims from various types of railcar incidents?

Discussion Questions

1. What types of outside resources or mutual aid exist in your area for special types of vehicle incidents, such as a vehicle in water or a hanging vehicle?
2. What types of industrial and agricultural equipment is common in your jurisdiction?
3. How do local SOPs dictate that railcar incidents be handled in your jurisdiction?

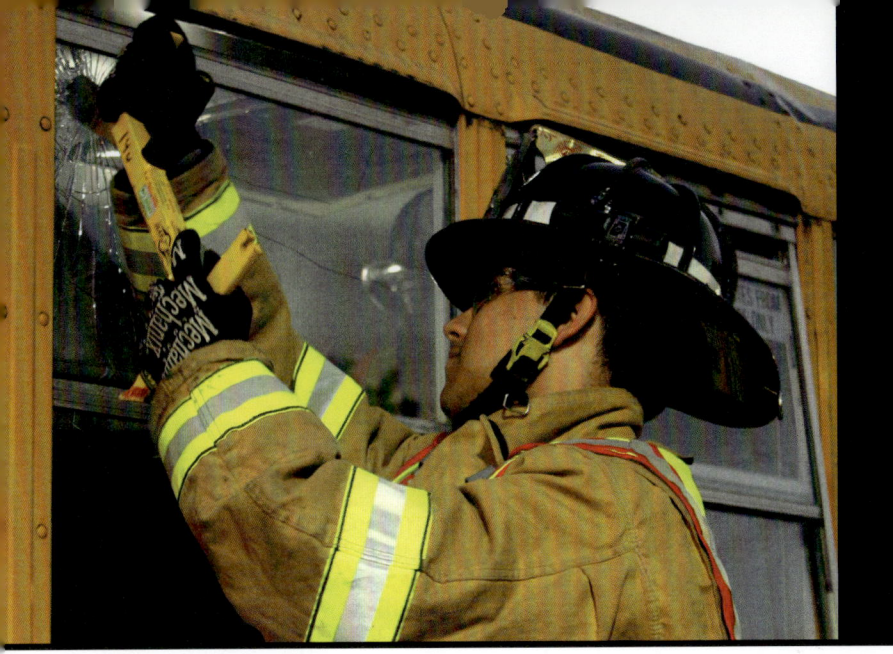

Appendices

Contents

Appendix A

Chapter and Page Correlation to NFPA Competencies 490

Appendix A

Chapter and Page Correlation to NFPA 1006, Standard for Technical Rescuer Professional Qualifications, 2017 Edition Chapter 8 Requirements

NFPA 472 Competency Number	Chapter References	Page Numbers
8.1.1	1	13-16, 22-30, 32, 40-47
8.1.2	1	24, 25, 27, 29-34, 41
8.1.3	1	11-13, 16-22, 24, 25, 29, 30, 33-47
8.1.4	1	13-22, 40-47
8.2.1	2, 3, 6, 8	61-84, 95-98, 99-106, 111, 191-219
8.2.2	2, 3	74-79, 86, 87, 90, 91
8.2.3	4, 7, 8, 12	127-133, 235-262, 264-274, 440-446
8.2.4	2	55-74
8.2.5	3, 6, 8	106, 107, 197-229, 279-281, 287-290, 309-327, 440-446
8.2.6	4, 5, 6, 8	133-161, 184-186, 197-229, 287-302, 440-446
8.2.7	4, 7, 8, 12	117-161, 242-262, 279-287, 303-308, 328-334, 440-446
8.2.8	5	167-186
8.2.9	2, 3	55-74, 107-110, 112
8.3.1	2, 3, 9	61-84, 98-106, 111, 339-349, 356-367
8.3.2	4, 10	127-133, 383-393, 440-446
8.3.3	9, 11, 12	350-355, 360-377, 402-406, 408-410, 423, 440-486
8.3.4	3, 4, 5, 9, 11, 12	106, 107, 133-161, 184-186, 350-355, 360-377, 402-418, 425-433, 440-486
8.3.5	4, 10, 11, 12	117-161, 383-393, 401, 407, 418-421, 434, 440-486
8.3.6	2	55-74, 86-89

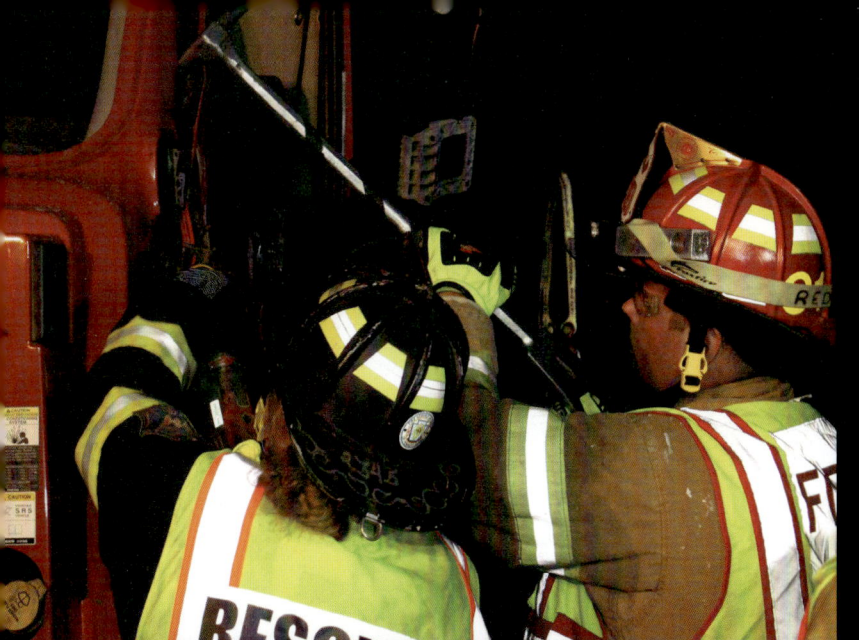

Glossary

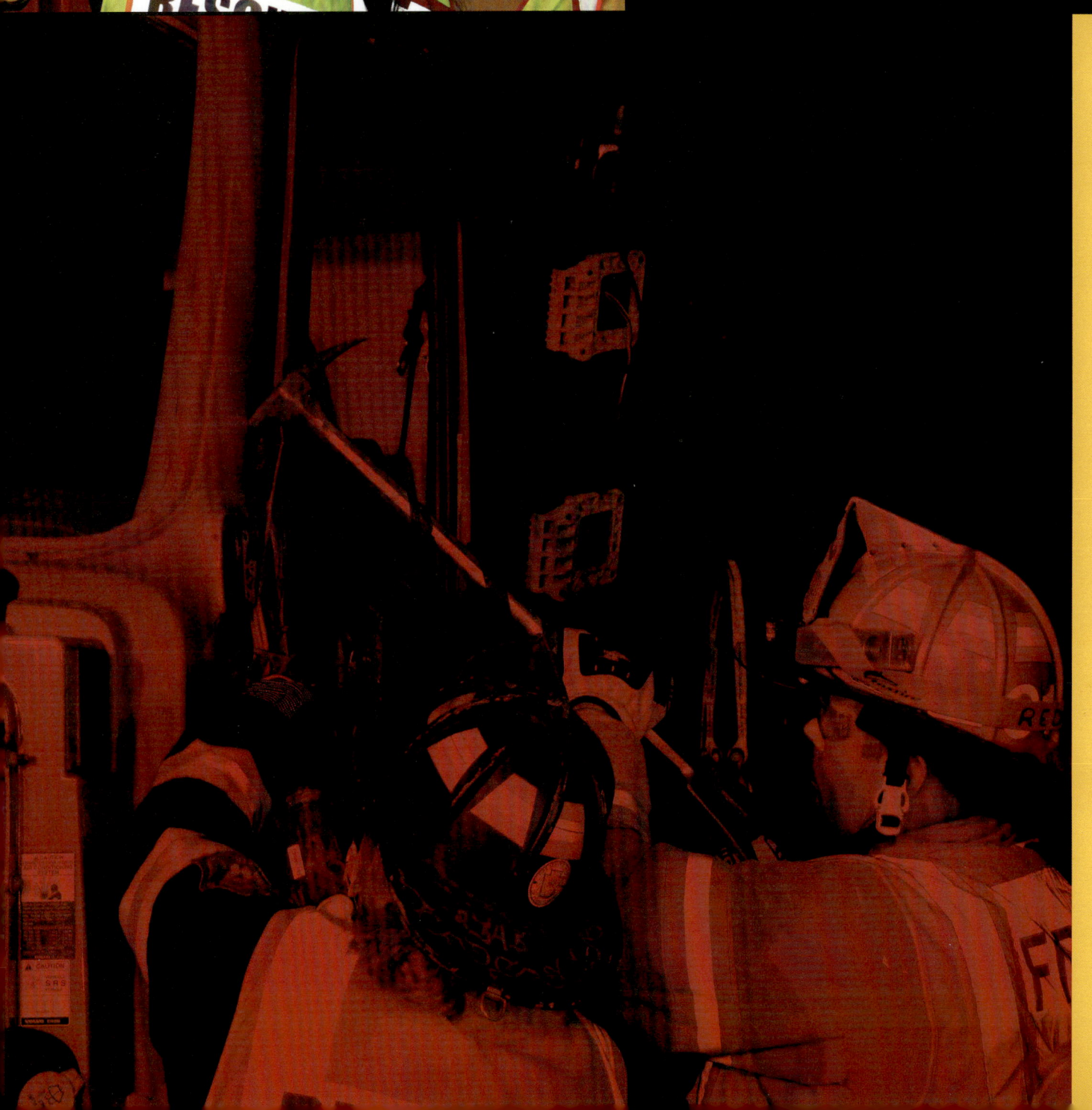

Glossary

A

Access — (1) Place or means of entering a structure or vehicle. (2) Roadways allowing fire apparatus to travel to an emergency. *See* Egress.

A-Frame — Vertical lifting device that can be attached to the front or rear of the apparatus; consists of two poles attached several feet (meters) apart on the apparatus and whose working ends are connected to form the letter A. A pulley or block and tackle through which a rope or cable is passed is attached to the end of the frame.

A-Post — Front post area of a vehicle where the door is connected to the body.

Advanced Life Support (ALS) — Advanced medical skills performed by trained medical personnel, such as the administration of medications, or airway management procedures to save a patient's life.

After Action Reviews (AAR) — Learning tools used to evaluate a project or incident to identify and encourage organizational and operational strengths and to identify and correct weaknesses.

Aorta — Largest artery in the body; originates at the left ventricle of the heart.

Apparatus Engine — Diesel or gasoline engine that powers the apparatus drive train and associated fire equipment. *Also known as* Power Plant.

Assistant Incident Safety Officer (AISO) — Individual(s) who reports to the Incident Safety Officer and assist with monitoring hazards and safe operations for designated portions of the operation at large or complex incidents.

Authority Having Jurisdiction (AHJ) — An organization, office, or individual responsible for enforcing the requirements of a code or standard, or approving equipment, materials, an installation, or a procedure.

B

B-Post — Post between the front and rear doors on a four-door vehicle, or the door-handle-end post on a two-door car.

Basic Life Support (BLS) — Emergency medical treatment administered without the use of adjunctive equipment; includes maintenance of airway, breathing, and circulation, as well as basic bandaging and splinting.

Berm — Outside or downhill side of a ditch or trench; a mound or wall of earth.

Bloodborne Pathogens — Pathogenic microorganisms that are present in the human blood and can cause disease in humans. These pathogens include (but are not limited to) hepatitis B virus (HBV) and human immunodeficiency virus (HIV).

Boiling Liquid Expanding Vapor Explosion (BLEVE) — Rapid vaporization of a liquid stored under pressure upon release to the atmosphere following major failure of its containing vessel. Failure is the result of overpressurization caused by an external heat source, which causes the vessel to explode when the temperature of the liquid is well above its boiling point at normal atmospheric pressure.

Bombproof Anchor Point — (1) Slang reference to an anchor that is immovable, such as a huge boulder, a large tree, or a fire engine. (2) Any anchor point capable of withstanding forces in excess of those that might be generated by the rescue operation or even catastrophic failure (and resultant shock load) of a raising or lowering system.

C

Cascade System — Three or more large, interconnected air cylinders, from which smaller SCBA cylinders are recharged; the larger cylinders typically have a capacity of 300 cubic feet (8 490 L).

Catenary System — Overhead wires used to transmit electrical power to buses, locomotives, and trams at a distance from the energy supply point.

Center of Gravity — Point through which all the weight of a vessel and its contents may be considered as concentrated, so that if supported at this point, the vessel would remain in equilibrium in any position.

Cervical Spine — First seven bones of the vertebral column, located in the neck.

Chassis — Basic operating system of a motor vehicle consisting of the frame, suspension system, wheels, and steering mechanism, but not the body.

Coil Spring Suspension — Suspension system consisting of numerous spirally bound, elastic steel bodies that recover their shape after being compressed, bent, or stretched.

Compartment Syndrome — Result of traumatic injury where the patient's muscle tissue becomes swollen and tightly encased. At four to six hours, crushed tissue begins to die and release toxins, which decreases the potential for saving the limb.

Compressed Natural Gas — Natural gas that is stored in a vessel at pressures of 2,400 to 3,600 psi (16 800 kPa to 25 200 kPa).

Consist — Rail shipping paper that contains a list of cars in the train by order; indicates the cars that contain hazardous materials. Some railroads include information on emergency operations for the hazardous materials on board with the consist. *Also known as* Train Consist.

Cribbing — Wooden or plastic blocks used to stabilize a vehicle during vehicle extrication or debris following a structural collapse; typically 4 X 4 (100 x 100 mm) inches or larger and 16 to 26 inches (400 to 650 mm) long.

Critical Incident Stress (CIS) — Physical, mental, or emotional tension caused when persons have been exposed to a traumatic event where they have experienced, witnessed, or been confronted with an event or events that involve actual death, threatened death, serious injury, or threat of physical integrity of self or others.

Crush Syndrome — Potentially fatal condition that occurs as a result of crushing pressure on a part of the body, typically the lower extremities. When blood flow to and from the injured area is absent for four to six hours, the injured tissue begins to die, giving off toxins; a sudden release of pressure may allow the toxins to flow into the bloodstream and to have an effect on other bodily organs.

D

Disentanglement — Aspect of vehicle extrication relating to the removal and/or manipulation of vehicle components to allow a properly packaged patient to be removed from the vehicle.

E

Egress — Place or means of exiting a structure or vehicle.

Entrapment — When the victim or part of the victim is being mechanically restrained, or has restricted means of egress, by a damaged vehicle or machinery component.

Extrication Group — Group within the Incident Management System that is responsible for extricating victims.

F

Fairing — An auxiliary structure or the external surface either attached to, or a part of the roof of a large truck that serves to reduce drag.

Flash Fire — Type of fire that spreads rapidly through a vapor environment.

Four-Point Box Crib — Cribbing constructed with four points that is made to look like a box.

Freelancing — To operate independently of the Incident Commander's command and control.

Fulcrum — Support or point of support on which a lever turns in raising or moving a load.

G

Gin Pole — Vertical lifting device that may be attached to the front or the rear of the apparatus; consists of a single pole attached to the apparatus at one end and has a working pulley at the other. Guy wires may also be used to stabilize the pole.

Gross Decontamination — Quickly removing the worst surface contamination, usually by rinsing with water from handheld hoselines, emergency showers, or other water sources.

Gross Vehicle Weight Rating (GVWR) — Maximum weight at which a vehicle can be safely operated on roadways; includes the weight of the vehicle itself plus fuel, passengers, cargo, and trailer tongue weight.

Ground Fault Circuit Interrupter (GFCI) — Device designed to protect against electrical shock; when grounding occurs, the device opens a circuit to shut off the flow of electricity. *Also known as* Ground Fault Indicator (GFI) Receptacle.

H

Halligan Tool — Prying tool with a claw at one end and a spike or point at a right angle to a wedge at the other end. *Also known as* Hooligan Tool.

Hazardous Material — Any substance or material that poses an unreasonable risk to health, safety, property, and/or the environment if it is not properly controlled during handling, storage, manufacture, processing, packaging, use, disposal, or transportation.

High-Strength Low-Alloy (HSLA) Steel — Alloy steel developed to provide better mechanical properties or greater resistance to corrosion than carbon steel; different from other varieties of steels in that it is designed to possess specific mechanical properties.

I

Incident Commander (IC) — Person in charge of the Incident Command System and responsible for the management of all incident operations during an emergency.

Incident Command Post (ICP) — Location at which the Incident Commander and Command Staff direct, order, and control resources at an incident; may be co-located with the incident base.

Incident Command System (ICS) — Standardized approach to Incident Management that facilitates interaction between cooperating agencies; adaptable to incidents of any size or type.

Incident Safety Officer (ISO) — Member of the Command staff responsible for monitoring and assessing safety hazards and unsafe conditions during an incident, and developing measures for ensuring personnel safety. The ISO is responsible for the enforcement of all mandated safety laws and regulations and departmental safety-related standard operating procedures. On very small incidents, the Incident Commander may act as the ISO.

J

Jack Plate — Unattached flat metal plate that is larger in area than the stabilizer foot; placed on the ground beneath the intended resting point of the stabilizer foot, in order to provide better weight distribution. *Also known as* Jack Pad or Stabilizer Pad.

K

Kingpin — Attaching pin on a semitrailer that connects with pivots within the lower coupler of a truck tractor or converter dolly while coupling the two units together.

Kneeling — Ability of some buses to lower the front end of the bus to curb level for ease of passenger boarding.

L

Leaf Spring Suspension — Type of suspension system consisting of several long, narrow, layers of elastic metal bracketed together.

Lever — Device consisting of a bar pivoting on a fixed point (fulcrum), using power or force applied at a second point to lift or sustain an object at a third point.

Lexan® — Polycarbonate plastic used for windows; has one-half the weight of an equivalent-sized piece of glass, yet is 30 times stronger than safety glass and 250 times stronger than ordinary glass. It cannot be broken using standard forcible entry techniques.

Limited Access (Warm) Zone — Large geographical area between the support zone and the restricted zone, for personnel who are directly aiding rescuers in the restricted zone. This includes personnel who are handling hydraulic tool power plants, fire personnel handling standby hoselines, and so on. Personnel in this zone should not get in the way of rescuers working in the restricted zone.

Liquefied Compressed Gas — Gas that under the charging pressure is partially liquid at 70°F (21° C). *Also known as* Liquefied Gas.

Liquefied Natural Gas (LNG) — Natural gas that has been converted to a liquid form for storage or transport.

M

Mass Casualty Incident (MCI) — Incident that results in a large number of casualties within a short time frame, as a result of an attack, natural disaster, aircraft crash, or other cause that is beyond the capabilities of local logistical support.

Mechanical Advantage —Advantage created when levers, pulleys, and other tools make work easier during rope rescue or while lifting heavy objects.

Monocoque — Construction technique in which an object's external skin supports the structural load of the object.

N

Nader Pin — Bolt on a vehicle's door frame that the door latches onto in order to close.

National Highway Traffic Safety Administration (NHTSA) — Agency within the U.S. Department of Transportation (DOT) that publishes annual summary reports of fatal highway accidents.

National Incident Management System - Incident Command System (NIMS-ICS) — The U.S. mandated incident management system that defines the roles, responsibilities, and standard operating procedures used to manage emergency operations; creates a unified incident response structure for federal, state, and local governments.

O

Operations Section Chief — Person responsible to the Incident Commander for managing all tactical operations directly applicable to accomplishing the incident objectives. Also known as Ops Chief or Ops Section Chief.

P

Pantograph — Mechanical linkage device that maintains electrical contact with a contact wire and transfers power from the wire to the traction unit of electric buses, locomotives, and trams.

Personnel Accountability System — Method for identifying which emergency responders are working on an incident scene.

Pike Pole — Sharp prong and hook of steel, on a wood, metal, fiberglass, or plastic handle of varying length, used for pulling, dragging, and probing.

Placard — Diamond-shaped sign that is affixed to each side of a structure or a vehicle transporting hazardous materials to inform responders of fire hazards, life hazards, special hazards, and reactivity potential. The placard indicates the primary class of the material and, in some cases, the exact material being transported.

Pneumatic — Operated by air or compressed air.

Pneumatic Chisel — Tool designed to operate at air pressures between 100 and 150 psi (700 kPa and 1 050 kPa); during periods of normal consumption, it will use about 4 to 5 cubic feet (113 L to 142 L) of air per minute. It is useful for extrication work. *Also known as* Air Chisel, Impact Hammer, or Pneumatic Hammer.

Power Take-Off (PTO) System — Mechanism that allows a vehicle engine to power equipment such as a pump, winch, or portable tool; it is typically attached to the transmission. Farm tractors are designed to operate the PTO shaft at either 540 or 1,000 revolutions per minute.

R

Reciprocating Saw — Electric saw that uses a short, straight blade that moves back and forth.

Rehabilitation — Allowing firefighters or rescuers to rest, rehydrate, and recover during an incident; also refers to a station at an incident where personnel can rest, rehydrate, and recover. *Also known as* Rehab.

Restricted (Hot) Zone — In a rescue or extrication operation, the area where the extrication is taking place. Only personnel who are attending directly to the victims should be in this zone; this avoids crowding and confusion among rescuers.

Rigging — Ropes or cables used with lifting or pulling devices such as block and tackle.

Risk-Benefit Analysis – Comparison between the known hazards and potential benefits of any operation; used to determine the feasibility and parameters of the operation.

Rollover Protection — Roll bars and cages within automobiles that protect passengers in the event of a rollover.

S

Seat Belt Pretensioners — Protective devices designed to tighten the belts as the front-impact airbags deploy.

Self-Contained Underwater Breathing Apparatus (SCUBA) — Protective breathing apparatus designed to be used underwater by divers to allow the exploration of underwater environments. *Also known as* SCUBA Gear *or* Underwater Breathing Gear.

Shoring — General term used for lengths of timber, screw jacks, hydraulic and pneumatic jacks, and other devices that can be used as temporary support for formwork or structural components or used to hold sheeting against trench walls. Individual supports are called shores, cross braces, and struts. Commonly used in conjunction with Cribbing.

Simple Triage and Rapid Treatment (START) — Triage evaluation method for checking respiratory, circulatory, and neurological function, with the intention of categorizing patients in one of the four care categories: minor, delayed, immediate, and expectant. The START method is recommended for use by first-arriving responders for initial and secondary field triage.

Size-Up — Ongoing evaluation of influential factors at the scene of an incident.

Sleeper — Compartment built into or behind the cab of a large truck, to be used by the driver for rest and relaxation.

Sling — Assembly that connects the load to the material handling equipment. There are four common types of slings: chain, wire rope, synthetic round, and synthetic web.

Standard Operating Procedure (SOP) — Formal methods or rules to guide the performance of routine functions or emergency operations. Procedures are typically written in a handbook, so that all firefighters can consult and become familiar with them. *Also known as* Operating Instruction (OI), Predetermined Procedures, *or* Standard Operating Guideline (SOG).

Support (Cold) Zone — Area that surrounds the limited access (warm) zone and is restricted to emergency response personnel who are not working in either the restricted (hot) zone or the limited access (warm) zone. This zone may include the portable equipment and personnel staging areas and the Command Post; cordon off the outer boundary of this area to the public.

T

Tactical Worksheet — Document that the IC may use on the fireground to track units and record field notes during an incident, could evolve into a written IAP if an incident escalates in size or complexity.

Traffic Control — Important function of scene management that helps to control scene access and vehicular traffic in and out of the area. This function is generally handled by law enforcement personnel.

Trailer — Highway or industrial-plant vehicle designed to be hauled/pulled by a tractor unit.

Triage — System used for sorting and classifying accident casualties to determine the priority for medical treatment and transportation.

U

Unified Command (UC) — In the Incident Command System, a shared command role in which all agencies with geographical or functional responsibility establish a common set of incident objectives and strategies. In unified command there is a single incident command post and a single operations chief at any given time.

V

Vehicle Stabilization —Providing additional support to key places between a vehicle and the ground or other solid anchor points to prevent unwanted movement.

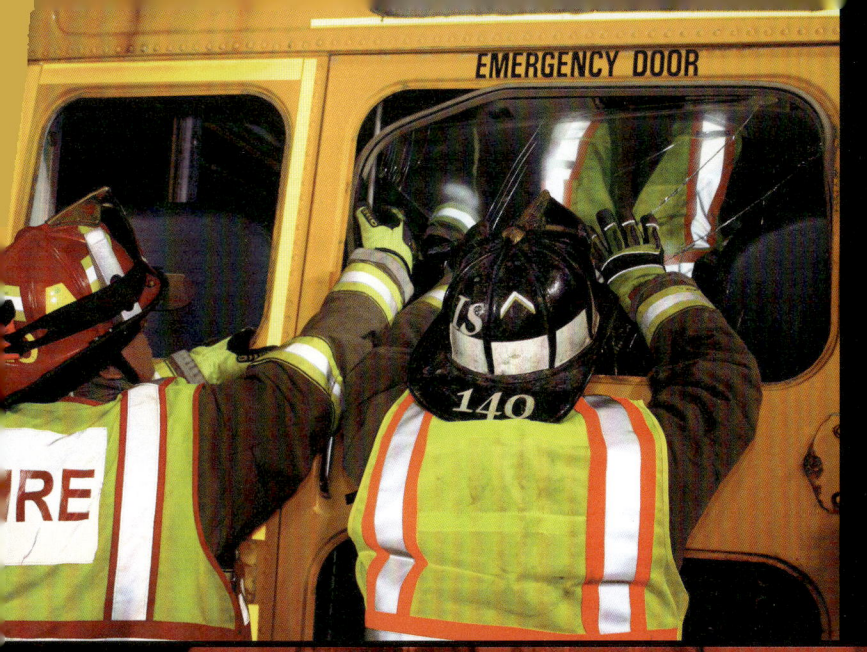

Index

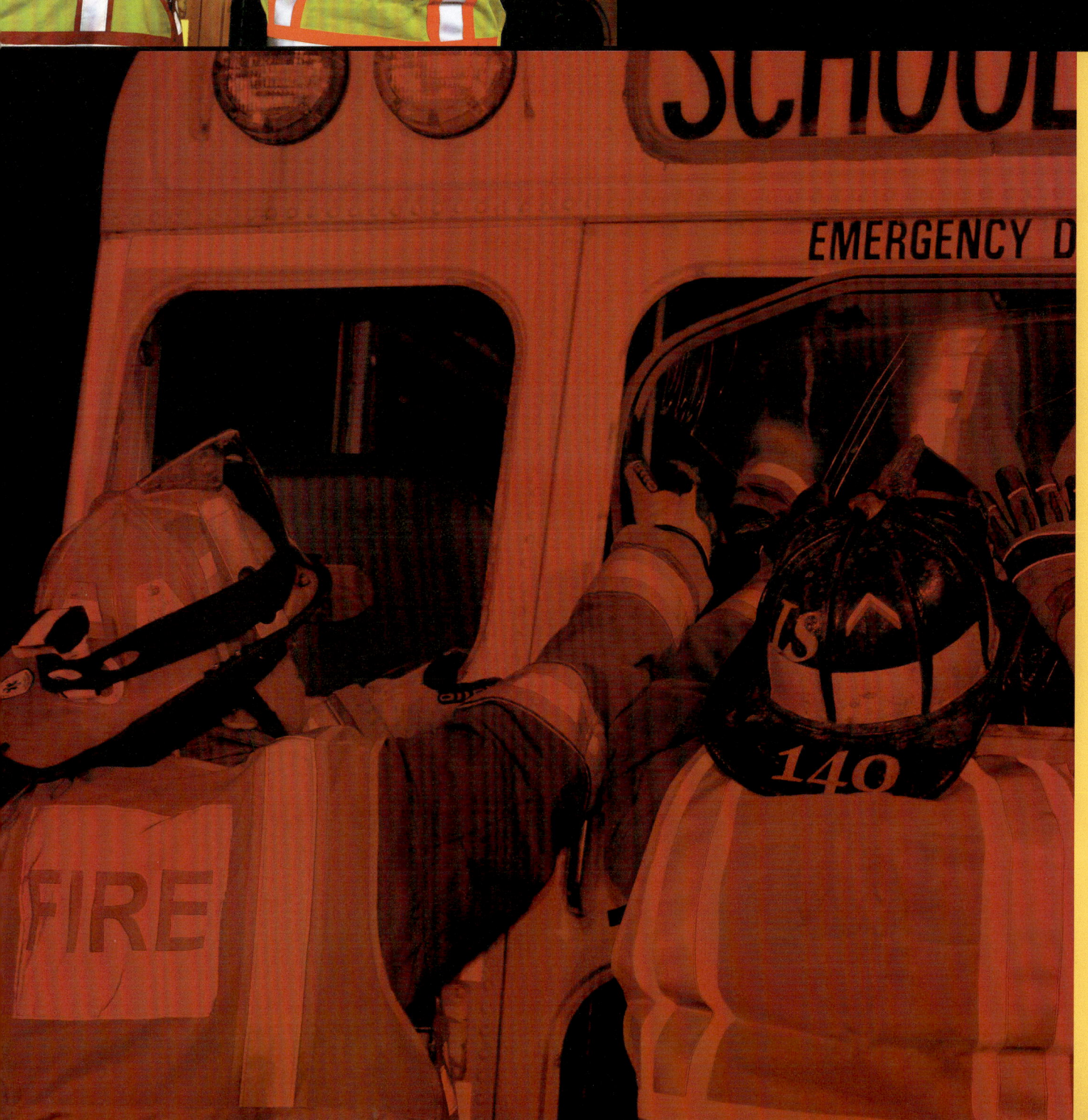

Index

A

AAR (after action review), 109, 182
Abdominal injuries, 171, 172
Access and egress
    buses, 408–410
    defined, 288
    disentangling victims, 303–308
        B-post displacement, 305
        dashboard displacement, 303–304, 330–331
        floor pan, dropping, 304–305
        pedal displacement and removal, 306–308
        seat displacement and removal, 305–306, 333–334
        steering column displacement, 303
        windshield removal, 303
    door removal, 293–297, 314–320
    entry points, 287–290
        determination of, 309
        doors, 289
        floor panels, 290
        windows, 288–289
    factory third and fourth doors, 297–298, 317
    floor entry, 300–301, 325–326
    fourth-door conversion, 299, 320
    glass removal, 291–293
    industrial and agricultural vehicles, 461–462
    kick panel removal, 300, 324
    medium and heavy trucks, 402–403, 423–424
    passenger vehicles, 288
    railcars, 479–483, 484
    roof, 299–300, 321–323
    third-door conversion, 298, 319
    total sidewall removal, 298, 318
    trunk tunneling, 301, 327
    vehicle stabilization and, 28
    vehicles with advanced steel, 301–302
        B-post lift, 302
        cross ramming, 302
        pie cut, 302
        ramming the roof off, 302
        sunroof, 302
Accountability Officer, 32
Acetone, extinguishing agent for fires, 79
Acids, extinguishing agent for fires, 79
Adapters, 144
Adaptive cruise control, 220
Advanced life support (ALS), 41, 173
Aerial apparatus (truck) companies, 120
AFFF (aqueous film forming foam), 79
A-frame, 125, 126
After action review (AAR), 109, 182
Agricultural vehicles. *See* Industrial and agricultural vehicles
AHJ. *See* Authority having jurisdiction (AHJ)
Air brakes on trucks, 353
Air chisels, 152, 416
Air compressors, 126–127
Air hammers, 152
Air supply systems, 126–127
Air suspension systems
    functions, 73
    medium and heavy trucks, 354
    securing the suspension, 88
    trailers, 347
Airbags
    accidental deployment, 70
    center-mounted, 223–224
    detection devices, 69
    disarming, 71, 222
    door removal with, 295
    examples, 68
    frontal- and side-impact, 70–71, 221, 222
    functions, 221
    head protection systems (HPS), 72, 222–223
    inflatable tubes, 223
    inflation materials, 71–72
    knee bolsters, 224
    neck protection system, 223
    peel and peek behind interior trim, 70
    reserve energy supply, 71, 222
    safety precautions for rescuers, 69–70
    safety zone distances, 69
    seat belt airbags, 223
    side-impact protection system (SIPS), 222
    sodium azide, 71
    stability during deployment, 28
    vehicle construction knowledge for responder safety, 27
    window curtains, 223
Air-purifying respirator (APR)
    air-purifying filters, 59–61
    factors in choice of, 60
    limitations, 60
    oxygen requirements, 60
    powered or non-powered, 60
    precautions for use, 61
Air-ride cab, 74, 89, 344
Air-suspension systems, 219
Aisles on buses, 366–367
AISO (Assistant Incident Safety Officer), 33–34
Alcohol/gasoline blended fuel, 80, 212
Alcohol-resistant aqueous film forming foam (AR-AFFF), 79, 80
Alloy construction materials, 205
All-terrain vehicles (ATV), 194
All-wheel drive powertrain, 218, 454
All-wheel drive rescue vehicles, 122
ALS (advanced life support), 41, 173
Alternative fuels
    alcohol/gasoline blended mixtures, 80, 212
    auxiliary fuel cells, 211–212
    biodiesel, 81, 212
    ethanol, 212. *See also* Ethanol
    fire suppression operations, 80–81
        alcohol/gasoline blends, 80
        biodiesel, 81
        hybrid and electric vehicles, 81
        hydrogen, 81
        natural gas, 80–81
        propane, 81
    hazards, 63
    hydrogen, 212. *See also* Hydrogen
    jet propellant-8 (JP-8), 212
    LNG. *See* Liquefied natural gas (LNG)
    LPG. *See* Liquefied petroleum gas (LPG, LP-Gas)
    propane, 79, 81, 211
Alternators on rescue vehicles, 123
Aluminum construction material, 204
Amphetamine, as on-scene hazard, 19
Amputations, 178
Anchor point, 389
ANSI
    ANSI/CGA G7.1, *Commodity Specification for Air*, 29
    Class 3 safety vests, 36, 58
    foot protection standards, 58
Aorta, 171
A-post, 407

Apparatus
    engine, 123
    ladder trucks, 120
    positioning at emergency scenes, 36
    rescue engines, 119
    standard engines, 120
    used for traffic control, 35
APR. *See* Air-purifying respirator (APR)
Aqueous film forming foam (AFFF), 79
AR-AFFF (alcohol-resistant aqueous film forming foam), 79, 80
Arcair®, 159
Artics, 341
Articulated lorries, 341
Articulated transit buses, 358, 359
Articulating vehicles, 448, 455
Assessment of the scene. *See* Scene assessment
Assignments in the Incident Action Plan (ICS 204 Form), 42, 106
Assistant Incident Safety Officer (AISO), 33–34
Atmospheric monitoring, 64
ATV (all-terrain vehicle), 194
Australia, truck/semitrailer combinations, 341
Authority having jurisdiction (AHJ)
    beneficial vehicle systems, 67
    bloodborne pathogens, 21
    chain of command, 104
    commercial/heavy vehicle stabilization, 383
    defined, 11
    evacuation and accountability measures, 107
    hazard and risk assessment surveys, 16
    Incident Management Coalition Team, 15
    level of capability for operations, 11
    operational protocols, 41–42
    personnel shelter and thermal control, 30
    rescue organization performance standards, 99
    traffic control, 19, 34
    vehicle access and egress points, 288
    vehicle energy source isolation and management, 62
    vehicle stabilization, 255–256
    victim care, 168
Auxiliary electrical equipment, 144
Auxiliary fuel cells, 211–212
Auxiliary lift axles on trucks, 354–355
Auxiliary power systems
    industrial and agricultural vehicles, 456
    trucks, 351–352
        hydraulic systems, 352
        mechanical systems, 352
        pneumatic systems, 353
Awareness Level
    NFPA 1006 requirements, 12
    risk-benefit analysis, 17
    size-up duties, 16–17
Axe, 137

B

Baggage cars, 468, 483
Band saws, 148
Bar screw jack, 141
Basic life support (BLS), 41
Basket hitch, 248
Batteries
    battery packs, 214, 215
    commercial buses, 372
    disabling, 87
    electric vehicles, 207, 210
    extended range electric vehicle (EREV), 210–211
    fire extinguishment, 81
    hazards, 65, 213
    hybrid electric vehicle (HEV), 64, 206–207
    location of, 215
    medium and heavy trucks, 350
    multiple batteries, 215
    Plug-In Hybrid Electric Vehicle (PHEV), 207
    purpose of, 214
    school buses, 372
    shut off switch, 372
    transit buses, 372
    types, 215
Beneficial vehicle systems, 67–74
    defined, 67
    examples, 68
    seat adjustment or positioning controls, 74
    supplemental restraint systems, 67–73. *See also* Supplemental restraint system (SRS)
    suspension system hazards, 73–74, 88, 89
Berm, 480
Big-rigs, 341
Biodiesel
    alternative fuels, 212
    fuel fires, 81
Biohazards, 21
BLEVE (boiling liquid expanding vapor explosion), 76
Blood, precautions to prevent contact with, 56
Blood loss (hypovolemia), 176
Bloodborne pathogens, 21
BLS (basic life support), 41
Blunt trauma, 171
Bodily fluids, precautions to prevent contact with, 56
Body armor, 61
Body protective clothing, 57–58
Body-on-chassis construction, 368, 390
Boiling liquid expanding vapor explosion (BLEVE), 76
Bolt cutters, 137
Bombproof anchor point, 389
Book organization, 2–3
Booms, 451–452
Box crib
    four-point, 386, 387
    uses for, 128–129, 243
Box trailers, 348
B-post displacement, 305, 407
B-post lift, 302
Braided wire rope, 250
Brain injury, 178
Brake systems
    industrial and agricultural vehicles, 455–456
    railcars, 471
    trucks, 353–354
Breathing air compressors, 126–127
Breathing protection. *See* Respiratory protection
Bridle hitch, 248
Briefing in the Incident Action Plan, 42, 105
Bullnose cab, 344
Bumpers
    crushable, 66, 225
    struts, 76, 225–226
Burning bars, 159
Buses, 356–377
    access and egress points, 408–410
    anatomy, 360–367
        aisles, 366–367
        doors, 361–363
        seats, 365–366
        windows, 363–365
    commercial buses
        aisles, 367
        batteries, 372
        construction, 371
        conversions, 360
        doors, 362–363
        electrical systems, 372–373
        generally, 358–359

seats, 366
stabilization, 391
windows, 365
construction, 368–377
batteries, 371–372
commercial buses, 371
electric buses, 375–376
electrical systems, 372–373
fuel systems, 374–376
hydraulic lifts, 371
school buses, 368–370
suspension systems, 376–377
transit buses, 370–371
extrication operations, 410–421
access and egress openings, 410–418
disentangling victims, 418–421
doors, 411–413
floors, 417–418
roofs, 416–417, 431–432
stair removal, 410
windows, 413–415, 429
floor as entry point, 410, 433
fuel systems, 374–376
haz mat incidents, 84
kneeling, 377
partitions, 419–420
rear wall access, 416
roof as entry point, 409–410
school buses
aisles, 366–367
batteries, 372
characteristics, 356
construction, 368–370
conversions, 360
defined, 356
door access opening, 427–428
doors, 361–362, 409, 412–413
electrical systems, 372–373
floor as entry point, 410, 433
roof as entry point, 409–410
seats, 365
stabilization, 390
Type A. *See* Type A school bus
Type B. *See* Type B school bus
Type C. *See* Type C school bus
Type D. *See* Type D school bus
windows, 363–364, 409
shutdown operations, 373
sidewall access, 409, 415–416, 430
specialty buses, 359–360
stabilizing, 389–393
suspension systems, 376–377
transit buses
aisles, 367
articulated, 358, 359
batteries, 372
construction, 370–371
disentanglement, 402
doors, 362
electrical systems, 372–373
generally, 357–358
seats, 365–366
stabilization, 391
windows, 364–365

C
Cab-beside-engine units, 344
Cable laid rope, 250
Cab-over units, 344
Cabs on trucks, 343–346
air-ride cab, 74, 89, 344

cab-beside-engine, 344
cab-over units, 344
conventional cabs, 344
described, 343
doors, 345
roof/fairing, 346, 350
sleepers, 344–345
windows, 346
Canada
metric conversions, 4–6
truck/semitrailer combinations, 341
Underwriters Laboratories of Canada (ULC), 137
Car carrier/haulers, 349
Cascade air supply systems, 126, 127
Cast iron construction materials, 205
Catalytic converters, 216
Catenary systems
defined, 466
functions, 472–473
hazards, 477
mechanics, 473
poles and wires illustrated, 474
Cell phone calls to dispatch, 45
Cement mixer, 343
Center of gravity, 236–237
Center punches, 140
Center-mounted airbags, 223–224
Cervical collar, 179, 184
Cervical spine
collision injuries, 172
defined, 171
injuries, 171, 176
Chain hoist, 254
Chain saws, 147
Chains
rescue chain, 249
safety rules, 131–132, 249
stabilizing a commercial truck, 383
uses for, 131
Charter bus, 358. *See also* Commercial buses
Chassis
defined, 200
rescue vehicle, 121
strength after a collision, 200
Cheater, 136
Chemical agent incidents, hazard and risk assessment surveys, 16
Chest injuries, 171, 172
Child safety restraint devices, 224
Chisels, 152
Chocking a vehicle
flat or sloped surface, 237
purpose of, 238
for roof-resting vehicle, 241
stabilization tools, 242, 264
step chocks, 129–130, 258, 268
wheel chocks, 242, 243, 264
wheel-resting vehicles, 258, 268
Choker hitch, 248
Chopping tools, 137
Circular saws, 147
CIS (critical incident stress), 109–110
CISD (Critical Incident Stress Debriefing), 109
CISM (Critical Incident Stress Management), 109
Class I lever, 246, 267
Class II lever, 247
Class III lever, 247
Clothing. *See also* Personal protective equipment (PPE)
NFPA 1999 standards, 58
reflective clothing, 36–37, 38, 57
safety vests
for flaggers, 38

for increased visibility, 36, 58
  for personnel identification, 101
Club cars, 469
CNG. *See* Compressed natural gas (CNG)
Coil springs
  hazards, 73
  suspension systems, 218, 354
Cold (support) zone, 31, 32
Collision avoidance systems, 219-220
Collision beams, 227-228
Collisions
  front impact. *See* Front-impact collision
  rear impact. *See* Rear-impact collision
  rollover. *See* Rollovers
  rotational impact, 173, 283
  train/highway, 485
  underrides and overrides, 257, 284-285
Colors
  hybrid electric vehicle coding, 206
  placards, 83, 342
  triage categories, 175
Combination compartmentation, 121-122
Combines, 450-451
Combustible metals, 75, 79
Combustible substances, 74-75
Come-alongs
  lifting a vehicle, 241
  manual cable winch, 253
  mechanical advantage systems, 157
  mechanism, 156, 157
Commercial buses
  aisles, 367
  batteries, 372
  construction, 371
  conversions, 360
  doors, 362-363
  electrical systems, 372-373
  generally, 358-359
  seats, 366
  stabilization, 391
  windows, 365
Commercial chassis, 121
Commercial vehicle stabilization, 383-396
  buses, 389-393
  considerations for, 384, 385-393
  gross vehicle weight rating (GVWR), 191, 385
  medium and heavy trucks, 385-389, 395-396
  tools and equipment, 383
Commodity Specification for Air (ANSI/CGA G7.1), 29
Common chain, 131
Communication
  dispatch, 45
  of hazards, 45-46
  patient transfer, 182
  radio communication of hazards, 107
  rescue strategy and objectives, 43-44
  response plans, 15
  signaling devices, 144
  telecommunications, 45
Compact cars, 195
Compartment syndrome, 177
Compartmentation, rescue vehicle, 121-122
Composite materials, 205
Compressed natural gas (CNG)
  bus fuel, 374-375
  defined, 81
  example, 80
  passenger vehicle use, 82
  truck fuel, 351
Compressors, air, 126-127
Consist, train, 464

Construction
  batteries, 371-372
  commercial buses, 371
  electric buses, 375-376
  electrical systems, 372-373
  fuel systems, 374-376
  hydraulic lifts, 371
  material hazards, 65-66
    crushable bumpers, 66
    vehicle components, 66
    windows, 65-66
  medium and heavy trucks, 350-355
    auxiliary lift axles, 354-355
    batteries, 350
    brake systems, 353-354
    components, 350
    electrical systems, 351
    fuel systems, 350-351
    hydraulic systems, 351-353
    suspension systems, 354
  passenger vehicle, 204-219
    electrical systems, 213-216
    exhaust systems, 216
    fuel systems, 205-212
    materials, 204-205
    powertrain, 216-218
    suspension systems, 218-219
  school buses, 368-370
  suspension systems, 376-377
  transit buses, 370-371
Contents of vehicle, hazards of, 19
Conventional cabs, 344
Conventional fuel hazards, 62-63
Convertibles, 196
Cooling fans, 215-216
Copper construction material, 205
Cordon off
  downed power lines, 20
  truck haz mat incidents, 84
  zone boundaries, 32
Coup contrecoup brain injury, 178
Crane
  hydraulic, 125-126
  industrial, 452
  rescue crane, 255
Crash dynamics, 27-28
Crew resource management, 22-23
Cribbing
  for airbag deployment stabilization, 28
  applications, 128-129
  box crib
    four-point, 386, 387
    uses for, 128-129, 243
  bus stabilization, 391
  defined, 127
  materials, 242-243
  plastic, 128, 129
  railroad ties, 478
  roof-resting vehicles, 241
  wheel-resting vehicles, 258, 269
  wooden, 127-128
Critical incident stress (CIS), 109-110
Critical Incident Stress Debriefing (CISD), 109
Critical Incident Stress Management (CISM), 109
Cross braces, 440
Cross ramming, 302
Crumple zones, 228
Crush syndrome, 177-178
Crushable bumpers, 66, 225
Cryogenic liquid hazards, 63
Custom chassis, 121

Cutting tools, 137–139
    bolt cutters, 137
    chopping tools, 137
    cutting flares, 159
    electric spreaders and cutters, 142
    hot wire cutters, 137
    hydraulic, 13, 149–150
    insulated wire cutters, 137
    knives, 139
    pedal cutters, 150, 307
    plasma-arc cutters, 160
    saws, 138, 139
    snipping tools, 137
    thermal cutting devices, 158–161
    windshield, 138, 139

D

Dashboard
    displacement, 303–304, 330–331
    as entrapment point, 281
    support beam, 227
Day of the week, scene assessment consideration, 97
Decontamination, gross, 177
Defoggers
    electronics, 216
    hazards, 65, 213
Delivery truck, 340
Department of Health and Human Services, 182
Department of Transportation (DOT)
    dump trailer gross vehicle weight, 349
    Emergency Response Guidebook, 82
    Manual on Uniform Traffic Control Devices (MUTCD), 19, 37
    passenger vehicle classification, 191
    safety vests, 36, 58
    support operations, 47
Diesel fuel
    bus fuel systems, 374
    fuel systems, 206
    locomotives, 465–466, 476
    truck fuel systems, 350
Dining cars, 469
Directional movement, 237–238
Disentanglement. *See also* Access and egress; Victim entrapment
    B-post displacement, 305
    buses, 418–421
    dashboard displacement, 303–304, 330–331
    defined, 279
    disentanglement point, 280
    Extrication Group responsibilities, 102
    floor pan, dropping, 304–305
    industrial and agricultural vehicles, 462–463
    medium and heavy trucks, 402–407
        access and egress routes, 402–403, 423–424
        entry points, 403–404, 423–424
        extrication operations, 407
        pneumatic lifting bags for lifting, 434
    pedal displacement or removal, 306–308
    railcars, 484
    seat displacement and removal, 305–306, 333–334
    steering column displacement, 303, 329
    windshield removal, 303, 328
Dispatch, 45
Documentation, postincident, 110
Dolly, 346
Doors
    beams, 227, 228
    box trailers, 348
    bus extrication operations, 411–413, 427–428
    door posts, 199
    as entrapment point, 281
    entry points, 289
    factory third and fourth doors, 297–298, 317
    fourth-door conversion, 299, 320
    industrial and agricultural vehicles, 462
    medium and heavy truck access and egress, 403, 404–405, 425
    Nader pin, 405
    railcars, 469–470, 481–483
    rear cargo doors, 348
    removal for access and egress, 293–297
        Halligan tool or pry bar, 296, 412
        hydra ram or rabbit tool, 296
        hydraulic spreaders, 295–296
        procedures, 314–320
    school buses, 361–362, 409
    side cargo doors, 348
    third door conversion
        access and egress techniques, 406
        door removal, 293
        extrication operations, 298, 319
    total sidewall removal, 298, 318
    truck cabs, 345
DOT. *See* Department of Transportation (DOT)
Double basket hitch, 248
Double choker hitch, 249
Drills, 143
Drivers, 140, 143
Driver's side of the vehicle, 199
Drivetrain of industrial and agricultural vehicles, 454
Dry bulk trailers, 349
Dual phase (DP) steel construction material, 204
Dump trailers, 349
Dump truck, 340, 448

E

E85 fuel, 212
Ear protection, 57
Earthmovers, 447, 448, 455
Egress. *See* Access and egress
18-wheelers, 341
Electric tools and equipment, 142–145
    auxiliary electrical equipment, 144
    drills and drivers, 143
    impact wrenches, 143
    portable lights, 143
    saws, 146
    signaling devices, 144
    spreaders and cutters, 142
    voltage detection devices, 145
Electric vehicles
    buses, 376
    fires, 81
    fuel systems, 207, 210
    locomotives, 465–466, 476
Electrical equipment on rescue vehicles, 123–124
Electrical lines as on-scene hazard, 20
Electrical systems
    airbag hazards, 71, 72
    batteries, 214–215. *See also* Batteries
    buses, 372–373
    components, 213
    defoggers, 213, 216
    electric engine cooling fans, 215–216
    extrication operation procedures, 213
    functions, 213
    ground fault circuit interrupter (GFCI), 143
    hazards, 65
    headlights, 214
    keyless entry ignition, 214
    medium and heavy trucks, 351
    power inverters, 213
    railcars, 472
    smart key ignitions, 214

Emergency Response Guidebook, 82
Endless sling, 252, 253
Energy sources for vehicles
    construction materials, 65–66
        crushable bumpers, 66
        vehicle components, 66
        windows, 65–66
    conventional electrical systems, 65
    procedures to secure and disable hazards, 86
    propulsion power, 62–64
        alternative fuels, 63
        atmosphere, monitoring, 64
        conventional fuels, 62–63
        hybrid electric vehicles, 64, 87
Energy-absorbing features, 224–228
    bumper struts, 225–226
    collision beams, 227–228
    crumple zones, 228
    crushable bumpers, 225
    steering column, 227
Engines
    apparatus, 123
    cooling fans, 215–216
    rescue, 119
    standard, 120
Enhanced protective glass (EPC), 203
Entrapment, defined, 280. *See also* Victim entrapment
Entry suits, 61
Environment
    conservation, 44
    size-up considerations, 17–18
        terrain, 18
        time of day, 17–18
        weather, 17
    uneven terrain, 180, 181
EPC (enhanced protective glass), 203
Equipment. *See* Tools and equipment
EREV (extended range electric vehicle), 210–211
Escape, routes of, 107
Esters, extinguishing agent for fires, 79
Ethanol
    alternative fuels, 212
    E85 fuel, 212
    extinguishing agents for fires, 79
    hazards, 63
Ethers, extinguishing agent for fires, 79
Evacuation, routes of, 107
Exclusive exterior compartment, 121, 122
Exclusive interior compartment, 121, 122
Exhaust piping, 216
Exhaust systems, 216
Exothermic cutting devices, 159
Explosion hazards, 76
Extended range electric vehicle (EREV), 210–211
Exterior of the vehicle, 198
Extinguishing devices and agents, 79
Extrication. *See also* Access and egress; Special extrication situations
    buses, 410–421
    defined, 1
    hanging vehicles, 444–446
    industrial and agricultural vehicles, 461–464
    medium and heavy trucks, 404–407, 425–426
    passenger vehicles, 290–308
    railcars, 483–486
    recreational vehicles, 446–447
    vehicles in a structure, 440–442
    vehicles in water, 442–444
Extrication Group, 101–102
Extrication Team Leader, 22–23
Extrication tools and equipment, 133–161
    come-alongs, 156–157

electric tools and equipment, 142–145
    auxiliary electrical equipment, 144
    drills and drivers, 143
    impact wrenches, 143
    portable lights, 143
    saws, 146
    signaling devices, 144
    spreaders and cutters, 142
    voltage detection devices, 145
hand tools, 133–142
    categories, 134
    center punches, 140
    cutting tools, 137–139
    glass hammers, 140, 141, 292
    handsaws, 138, 139
    lifting tools, 140–141
    mechanic's tools, 139–140
    prying tools, 136
    striking tools, 135–136
    trench tools, 142
hydraulic tools and equipment, 148–152
    manual, 151–152
    power-driven, 148–152
lifting or pulling tools, 155–156
pneumatic tools and equipment, 152–155
    chisels and hammers, 152
    lifting bags and cushions. *See* Lifting bags and cushions
    saws, 153
    wrenches, 153
power saws, 145–148
    chain saws, 147
    circular saws, 147
    portable band saws, 148
    reciprocating saws, 146–147, 417
    removing a heavy vehicle door, 404
    rotary saws, 147
    safety rules, 145
thermal cutting devices, 158–161
    cutting flares, 159
    exothermic cutting devices, 159
    oxyacetylene cutting torches, 160
    oxygasoline cutting torches, 160–161
    plasma-arc cutters, 160
    safety rules, 158–159
Eye protection, 56–57

F

Face injuries, 171, 172
Face protection, 56–57
Fairing, 346, 350
Farm implements. *See* Industrial and agricultural vehicles
Fatality in the same vehicle, 169
FCW (forward collision warning) system, 355
Federal Motor Carrier Safety Administration (FMCSA), 355
Federal Motor Vehicle Safety Standards, 205, 301, 362
Federal Response Plan, 40, 99
Fenders
    fender crush technique, 295–296
    functions, 199
Field amputations, 178
Fifth wheel, 341, 355
Fire extinguishers, ABC dry-chemical, 79
Fire fighter professional qualifications (NFPA 1001), 2
Fire hazards, 74–76
    flammable and combustible substances, 74–75
    foam to extinguish, 75, 79
    ignition sources, 75–76
Fire suppression operations, 77–81
    alternative fuels, 80–81
        alcohol/gasoline blends, 80
        biodiesel, 81

hybrid and electric vehicles, 81
hydrogen, 81
natural gas, 80-81
propane, 81
extinguishing devices and agents, 79
fire control strategies, 78
fire control support, 77-78
foam for vehicle fires, 75, 79
liquefied natural gas (LNG), 77, 80
procedures for establishing, 90-91
Firewall of the vehicle, 199
Flaggers, 38, 476
Flammable substances, 74-75
Flapping a roof, 300, 322, 432
Flash fire, 418
Flash hoods, 57
Flemish eye, 250
Floor
    access points, 300-301, 325-326
    bus entry points, 409-410, 417-418, 433
    entry points, 290
    floor pan drop, 304-305, 332
    industrial and agricultural vehicle entry point, 462
    medium and heavy truck entry points, 403
    railcars, 470, 471
    school bus construction, 369-370
FM Global, 137
FMCSA (Federal Motor Carrier Safety Administration), 355
Foam
    alcohol-resistant aqueous film forming foam (AR-AFFF), 79, 80
    aqueous film forming foam (AFFF), 79
    for vehicle fires, 75, 79
Folding screw jack, 141
Food service/lounge cars, 469, 483
Foot protection, 58
Fork trucks, 452
Forklifts, 452-453, 455
Forward collision warning (FCW) system, 355
Forward-looking collision-avoidance systems, 219
Four points of contact, 258
Four-point box crib, 386, 387
Four-point support, 258
Fourth-door conversion, 299, 320
Four-wheel drive powertrain, 218
Fractures, 176
Frame of the vehicle, 200-201
Freelance, 22, 255
Freight cars, 468
Front of the vehicle, 198
Frontal impact airbags, 222
Front-impact collision
    illustrated, 240
    injuries sustained from, 170-171, 281-282
    structural damage, 256
    victim entrapment, 281-282
Fuel cells, 211-212
Fuel hazards
    alcohol/gasoline blended fuel fires, 80
    alternative fuels, 63
    atmospheric monitoring, 64
    conventional fuels, 62-63
    hybrid electric vehicles, 64, 87
Fuel spills, 20, 21
Fuel systems
    alcohol/gasoline blended mixtures, 212
    auxiliary fuel cells, 211-212
    biodiesel, 212
    buses, 374-376
    compressed natural gas (CNG)
        bus fuel, 374-375
        defined, 81
        example, 80
        passenger vehicle use, 82
        truck fuel, 351
    conventional fuels, 206
    electric vehicles, 207, 210
    extended range electric vehicle (EREV), 210-211
    fuel tanks, 212
    hybrid car examples, 208-210
    hybrid electric vehicle (HEV), 205, 206-207
    hydrogen, 212
    industrial and agricultural vehicles, 455
    jet propellant-8 (JP-8), 212
    liquefied natural gas (LNG), 211
    liquefied petroleum gas (LPG, LP-Gas)
        bus fuel, 374-375
        as ignition source, 211
        truck fuel, 351
        uses for, 211
    locomotives, 465
    medium and heavy trucks, 350-351
    Plug-In Hybrid Electric Vehicle (PHEV), 207
    propane, 211
    saddle tanks on trucks, 350-351
Fulcrum, 246
Full frame, 200-201
Full size van, 197

G

Gasoline
    alcohol/gasoline blended mixtures, 80, 212
    bus fuel systems, 374
    containers as on-scene hazard, 19
    extinguishing agents for fires, 79
    fire extinguishment, 80
    fuel systems, 206
Generators on rescue vehicles, 123-124
GFCI (ground fault circuit interrupter), 143
GFI (ground fault indicator) receptacle, 143
Gin poles, 125
Glad-hand connection, 353, 387
Glass. *See also* Windows
    alternative glass removal, 293, 313
    construction materials, 205
    enhanced protective glass (EPC), 203
    glass hammer, 140, 141, 292
    glass saw, 138, 139
    hazards to victims, 176
    laminated safety glass
        characteristics, 202-203
        hazards, 65
        removal for access and egress, 291-292, 311
    removal for access and egress, 291-293, 310-313
    tempered glass
        characteristics, 203
        hazards, 65
    Lexan®, 470
    railcar windows, 470
    removal for access and egress, 292-293, 312
    vehicle windows, 65-66
Global positioning system (GPS), 45
Gloves, 58
Golden Hour, 168, 169
Government
    adoption of NIMS-ICS, 11
    state/provincial government, defined, 3
GPS (global positioning system), 45
Graders, 451
Griphoist®
    characteristics, 156
    functions, 241
    manual cable winch, 253

Index **507**

Gross decontamination, 177
Gross vehicle weight rating (GVWR), 191, 385
Ground fault circuit interrupter (GFCI), 143
Ground fault indicator (GFI) receptacle, 143
Groups
    Extrication Group, 101-102
    Group Supervisor, 100
    incident operation groups, 100-102
    Medical Group, 33, 102, 103
    Rescue Group, 33
    Suppression Group, 33
GVWR (gross vehicle weight rating), 191, 385

H

Half-cab, 344
Halligan tool, 296, 412
Hand protection, 58
Hand tools, 133-142
    categories, 134
    center punches, 140
    cutting tools, 137-139
    glass hammers, 140, 141, 292
    handsaws, 138, 139
    lifting tools, 140-141
    mechanic's tools, 139-140
    prying tools, 136
    striking tools, 135-136
    trench tools, 142
Hanging vehicle incidents, 444-446
Hardware chain, 131
Harvesters, 450-451
Hatchback struts, 226
Hazardous materials (haz mat)
    bus incidents, 84
    defined, 82
    DOT placards, 83
    environmental protections, 44
    fuel spills, 20, 21
    gross decontamination, 177
    industrial and agricultural vehicle hazards, 459
    inhalation protection from, 59
    medium and heavy truck incidents, 82, 84
    NFPA 472 incident standards, 12
    operational protocols, 41, 42
    passenger vehicle incidents, 82
    personal protective equipment for, 61
    pyrotechnic devices on seat belt pretensioners, 69
    sodium azide, 71
    victim exposure to, 177
Hazards
    industrial and agricultural vehicles, 459
    potential, 24-25
    railcars, 476-477
    risk assessment survey, 16
    scene assessment considerations, 97-98
HBV (hepatitis B virus), 21
Head injuries, 171, 172
Head protection, 56-57
Head protection system (HPS), 72, 222-223
Headlights, 214
Head-on impact collision
    injuries sustained from, 170-171
    structural damage, 256
Health Insurance Portability and Accountability Act (HIPAA), 182
Hearing protection, 57
Heavy rescue vehicles, 118-119
Heavy trucks. See Medium and heavy trucks
Heavy vehicle stabilization, 383-396
    buses, 389-393
    considerations for, 384, 385-393
    gross vehicle weight rating (GVWR), 385
    medium and heavy trucks, 385-389, 395-396
    tools and equipment, 383
Heavy-duty trailers, 349
Helmets, 56
Hepatitis B virus (HBV), 21
HEV. See Hybrid electric vehicle (HEV)
HID (high-intensity discharge) headlights, 214
High strength/low alloy steel (HSLA), 204, 228
High-intensity discharge (HID) headlights, 214
High-pressure lifting bags, 154-155, 244-245
Hi-Lift® jacks, 141, 296-297, 314
Hinges on the vehicle, 199
HIPAA (Health Insurance Portability and Accountability Act), 182
Hitches, 247-249
    basket, 248
    bridle, 248
    choker, 248
    double basket, 248
    double choker, 249
    sling, 247
    vertical, 247-248
HIV (human immunodeficiency virus), 21
Hoists
    chain joist, 254
    Griphoist®, 156, 241, 253
Homeland Security Presidential Directive-5 (HSPD-5), 11
Hood struts, 226
Hooligan tool, 412. See also Halligan tool
Horizontal axis, 237
Hot (restricted) zone, 31
Hot wire cutters, 137
HPS (head protection system), 72, 222-223
HSLA (high strength/low alloy) steel, 204, 228
HSPD-5 (Homeland Security Presidential Directive-5), 11
Human immunodeficiency virus (HIV), 21
Hybrid electric vehicle (HEV)
    battery hazards, 64
    buses, 375-376
    disabling a battery, 87
    examples, 208-210
    fire extinguishment, 81
    fuel systems, 205, 206-207
    voltage, 207
Hydra ram, 296
Hydraulic lifts on buses, 371
Hydraulic systems on trucks, 351-353
Hydraulic tools and equipment, 148-152
    cranes, 125-126
    cutters, 13, 149-150
    for door removal, 297, 316
    jacks, 151, 152
    manual, 151-152
    pedal cutters, 150
    Porta-Power®, 151, 152
    power-driven, 148-152
    rams
        characteristics, 150-151
        for school bus access point, 412
        uses for, 304, 407
    spreaders, 149, 150
Hydrofluoric acid (HF) from crushable bumpers, 66
Hydrogen
    alternative fuels, 212
    auxiliary fuel cells, 211-212
    bus fuel cells, 375
    fuel fires, 81
    truck fuel, 351
Hyperthermia, 177
Hypothermia, 177
Hypovolemia (blood loss), 176

I

IAP. *See* Incident Action Plan (IAP)
IC. *See* Incident Commander (IC)
ICP (Incident Command Post), 101
ICS. *See* Incident Command System (ICS)
IFSTA, NIMS-ICS applicability, 99-100
Ignition sources, 75-76
Immobilization of victims
    cervical collar, 179, 184
    cervical spine, 167
    devices, 179
    long board, 179
    procedures, 180
    for removal, 168
    seated spinal immobilization device, 179, 186
    vacuum mattress, 179
Impact hammers, 152, 416
Incident Action Plan (IAP)
    assigned tasks, 44
    Assignments in the Incident Action Plan (ICS 204 Form), 42, 106
    communicating rescue strategy and objectives, 43-44
    elements, 42-43
    incident stabilization, 44
    initial response plan, 14
    NIMS-ICS planning process, 104-106
    operational capability, 49
    personnel protection and life safety, 43
    property and environmental conservation, 44
    safety message (ICS 208 or 208H Form), 43, 106
    tactical worksheet, 42, 105
    terminating an incident, 107-108, 111
    transition from verbal to written IAP, 105
    verbal, 43
    written, 105, 106
Incident briefing (ICS 201 Form), 42, 105
Incident Command Post (ICP), 101
Incident Command System (ICS)
    announcement example, 104
    Assignments in the Incident Action Plan (ICS 204 Form), 42, 106
    command and control, 100
    defined, 99
    ICS forms, purpose of, 105
    incident briefing (ICS 201 Form), 42, 105
    Incident Command Post (ICP), 101
    Incident Commander in charge or, 25
    incident objectives (ICS 202 Form), 42, 106
    incident operation groups, 100-102
        Extrication Group, 101-102
        Group Supervisor, 100
        Medical Group, 102
    Incident Safety Analysis (ICS form 215A), 105, 106
    Operations Section Chief, 100
    operations within, 103-104
    organization (ICS 203 Form), 106
    performance standards, 99-100
    planning process, 104-106
    purpose of, 103
    resource status information, 106
    safety message (ICS 208 or 208H Form), 43, 106
    situation status information, 106
    support materials, 43, 106
Incident Commander (IC)
    assigned incident tasks, 44
    command and control, 100, 101
    communicating hazards, 45
    defined, 25
    evacuation methods, 107
    expert assistance needs, 46-47
    NIMS-ICS planning process, 105
    pedestrian control, 36
    Personnel Accountability Report (PAR), 106
    PPE choices, 55
    responsibilities during extrication operations, 25
    scene control, 255
    span-of-control, 100
    traffic control, 36
    verbal Incident Action Plan, 43
    zone boundaries, establishment of, 32
Incident Management Coalition Team, 15
Incident management standards (NFPA 1561), 11, 41
Incident operation groups, 100-102
    Extrication Group, 101-102
    Group Supervisor, 100
    Medical Group, 102
Incident Safety Analysis (ICS form 215A), 105, 106
Incident Safety Officer (ISO)
    assigned incident tasks, 44
    defined, 25
    evacuation methods, 107
    monitoring hazard zones, 33-34
    personnel accountability, 26
    PPE choices, 55
    responsibilities during extrication operations, 25-26
    verbal Incident Action Plan, 43
Incident stability
    Incident Action Plan (IAP), 44
    resource capabilities and limitations, 27
    restoring the scene, 29
    scene control and protection, 27
    on-scene medical care, 28-29
    vehicle crash dynamics, 27-28
    vehicle stabilization and access, 28
Industrial and agricultural vehicles, 447-464
    anatomy, construction, and features, 453-457
        articulating and telescoping vehicles, 455
        auxiliary power sources, 456
        brake systems, 455-456
        drivetrain, 454
        fuel systems, 455
        jacks, 456-457
        operational controls, 454
        rollover protection systems, 456
        tires, 455
        tracked vehicles, 454
    booms, 451-452
    cranes, 452
    extrication operations, 461-464
    forklifts, 452-453, 455
    graders, 451
    harvesters, 450-451
    hazards, 459
    incident size-up, 457-459
    tractors, 448-450
    vehicle stabilization, 459-461
Inflatable tubes, 223
Infrared night vision systems, 220
Initial size-up, 95
Injuries
    compartment syndrome, 177
    crush syndrome, 177-178
    field amputations, 178
    fractures, 176
    front-impact collisions, 170-171, 281-282
    hazardous materials exposure, 177
    hypothermia and hyperthermia, 177
    hypovolemia (blood loss), 176
    internal injuries, 178
    lacerations, 176
    mechanisms of, 168-173
        blunt and penetrating trauma, 171
        fatality in the same vehicle, 169
        head-on impact collision, 170-171

rear impact collision, 172-173
rollover, 173
rotational impact collisions, 173
side impact collision, 171-172
prevention of, 175-176
rear-impact collisions, 172-173, 282
rollovers, 283-284
rotational collisions, 283
side-impact collisions, 171-172, 282-283
traumatic brain injury (TBI), 178
underrides and overrides, 284-285
Insulated wire cutters, 137
Integral body construction
anatomy, 390
commercial buses, 371
school buses, 368
transit buses, 370-371
Interior of the vehicle, 198
Internal injuries, 178
Inverters
passenger vehicle, 213
remote power outlets, 65, 213
rescue vehicle, 123
Ireland, truck/semitrailer combinations, 341
ISO. *See* Incident Safety Officer (ISO)

J
Jacks
bus disentanglement, 420-421
commercial/heavy truck stabilization, 391
Hi-Lift® jacks, 141, 296-297, 314
hydraulic, 151, 152
industrial and agricultural vehicles, 456-457
jack pad, 391
jack plate, 391
lifting a wheel-resting passenger vehicle, 266
procedures, 245, 246
ratchet-lever, 141
screw jacks, 140-141
for vehicle stabilization, 245, 246, 266
Jargon, 3
Jet propellant-8 (JP-8), 212
Job performance requirements (JPRs), 2
JP-8 (jet propellant-8), 212
JPRs (job performance requirements), 2
Junction boxes, 144

K
KED® (Kendrick Extrication Device), 179
Kendrick Extrication Device (KED®), 179
Kenworth cab-beside-engine, 344
Key information in this book, 3-4
Keyless entry ignitions, 214
Kick panel
defined, 200
removal for access and egress, 300, 324
Kingpin, 387
Kit cars, 196
Knee bolsters, 224
Kneeling of buses, 377
Knives, 139

L
Lacerations, 176
Ladder trucks, 120
Ladders used for access
buses, 408, 409
medium and heavy trucks, 403
Laminated safety glass
characteristics, 202-203

hazards, 65
removal for access and egress, 291-292, 311
Land trains, 341
Landing gear, 346-347
Lane departure warning (LDW) system, 355
Large cars, 195
Latches on the vehicle, 199
Lateral axis, 237
Law enforcement
safety zone responsibilities, 33
for traffic control, 34
LDW (lane departure warning) system, 355
Leaf spring suspension, 390
Leaf springs, 218
Levers
Class I, 246, 267
Class II, 247
Class III, 247
defined, 246
fulcrum, 246
Lexan®, 470
Lift trucks, 452
Lifting bags and cushions
bus entanglement operations, 420, 434
high-pressure, 154-155
industrial and agricultural vehicle incidents, 459
low- and medium-pressure, 155
safety rules for using, 153-154
uses for, 153, 383
Lifting techniques
commercial/heavy vehicles, 384
passenger vehicle, 239, 241-242
Lifting tools
Griphoist®, 156, 241, 253
lifting bags and cushions. *See* Lifting bags and cushions
pneumatic lifting bags and cushions, 243-245, 265, 383
ratchet-lever jacks, 141
safety rules, 156
screw jacks, 140-141
uses for, 155
Light rescue vehicles, 117-118
Lighting
emergency vehicles and equipment, 36
headlights, 214
low-light incidents, 17-18
portable lights, 143
stationary lights on rescue vehicles, 124
Limited access (warm) zone, 31, 32
Limousines, 196
Liquefied natural gas (LNG)
alternative fuels, 211
bus fuel, 374-375
defined, 77
fire suppression, 77, 80
truck fuel, 351
Liquefied petroleum gas (LPG, LP-Gas)
bus fuel, 374-375
as ignition source, 211
truck fuel, 351
uses for, 211
Livestock trailers, 348
LNG. *See* Liquefied natural gas (LNG)
Load binder, 254
Load limiters, 221
Loading platform incidents, 484-485
Lock-out/tag-out procedures, 352
Locks on the vehicle, 199
Locomotives
diesel and diesel/electric, 465-466, 476
electric, 466

entry into, 480
steam, 466, 467
Long board, 179, 185
Longitudinal axis, 237
Lounge/food service cars, 469, 483
Lowboy trailers, 349
Low-pressure lifting cushions, 155, 245
LPG. *See* Liquefied petroleum gas (LPG, LP-Gas)

M

Magnesium
combustibility, 75
construction materials, 204
vehicle component material, 66, 75
Maintainers, 451
Manual cable winch, 253
Manual hydraulic tools, 151–152
Manual on Uniform Traffic Control Devices (MUTCD), 19, 37
Marrying vehicles or objects together, 262, 274
Mass casualty incident (MCI), 174–175, 285, 476
Material handling cars, 468, 483
MCI (mass casualty incident), 174–175, 285, 476
Measurement, metric conversions, 4–6
Mechanical advantage, 136, 157
Mechanical systems on trucks, 352
Mechanic's tools, 139–140
Mechanism of movement, 236–238, 384
Medical
Medical Group, 33, 102, 103
safety measures, 24
on-scene care, 28–29
Medium and heavy trucks, 339–355
access and egress points, 402–404, 423–424
anatomy, 343–349
cabs, 343–346
trailers, 346–349
characteristics, 339
construction, 350–355
auxiliary lift axles, 354–355
batteries, 350
brake systems, 353–354
components, 350
electrical systems, 351
fuel systems, 350–351
hydraulic systems, 351–353
suspension systems, 354
door, open or removing, 425
extrication operations, 404–407, 425–426
fifth wheels, 341, 355
placards, 341, 342
roof access point, 426
safety features, 355
specialty trucks, 341
stabilization, 385–389
disconnecting glad hands, 387
other positions, 388–389
roof-resting trucks, 388
side-resting trucks, 387–388
wheel-resting trucks, 386–387
straight trucks, 340, 354
truck/semitrailer combinations, 341
wall access point, 426
weights, 339
Medium rescue vehicles, 118
Medium-pressure lifting cushions, 155, 245
Metals, combustible, 75, 79
Meth laboratories, as on-scene hazard, 19
Methanol, extinguishing agent for fires, 79
Metric conversions, 4–6
Micro-alloy (MA) steel, 228
Midsize cars, 195

Mild steel construction materials, 204
Minicompact cars, 194
Minivans, 196–197, 298
Monocoque frame construction, 200
Motor coach, 358, 418. *See also* Commercial buses
Motor homes, 446–447
Movement, mechanism of, 236–238, 384
MPI (Multiple Patient Incident), 174
Mufflers, 216
Multiple Patient Incident (MPI), 174
Multiple vehicle incident (MVI), 285–287
MUTCD (*Manual on Uniform Traffic Control Devices*), 19, 37
MVI (multiple vehicle incident), 285–287

N

Nader pin, 405
National Fire Protection Association (NFPA) performance standards, 40, 99. *See also specific NFPA*
National Highway Traffic Safety Administration (NHTSA)
airbag safety, 70
defined, 70
passenger car classifications, 194–195
passenger vehicle classification, 191
National Incident Management System (NIMS)
defined, 40
performance standards, 99
Planning "P" form, 105, 106
National Incident Management System-Incident Command System (NIMS-ICS)
adoption by state and local government, and tribal entities, 11
defined, 40
IAP planning process, 104–106
operational protocols, 41
purpose of, 99
National Search and Rescue Plan, 40, 99
NATO (North Atlantic Treaty Organization), 212
Natural gas fire extinguishment, 79, 80–81
Neck injuries, 171, 172
Neck protection system, 223
New Zealand, truck/semitrailer combinations, 341
NFPA. *See* National Fire Protection Association (NFPA) performance standards
NFPA 472, *Standard for Competence of Responders to Hazardous Materials/Weapons of Mass Destruction Incidents*, 12
NFPA 1001, *Standard for Fire Fighter Professional Qualifications*, 2
NFPA 1006, *Standard for Technical Rescuer Professional Qualifications, 2017 Edition*
Awareness Level, 12
incident safety, 11
job performance requirements, 2
operating levels, 12
Operations Level, 12–13
organization responsibilities, 40
performance standards, 99
Technician Level, 13
NFPA 1500, *Standard on Fire Department Occupational Safety and Health Program*
critical incident stress, 109
eye protection, 57
fit-testing self-contained breathing apparatus, 59
hand protection, 58
operational protocols, 41
operations management, 11
NFPA 1521, *Standard for Fire Department Safety Office Professional Qualifications*, 33–34, 41
NFPA 1561, *Standard on Emergency Services Incident Management System and Command Safety*, 11, 41
NFPA 1670, *Standard on Operations and Training for Technical Rescue Incidents*
extrication, defined, 1
incident safety, 11

organization responsibilities, 40
performance standards, 99
scope of this manual, 2
NFPA 1936, *Standard on Powered Rescue Tools*, 150
NFPA 1971, *Standard on Protective Ensembles for Structural Fire Fighting and Proximity Fire Fighting*
    foot protection, 58
    hand protection, 58
    helmet requirements, 56
    reflective striping, 57
    turnout gear, 57
NFPA 1981, *Standard on Open-Circuit Self-Contained Breathing Apparatus (SCBA) for Emergency Services*, 29, 59
NFPA 1999, *Standard on Protective Clothing for Emergency Medical Operations*, 58
NHTSA. *See* National Highway Traffic Safety Administration (NHTSA)
NIMS. *See* National Incident Management System (NIMS)
NIMS-ICS. *See* National Incident Management System-Incident Command System (NIMS-ICS)
Non-breathing air compressors, 127
North Atlantic Treaty Organization (NATO), 212
Nuclear incidents, hazard and risk assessment surveys, 16

O

Objectives, incident (ICS 202 Form), 42, 106
OBSS (on-board safety system), 355
Occupant position sensors, 68
Occupant weight sensors, 68
Occupational Safety and Health Administration (OSHA)
    forklifts, 452
    rollover protection systems, 449, 456
    tractor safety requirements, 449
OI (operating instruction), 55
On-board safety system (OBSS), 355
Ongoing size-up, 99
Operating instruction (OI), 55
Operational readiness, restoring, 109
Operations at vehicle incidents, 40–47
    communication, 44–46
    Incident Action Plan (IAP), 42–44. *See also* Incident Action Plan (IAP)
    protocols, 40–42
    resources, 46–47
    support operations, 46
Operations Level
    emergency escape and evacuation, 106–107
    Incident Command System, 99–106
    NFPA 1006 requirements, 12–13
    postincident responsibilities and analysis, 108–110
    scene size-up, 95–99
    stabilization, 383–396
        buses, 389–393
        considerations for, 384, 385–393
        medium and heavy trucks, 385–389, 395–396
        tools and equipment, 383
    terminating an incident, 107–108
Operations Section Chief, 100
Opposite-side, independent stabilization system, 261
Ops Chief, 100
Ops Section Chief, 100
Organization
    ICS 203 Form, 106
    Incident Action Plan (IAP), 42, 106
    of this book, 2–3
OSHA. *See* Occupational Safety and Health Administration (OSHA)
Outer perimeter of incidents, 32
Outriggers on industrial and agricultural vehicles, 456–457
Overrides, 257, 284–285
Oxyacetylene cutting torches, 160
Oxygasoline cutting torches, 160–161

P

Packaging a patient
    cervical collar, 179
    immobilizing and, 167, 168, 180
    long board, 179, 185
    removing a packaged patient, 180–181
    seated spinal immobilization device, 179, 186
    vacuum mattress, 179
Pantograph
    defined, 376, 466
    functions, 472
    hazards, 476–477
PAR (Personnel Accountability Report), 106
Passenger cars, 194–196
    compact cars, 195
    convertibles, 196
    door entry, 481
    kit cars, 196
    large cars, 195
    limousines, 196
    midsize cars, 195
    minicompact cars (station cars), 194
    railcars, 465, 466–467
    roadsters, 196
    sports cars/sports coupes, 196
    station wagons, 195
    subcompact cars, 194–195
    window entry, 481–482
Passenger vehicles, 191–229
    anatomy, 197–204
        frame, 200–201
        terminology, 198–200
        windows, 201–204
    construction, 204–219
        electrical systems, 213–216
        exhaust systems, 216
        fuel systems, 205–212
        materials, 204–205
        powertrain, 216–218
        suspension systems, 218–219
    examples, 192–193
    haz mat incidents, 82
    safety features, 219–229
        collision avoidance systems, 219–220
        energy-absorbing features, 224–228
        rollover protection systems, 229
        supplemental restraint systems, 220–224
    stabilization, 235–274
        defined, 235
        lifting, 239, 241–242
        mechanism of movement, 236–238
        operations, 255–262, 268–274
        points and surfaces/terrain, 238–239, 240
        tools and equipment, 242–255, 264–267
    types of, 191–197
        all-terrain vehicles (ATV), 194
        gross vehicle weight rating (GVWR), 191
        passenger cars, 194–196
        pickup trucks, 192–193, 197
        sport utility trucks, 197
        sport utility vehicle (SUV), 197
        vans, 196–197
Passenger's side of the vehicle, 199
Passive restraint devices, neck protection systems, 223
Patient
    defined, 26
    follow up, 182
Pedals
    cutters, 150, 307
    displacement and removal, 306–308
    as entrapment point, 281

medium and heavy truck disentanglement, 407
Pedestrians
    collisions with trains, 485
    control of, 36, 84
    scene assessment, 97
Peel and peek for supplemental restraint system information, 67–68, 70, 293
Penetrating trauma, 171
Performance standards, Incident Command System, 99–100
Personal protective equipment (PPE)
    body armor, 61
    body protection, 57–58
    body substance isolation, 56
    foot protection, 58
    hand protection, 58
    hazardous materials suits, 61
    head, eyes, and face protection, 56–57
    hearing protection, 57
    proximity or entry suits, 61
    reflective clothing, 36–37, 38, 57
    respiratory protection, 58–61. *See also* Respiratory protection
    response preparation, 16
    safety standards. *See* NFPA 1971, *Standard on Protective Ensembles for Structural Fire Fighting and Proximity Fire Fighting*
    safety vests
        for flaggers, 38
        for increased visibility, 36, 58
        for personnel identification, 101
    standard operating procedures for choosing, 55
    training for use of, 29–30
    wet suits, 61
Personnel, responders to vehicle extrication incidents, 1
Personnel Accountability Report (PAR), 106
Personnel accountability system, 26
Petroleum-based materials, 75
PHEV (Plug-In Hybrid Electric Vehicle), 207
PIA (postincident analysis), 109
Picks, 137
Pickup trucks, 197
Pie cut for access, 302
Piggyback chambers, 353
Pike pole, 385, 411
Pitch of a vehicle, 238
Placard
    biohazards, 21
    defined, 341
    industrial and agricultural labeling, 458
    parts, colors, symbols, 83, 342
    tractor/trailer labeling, 341
Planning "P," 105, 106
Plans. *See* Preincident planning
Plasma-arc cutters, 160
Plastics
    construction materials, 205
    cribbing, 128, 129
    fuel tanks, 212
    health hazards, 75
    step chocks, 130, 258
Pliers, 139, 140
Plug-In Hybrid Electric Vehicle (PHEV), 207
Pneumatic, defined, 354
Pneumatic lifting bags and cushions, 243–245, 265, 383
Pneumatic stringers on trucks, 354–355
Pneumatic systems on trucks, 353
Pneumatic tools and equipment, 152–155
    chisels and hammers, 152, 416
    lifting bags and cushions
        bus entanglement operations, 420, 434
        high-pressure, 154–155
        industrial and agricultural vehicle incidents, 459

low- and medium-pressure, 155
safety rules for using, 153–154
uses for, 153, 383
saws, 153
wrenches, 153
Pogo stick, 353
Polycarbonate, 203
Portable band saws, 148
Portable lights, 143
Porta-Power®, 151, 152
Postincident analysis (PIA), 109
Postincident responsibilities and analysis, 108–110
Post-traumatic stress disorder (PTSD), 110
Potential hazards, 24–25
Power inverters, 213
Power lines, on-scene hazards, 20
Power plant, 123
Power saws, 145–148
    chain saws, 147
    circular saws, 147
    portable band saws, 148
    reciprocating saws, 146–147, 417
    removing a heavy vehicle door, 404
    rotary saws, 147
    safety rules, 145
Power take-off (PTO) system
    controlling, 456
    defined, 123
    entanglement dangers, 352
    functions, 352
    industrial and agricultural vehicle incidents, 464
Power transference, 217
Power unit, 148
Power-driven hydraulic tools, 148–152
Powered cable winch, 253–254
Powertrain systems, 216–218
PPE. *See* Personal protective equipment (PPE)
Predetermined procedures, 55
Preincident planning
    fire control strategies, 78
    purpose of, 14
    special extrication situations, 439
Pre-tensioners, 68–69
Proof coil chain, 131
Propane
    alternative fuels, 211
    characteristics, 81
    fire extinguishment, 79, 81
Property conservation, 44
Propulsion power, 62–64
    alternative fuels, 63
    atmosphere, monitoring, 64
    conventional fuels, 62–63
    hybrid electric vehicles, 64, 87
Protected Health Information, 182
Protecting personnel and the public, 107–108
Protocols, operational, 40–42
Proximity suits, 61
Prying tools
    Halligan tool, 296, 412
    pry bar, 296
    safety rules, 136
    uses for, 136
Psychological concerns of victims, 176
PTO. *See* Power take-off (PTO) system
PTSD (post-traumatic stress disorder), 110
Pulling tools, 155–156
Purchase point, 295–296
Purpose of this manual, 1
Pyrotechnic devices on seat belt pretensioners, 69

Index **513**

Q
Quarter panels of the vehicle, 199

R
Rabbit tool, 296
Radio for communicating hazards, 107
Railcars, 464–486
    access and egress, 479–483
    anatomy, construction, and features, 469–475
        brakes, 471
        catenary systems, 466, 472–474
        doors, 469–470
        electrical systems, 472
        floors, 470, 471
        roadbeds, 475
        third-rail systems, 475
        trucks, 471
        walls and roofs, 470–471
        windows, 470
    collisions with highway vehicles, 485
    collisions with pedestrians, 485
    disentanglement/tunneling, 484
    extrication operations, 483–486
    hazards, 476–477, 478
    incident size-up, 475–476
    loading platform incidents, 484–485
    passenger, 465, 467
    stabilization, 477–479
    trams, 485–486
    trolley, 466, 472–474
    types of, 464–469
        baggage cars, 468, 483
        consist, 464
        freight cars, 468
        locomotives, 465–466, 467
        lounge/food service cars, 469, 483
        material handling cars, 468, 483
        passenger cars, 466–467
        sleeping car, 482–483
Rams
    characteristics, 150–151
    for school bus access point, 412
    uses for, 304, 407
Ratchet, for door removal, 315
Ratchet straps, 132–133
Ratchet-lever jacks, 141
Rear of the vehicle, 198
Rear-impact collision
    illustrated, 240
    injuries sustained from, 172–173, 282
    neck protection systems, 223
    structural damage, 256
    victim entrapment, 282
Rear-looking collision-avoidance systems, 220
Reciprocating saws, 146–147, 417
Recovery vehicles, 255, 384, 385
Recreational vehicles (RVs), 446–447
Reflective clothing, 36–37, 38, 57
Refrigerated trailers, 348
Rehabilitation (rehab)
    defined, 24
    station, as safety measure, 24
Remote power outlet (RPO), 65, 213
Removal of wrecked vehicles, 107, 108
Rescue crane, 255
Rescue engines, 119
Rescue Group, 33
Rescue vehicles, 117–127
    chassis, 121
    compartmentation, 121–122
    features and equipment, 122–127
        air supply systems, 126–127
        all-wheel drive, 122
        electrical equipment, 123–124
        gin poles and A-frames, 125, 126
        hydraulic cranes, 125–126
        stabilizers, 126
        winches, 124–125
    heavy rescue vehicles, 118–119
    ladder trucks, 120
    light rescue vehicles, 117–118
    medium rescue vehicles, 118
    rescue engines, 119
    standard engines, 120
Rescuer control, 36
Rescuer protection, 108
Resources
    crew resource management, 22–23
    expert assistance, 46–47
    incident stability, 27
    safety operations, 46–47
    status information, 106
    support operations, 46–47
    traffic control, 40
Respiratory protection
    air-purifying respirator (APR)
        air-purifying filters, 59–61
        factors in choice of, 60
        limitations, 60
        oxygen requirements, 60
        powered or non-powered, 60
        precautions for use, 61
    breathing air compressors, 126–127
    hazards at vehicle extrication incidents, 58
    inhalation of hazardous materials, 59
    self-contained breathing apparatus (SCBA)
        cascade systems, 126
        fit-testing, 59
        NFPA 1981 requirements, 29, 59
        positive-pressure, 59
        training for use, 59
    self-contained underwater breathing apparatus (SCUBA), 443
Response plans, 14–15
Restoring the scene, 29
Restraint systems. *See* Supplemental restraint system (SRS)
Restricted (hot) zone, 31
Rigging, 130–132
    chains, 131–132
    commercial/heavy truck stabilization, 384, 389
    components, 253
    defined, 253
    fittings, 254–255
    rope, 131
    tighteners, 253–254
    webbing, 132, 133
Rigid frame, 200–201
Risk assessment survey, 16
Risk-benefit analysis, 17
Roadbed, railroad, 475
Roadsters, 196
Rocker panel/channel, 200
Roll stability control (RSC) system, 355
Rollovers
    end-over-end, 283–284
    industrial and agricultural vehicle incidents, 458–459
    injuries sustained from, 173
    rollover protection systems
        for convertibles, 73
        defined, 229
        driving mode and rollover mode, 229
        examples, 68
        industrial and agricultural vehicles, 456, 462–463

passenger vehicles, 229
tractors, 449
victim entrapment, 283-284
RollTek®, 355
Roof
bus access point, 416-417, 431-432
as entrapment point, 281
entry points, 289
flapping a roof, 300, 322, 432
industrial and agricultural vehicle entry point, 462
medium and heavy truck entry points, 403, 406, 426
posts, 199
railcars, 470-471, 482
ramming the roof off, 302
removal for access and egress, 299-300, 321-323
roof posts, 199
school bus emergency escape hatch, 369, 370
school bus entry point, 409-410
sunroof access, 302
truck cab/fairing, 346, 350
Roof-resting vehicle
bus stabilization, 392-393
buses, 421
commercial/heavy truck stabilization, 388
illustrated, 240
industrial and agricultural vehicles, 460-461
railcars, 479
stabilization, 261, 273
victim rescue, 280
Rope
commercial/heavy truck stabilization, 388
uses for, 131
utility rope, 131
for vehicle stabilization, 261
wire rope, 250-251, 253
Rotary saws, 147
Rotational collisions, 173, 283
Round slings, 252
RPO (remote power outlet), 65, 213
RSC (roll stability control) system, 355
Rubber construction materials, 205
RVs (recreational vehicles), 446-447

S

Saddle tanks, 350-351
Safety at vehicle incidents, 11-51
chain usage, 131-132, 249
crew resource management, 22-23
Incident Safety Analysis (ICS form 215A), 105, 106
ISO. *See* Incident Safety Officer (ISO)
jack, use of, 151
lifting bags and cushions, 153-154
medical personnel, 24
NFPA standards. *See* NFPA 1500, *Standard on Fire Department Occupational Safety and Health Program*
operational capability, 11-13
Awareness Level, 12
Incident Action Plan (IAP), 49
Operations Level, 12-13
Technician Level, 13, 14
operations, 40-47
communication, 44-46
Incident Action Plan (IAP), 42-44
protocols, 40-42
resources, 46-47
support operations, 46
personnel accountability, 26
potential hazards, 24-25
power saws, 145
prying tool use, 136
rehabilitation station, 24

rescuer protection, 108
response preparation, 13-16
hazard and risk assessment surveys, 16
personal protective equipment, 16
response plans, 14-15
safety zones, 30-34
boundaries, 32
limited access (warm) zone, 31, 32
monitoring, 33-34
procedures for establishing, 51
purpose of, 30-31
restricted (hot) zone, 31
staffing requirements, 32-33
support (cold) zone, 31, 32
scene safety, 26-30
incident stability, 27-29
personal safety equipment and techniques, 29-30
scene size-up, 16-22
environmental considerations, 17-18
procedures, 50
risk-benefit analysis, 17
on-scene hazards, 18-22
striking tool use, 136
thermal cutting devices, 158-159
traffic control, 34-40
concepts, 34-36
devices, 36-40
resources, 40
training for personnel, 22
turning down assignments, 23
vehicle stabilization, 235
winch danger zone, 125
Safety features, passenger vehicle, 219-229
collision avoidance systems, 219-220
energy-absorbing features, 224-228
bumper struts, 225-226
collision beams, 227-228
crumple zones, 228
crushable bumpers, 225
steering column, 227
rollover protection systems, 229. *See also* Rollovers, *subhead* rollover protection systems
supplemental restraint systems, 220-224
airbags, 221-224
child safety restraint devices, 224
seat belts, pretensioners, and load limiters, 220-221
Safety features, trucks, 355
Safety glasses, 56
Safety message in the Incident Action Plan (ICS 208 or 208H Form), 43, 106
Safety signals, 107
Safety zones, 30-34
airbags, 69
boundaries, 32
limited access (warm) zone, 31, 32
monitoring, 33-34
procedures for establishing, 51
purpose of, 30-31
restricted (hot) zone, 31
staffing requirements, 32-33
support (cold) zone, 31, 32
Same-side, opposing force system, 260, 271
Saws
glass saw, 138, 139
handsaws, 138
pneumatic, 153
power saws, 145-148
chain saws, 147
circular saws, 147
portable band saws, 148
reciprocating saws, 146-147, 417

Index **515**

removing a heavy vehicle door, 404
    rotary saws, 147
    safety rules, 145
  whizzer saw, 153
  windshield cutter, 138
SCBA. *See* Self-contained breathing apparatus (SCBA)
Scene assessment, 96–98
  day of the week, 97
  hazards, 97–98
  pedestrians, 97
  time of day, 97
  vehicles involved, 97, 98
  vehicular traffic, 97
  weather, 96
Scene control
  cordoning off the area, 20, 32, 84
  by the Incident Commander, 255
  incident stability, 27
Scene safety, 26–30
  incident stability, 27–29
  personal safety equipment and techniques, 29–30
Scene security barriers, 32
School buses
  aisles, 366–367
  batteries, 372
  characteristics, 356
  construction, 368–370
    body-on-chassis, 368
    floor and undercarriage, 369–370
    integral construction, 368
    skeletal system, 368–369
  conversions, 360
  defined, 356
  doors
    access opening, 427–428
    entry points, 409
    front doors, 361–362, 412
    rear doors, 362, 413
  electrical systems, 372–373
  roof emergency escape hatch, 369, 370
  seats, 365
  stabilization, 390
  Type A
    characteristics, 356, 357
    conversions, 360, 371
    doors, 362
    electrical systems, 372–373
    fuel systems, 374
    hydraulic lifts, 371
  Type B
    characteristics, 357
    conversions, 360, 371
    doors, 362
    electrical systems, 372–373
    fuel systems, 374
    hydraulic lifts, 371
    seat belts, 365
  Type C
    characteristics, 357, 358
    doors, 361, 362
    electrical systems, 372–373
    fuel systems, 374
    seat belts, 365
    windows, 364
  Type D
    characteristics, 357, 358
    doors, 361, 362
    electrical systems, 372–373
    fuel systems, 374
    seat belts, 365
    windows, 364

    windows, 363–364, 409
Scissor jack, 141
Scope of this manual, 2
Screw jacks, 140–141
SCUBA (self-contained underwater breathing apparatus), 443
Seat adjustment or positioning controls, 74
Seat belts
  airbags, 223
  knives, 139
  overview, 220–221
  pretensioners
    cutting to release pressure, 69
    defined, 221
    extrication precautions, 69
    functions, 68, 221
    pyrotechnic device for deployment, 69
    vehicle construction knowledge for responder safety, 27
  school buses, 365
Seated spinal immobilization device, 179, 186
Seats
  bus seat disentanglement, 418–420
  bus seat removal, 415
  commercial buses, 366
  displacement and removal, 305–306, 333–334
  as entrapment point, 281
  medium and heavy truck disentanglement, 407
  school buses, 365
  transit buses, 365–366
Security barrier, 32
Self-contained breathing apparatus (SCBA)
  cascade systems, 126
  fit-testing, 59
  NFPA 1981 requirements, 29, 59
  positive-pressure, 59
  training for use, 59
Self-contained underwater breathing apparatus (SCUBA), 443
Semis, 341
Semi-tractor trains, 341
Semitrailer trucks, 341
Semitrailers, 341, 346–347
Shackles, 254–255
Shelter for responders, 30
Shims, 129
Shock absorbers
  hazards, 73, 76
  suspension systems, 218
Shock from hypovolemia, 176
Shores, 440
Shoring, 440–441
Side Impact Protection System (SIPS), 222, 299
Side-impact (T-bone) collision
  injuries sustained from, 171–172, 282–283
  structural damage, 257
  victim entrapment, 282–283
Side-resting vehicle
  bus access opening, 431–433
  bus stabilization, 392
  commercial/heavy truck stabilization, 387–388
  illustrated, 240
  industrial and agricultural vehicles, 460
  railcars, 479
  roof removal, 300, 322–323
  stabilization, 259–261, 271–272
  victim rescue, 279
Side-sensing collision-avoidance systems, 220
Sidewalls as access point
  buses, 409, 415–416, 430
  procedures, 318
  total sidewall removal, 298
Signaling devices, 144
Signs, warning, 37–38, 39

Simple triage and rapid treatment (START), 173-174
SIPS (Side Impact Protection System), 222, 299
Situation status information, 106
Six points of contact, 258
Six-point support, 258
Size-up, 16-22
    Awareness Level duties, 16-17
    defined, 95
    environmental considerations, 17-18
        terrain, 18
        time of day, 17-18, 97
        weather, 17, 96
    fire control support, 77, 78
    industrial and agricultural vehicle incidents, 457-459
    initial size-up, 95
    ongoing size-up, 99
    procedures, 50
    railcar incidents, 475-476
    risk-benefit analysis, 17
    scene assessment, 96-98
        day of the week, 97
        hazards, 97-98
        pedestrians, 97
        time of day, 17-18, 97
        vehicles involved, 97
        vehicular traffic, 97
        weather, 17, 96
    on-scene hazards, 18-22
        biohazards, 21
        fuel spills, 20-21
        power lines/transformers, 20
        traffic, 18-19
        vehicle contents, 19
        vehicle occupants, 21-22
        vehicle stability, 19
Sleepers on trucks, 344-345
Sleeping car, 482-483
Sling
    defined, 247
    endless, 252, 253
    round, 252
    standard eye, 253
    synthetic, 251-253
    twisted eye, 253
    web slings, 253
Smart key ignitions, 214
Snipping tools, 137
Sockets, 139, 140, 315
Sodium azide, 71
SOG (standard operating guideline), 55
SOP. *See* Standard operating procedures (SOPs)
Space frame, 201
Span-of-control if the Incident Commander, 100
Special extrication situations, 439-486
    hanging vehicles, 444-446
    industrial and agricultural vehicles, 447-464
        anatomy, construction, and features, 453-457
        booms, 451-452
        cranes, 452
        extrication operations, 461-464
        forklifts, 452-453, 455
        graders, 451
        harvesters, 450-451
        hazards, 459
        incident size-up, 457-459
        tractors, 448-450
        vehicle stabilization, 459-461
    railcars, 464-486
        access and egress, 479-483
        anatomy, construction, and features, 469-475
        extrication operations, 483-486
        hazards, 476-477, 478
        incident size-up, 475-476
        stabilization, 477-479
        third-rail systems, 478
        types of, 464-469
    recreational vehicles, 446-447
    vehicles in a structure, 440-442
    vehicles in water, 442-444
Specialized unit vehicles, 118
Specialty trucks, 341, 343
Spinal injuries, 179, 186
Sport utility trucks, 197
Sport utility vehicle (SUV), 197
Sports cars/sports coupes, 196
Spreaders
    charactcristics, 142
    combination spreader/cutters, 150
    gain a purchase point, 295-296
    hydraulic, 149
    opening school bus doors, 412, 413
    removing heavy vehicle doors, 404
Springs
    coil springs, 73, 218, 354
    hazards, 73
    leaf springs, 218, 390
    suspension systems, 218
    truck brake systems, 353
Stability of the incident, 27-29
Stability of the vehicle, 19, 28
Stabilization
    defined, 235
    Incident Action Plan (IAP), 44
Stabilization tools and equipment, 127-133, 242-255
    chains, 249
    chocking, for roof-resting vehicle, 241
    cribbing, 127-129
        airbag deployment stabilization, 28
        applications, 128-129
        box crib. *See* Box crib
        bus stabilization, 391
        defined, 127
        materials, 242-243
        plastic, 128
        railroad ties, 478
        for roof-resting vehicle, 241
        wheel-resting vehicles, 258, 269
        wooden, 127-128
    hitches, 247-249
    jacks, 245, 246, 266. *See also* Jacks
    levers, 246-247
    lifting bags and cushions. *See* Lifting bags and cushions
    ratchet straps and tie downs, 132-133
    recovery vehicles, 255, 384, 385
    rigging, 130-132
        chains, 131-132
        commercial/heavy truck stabilization, 384, 389
        components, 253
        defined, 253
        fittings, 254-255
        rope, 131
        tighteners, 253-254
        webbing, 132, 133
    step chocks, 129-130, 258, 268
    struts, 130, 255
    synthetic slings, 251-253
    uses for, 383
    wheel chocks, 242, 243
    wire rope, 250-251
Stabilizer pad, 391
Stabilizers on industrial and agricultural vehicles, 456-457
Stabilizers on rescue vehicles, 126

Stabilizing a vehicle, 383–396
    buses, 389–393
    chocking, 237, 238
    considerations for, 384, 385–393
    defined, 235
    hanging vehicles, 445
    industrial and agricultural vehicles, 459–461
    lifting, 239, 241–242
    mechanism of movement, 236–238, 384
    medium and heavy trucks, 385–389, 395–396
    operations, 255–262
        fire protection, 256
        maintaining vehicle stability, 257, 384
        other vehicle positions, 261–262, 274
        roof-resting vehicles, 261, 273
        side-resting vehicles, 259–261, 271–272
        vehicle structural damage, 256–257
        wheel-resting vehicles, 257–258, 268–270
    override incidents, 285
    phases, 235
    points and surfaces/terrain, 238–239, 240, 384
    railcars, 477–479
    recreational vehicles, 446–447
    safety rules, 235
    tools and equipment. *See* Stabilization tools and equipment
Stair removal, buses, 410
Standard engines, 120
Standard eye sling, 253
Standard for Competence of Responders to Hazardous Materials/Weapons of Mass Destruction Incidents (NFPA 472), 12
Standard for Fire Department Safety Office Professional Qualifications (NFPA 1521), 33–34, 41
Standard for Fire Fighter Professional Qualifications (NFPA 1001), 2
Standard for Technical Rescuer Professional Qualifications, 2017 Edition. See NFPA 1006, *Standard for Technical Rescuer Professional Qualifications, 2017 Edition*
Standard on Emergency Services Incident Management System and Command Safety (NFPA 1561), 11, 41
Standard on Fire Department Occupational Safety and Health Program. See NFPA 1500, *Standard on Fire Department Occupational Safety and Health Program*
Standard on Open-Circuit Self-Contained Breathing Apparatus (SCBA) for Emergency Services (NFPA 1981), 29, 59
Standard on Operations and Training for Technical Rescue Incidents. See NFPA 1670, *Standard on Operations and Training for Technical Rescue Incidents*
Standard on Powered Rescue Tools (NFPA 1936), 150
Standard on Protective Clothing for Emergency Medical Operations (NFPA 1999), 58
Standard on Protective Ensembles for Structural Fire Fighting and Proximity Fire Fighting. See NFPA 1971, *Standard on Protective Ensembles for Structural Fire Fighting and Proximity Fire Fighting*
Standard operating guideline (SOG), 55
Standard operating procedures (SOPs)
    defined, 55
    evacuation methods, 107
    fire control strategies, 78
    operational protocols, 40–42
    personal protective equipment choices, 55
    tires, deflating, 258
START (simple triage and rapid treatment), 173–174
State/provincial government, defined, 3
Station cars, 194
Station wagons, 195
Stationary lights on rescue vehicles, 124
Steam locomotives, 466, 467
Steel
    access and egress openings on vehicles with advanced steel, 301–302
    dual phase (DP), 204
    high strength/low alloy steel (HSLA), 204, 228
    micro-alloy (MA), 228
    mild steel, 204
    transformation induced plasticity (TRIP), 204
    ultra high strength steel (UHSS), 204, 228
Steering column
    displacement, 303, 329
    energy-absorbing, 227
    medium and heavy truck disentanglement, 407
Steering wheel
    bus disentanglement, 419
    as entrapment point, 281
Step chocks, 129–130, 258, 268
Straight trucks, 340, 354
Strand laid rope, 250
Stress, 109–110
Striking tools, 135–136
Stringers, 354
Structure, vehicles in a, 440–442
Struts
    bumper struts, 76, 225–226
    gas-filled, 226
    hatchback and hood struts, 226
    hazards, 73, 76
    opposite-side, independent stabilization system, 261
    shoring, 440
    side-resting vehicle stabilization, 259
    stabilization tools, 130
    stabilizing a vehicle, 241, 255
    suspension systems, 218, 226
    tensioned buttress system of stabilization, 260–261, 272, 274
Subcompact cars, 194–195
Sunroof, 302
Supplemental restraint system (SRS), 67–73, 220–224
    ABCs of dealing with, 67
    airbags, 69–72, 221–224. *See also* Airbags
    child safety restraint devices, 224
    load limiters, 221
    peel and peek behind interior trim, 67–68
    rollover protection systems, 73
    seat belt pretensioners, 68–69, 221
    seat belts, 220–221
    vehicle construction knowledge for responder safety, 27
Support (cold) zone, 31, 32
Support materials in the Incident Action Plan, 43, 106
Support operations and resources, 46–47
Suppression Group, 33
Survey, hazard and risk assessment, 16
Suspension systems
    air-suspension systems, 219
    buses, 376–377
    hazards
        air-ride cab, securing, 89
        explosions, 76
        securing the suspension, 88
        various hazards, 73–74
    leaf springs, 390
    medium and heavy trucks, 354
    shock absorbers, 218
    springs, 218
    struts, 218, 226
    tires, 219
SUV (sport utility vehicle), 197
Symbols, placard, 83, 342
Synthetic slings, 251–253

T

Tactical worksheet, 42, 105
Tanker trailers, 348
TBI (traumatic brain injury), 178
T-bone collision. *See* Side-impact (T-bone) collision
Teamwork
    Extrication Team Leader, 22–23

freelance, 22, 255
Incident Management Coalition Team, 15
response plans, 15
training for personnel, 22
Technical rescuer professional qualifications. *See* NFPA 1006, *Standard for Technical Rescuer Professional Qualifications, 2017 Edition*
Technician Level
commercial and heavy vehicle techniques, 13, 14
emergency escape and evacuation, 106–107
Incident Command System, 99–106
NFPA 1006 requirements, 13
postincident responsibilities and analysis, 108–110
scene size-up, 95–99
terminating an incident, 107–108
Telecommunicators, 45
Telephone calls to dispatch, 45
Telescoping rams, 151
Telescoping vehicles, 455
Tempered glass
characteristics, 203
hazards, 65
railcar windows, 470
removal for access and egress, 292–293, 312
Tensioned buttress system of stabilization, 260–261, 272, 274
Terminating an incident, 107–108, 111, 112
Terminology
international terms, 3
patient, defined, 26
vehicle, 198–200
victim, defined, 26
Terrain, uneven, 180, 181
Terrain considerations during scene size-up, 18
Thermal control for responders, 30
Thermal cutting devices, 158–161
cutting flares, 159
exothermic cutting devices, 159
oxyacetylene cutting torches, 160
oxygasoline cutting torches, 160–161
plasma-arc cutters, 160
safety rules, 158–159
Thimble, 250
Third door conversion
access and egress techniques, 406
door removal, 293
extrication operations, 298, 319
Third-rail systems, 475, 477, 478
Tie downs, 132–133
Tighteners, rigging, 253–254
Time of day, scene assessment consideration, 17–18, 97
Tires
deflating for stabilizing vehicles, 258, 270
explosion hazard, 73
functions, 219
hazards, 66
industrial and agricultural vehicles, 455
Tools and equipment, 117–162
door removal, 296–297
electric, 142–145
extrication, 133–161
come-alongs, 156–157
electric tools and equipment, 142–145
hand tools, 133–142
hydraulic tools and equipment, 148–152
lifting or pulling tools, 155–156
pneumatic tools and equipment, 152–155
power saws, 145–148, 404
thermal cutting devices, 158–161
Halligan tool, 296, 412
heavy vehicle stabilization, 383
hydra ram, 296
hydraulic, 148–152

lifting. *See* Lifting tools
lighting, 17–18
operational checks and maintenance, 161
passenger vehicle stabilization, 242–255, 264–267
pike pole, 385, 411
pneumatic, 152–155
power tool standards (NFPA 1936), 150
PPE. *See* Personal protective equipment (PPE)
pry bar, 296
rabbit tool, 296
rescue vehicles, 117–127
chassis, 121
compartmentation, 121–122
features and equipment, 122–127
heavy rescue vehicles, 118–119
ladder trucks, 120
light rescue vehicles, 117–118
medium rescue vehicles, 118
rescue engines, 119
standard engines, 120
stabilization. *See* Stabilization tools and equipment
Torches, 160–161
Torsion bar, 218
Total sidewall removal, 298, 318
Touring bus, 358. *See also* Commercial buses
Tow bar, 346
Tow truck, 255
Tracked vehicles, 449–450, 454
Tractors, 448–450
attachments and implements, 450
rollovers, 458, 459
tracked, 454, 4449–4450
wheeled, 448–449
Tractor-trailers, 341
Traffic control, 34–40
apparatus positioning, 34, 35
conditions for use of, 34
defined, 34
devices, 36–40
equipment, 37
positioning, 38
setting up, 38, 40
traffic channeling taper, 38–39
traffic cones, 39
warning signs, 37–38
emergency vehicle and equipment control, 36
flaggers, 38, 476
hanging vehicle incidents, 444
pedestrian control, 36
rescuer control, 36
resources, 40
Traffic incident hazards, 18–19
Traffic scene assessment, 97
Trailers
air brakes, 353
air suspension systems, 347
axle track/frame, 347
box trailers, 348
car carrier/haulers, 349
configurations, 347
defined, 346
dry bulk, 349
dump trailers, 349
livestock, 348
lowboys, 349
semitrailer, 341, 346–347
tanker, 348
travel trailers, 446–447
types of, 346
Training
Awareness Level personnel, 12

Index **519**

hazardous materials/weapons of mass destruction, 12
minimum entrance and fitness requirements, 41–42
NFPA standards. *See* NFPA 1670, *Standard on Operations and Training for Technical Rescue Incidents*
Operations Level personnel, 12–13
personal protective equipment, 29–30
safety measures, 22
self-contained breathing apparatus (SCBA), 59
Technician Level personnel, 13
Trains. *See* Railcars
Trams, 485–486
Transferring a victim, 181–182
Transformation induced plasticity (TRIP) steel construction material, 204
Transformer hazards, 20
Transit buses
    aisles, 367
    articulated, 358, 359
    batteries, 372
    construction, 370–371
    disentanglement, 402
    doors, 362
    electrical systems, 372–373
    generally, 357–358
    seats, 365–366
    stabilization, 391
    windows, 364–365
Transparent armor, 204
Transportation of victims
    Medical Group responsibilities, 102, 103
    on-scene medical care, 29
Trauma
    blunt, 171
    penetrating, 171
    traumatic brain injury (TBI), 178
Travel trailers, 446–447
Treatment by the Medical Group, 102
Trench tools, 142
Triage
    advanced life support (ALS), 41, 173
    categories, 175
    defined, 173
    mass casualty incident (MCI), 174–175, 476
    Medical Group responsibilities, 102
    multiple vehicle incidents, 286
    simple triage and rapid treatment (START), 173–174
    triage tag, 175
Tribal entities, adoption of NIMS-ICS, 11
Trolley, 466, 472–474
Trucks. *See also* Medium and heavy trucks
    dump trucks, 340, 448
    haz mat incidents, 82, 84
    lift or fork trucks, 452
    railcars, 471
    trailers and, 341
Trunk tunneling, 301, 327
Tunneling
    railcars, 484
    trunk, 301, 327
Turnbuckles, 254
Turning down assignments, 23
Turnout gear standards, 57
29 CFR 1910.178, forklifts, 452
Twisted eye sling, 253
Two-wheel drive powertrain, 218, 454
Type A school bus
    characteristics, 356, 357
    conversions, 360, 371
    doors, 362
    electrical systems, 372–373
    fuel systems, 374

    hydraulic lifts, 371
Type B school bus
    characteristics, 357
    conversions, 360, 371
    doors, 362
    electrical systems, 372–373
    fuel systems, 374
    hydraulic lifts, 371
    seat belts, 365
Type C school bus
    characteristics, 357, 358
    doors, 361, 362
    electrical systems, 372–373
    fuel systems, 374
    seat belts, 365
    windows, 364
Type D school bus
    characteristics, 357, 358
    doors, 361, 362
    electrical systems, 372–373
    fuel systems, 374
    seat belts, 365
    windows, 364

U

UATV (utility all-terrain vehicle), 194
UC (Unified Command), 104
UHSS (ultra high strength steel), 204, 228
UL (Underwriters Laboratories), 137
ULC (Underwriters' Laboratories of Canada), 137
Ultra high strength steel (UHSS), 204, 228
Undercarriage of the vehicle, 199, 369–370
Underrides, 257, 284–285
Underwriters' Laboratories of Canada (ULC), 137
Unibody frame, 201
Unified Command (UC), 104
United Kingdom, truck/semitrailer combinations, 341
United States
    Department of Health and Human Services, 182
    DOT. *See* Department of Transportation (DOT)
    HSPD-5 functions, 11
    metric conversions, 4–6
    NHTSA. *See* National Highway Traffic Safety Administration (NHTSA)
    truck/semitrailer combinations, 341
Unitized body frame, 201
Utility all-terrain vehicle (UATV), 194
Utility rope, 131

V

Vacuum mattress, 179
Vans, 196–197
V-blade (seat belt) knives, 139
Vehicle construction, incident stability, 27–28
Vehicle contents, hazards of, 19
Vehicle energy sources, 61–66
Vehicle stability, 19, 28
Vehicle stabilization, 101, 102
Vehicle terminology, 198–200
Vehicles, rescue. *See* Rescue vehicles
Vehicles in a structure, 440–442
Vehicles in water, 442–444
Vehicles involved, scene assessment consideration, 97, 98
Verbal Incident Action Plan, 43
Vertical axis, 237
Vertical hitch, 247–248
Vests, safety
    for flaggers, 38
    for increased visibility, 36, 58
    for personnel identification, 101

Victim entrapment, 279-287
    disentanglement, 281-285
        front-end collisions, 281-282
        rear-impact collisions, 282
        rollovers, 283-284
        rotational collisions, 283
        side-impact collisions, 282-283
        underrides and overrides, 257, 284-285
    entrapment, defined, 280
    locations of victim, 279-280
    minimizing hazards, 287
    multiple vehicle incidents, 285-287
    points of, 280-281
Victims
    administering care, 167-178
        compartment/crush syndrome, 177-178
        field amputations, 178
        fractures and lacerations, 176
        hazardous materials exposure, 177
        HIPAA regulations, 182
        hypothermia and hyperthermia, 177
        hypovolemia, 176
        internal injuries, 178
        mechanisms of injury, 168-173
        preventing further injury, 175-176
        triage, 173-175
    defined, 26
    follow up, 182
    immobilization
        cervical collar, 179, 184
        cervical spine, 167
        devices, 179
        procedures, 180
        for removal, 168
        seated spinal immobilization device, 179, 186
    mechanisms of injury, 168-173
        blunt and penetrating trauma, 171
        fatality in the same vehicle, 169
        head-on impact collision, 170-171
        rear impact collision, 172-173
        rollover, 173
        side impact collision, 171-172
    occupant on-scene hazards, 21-22
    packaging, 178-181, 185-186
    psychological concerns, 176
    removal from industrial and agricultural vehicles, 463
    shelter from inclement weather, 30
    transfer, 181-182
Voltage, hybrid electric vehicle, 207
Voltage detection devices, 145

W

Walls
    firewall, 199
    medium and heavy truck entry points, 406, 426
    railcars, 470-471, 482
    rear wall access, 416
    sidewalls as access point
        buses, 409, 415-416, 430
        procedures, 318
        total sidewall removal, 298
    total sidewall removal, 298, 318
Warm (limited access) zone, 31, 32
Warning signs, 37-38, 39
Water, vehicles in, 442-444
Water as extinguishing agent, 79
Weapons of mass destruction (WMDs)
    hazard and risk assessment surveys, 16
    NFPA 472 incident standards, 12
Weather
    personnel shelter and thermal control, 30

    scene assessment, 96
    scene size-up considerations, 17
Web slings, 253
Webbing
    characteristics, 132
    commercial/heavy truck stabilization, 388
    door removal, 294
    pedal displacement, 307
    uses for, 133
    for vehicle stabilization, 261
Wedge socket, 250
Wedges, 129
Wet suits, 61
Wheel chocks, 242, 243, 264. *See also* Chocking a vehicle
Wheeled tractors, 448-449
Wheel-resting vehicle
    bus stabilization, 389-391
    chocking a vehicle, 258
    commercial/heavy truck stabilization, 386-387
    illustrated, 240
    industrial and agricultural vehicles, 460
    lifting with a jack, 266
    passenger vehicle stabilization, 257-258
    railcars, 478-479
    roof removal, 299, 321
    stabilization operations, 268-270
Wheels, 66
Whizzer saw, 153
Winch
    lifting a vehicle, 241
    manual cable winch, 253
    powered cable winch, 253-254
    vehicle-mounted, 124-125
Window curtains, 223
Windows. *See also* Glass
    bus extrication operations, 413-415, 429
    commercial buses, 365
    construction materials, 65-66
    controlling breaking glass, 65-66
    defoggers
        electronics, 216
        hazards, 65, 213
    enhanced protective glass (EPC), 203
    entry points, 288-289
    glass construction materials, 205
    industrial and agricultural vehicles, 462
    laminated safety glass
        characteristics, 202-203
        hazards, 65
        Lexan®, 470
        removal for access and egress, 291-293, 310-313
    medium and heavy truck entry points, 403, 405
    polycarbonate, 203
    purpose of, 201-202
    railcars, 470, 481-482
    school buses, 363-364, 409
    tempered glass, 65, 203, 470
    transit buses, 364-365
    transparent armor, 204
    truck cabs, 346
Windshield
    bus extrication operations, 413-414
    cutter, 138, 139
    removal from around a victim, 303, 328
Wire rope, 250-251
Wire rope tighteners, 253
WMDs. *See* Weapons of mass destruction (WMDs)
Wooden cribbing, 127-128
Wooden step chocks, 130, 258
Wrenches
    for door removal, 297, 315

electric impact, 143
   pneumatic, 153
   types of, 139

Y
Yaw of a vehicle, 238

Z
Zones. *See also* Safety zones
   airbag safety zones, 69
   boundaries, 32
   crumple zones, 228
   hazard zone monitoring, 33–34
   limited access (warm) zone, 31, 32
   purpose of, 30–31
   restricted (hot) zone, 31
   staffing requirements for safety zones, 32–33
   support (cold) zone, 31, 32
   winch danger zone, 125

NOTES

NOTES

NOTES

NOTES